HOLISTIC APPROACHES FOR WOMEN'S SUSTAINABLE HEALTH

Volume 2

Advancements, Socioeconomic Impacts, and Innovative Strategies

Holistic Approaches for Women's Sustainable Health, 4-volume set
ISBN: 978-1-77964-170-0 (hbk)

Volume 1: Foundations, Innovations, Challenges, and Management
ISBN: 978-1-77964-162-5 (hbk)
ISBN: 978-1-77964-163-2 (ebk)

Volume 2: Advancements, Socioeconomic Impacts, and Innovative Strategies
ISBN: 978-1-77964-164-9 (hbk)
ISBN: 978-1-77964-165-6 (ebk)

Volume 3: Herbs, Spices, Phytochemicals, and Cereals: Body Care, Cancer Prevention, and Hormonal Health
ISBN: 978-1-77964-166-3 (hbk)
ISBN: 978-1-77964-167-0 (ebk)

Volume 4: Benefits of Vegetables and Medicinal Plants and Trees
ISBN: 978-1-77964-168-7 (hbk)
ISBN: 978-1-77964-169-4 (ebk)

HOLISTIC APPROACHES FOR WOMEN'S SUSTAINABLE HEALTH

Volume 2

Advancements, Socioeconomic Impacts, and Innovative Strategies

Junaid Ahmad Malik, PhD
Anamika Chauhan, PhD
Megh R. Goyal, PhD
Editors

AAP | APPLE ACADEMIC PRESS

First edition published 2027

Apple Academic Press Inc.
1265 Goldenrod Circle, NE,
Palm Bay, FL 32905 USA

760 Laurentian Drive, Unit 19,
Burlington, ON L7N 0A4, Canada

CRC Press
2385 NW Executive Center Drive,
Suite 320, Boca Raton FL 33431

4 Park Square, Milton Park,
Abingdon, Oxon, OX14 4RN UK

Library and Archives Canada Cataloguing in Publication

Title: Holistic approaches for women's sustainable health / Megh R. Goyal, PhD, Anamika Chauhan, PhD, Junaid Ahmad Malik, PhD, editors.
Names: Goyal, Megh R., editor | Cauhāna, Anāmikā, 1985- editor. | Malik, Junaid Ahmad, 1987- editor
Description: First edition. | Includes bibliographical references and indexes. | Contents: Volume 2: Advancements, socioeconomic impacts, and innovative strategies.
Identifiers: Canadiana (print) 20260181994 | Canadiana (ebook) 20260182001 | ISBN 9781779641700 (set) | ISBN 9781779641649 (v. 2 ; hardcover) | ISBN 9781779641656 (v. 2 ; ebook)
Subjects: LCSH: Women—Health and hygiene. | LCSH: Holistic medicine.
Classification: LCC RA778 .H65 2026 | DDC 613/.04244—dc23

Library of Congress Cataloging-in-Publication Data

CIP data on file with US Library of Congress

ISBN: 978-1-77964-164-9 (hbk)
ISBN: 978-1-77964-165-6 (ebk)
DOI: 10.1201/9781779641656

Dedication

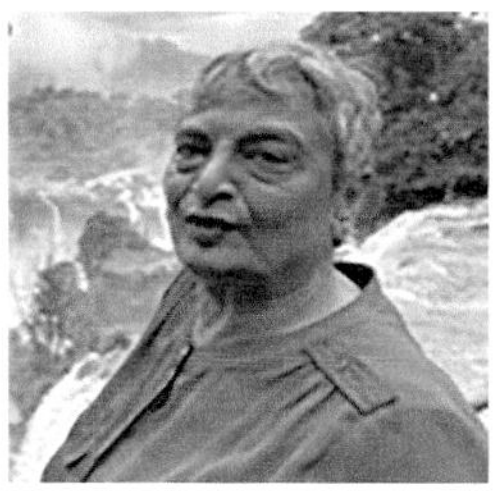

In the sacred verses of Proverbs 31, we find a timeless ode to the essence of womanhood—a testament to strength, wisdom, and compassion. It is within these words that we uncover the embodiment of virtues celebrated in the life of Subhadra Devi Goyal—a remarkable woman whose journey resonates with the noblest qualities of a daughter, wife, mother, pastor, and social worker.

From her earliest days, Subhadra Devi Goyal has exemplified the profound bond of filial love and respect. Her reverence for family, her unwavering support, and her tender care stand as a testament to the enduring legacy of familial ties.

In the sacred covenant of marriage, Subhadra Devi Goyal has shown boundless strength and unwavering commitment. Her partnership with her beloved spouse is marked by resilience, mutual respect, and a shared journey toward growth and understanding.

As a mother, Subhadra's love knows no bounds. Her nurturing embrace, her guiding hand, and her boundless affection shape the lives of her three children, instilling in them the values of integrity, empathy, compassion, and love for God, others, country, and nature.

In her role as a pastor, Subhadra serves as a beacon of light and hope for her congregation and community. Her wisdom, her faith, and her compassionate guidance inspire others to seek solace, understanding, and spiritual growth.

As a social worker, Subhadra's heart knows no bounds. Her selfless service, her tireless advocacy, and her unwavering commitment to justice uplift the marginalized, empower the oppressed, and transform communities with love, compassion, and dedication.

In recognition of her exemplary life, filled with service, devotion, and unwavering faith, we dedicate this book to Subhadra Devi Goyal—a living embodiment of the timeless wisdom of Proverbs 31. May her legacy continue to inspire and uplift all, who are touched by her remarkable spirit!

About the Editor

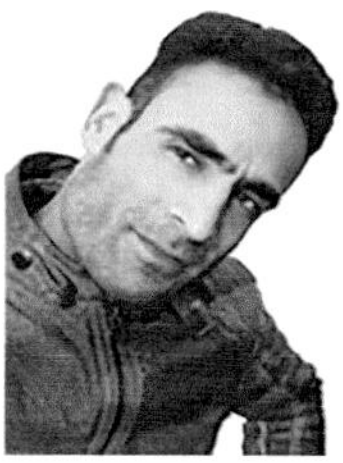

Junaid A. Malik, PhD
Lecturer, Department of Zoology, Government Degree College, Kulgam, Kashmir (J&K), India

Junaid A. Malik, PhD, received BSc (2008) in Science from the University of Kashmir, Srinagar, J&K; MSc (2010) in Zoology from Barkatullah University, Bhopal, Madhya Pradesh; and PhD (2015) in Zoology from the same university. He completed his BEd program in 2017 from the University of Kashmir, Srinagar, J&K. He started his career as Lecturer in the School Education Department, Government of J&K for two years. Dr. Malik is now working as a Lecturer in the Department of Zoology, Government Degree College, Bijbehara, Kashmir (J&K), and is actively involved in teaching and research activities. He has more than eight years of research experience. His areas of interest are ecology, soil macrofauna, wildlife biology, conservation biology, etc.

Dr. Malik has published more than 20 research papers in various national and international peer-reviewed journals. He has authored four books, 33 book chapters, edited 16 books, and more than 10 popular editorial articles. He is also serving as editor and reviewer of several journals. He has participated in several state, national, and international conferences, seminars, workshops, and symposia and more than 20 conference papers are to his credit. He is a life member of SBBS (Society for Bioinformatics and Biological Sciences).

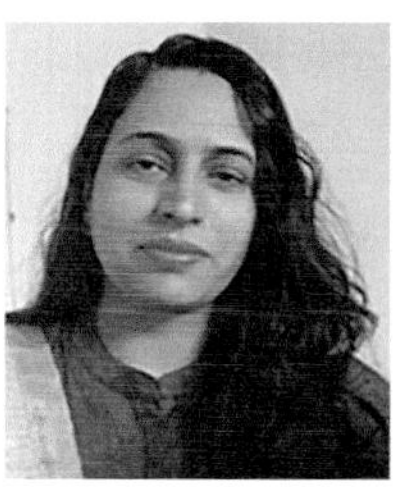

Anamika Chauhan, PhD
Chaman Lal Mahavidhyalya Haridwar (Sri Dev Suman University, Tehri, Uttarakhand), Haridwar, Uttarakhand, India

Anamika Chauhan, PhD, is an accomplished academician who holds a master's degree and a PhD from HNB Garhwal Srinagar, Central University,

Uttarakhand, India. In addition to her impressive academic credentials, she boasts master's degrees in English and Education, showcasing the breadth of her intellectual pursuits.

Furthermore, Dr. Chauhan has proven her academic prowess by successfully qualifying for UGC-NET, USET, and MPhil. Her dedication and excellence in the field have earned her the prestigious "Young Scientist Award" from the Uttarakhand State Council for Science and Technology and the esteemed "Teacher's Excellence Award" from Motherhood University in Uttarakhand. Notably, she was also recognized with the distinguished "Dr. Sarvepalli Radhakrishnan Global Educator Award-2022" by the International Council for Education, Research, and Training Delhi, India and Teacher of the Year 2023 by the Government of Uttarakhand, India.

Dr. Chauhan's contributions extend beyond accolades, as she holds a patent for her groundbreaking work on "Gold Nanoparticles with *Albizia lebbeck* (L.) Benth Leaves Extract for Dermal Cancer." This patent exemplifies her commitment to advancing scientific knowledge in the field.

Her involvement in academia is not only recognized through awards and patents but is also evident in her role as a valuable member of the Board of Studies at the University. Dr. Chauhan's commitment to academic excellence is further underscored by her lifetime memberships in esteemed organizations, including the Indian Science Congress Association Kolkata, Scientific and Technical Research Association (STRA), and Home Science Association of India.

A prolific researcher, Dr. Chauhan has authored numerous research papers published in peer-reviewed national and international journals. Additionally, she has contributed to academia through the publication of eight edited books and a textbook. Her intellectual engagement extends to active participation in workshops and conferences, further showcasing her dedication to the dissemination of knowledge.

Dr. Chauhan's research interests span a wide spectrum, encompassing critical areas such as the food and nutrition, human health, and social issues. Her multifaceted expertise and commitment to advancing knowledge make her a distinguished figure in the academic community.

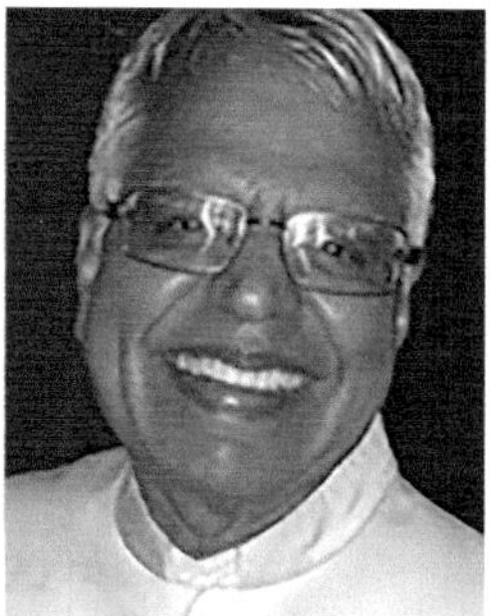

Megh R. Goyal, PhD, PE
Retired Professor in Agricultural and Biomedical Engineering, University of Puerto Rico, Mayaguez Campus; Senior Acquisitions Editor, Biomedical Engineering and Agricultural Science, Apple Academic Press, Inc.

Megh R. Goyal, PhD, PE, is, at present, a Retired Professor in Agricultural and Biomedical Engineering from the General Engineering Department in the College of Engineering at the University of Puerto Rico—Mayaguez Campus (UPRM); and Senior Acquisitions Editor and Senior Technical Editor-in-Chief in Agricultural and Biomedical Engineering for Apple Academic Press, Inc.

He received his BSc degree in engineering from Punjab Agricultural University, Ludhiana, India; his MSc and PhD degrees from the Ohio State University, Columbus; his Master of Divinity degree from Puerto Rico Evangelical Seminary, Hato Rey, Puerto Rico, USA.

Since 1971, he has worked as Soil Conservation Inspector (1971); Research Assistant at Haryana Agricultural University (1972–1975) and the Ohio State University (1975–1979); Research Agricultural Engineer/Professor at the Department of Agricultural Engineering of UPRM (1979–1997); and Professor (Agricultural and Biomedical Engineering) at UPRM (1997–2012). He spent one-year sabbatical leave in 2002–2003 at Biomedical Engineering Department, Florida International University, Miami, USA.

He was the first agricultural engineer to receive the professional license in Agricultural Engineering in 1986 from the College of Engineers and Surveyors of Puerto Rico. On September 16, 2005, he was proclaimed as "Father of Irrigation Engineering in Puerto Rico for the twentieth century" by the American Society of Agricultural and Biological Engineers, Puerto Rico Section, for his pioneer work on micro-irrigation, evapotranspiration, agroclimatology, and soil and water engineering.

During his professional career of 52 years, he has received awards such as: Scientist of the Year, Blue Ribbon Extension Award, Research Paper Award, Nolan Mitchell Young Extension Worker Award, Agricultural Engineer of the Year, Citations by Mayors of Juana Diaz and Ponce, Membership Grand Prize for ASAE Campaign, Felix Castro Rodriguez

Academic Excellence, Rashtrya Ratan Award and Bharat Excellence Award and Gold Medal, Domingo Marrero Navarro Prize, Adopted son of Moca, Irrigation Protagonist of UPRM, Man of Drip Irrigation by Mayor of Municipalities of Mayaguez/Caguas/Ponce and Senate/Secretary of Agriculture of ELA, Puerto Rico.

The Water Technology Centre of Tamil Nadu Agricultural University in Coimbatore, India recognized Dr. Goyal as one of the experts "who rendered meritorious service for the development of micro-irrigation sector in India" by bestowing *Award of Outstanding Contribution in Micro Irrigation.* This award was presented to Dr. Goyal during the inaugural session of the National Congress on "New Challenges and Advances in Sustainable Micro Irrigation" on March 1, 2017, held at Tamil Nadu Agricultural University.

At the Annual Meeting on August 01, 2018 in Detroit, MI, ASABE bestowed on him Netafim Microirrigation Award for his unselfish contribution. VDGOOD Professional Association of India awarded Lifetime Achievement Award at 12th Annual Meeting on Engineering, Science and Medicine that was held on 20–21 of November of 2020 in Visakhapatnam, India.

He has authored more than 200 journal articles and more than 150 books including: *Elements of Agroclimatology (Spanish)* by UNISARC, Colombia; two *Bibliographies on Drip Irrigation.* Apple Academic Press, Inc. (AAP) has published his books, namely: "Management of Drip/Trickle or Micro Irrigation," and "Evapotranspiration: Principles and Applications for Water Management," 10-volume set on *Research Advances in Sustainable Micro Irrigation.* During 2016–2025, AAP will be publishing book volumes on emerging technologies/issues/challenges under book series, *Innovations and Challenges in Micro Irrigation,* and *Innovations in Agricultural & Biological Engineering.*

Contents

Contributors

Amal Abdellaoui
Cardiovascular Surgery Department, Ibn Roch University Hospital Center, Casablanca, Morocco

Didhiti Agarwal
Symbiosis School of Biological Sciences, Symbiosis International University, Maharashtra, Lavale, Pune, Maharashtra, India

Shervin Assari
Marginalization-Related Diminished Returns (MDRs) Research Center,
Charles R Drew University of Medicine and Science, Los Angeles, CA, USA;
Department of Family Medicine and Department of Urban Public Health,
Charles R Drew University of Medicine and Science, Los Angeles, CA, USA

Mohammad Awde
Faculty of Medicine, Damascus University, Damascus, Syria

Mahbube Askari Azad
University of Medicine and Science, Los Angeles, CA, USA;
Department of Family Medicine and Department of Urban Public Health,
Charles R Drew University of Medicine and Science, Los Angeles, CA, USA

Sagar Barage
Amity Institute of Biotechnology, Amity University, Mumbai-Pune Expressway, Bhatan, Panvel, Mumbai, India

Aditi Bhardwaj
Department of Computer Science, ShriRam Institute of Information Technology, Banmore, Morena, Madhya Pradesh, India

Ayan Chatterjee
Department of Allied Health, School of Health and Medical Sciences, Adamas University, West Bengal, India

Anamika Chauhan
Department of Home Science, Chaman Lal Mahavidhyalya, Landhaura, Haridwar, Uttarakhand, India

Moumita Das
Department of Applied Nutrition and Dietetics, Sister Nivedita University, Newtown, Kolkata, India

Sasmita Dash
Department of Electronics and Communication Engineering, GIET University, Odisha, India

Danielle Gilmore
Department of Health, Behavior, and Society, Johns Hopkins Bloomberg School of Public Health, Baltimore, Maryland, USA

Priya Gogia
Department of Pediatrics, All India Institute of Medical Sciences, Bhopal, Madhya Pradesh, India

Emi Grace Mary Gowshika R.
Department of Home Science, Women's Christian College, Chennai, Tamil Nadu, India

Megh R. Goyal
Apple Academic Press Inc.; and Retired Faculty in Agricultural and Biomedical Engineering, University of Puerto Rico, Mayaguez Campus, USA

Sanjib Kumar Haldar
Mukundabagh High School, Murshidabad, West Bengal, India

Rukshana Irani
Department of Food and Nutrition, Raidighi College (Affiliated to the University of Calcutta), West Bengal, India

Saloni Jain
Department of Pharmacology, ShriRam College of Pharmacy, Banmore, Morena, MP, India
Muzamil Jan, Institute of Home Science, University of Kashmir, Srinagar, India

Vinay Jain
Department of Pharmacognosy, ShriRam College of Pharmacy, Banmore, Morena, Madhya Pradesh, India

Ali Jawad
Faculty of Medicine, Damascus University, Damascus, Syria

Poonam Joshi
Uttaranchal Institute of Pharmaceutical Sciences, Uttaranchal University, Dehradun, Uttarakhand, India

Haidar Kanso
Faculty of Medicine, Damascus University, Damascus, Syria

Aya Kawssan
Faculty of Medical Sciences, Lebanese University, Beirut, Lebanon

Shweta Keswani
Department of Foods and Nutrition, Shri Vaishnav Institute of Home Science, Shri Vaishnav Vidyapeeth Vishwavidyalaya, Indore, Madhya Pradesh, India

Indresh Kumar
Regional Center of Excellence for Nutrition Rehabilitation Resource and Training, Department of Pediatrics, All India Institute of Medical Sciences, Bhopal, Madhya Pradesh, India

Neeti Kushwaha
Centre for Panchayati Raj, Decentralized Planning and Social Service Delivery (CPRDP&SSD), National Institute of Rural Development and Panchayati Raj (NIRDPR), Rajendranagar, Hyderabad, India

Jad Majed
Dipartimento di Medicina Molecolare, Università degli Studi di Pavia, Pavia, Italy

Shikha Malik
Department of Pediatrics, All India Institute of Medical Sciences, Bhopal, Madhya Pradesh, India

Neelesh Kumar Maurya
Department of Nutrition and Dietetics, School of Allied Health Science, Sharda University, Greater Noida, India

Chinmoy Kumar Mondal
Anderson Centre for Autism, Hyde Park, New York, USA

Mohammad Ali Mtairek
Faculty of Medicine, Damascus University, Damascus, Syria

Vrushali Neve
Department of Pharmacology, Dr. D.Y. Patil Institute of Pharmaceutical Sciences and Research, Savitribai Phule Pune University, Pimpri, Pune, Maharashtra, India

Jayanta Kumar Panda
Department of Journalism and Mass Communication, Berhampur University, Odisha, India
Jaymala Kumawat, Vishwakarma University School of Pharmacy, Pune, Maharashtra, India

Afrima Parven
Department of Psychology, Biam Laboratory School and College, Noughan, Bangladesh
Nisha Rana, Swami Vivekanand Subharti University, Meerut, Uttar Pradesh, India

Priya
Uttaranchal Institute of Pharmaceutical Sciences, Uttaranchal University, Dehradun, Uttarakhand, India

Ritika Rasaily
Department of Applied Nutrition and Dietetics, Sister Nivedita University, Newtown, Kolkata, West Bengal, India

Arpan Ray
Manicktala ESI Hospital, West Bengal, India

Ropak Roy
Department of Physiotherapy, Gono Bishwabidyalay, Savar, Dhaka, Bangladesh

Asoke Kumar Saha
Department of Psychology, Jagannath University, Dhaka, Bangladesh

Dipali Saxena
Department of Foods and Nutrition, Shri Vaishnav Institute of Home Science, Shri Vaishnav Vidyapeeth Vishwavidyalaya Indore, Madhya Pradesh, India

Rahul Saxena
Department of Biochemistry, SSAHS, Sharda University, Greater Noida, Uttar Pradesh, India

Suyash Saxena
Department of Biochemistry, SSAHS, Sharda University, Greater Noida, Uttar Pradesh, India

Archana Shaha
Vishwakarma University School of Pharmacy, Pune, Maharashtra, India

Pankaj Sharma
Department of Pharmaceutics, ShriRam College of Pharmacy, Banmore, Morena, Madhya Pradesh, India

Sandeep Sharma
Department of Computer Science, ShriRam Institute of Information Technology, Banmore, Morena, MP, India

Simple Sharma
Department of Food Science and Technology, I. K. Gujral Punjab Technical University, Kapurthala, Punjab, India

Swati Sharma
Research and Development Cell, Swami Vivekanand Subharti University, Meerut, Uttar Pradesh, India

Yogita Shinde
Vishwakarma University School of Pharmacy, Pune, Maharashtra, India

Ajit Pal Singh
Department of Medical Lab Technology, School of Medical and Allied Sciences, Galgotias University, Sharda University, Greater Noida, Uttar Pradesh, India

Rajshri Singh
Amity Institute of Biotechnology, Amity University, Mumbai–Pune Expressway, Bhatan, Panvel, Mumbai, India

Zoomi Singh
School of Health Sciences, UPRTOU, Prayagraj, Uttar Pradesh, India

Prachi Sinha
Department of Pediatrics, All India Institute of Medical Sciences, Bhopal, Madhya Pradesh, India

Jyoti Srivastava
Uttaranchal Institute of Pharmaceutical Sciences, Uttaranchal University, Dehradun, Uttarakhand, India

Dipali Talele
Vishwakarma University School of Pharmacy, Pune, Maharashtra, India

Ananya Verma
Amity Institute of Biotechnology, Amity University, Mumbai–Pune Expressway, Bhatan, Panvel, Mumbai, India

Hossein Zare
Department of Health Policy and Management,
Johns Hopkins Bloomberg School of Public Health, Baltimore, Maryland, USA;
University of Maryland Global Campus, Health Services Management, Adelphi, MD, USA

Mohd Younus Zaroo
Government Medical College, Sher-i-Kashmir Institute of Medical Sciences, Srinagar, India

Hamida Zinat
Department of Psychology, Jagannath University, Dhaka, Bangladesh

Abbreviations

5 HT	5-hydroxy tryptamine
ACOG	American College of Obstetricians and Gynaecologists
AD	Alzheimer's disease
ADHD	attention deficit hyperactivity disorder
AI	artificial intelligence
AMP	adenosine monophosphate
ANC	antenatal care
APH	ante partum hemorrhage
ART	assisted reproductive technology
ART	antiretroviral
ARVs	antiretroviral drugs
ATAC-seq	assay for transposase-accessible chromatin with sequencing
BDNF	brain derived neurotrophic factor
BMI	body–mass index
BMPs	bone morphogenetic proteins
CAG	cytosine-adenine-guanine
CAM	complementary and alternative medicine
cAMP	cyclic adenosine monophosphate
Cas9	crispr-associated protein 9
CBAs	carbamates
CBT	cognitive behavioral therapy
CD 8 and 16	cluster of differentiation 8 and 16
CD38	cyclic ADP ribose hydrolase
CDC	centers for disease control and prevention
CGRP	calcitonin gene-related peptide
ChIP-seq	chromatin immunoprecipitation sequencing
CIN	cervical intraepithelial neoplasia
CL	conventional laparoscopy
CNS	central nervous system
COVID	coronavirus
COVID-19	coronavirus-2019
CREB	camp response element-binding protein
CRH	corticotropin-releasing hormone
CRISPR	clustered regularly interspaced palindromic repeats
CS	cesarean section
CSD	cortical spreading depression

CT	computed tomography
D&C	dilatation and curettage
D&E	dilatation and evacuation
DA	dopamine
DAG	diacylglycerol
DALYs	disability-adjusted life-years
DBCA	drug-based cellular assay
DDT	dichlorodiphenyltrichloroethane
DHA	docosahexaenoic acid
DSD	decreased sexual desire
EBP	evidence-based practice
ECT	electroconvulsive therapy
EGFR	epidermal growth factor receptor
EMS	endometriosis
ENDS	electronic nicotine delivery systems
EPA	eicosapentaenoic acid
EpiLCs	epiblast-like cells
ER β	estrogen receptor β
ERK2	extracellular signal regulated kinase 2
ESC	embryonic stem cells
FAS	fetal alcohol syndrome
FASD	fetal alcohol spectrum disorder
FMEA	failure mode and effects analysis
fMRI	functional magnetic resonance imaging
FOBT	fecal occult blood testing
GABA	gamma amino butyric acid
GAD	generalized anxiety disorder
GDP	gross domestic product
GMCs	general medical conditions
HD	hypothalamic dysfunction
HD	Huntington's disease
HER	electronic health record
hESCs	human embryonic stem cells
HIPAA	health insurance portability and accountability act
HIV	human immunodeficiency virus
HLD	high level disinfection
HPA	hypothalamic pituitary adrenal axis
HPE	holoprosencephaly
HPL	hyperprolactinemia
HPV	human papillomavirus
HRT	hormone replacement therapy
HSG	hysterosalpingography

ICPD	international conference on population and development
IP3	inositol triphosphate
iPSCs	induced pluripotent stem cells
IUCD	intrauterine contraceptive device
IV	intravenous
IVF	*in vitro* fertilization
LBW	low birth weight
LMICs	low- or middle-income country
MAOIs	monoamine oxidase inhibitors
MAPK	mitogen activated protein kinase
MAT	medication-assisted treatment
MBCT	mindfulness-based cognitive therapy
MBI	mindfulness-based interventions
MBSR	mindfulness-based stress reduction
MEK2	mitogen activated protein kinase 2
MICP	migraine interactive care plan
ML	machine learning
MOUD	medications for opioid use disorder study
MRI	magnetic resonance imaging
MS	menopausal symptoms
MTCT	mother-to-child transmission
Myd88	myeloid differentiation primary response 88
NAS	neonatal abstinence syndrome
NF-κB	nuclear factor kappa b
NICU	neonatal intensive care unit
NLP	natural language processing
NOWS	neonatal opioid withdrawal syndrome
OCs	organochlorines
OHCs	online health communities
OPD	out-patient department
Ops	organophosphates
OPS	osteoporosis
OTC	over-the-counter
OXTR	oxytocin receptor
PAP smear	Papanicolaou smear test
PCOS	polycystic ovarian syndrome
PCPs	primary care physicians
PCR	polymerase chain reaction
PD	Parkinson's disease
PID	polyphenol-induced disease
PID	pelvic inflammatory disease
PKA	protein kinase a

PLC	phospholipase c
PMS	premenstrual syndrome
POD	polypeptide disorder
PPH	post-partum hemorrhage
PTSD	post-traumatic stress disorder
PYRs	pyrethroids
RALP	robot assisted laparoscopic prostatectomy
RAS	robotic-assisted surgery
RAS	reticular activating system
RBCs	red blood cells
RCTs	randomized controlled trials
RLRS	real-life risk simulation
RNA	ribonucleic acid
SDG	sustainable development goals
SIDS	sudden infant death syndrome
s-IgA	salivary immunoglobulin a
SNRIs	serotonin and noradrenaline reuptake inhibitors
SOD	superoxide dismutase
SOL	space occupying lesion
SSA	sub-Saharan Africa
SSRIs	selective serotonin reuptake inhibitor
STD	sexually transmitted disease
STI	sexually transmitted infection
TAU	treatment as usual
TCAs	tricyclic antidepressants
tDCS	transcranial direct current stimulation
TLR4	toll-like receptor
tMS	transcranial magnetic stimulation
TQM	total quality management
TRD	treatment-resistant depression
UNGASS	special session of the united nations general assembly
VVF	vesico vaginal fistula
WHI	women's health initiative
WHO	world health organization
WITS	women and newborns transmission study

Preface

The topic of women's health is complex and impacted by social, cultural, psychological, and biological elements. Even if the medical and health fields have seen tremendous advancements, the particular difficulties faced by women are still changing, calling for creative solutions and a better comprehension of the socioeconomic elements influencing their well-being. These complexities are covered in this Volume 2 of *Holistic Approaches for Women's Sustainable Health,* which builds on the conversations started in the first volume and examines recent developments, socioeconomic effects, and creative approaches to improving female health globally.

This volume is divided into four comprehensive parts, each addressing a distinct aspect of women's health.

Part I (Socioeconomic and Social Impacts on Women's Health) looks at how women's experiences with healthcare are influenced by social and economic variables. This section highlights the external factors that impact women's health outcomes, especially in marginalized and disadvantaged communities, ranging from the impact of marital relations and social problems to the implications of socioeconomic position on healthcare access.

The psychological aspects of female health are examined in Part II (Psychological and Emotional Well-Being), with particular attention paid to problems like stress, mental health, and the psychological effects of certain medical illnesses like breast cancer. The importance of social and professional support networks in enhancing women's mental health outcomes is also covered, highlighting the necessity of taking a comprehensive approach to women's emotional health.

Modern developments in women's healthcare are covered in detail in Part III (Technological and Innovative Solutions). This section demonstrates the revolutionary potential of technology in tackling the health difficulties faced by women, ranging from digital ecosystems and the use of IoT and artificial intelligence in diagnostics to machine-learning approaches for illness detection. New avenues for individualized and preventative care are made possible by the incorporation of cutting-edge technologies like chatbots and ChatGPT into the healthcare industry.

The holistic methods and traditional knowledge that have benefited women's health for ages are revisited in Part IV (Holistic and Traditional Approaches to Female Health). The use of yoga, meditation, and religion as supplementary treatments is being investigated, especially in the treatment of diseases such as polycystic ovary syndrome. Additionally, time management techniques, health education, and outreach are included in this part as essential resources for enabling women to take charge of their own health.

The contributors to this volume offer their distinct viewpoints and areas of expertise to illuminate the complex aspects of women's health. The goal is to provide readers a thorough grasp of how traditional, social, and technical approaches may come together to treat women's health holistically.

We hope that this second volume will stimulate more study, discussion, and action to enhance women's health and well-being throughout the world. We may strive toward a day when women's health is completely recognized and treated holistically by taking into account both the insights of traditional methods and the developments in contemporary medicine.

The entire 4-volume set consists of:

Holistic Approaches for Women's Sustainable Health

Volume 1: Foundations, Innovations, Challenges, and Management

Volume 2: Advancements, Socioeconomic Impacts, and Innovative Strategies

Volume 3: Herbs, Spices, Phytochemicals, and Cereals: Body Care, Cancer Prevention, and Hormonal Health

Volume 4: Benefits of Vegetables, Medicinal Plants, and Trees

—Editors

PART I

SOCIOECONOMIC AND SOCIAL IMPACTS ON WOMEN'S HEALTH

CHAPTER 1

Holistic Approach to Female Health Issues: An Introduction

AJIT PAL SINGH,[1*] NEELESH KUMAR MAURYA,[2]
RAHUL SAXENA,[3] SUYASH SAXENA,[3] and NEETI KUSHWAHA[4]

*Corresponding author

ABSTRACT

A holistic approach to women's health empowers all ages to manage the intricate aspects of their physical and emotional well-being. This approach acknowledges the multidimensional character of women's health, including the effects of hormone cycles, social issues, and environmental exposure. However, the voyage goes beyond the physical. Understanding the relationship between stress, anxiety, depression, and emotional resilience is critical. Women can develop coping skills and negotiate life's obstacles more easily by using techniques such as cognitive–behavioral therapy, mindfulness practices, and cultivating strong social connections. Furthermore, reducing exposure to environmental contaminants and cultivating a supportive atmosphere can have considerable long-term benefits. Finally, a comprehensive approach promotes self-awareness and encourages women to develop individualized well-being strategies. This includes incorporating holistic practices into daily life, recognizing accomplishments, and seeking professional assistance if needed.

Holistic Approaches for Women's Sustainable Health, Volume 2: Advancements, Socioeconomic Impacts, and Innovative Strategies. Junaid Ahmad Malik, Anamika Chauhan, and Megh R. Goyal (Eds)

DOI: 10.1201/9781779641656-2

1.1 INTRODUCTION

The traditional healthcare model has been criticized for its reactive approach to illness, which often treats symptoms in isolation and neglects the intricate web of connections that influence a woman's overall health. This approach is a journey toward wholeness, where each element supports and harmonizes with the others [1]. Traditional medicine often treats these pulled threads individually, neglecting the underlying pattern of the entire tapestry. A holistic approach to women's health recognizes the interconnectedness of all aspects of being and seeks to create a symphony of well-being, where each element supports and harmonizes with the others. By embracing a holistic approach, women can empower themselves to take charge of their health and create a foundation for a vibrant and fulfilling life [3]. A holistic approach offers a more comprehensive and empowering alternative, acknowledging that physical, mental, emotional, and spiritual well-being are intricately connected. Prevention is key, as focus on healthy lifestyle choices and stress management can significantly reduce the risk of future health complications. Each woman is unique, with distinct needs and experiences, and a holistic approach allows for personalized strategies tailored to each woman's journey [4]. Empowerment is essential, as women are active participants in their health journey [6]. This holistic approach incorporates various elements to create a symphony of well-being, including diet and nutrition; mind–body practices such as yoga, meditation, mindfulness, exercise, and movement; complementary and alternative therapies; and spiritual connection.

1.1.1 SPECIFIC SYSTEMS AND LIMITATIONS

- **Mental health:** Persons often overlook or misunderstand the symptoms of anxiety, depression, and postpartum depression. Most people tend to overlook the emotional and psychological components of women's health.
- **Musculoskeletal system:** The prevention of osteoporosis, which poses a substantial threat to the bone health of women, has not been fully addressed or addressed adequately [10].

- **Reproductive system:** While necessary, this attention may overshadow other critical systems. Hormonal changes, menstrual irregularities, and reproductive issues were prioritized over other issues, such as cardiovascular health, which is a significant cause of death for women worldwide [9].

1.1.2 CONSEQUENCES OF TRADITIONAL APPROACHES

- **Disempowerment:** Ignoring women's health concerns can lead to frustration and a loss of control over their well-being [11].
- **Incomplete treatment:** Treatment procedures frequently ignore emotional and social factors that influence women's health [12].
- **Limited diagnosis:** The narrow focus on the reproductive domain may result in overlooked or inaccurate diagnoses of other disorders.

Today's understanding of women's health recognizes a multifaceted interaction of physical, mental, emotional, and social elements, evolving beyond a sole focus on reproduction. Current research reinforces this comprehensive approach by highlighting the correlation between improved sleep quality and reduced depression in menopausal women. This empowers women to take charge of their overall health throughout their lifespan. A holistic approach, which incorporates stress reduction techniques such as mindfulness meditation and explores complementary therapies such as acupuncture (endorsed by the National Centre for Complementary and Integrative Health), can effectively enhance overall health outcomes, prevent chronic diseases, and improve emotional well-being. While challenges such as accessibility and time commitment exist, women can achieve a healthier and more empowered future by prioritizing healthy behaviors, cultivating strong social connections, and seeking support from a healthcare provider.

This chapter focuses on holistic approach that acknowledges multidimensional character of women's health, including the effects of hormone cycles, social issues, and environmental factors. However, today's understanding of women's health recognizes a multifaceted interaction of physical, mental, emotional, and social elements.

1.2 PARADIGM SHIFT: THE HOLISTIC APPROACH

Holistic medicine offers a more comprehensive approach to women's health, recognizing the interconnectedness of mind, body, and spirit. This approach fosters the creation of individualized healthcare plans that consider a woman's physical health, mental and emotional well-being, social environment, and spiritual values [14].

1.2.1 BENEFITS OF A HOLISTIC APPROACH

- **Comprehensive care** addresses a woman's health requirements holistically, encouraging total well-being.
- **Empowerment:** Women participate in decision-making and feel heard about their health concerns.
- **Improved diagnosis** identifies all contributing factors for a more accurate diagnosis and treatment approach [17].
- **Preventative focus** promotes long-term health and disease prevention through healthy lifestyle habits.

1.2.2 IMPLEMENTING HOLISTIC APPROACH

- **Emphasis on preventative care:** Regular checkups, good food, exercise, and stress management promote general well-being.
- **Integrative medicine** may combine alternative therapies such as acupuncture, massage therapy, or herbal remedies with traditional medicine when necessary.
- **Mind–body connection:** Mindfulness meditation and yoga can promote stress reduction and emotional well-being [18, 21].
- **Patient-centered care** involves physicians actively listening to and addressing a woman's specific wants and preferences.

1.3 POWER OF THE INTERCONNECTED SELF: BODY, MIND, AND SPIRIT

- **Body:** Engaging in physical activity is not just about physical health; it also enhances mental well-being and emotional resilience.

- **Mind:** Stress, anxiety, and depression can manifest as physical symptoms. Conversely, chronic physical conditions can take a toll on mental health.
- **Spirit:** A sense of purpose, spiritual connection, or strong social bonds can positively impact overall health and well-being [12].

A holistic approach promotes optimal health since it addresses all aspects. For example, controlling stress with meditation can improve sleep quality, which boosts energy and emotional well-being. This has a good ripple effect on a woman's physical and emotional well-being. The old approach to women's health served its purpose, but it provided an incomplete picture [20]. A holistic approach, which recognizes the interdependence of mind, body, and spirit, encourages women to take control of their health and build a symphony of health that lasts their entire lives [22].

1.4 PILLARS OF A HOLISTIC APPROACH

- **Physical health:** Women's health is a unique landscape shaped by a complex interplay of biological and social factors: hormonal fluctuations, from puberty through menopause and beyond, significantly impact both physical and mental well-being. However, women can take charge of their health across their lifespan by prioritizing key lifestyle behaviors. This comprehensive approach emphasizes four pillars: (1) balanced nutrition, (2) regular exercise, (3) healthy sleep hygiene, and (4) proactive participation in preventive health screenings [23].
- **Nutrition and dietary considerations for women:** A healthy body begins with a well-balanced diet rich in important nutrients. Women's nutritional demands change throughout their lives, influenced by hormonal shifts and individual health concerns. Here is an overview of the important considerations: Nutrition plays a fundamental role in women's health across all life stages. Taking a holistic approach to diet transcends mere calorie counting. It prioritizes providing the body with the essential nutrients it requires for optimal functioning. This chapter explores the distinct

nutritional requirements of women and investigates how dietary choices can profoundly influence physical, mental, and emotional well-being [24].

- **Understanding the female body:** Women's bodies experience hormonal fluctuations throughout their lives, from menstruation and pregnancy to menopause. These hormonal shifts create specific nutritional needs that differ from men's. For example, women generally require less total energy intake due to differences in muscle mass and basal metabolic rate. However, their needs for certain micronutrients such as iron, calcium, and folate are often higher [27].
- **Essential nutrients for women:** Throughout their whole lives, women should strive to maintain maximum health by adhering to a diet that is both well-balanced and abundant in whole foods. However, due to the specific physiological requirements of women, certain nutrients play an even more important role than they already do. This chapter presents a comprehensive overview of several vital nutrients, focusing on their functions, the hazards associated with deficiency, and the sources of diet. This chapter also provides a comprehensive overview of essential nutrients for women, focusing on their functions, risks associated with deficiency, and sources of diet. Iron is a crucial component in the transportation of oxygen within red blood cells, energy generation, and brain functioning. Women are more likely to experience menstruation and childbirth, which can result in anemia, which is characterized by symptoms such as loss of strength, weariness, and shortness of breath [28].

Lean meats, poultry, fish, beans, lentils, and cereals that have been fortified with iron are particularly beneficial for women. Vitamin C can improve the absorption of nonheme iron, so it is good to consume plant-based iron sources in conjunction with fruits and vegetables abundant in vitamin C. The risk of osteoporosis, a disorder characterized by bone loss and increased fracture risk, is enhanced when there is a shortage in *calcium*. This risk is especially significant for women who have gone through menopause due to hormonal changes [29]. Dairy products (milk, yoghurt, cheese), vegetables with dark green leaves (kale, collard greens), and fortified meals (plant-based milks, tofu) are important sources of vitamin D. Folate (folate and folic acid) is essential for DNA production and cell division, and its deficiency can raise the risk of neural tube abnormalities in the growing baby, particularly during pregnancy. Vitamin D works in conjunction with calcium for bone health and absorption, increasing the immune system's function and controlling mood. Fattening fish, egg yolks, and fortified foods are some of the few dietary sources of vitamin D. Inadequate consumption of omega-3 fatty acids may be a contributing factor in various health problems, but it is not a standard definition of insufficiency [31].

1.5 DIETARY CONSIDERATIONS ACROSS LIFE STAGES

- **Lactation:** Women who are breastfeeding require additional calories and nutrients to support milk production. A healthy diet with a focus on fruits, vegetables, whole grains, and lean protein is essential.
- **Menopause:** Hormonal shifts that occur during menopause have been shown to raise the chance of developing chronic diseases such as osteoporosis and cardiovascular disease. It is possible to mitigate these risks by consuming a diet that is abundant in fruits, vegetables, whole grains, and healthy fats.
- **Menstruation:** During menstruation, women may experience iron loss and premenstrual syndrome (PMS) symptoms. A diet rich in iron, complex carbohydrates, and healthy fats can help manage these issues.
- **Pregnancy:** Nutritional needs significantly increase during pregnancy to support fetal development. A balanced diet rich in essential nutrients and adequate hydration is crucial.

1.5.1 HOLISTIC DIETARY PRACTICES

Beyond specific nutrients, a holistic approach to diet incorporates mindful eating practices and emphasizes the social and emotional aspects of food. Some key considerations are given as follows:

- **Cultural and familial influences:** Acknowledge how cultural traditions and family habits shape dietary choices. Consider adapting these influences to promote a healthy eating pattern.
- **Emotional awareness:** Identify emotional triggers that lead to unhealthy eating habits. Develop coping mechanisms to address these emotions without resorting to food.

1.5.2 IMPORTANCE OF EXERCISE AND MOVEMENT FOR OVERALL HEALTH

Exercise on a regular basis helps to promote cardiovascular health by strengthening the heart and boosting circulation. This is essential for maintaining physical health. Furthermore, it helps in the management of weight by assisting in the burning of calories and the development of lean muscle mass. Exercise is beneficial to the health of the musculoskeletal system because it helps to maintain strong bones and muscles, which in turn reduces the risk of osteoporosis and promotes improved posture and balance. Specifically, weight-bearing workouts are excellent for bone density because of their positive effects [21]. These endorphins can alleviate adverse emotions such as stress, anxiety, and despair. There is a correlation between engaging in regular physical activity and enhanced cognitive performance as well as the quality of sleep. The prevention of disease can be accomplished by engaging in regular physical activity, which can reduce the risk of a variety of chronic diseases, such as cardiovascular disease, stroke, some types of cancer, and metabolic disorders. Additionally, it can assist in the management of preexisting health issues such as arthritis and persistent pain. The results of numerous studies have repeatedly demonstrated that those who engage in physical activity have a greater propensity to live longer and healthier lives in comparison to those who lead sedentary lifestyles. Participating in regular physical activity is linked to a lower chance of dying prematurely from several causes. Being physically active can improve one's overall quality of life by boosting one's energy levels, elevating one's mood, and fostering a sense of well-being. In addition to this, it offers an opportunity for social interaction, which can be beneficial to one's self-esteem and confidence.

1.5.3 SLEEP HYGIENE AND ITS IMPACT ON FEMALE HEALTH

Even though it may appear to be a state of inactivity, sleep is an essential component of general health and well-being. Therefore, it is necessary for women to engage in appropriate sleep hygiene activities. The following is an in-depth examination of the significance of proper sleep hygiene for the health of women, focusing on the impact that it has on several elements of well-being. The term "sleep hygiene" refers to the routines that support the quality of one's sleep. The creation of a regular sleep schedule, the establishment of a pleasant nighttime routine, the optimization of the sleeping environment, and the avoidance of behaviors that interrupt sleep are all activities that fall under this category; for the purpose of preserving emotional fortitude and mental clarity, it is essential to get enough quality sleep. Sleep deprivation can have a negative impact on cognitive function, which can include memory, focus, and the ability to make decisions. Studies have shown that there is a connection between insufficient sleep and menstruation irregularities as well as fertility problems. Sleep deprivation that lasts for an extended period of time can cause persistent weariness, which can have an effect on overall energy levels and everyday functioning (National Academies of Sciences, Engineering, and Medicine). Because of the hormonal shifts and biological processes that occur, it is essential for women to practice excellent sleep hygiene. The establishment of a regular sleep schedule, the development of a calming nighttime routine, the optimization of the environment in which one sleeps, and the formation of healthy habits are all essential practices. To maintain the natural sleep–wake cycle of the body, it is necessary to establish a constant sleep pattern, even on weekends. Melatonin production, which is responsible for regulating sleep, is stimulated when a bedroom is made to be cold, calm, dark, and free of clutter. Additionally, limiting blue light from electronic devices and avoiding use of screens for at least an hour before going to bed can be beneficial. Exercising on a regular basis can increase the quality of sleep, but you should avoid doing intensive activities close to bedtime [22]. Additionally, following a diet that is well-balanced and reducing the amount of caffeine and alcohol consumed, particularly at nights, can be of assistance. These behaviors contribute to the facilitation of a good sleeping environment for females.

1.6 STRESS–HEALTH TANGO: A TWO-WAY STREET

Stress, a normal reaction to difficult conditions, can appear both physically and emotionally. When managed properly, stress can push us to act. However, persistent or mismanaged stress can harm both mental and physical health.

- **Stress and physical health:** Chronic stress weakens the immune system, increasing vulnerability to sickness. It increases the risk of chronic diseases such as heart disease, high blood pressure, type 2 diabetes, and certain malignancies. Musculoskeletal issues and digestive issues can also result from stress.
- **Stress and mental health:** Irritability, anger, and difficulty in concentrating are common effects of stress. Stress can sap energy and disrupt sleep patterns.

1.6.1 ANXIETY AND DEPRESSION: UNDERSTANDING COMMON ISSUES IN WOMEN

- **Anxiety:** Symptoms of anxiety are excessive worry; racing thoughts; restlessness; irritability; fatigue; difficulty in concentrating; and physical symptoms such as sweating, rapid heartbeat, and shortness of breath. Hormonal fluctuations, life transitions (e.g., childbirth, menopause), social pressures, and genetics can all play a role as contributing factors of anxiety.
- **Depression** is a condition characterized by persistent sadness, hopelessness, loss of interest in activities, changes in appetite and sleep, feelings of worthlessness, and difficulty in concentrating or making decisions and can be influenced by hormonal changes, stressful life events, genetics, and certain medical conditions.

1.6.2 BUILDING COPING MECHANISMS AND EMOTIONAL RESILIENCE

Developing coping mechanisms and emotional resilience empowers women to navigate stress, anxiety, and depression. Here are some effective strategies: cognitive–behavioral therapy helps identify negative thought patterns and develop healthier coping mechanisms. Mindfulness and meditation cultivate present-moment awareness and emotional regulation. Building strong social support provides understanding. Regular exercise releases endorphins and promotes well-being. Relaxation techniques such as deep breathing and yoga manage stress. Last, prioritizing good sleep hygiene is crucial for optimal mental and physical health.

1.6.3 POWER OF SELF-CARE AND STRESS MANAGEMENT TECHNIQUES

Self-care is not a luxury but a necessity for emotional well-being. By prioritizing self-care, women nurture their emotional needs and strengthen their resilience against stress.

- **Disconnecting to reconnect:** Limit screen time and social media use before bed to promote restful sleep and reduce stress.
- **Healthy eating:** Nourish the body with nutritious foods to support emotional well-being and energy levels.
- **Mindfulness practices:** Meditation, yoga, and deep breathing techniques can enhance self-awareness and manage stress.
- **Setting boundaries:** Saying no to additional commitments when overwhelmed protects your mental and emotional space.

1.6.4 STRESS MANAGEMENT TECHNIQUES

This summary discusses various techniques for promoting calmness and relaxation, including progressive muscle relaxation, visualizing a peaceful place, deep breathing exercises, and journaling. It emphasizes the importance of releasing tension, creating a mental image of a relaxing place, and focusing on slow, controlled breaths to reduce anxiety.

1.7 SEEKING PROFESSIONAL HELP

A therapist can provide valuable guidance and support in managing stress, anxiety, and depression. Women's mental and emotional well-being is multifaceted. In gaining insights and understanding on how stress impacts them, the most common types of mental health issues seen in women, the importance of self-care and that stress management should be a priority for everything else, women can develop emotional strength so they feel greater confidence to handle what life throws at them.

1.7.1 SOCIAL AND ENVIRONMENTAL HEALTH

Social and environmental factors significantly impact women's health, influencing everything from mental well-being to physical health outcomes. This section explores the importance of strong social connections, the impact of healthy relationships, the influence of environmental toxins, and strategies for creating a supportive and healthy environment.

1.7.2 POWER OF CONNECTION: SOCIAL RELATIONSHIPS AND WOMEN'S WELL-BEING

Humans are social creatures, and strong social connections are essential for emotional and physical health. Women often thrive in supportive social networks. The impact of social relationships is given as follows:

- **Improved physical health:** Strong social connections can lower blood pressure, strengthen the immune system, and even increase longevity.
- **Increased happiness:** Social interaction releases endorphins, natural mood lifters, promoting feelings of happiness and well-being.
- **Reduced stress:** Social support buffers the negative effects of stress. Sharing burdens and receiving encouragement foster resilience.
- **Sense of belonging:** Feeling valued and understood by a supportive network fosters self-esteem and purpose.

1.7.3 BUILDING A STRONG SUPPORT SYSTEM

- **Joining groups:** Find communities based on shared interests or hobbies to expand your social network.

- **Nurturing close relationships:** Invest time and energy in cultivating strong friendships and familial bonds.
- **Seeking professional help:** If you struggle to build or maintain healthy relationships, consider therapy for guidance and support.
- **Volunteering:** Helping others fosters a sense of connection and purpose while building new relationships.

1.7.4 CULTIVATING HEALTHY RELATIONSHIPS: BEYOND THE OBVIOUS

Healthy relationships, both romantic and platonic, contribute significantly to women's well-being. Following should be considered:

1.7.4.1 ROMANTIC RELATIONSHIPS

- **Healthy boundaries**: Maintaining healthy boundaries protects your emotional and physical well-being within the relationship.
- **Mutual respect and support**: A healthy partnership fosters open communication, trust, and emotional support in both directions.
- **Shared values and goals**: Compatibility on core values and life goals creates a foundation for a fulfilling relationship.

1.7.4.2 PLATONIC RELATIONSHIPS

- **Nonjudgmental support**: Friends who listen without judgment and offer encouragement create a safe space for emotional expression.
- **Reliability and trustworthiness**: Knowing you can depend on your friends strengthens the bonds of trust and support.
- **Shared interests and activities**: Engaging in activities you enjoy with friends fosters a sense of connection and shared experiences.

1.8 ENVIRONMENTAL HEALTH: THE SILENT THREAT

1.8.1 ENVIRONMENTAL FACTORS AFFECTING WOMEN'S HEALTH

The environment we live in plays a crucial role in women's health. Modern life unfortunately exposes us to various environmental toxins and pollutants that can have a detrimental impact.

- **Air and water pollution**: Exposure to air and water pollution can exacerbate respiratory problems, increase the risk of heart disease, and negatively impact fertility.
- **Endocrine-disrupting chemicals (EDCs)**: EDCs are found in many common household products and can interfere with hormonal processes, potentially contributing to reproductive issues and certain cancers.
- **Heavy metals**: Exposure to heavy metals such as lead and mercury can affect cognitive function, fertility, and fetal development.

1.8.2 CREATING A HEALTHY AND SUPPORTIVE ENVIRONMENT

While we cannot entirely control the environment, following strategies can minimize exposure to environmental toxins:

- **Consume organic produce**: When possible, choose organic fruits and vegetables to limit pesticide exposure.
- **Drink filtered water**: Filtering tap water can reduce exposure to certain contaminants.
- **Improve indoor air quality**: Open windows for ventilation and consider using air purifiers.
- **Reduce exposure to everyday toxins**: Choose cleaning products and personal care products labeled "natural" or "eco-friendly."
- **Stay informed**: Stay updated on environmental hazards and advocate for clean air and water policies.

1.8.3 A HOLISTIC APPROACH TO WELL-BEING

Understanding the interplay between social and environmental factors with women's health empowers you to make informed choices and prioritize a holistic approach to well-being. By nurturing strong social connections, cultivating healthy relationships, minimizing exposure to environmental toxins, and creating a supportive environment, women can navigate life's challenges with greater resilience and well-being. The journey toward optimal health is a continuous process. Celebrate your successes, seek help when needed, and embrace the power of social and environmental factors to create a life that nourishes your mind, body, and spirit [33, 35, 36].

1.9 IMPLEMENTING THE HOLISTIC APPROACH: A PRACTICAL GUIDE

The holistic approach to well-being may seem complex, but it can be broken down into manageable steps you can integrate into daily life. Following practical guide can be considered:

- **Minimize toxin exposure:** Choose natural cleaning products and personal care items whenever possible. Limit exposure to environmental pollutants by spending time outdoors in green spaces.
- **Prioritize self-awareness:** Tune into body's signals. Pay attention to energy levels, mood fluctuations, and physical sensations. Track sleep patterns, dietary habits, and emotional state. Identifying patterns can help to tailor the approach.
- **Start small and build gradually:** Do not overwhelm with drastic changes. Begin by incorporating one or two new practices each week. Celebrate the successes, no matter how small. Consistency is a key!
- **Support sustainability efforts:** Choose eco-friendly products and support businesses committed to sustainability.

1.9.1 BUILDING A PERSONALIZED WELLNESS PLAN: A MULTIFACETED APPROACH

- **Be flexible:** Adapt your plan as needed. Life is dynamic, and your wellness needs might change over time.
- **Focus on balance:** Include practices that address physical, mental, emotional, social, and environmental aspects of well-being.

- **Seek guidance:** Consider consultations with healthcare professionals such as registered dietitians, therapists, or holistic practitioners who can tailor their advice to your unique situation.
- **Start small:** Introduce changes gradually to avoid overwhelming. Celebrate your successes along the way.

1.10 QUALIFIED HEALTHCARE PRACTITIONERS TO SUPPORT A HOLISTIC APPROACH

In a world of fragmented medical model, seeking healthcare practitioners who embrace a holistic approach can feel like navigating a maze. This chapter delves into the analytical considerations involved in finding qualified professionals who support the holistic well-being journey.

1.11 EMBRACE THE JOURNEY: HOLISTIC WELLNESS IS A LIFELONG PURSUIT

This chapter delves into the analytical framework of holistic wellness, emphasizing its lifelong nature and the ongoing pursuit of optimal health. Tables 1.1–1.3 summarize components of a holistic approach to health issues of a female.

- **Adapting to challenges**: Life inevitably presents challenges and setbacks. A holistic approach equips us with the tools and resilience to navigate these difficulties and maintain a sense of well-being (techniques such as stress management and emotional processing can help us to maintain balance even during turbulent times).
- **Balance is key**: While all aspects of holistic wellness are important, focusing too heavily on any one area can create an imbalance. Striving for a balanced approach that prioritizes each component is essential.
- **Dynamic needs**: Our needs for physical activity, dietary intake, and social connection can change significantly throughout our lives. For example, the hormonal shifts experienced during menstruation, pregnancy, and menopause necessitate adjustments in self-care practices.

- **Evolving self-awareness**: As we navigate life experiences, our self-awareness deepens. We may discover new triggers for stress, identify unhealthy habits, or uncover areas where we can prioritize self-care. This ongoing process allows for continuous refinement of our holistic wellness strategies.
- **Lifelong pursuit—embracing the journey**: Life throws unexpected curveballs, and our needs and circumstances change over time. Here is why a lifelong approach is crucial.
- **Self-compassion**: The journey toward holistic wellness is not always linear. There will be setbacks and moments where self-care feels challenging. Cultivating self-compassion allows us to learn from setbacks and get back on track with kindness and understanding.

TABLE 1.1 Holistic Approach to Female Health Issues

Aspect of Holistic Approach	Description	Potential Benefits
Complementary and alternative medicine (CAM)	Therapies such as acupuncture or massage can provide additional support for specific health concerns [32]	Pain management Improved sleep Enhanced relaxation
Exercise and movement	Regular physical activity promotes cardiovascular health, strengthens bones, and boosts energy levels [34]	Weight management Improved mood Reduced risk of chronic diseases
Mind–body practices	Techniques such as yoga, meditation, and mindfulness help manage stress and promote emotional well-being [16]	Reduced stress and anxiety Improved sleep quality Increased emotional resilience
Nutrition and diet	Focuses on whole, unprocessed foods rich in essential nutrients tailored to women's specific needs across life stages [25, 26]	Hormone balance Improved energy levels Reduced risk of chronic diseases
Spiritual connection	Nurturing a sense of purpose and connection to something larger than oneself can contribute to overall well-being	Increased sense of peace and meaning Improved coping mechanisms for challenges

TABLE 1.2 Nutrition and Dietary Considerations for Women

Nutrients	Importance for Women	Dietary Sources
Calcium	Crucial for strong bones and teeth. Needs increase during pregnancy and lactation. Deficiency can increase the risk of osteoporosis later in life	Dairy products, green leafy vegetables, and fortified foods [8]
Folate	Plays a vital role in DNA synthesis and cell division. Adequate folate intake during pregnancy helps prevent neural tube defects in the baby	Green leafy vegetables, lentils, beans, and fortified grains [5]
Iron	Essential for oxygen transport, energy production, and red blood cell formation. Deficiency can lead to anemia, fatigue, and decreased cognitive function	Women are more susceptible to iron deficiency due to menstruation and childbirth [25]
Vitamin D	Aids in calcium absorption and bone health. Vitamin D deficiency can contribute to bone loss and increased risk of fractures	Fatty fish, egg yolks, fortified foods, and sunlight exposure [13]

TABLE 1.3 Additional Considerations Across Life Stages

Life Stages	Nutritional Considerations
Lactation	Women who are breastfeeding require additional calories and nutrients to support milk production. A healthy diet with a focus on fruits, vegetables, whole grains, and lean protein is essential [15]
Menopause	Hormonal changes during menopause can increase the risk of chronic diseases such as heart disease and osteoporosis. A diet rich in fruits, vegetables, whole grains, and healthy fats can help manage these risks [15]
Menstruation	Iron-rich foods and complex carbohydrates can help manage iron loss and PMS symptoms [30]
Pregnancy	Nutritional needs significantly increase to support fetal development. A balanced diet rich in essential nutrients and adequate hydration is crucial [2]

1.12 CHALLENGES AND CONSIDERATIONS

- **Defining "holistic"**: The term "holistic" can encompass various philosophies and practices. It is crucial to define what aspects of a holistic approach are most important.
- **Limited regulation**: Many CAM practitioners operate outside the traditional medical regulatory framework. This necessitates careful evaluation to ensure qualifications and safety.
- **Misinformation and unproven practices**: The landscape of CAM therapies is vast, and some lack strong scientific backing.

It is essential to be discerning and avoid practitioners promoting unproven or potentially harmful practices.

Finding a qualified holistic healthcare practitioner involves a multi-pronged approach given as follows:

- **Communication style**: Find a practitioner who fosters open communication and actively listens to your concerns. A collaborative approach is vital for a successful therapeutic relationship.
- **Patient reviews**: While online reviews should be taken with a grain of salt, they can offer some insight into other patients' experiences. Look for consistent themes and red flags.
- **Safety and integration**: Discuss potential interactions with conventional medications and the role of the practitioner in collaborating with your primary care physician to ensure a cohesive healthcare plan.
- **Treatment philosophy**: Discuss the practitioner's philosophy and treatment approach. Ensure it aligns with your definition of "holistic" and your specific health goals.
- **Understanding credentials**: Research the practitioner's training and qualifications. Look for board certification within their specific field, membership in reputable professional organizations, and evidence of continuing education.

Several resources can aid to search for qualified holistic practitioners given as follows:

- **Online directories**: Several online directories list holistic practitioners, often with user reviews. These can be a starting point, but thorough vetting is still necessary.
- **Professional associations**: Many CAM professions have national or regional professional organizations that maintain directories of certified practitioners. These organizations can also provide information on ethical standards and qualifications.
- **Importance of collaboration**: The ideal scenario involves collaboration between a qualified holistic healthcare practitioner and primary care physician. Open communication and information

sharing between all parties ensure a coordinated approach to your overall health and well-being [7].

- **Word-of-mouth recommendations**: Seek recommendations from friends, family, or healthcare providers familiar with holistic approaches.

1.13 SUMMARY

This chapter discusses the concept of a holistic approach to female health, emphasizing that it is a multifaceted approach that addresses the interplay of physical, mental, emotional, social, and spiritual factors. Traditional medical approaches often focus on treating specific symptoms, but a holistic approach aims to optimize overall well-being. This approach includes addressing women's unique physiological needs, incorporating mind–body practices such as yoga and meditation, encouraging regular exercise, exploring supplementary and alternative therapies, promoting sleep hygiene and rest, recognizing the importance of social support networks, and acknowledging the benefits of spirituality or a sense of purpose in fostering resilience and well-being. The chapter concludes that a holistic approach empowers women to take charge of their health and navigate the complexities of their well-being throughout life. It acknowledges that women's health is a journey, not a destination, and encourages continuous exploration and adaptation based on individual needs and circumstances.

KEYWORDS

- **anxiety**
- **depression**
- **diet**
- **emotional**
- **holistic approach**
- **stress**
- **women's health**
- **yoga**

REFERENCES

1. Adams, A. M., & White, B. C. (2020). *Integrative Therapies in Women's Health.* Health Press.
2. American College of Obstetricians and Gynecologists (2013). ACOG Committee opinion no. 548: Weight gain during pregnancy. *Obstetrics and Gynecology*, *121*(1), 210–212.
3. Baker, J. L., & Wilson, K. R. (2019). The impact of holistic practices on female reproductive health: A review. *Journal of Women's Health, 28*(4), 567–579.
4. Brown, E. R., & Davis, C. L. (2021). *Mind–body Approaches to Chronic Conditions in Women.* Wellness Publishing.
5. CDC (2020). *Centers for Disease Control (CDC) and Prevention.*
6. Cohen, T. J. (2018). Yoga and women's health: An integrative review. *International Journal of Yoga Therapy*, *28*(1), 35–46.
7. Coke, L. A., & Hayman, L. L. (2021). Women's awareness of heart disease and risk: Two steps forward and one step back. *Journal of Cardiovascular Nursing*, *36*(1), 6–7.
8. Dawson-Hughes, B., & National Osteoporosis Foundation Guide Committee. (2008). A revised clinician's guide to the prevention and treatment of osteoporosis. *The Journal of Clinical Endocrinology & Metabolism*, *93*(7), 2463–2465.
9. Duffy, S. H., & Lee, H. K. (2017). Nutritional interventions for female health: A holistic perspective. *Nutritional Science Review*, *42*(2), 125–142.
10. Edwards, J. F., & Wang, Y. (2022). *Holistic Medicine and Women's Wellness: Exploring Alternative Treatments*. Complementary Medicine Publications.
11. Fox, M. J. (2016). The role of acupuncture in managing menopause symptoms: A meta-analysis. *Journal of Alternative and Complementary Medicine*, *22*(8), 652–660.
12. Green, C. P. (2023). *Herbal remedies for women's health issues*. Herbal Health Books.
13. Grygorieva, N. V., Kovalenko, V. M., Korzh, M. O., Tatarchuk, T. F., Dedukh, N. V., Strafun, S. S., & Chaykivska, E. F. (2023). Guideline for diagnostic, prevention and treatment of postmenopausal osteoporosis. *Pain, Joints, Spine*, *13*(3), 128–154.
14. Harris, K. M. (2020). Integrative Approaches to Managing Female Cardiovascular Health. *Cardiovascular Wellness Journal*, *15(*3), 198–210.
15. Heymsfield, S., McCarthy, C., Wong, M., Brown, J., Ramirez, S., Yang, S., & Shepherd, J. (2024). Accurate prediction of three-dimensional humanoid avatars for anthropometric modeling. *International Journal of Obesity*, 48, 1741–1747.
16. Interview by, Weeks, J., & Editor-in-Chief, JACM. (2016). The new USA NIH strategic plan for complementary and integrative health (part I)): Interview with Josephine Briggs (Director, National Center for Complementary and Integrative Health). *Alternative and Complementary Therapies*, *22*(6), 251–254.
17. Jackson, R. L. (2018). *Mindfulness and Stress Reduction in Female Populations.* Mindful Living Publications.
18. Johnson, L. E., & Thompson, G. R. (2021). Holistic approaches to managing polycystic ovary syndrome. *Reproductive Health Insights*, *14*(1), 30–42.
19. Kim, D. Y., Hong, S. H., Jang, S. H., Park, S. H., Noh, J. H., Seok, J. M., & Lee, E. J. (2022). Systematic review for the medical applications of meditation in randomized

controlled trials. *International Journal of Environmental Research and Public Health*, *19*(3), 1244–1250.

20. Lee, N. A., & Davis, M. B. (2019). Alternative therapies in women's healthcare: A comprehensive review. *Integrative Medicine Review*, *27*(2), 121–137.
21. Lief, J. (2024). *Occupational Therapy Evidenced-Based Guide for the Treatment of Peripartum People.* Doctoral dissertation, Boston University.
22. Martinez, S. R. (2017). The benefits of aromatherapy for female wellness: A systematic review. *Journal of Holistic Medicine*, *12*(3), 275–284.
23. Mitchell, I., & Govias, G. (2021). Complementary and alternative medicine in asthma. In *Asthma education* (pp. 421–443). Springer.
24. Moore, D. P., & Liu, J. Y. (2020). Exploring the impact of dietary supplements on women's health issues. *Journal of Dietary Supplements*, *17*(4), 453–465.
25. National Academies of Sciences, Division of Behavioral, Social Sciences, Medicine Division, Board on Behavioral, Sensory Sciences, & Loneliness in Older Adults. (2020). *Social Isolation and Loneliness in Older Adults: Opportunities for the Health Care System*. National Academies Press.
26. National Academies of Sciences, Division of Behavioral, Social Sciences, Medicine Division, Board on Behavioral, Sensory Sciences, & Loneliness in Older Adults. (2021). *Social Isolation and Loneliness in Older Adults: Opportunities for the Health Care System* (Part II). National Academies Press.
27. Nelson, P. A. (2018). The role of holistic nutrition in managing premenstrual syndrome. *Women's Nutrition Journal*, *33*(2), 89–99.
28. Patel, R. K. (2022). *Herbal Medicine and Female Reproductive Health.* Traditional Medicine Publications.
29. Roberts, T. J., & Clark, H. S. (2019). Yoga and hormonal balance in women: An overview. *Journal of Yoga & Physical Therapy*, 29(3), 345–357.
30. Romero, R. (2022). Introduction to the guest editors of the *American Journal of Obstetrics & Gynecology* supplement on preeclampsia 2022. *American Journal of Obstetrics & Gynecology*, *226*(2), S781–S785.
31. Smith, A. D. (2020). The impact of holistic therapies on chronic female pain. *Chronic Pain Research Journal*, *11*(1), 55–67.
32. Sodders, M. D., Martin, A. M., Coker, J., Hammond, F. M., & Hoffman, J. M. (2023). Acupuncture use for pain after traumatic brain injury: A NIDILRR traumatic brain injury model systems cohort study. *Brain Injury*, *37*(6), 494–502.
33. Taylor, S. L., Hoggatt, K. J., & Kligler, B. (2019). Complementary and integrated health approaches: What do veterans use and want? *Journal of General Internal Medicine*, *34,* 1192–1199.
34. Warburton, D. E., & Bredin, S. S. (2017). Health benefits of physical activity: A systematic review of current systematic reviews. *Current Opinion in Cardiology*, *32*(5), 541–556.
35. Wilson, A. R., & Brown, L. M. (2021). Evaluating experiences of stress and coping among African American women during the COVID-19 pandemic to inform future interventions. *Health Education & Behavior*, *48*(6), 739–746.
36. Young, M. J. (2019). Essential oils and female health: Benefits and considerations. *Aromatherapy Journal, 25*(2), 189–202.

CHAPTER 2

Impact of Socioeconomic Status on Women's Healthcare: Factors, Clinical Stressors, Disease Conditions, and Solutions

HOSSEIN ZARE,* DANIELLE GILMORE, and SHERVIN ASSARI

*Corresponding author

ABSTRACT

This study explores the relationship between income inequality and health issues among women aged 20 years and older, highlighting the intersectionality of gender and income disparities. Women face unique challenges shaped by socioeconomic factors such as education, employment, and gender roles, which impact their health outcomes. In this study, we access the link between the poverty-to-income ratio (PIR) and five common health issues among US women: (1) obesity, (2) hypertension, (3) diabetes, (4) depression, and (5) clinical stress (measured by allostatic load). Data from the National Health and Nutrition Examination Survey (1999–2016) were analyzed using descriptive statistics and multivariate regression. The Lorenz curve analyzed income inequality distribution among women with obesity, hypertension, diabetes, depression, and high allostatic load, including 22,650 participants from diverse racial backgrounds. The findings showed that women in lower PIR groups had higher prevalence rates for obesity, diabetes, depression, and elevated stress compared to those in higher PIR groups, indicating a clear link between income inequality and health issues. This study emphasizes the need to address poverty

Holistic Approaches for Women's Sustainable Health, Volume 2: Advancements, Socioeconomic Impacts, and Innovative Strategies. Junaid Ahmad Malik, Anamika Chauhan, and Megh R. Goyal (Eds)

DOI: 10.1201/9781779641656-3

and income inequality as key drivers of poor health outcomes in women, advocating for policies that promote economic equity to improve health.

2.1 INTRODUCTION

The concept of the "American Dream," emblematic of the belief that every individual in the United States possesses an equal opportunity to achieve success and prosperity through perseverance, hard work, and initiative, stands as a cornerstone of the national ethos. This idea suggests a level playing field where success is attainable for all, regardless of their starting point [15, 34, 58]. However, the pervasive issue of income inequality sharply contrasts with this narrative, presenting significant barriers that prevent many from realizing this dream. Income inequality, characterized by a disproportionate distribution of wealth and income, erodes the foundation of economic stability and upward mobility that the "American Dream" promises to provide [5, 34, 58, 107, 159].

Over the last five decades, the United States has seen income inequality rise at rates unparalleled by other industrialized nations [5, 82, 85, 107]. This trend has persisted despite periods of economic growth both domestically and internationally. A 2019 Congressional Budget Office report revealed that the wealthiest 10% of individuals held almost three-quarters (72%) of the total wealth in the United States, while the bottom 50% only holds about 2% [30]. The COVID-19 pandemic not only amplified existing health disparities but also brought to the forefront the systemic barriers that perpetuate income inequality. Women and individuals from lower income backgrounds have borne the brunt of the pandemic's impact, facing disproportionate challenges in terms of job losses, reduced access to healthcare, and increased caregiving burdens, further amplifying existing health disparities and economic insecurities [8, 44, 63, 88, 149]. Income inequality detrimentally affects health outcomes by directly restricting access to healthcare and indirectly limiting essential resources such as education, employment, and housing. As a result, individuals and families with lower incomes face a higher risk of chronic diseases, mental health conditions, and shorter lifespans compared to wealthier individuals [3, 12, 67, 105, 124, 141, 161].

The impact of income inequality is even more pronounced for women, particularly women of color, who are more likely to experience poverty, earn lower wages, and carry a more significant burden of unpaid caregiving responsibilities. In this chapter, we will explore how these challenges, compounded by societal norms and gender roles, often prevent women from accessing well-paying, secure jobs, pushing them toward part-time or informal work with little to no health benefits [18, 28, 29, 79, 146]. This highlights the critical need for targeted interventions to overcome the unique barriers women face, promote health equity, and empower them economically. The COVID-19 pandemic underscored the vital intersections between economic disparity, health outcomes, and access to essential resources, spotlighting the urgent need for comprehensive policy and programmatic interventions to improve population health and economic well-being [8, 130, 147, 149, 194].

2.2 THEORETICAL FRAMEWORK: THE SOCIAL DETERMINANTS OF HEALTH

In the quest for women's health equity, the interplay between income inequality and health outcomes emerges as a critical area of concern, underscoring the profound impact of socioeconomic factors on individual and community well-being. The World Health Organization's (WHO's) social determinants of health (SDOH) framework, developed to understand these impacts, identifies vital areas such as economic stability, education access and quality, healthcare access and quality, neighborhood and built environment, and social and community context as fundamental determinants that shape health outcomes [183]. The framework elucidates how social determinants such as income level, employment status, education, and access to healthcare services collectively shape individuals' health and contribute to the health inequities observed across different populations [61, 66, 83, 155, 192].

This study employs the SDOH framework to explore how individual income levels and broader factors, including race/ethnicity, behaviors, and socioeconomic conditions, influence women's health outcomes (see Figure 2.1). Economic disparities, such as poverty and income inequality, intersect with race and gender to shape access to education, employment, healthcare, and social opportunities, creating a multifaceted network of influences on women's health. These interlocking factors collectively impact women's physical health, mental well-being, and stress levels, highlighting the need for a holistic approach to developing interventions and policies that tackle the societal roots of health disparities and champion equitable health outcomes for women, particularly women of color.

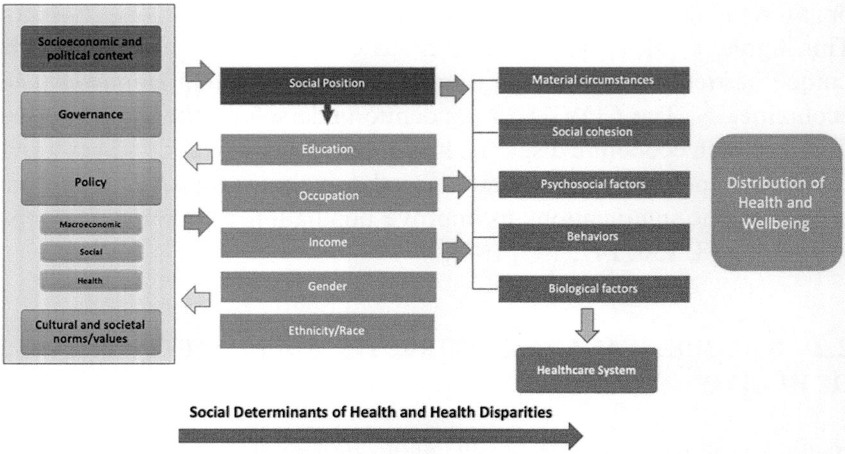

FIGURE 2.1 WHO's conceptual framework for SDOH.
Source: Reprinted from Ref. [144].

The SDOH framework demonstrates how gender and race intersect with other determinants to sculpt health outcomes, emphasizing the imperative to integrate gender and racial considerations in policy and intervention development. Key areas of focus include:

1. **Economic stability:** The gender wage gap, exacerbated by racial disparities, poses significant challenges to economic stability and access to health benefits for women, with women of color facing the most severe systemic barriers [22, 50, 121, 193].
2. **Education access and quality:** Systemic racism and gender bias amplify barriers to higher education and vocational training for women, particularly women of color, impacting their health outcomes due to caregiving responsibilities and economic constraints [88, 92, 100, 108].
3. **Healthcare access and quality:** Women face hurdles accessing comprehensive healthcare, including reproductive and mental health services. These challenges are magnified for women of

color by cost, insurance gaps, and entrenched biases within the healthcare system [35, 95, 116, 127, 140].

4. **Neighborhood and built environment:** Safe housing, access to nutritious food, and recreational spaces are critical for health. Women, especially those in low income and racially marginalized communities, face greater exposure to environmental hazards and limited access to health-promoting resources [42, 45, 143, 168, 172, 174].
5. **Social and community context:** Gender-based violence and discrimination, compounded by racial prejudice and transphobia, present unique stressors that negatively impact the health and well-being of women, with women of color experiencing these effects more acutely [19, 45, 60, 153, 158, 172].

2.3 RELATIONSHIP BETWEEN HEALTH AND INCOME INEQUALITY

The nexus of social determinants, race, and gender elucidates the mechanisms through which income inequality amplifies health disparities, particularly among women, underscoring the imperative for gender-sensitive strategies to advance health equity. Anchored in the SDOH framework, the authors critically examine the intricate relationship between income disparity and adverse health outcomes, with a specific focus on conditions such as obesity, hypertension, diabetes, depression, and allostatic load (AL). These conditions manifest disproportionately among women, especially those from socioeconomically marginalized and racially diverse backgrounds, accentuating the critical need for targeted interventions and policy reforms.

2.3.1 OBESITY

Obesity, defined as an abnormal or excessive fat accumulation that presents a health risk, is a growing concern worldwide [35, 41, 118, 156]. The prevalence of obesity among low-income women is notably higher, a disparity that underscores the intersection of economic hardship with limited access to nutritious food and safe recreational facilities

[10, 20, 119, 197, 198]. For women of color, these challenges increase the likelihood of residing in neighborhoods lacking essential resources for a healthy lifestyle, such as green spaces or farmers' markets [40, 84, 143, 168, 174, 187]. Studies have shown that women of color have higher obesity rates than white women [139]. According to the National Institutes of Health (2021) [10, 20, 118, 197, 198], the obesity rate among non-Hispanic (NH) Black women (56.8%) and Hispanic women (43.7%) significantly surpassed that of NH White women (38.9%), illustrating a clear link between race, income, and health outcomes [137].

2.3.2 HYPERTENSION

Hypertension, or high blood pressure, is the leading cause of premature cardiovascular morbidity. Low-income women experience higher rates of hypertension, a trend that is exacerbated for women of color due to the stressors associated with financial instability and limited healthcare access [2, 38, 39, 59, 75]. Substantial evidence has confirmed that hypertension prevalence is significantly higher among individuals with lower socio-economic status (SES), highlighting the need for targeted public health interventions that address these underlying determinants [2, 59, 65, 78, 89, 145, 197, 198].

2.3.3 DIABETES

Type 2 diabetes, a chronic condition characterized by elevated levels of blood sugar, poses a significant health risk and is closely linked to obesity and physical inactivity [9, 97, 189, 200]. The risk of developing diabetes is markedly higher in lower income populations, with economic barriers limiting access to diabetes management and preventive care [46, 81, 104, 182]. While the overall prevalence of diabetes among US women stands at approximately 14.1% compared to 15.4% in men, a closer examination by race reveals stark health disparities among women. Approximately 17.4% of NH Black women and 15.5% of Hispanic women are diagnosed with diabetes, compared to Asian and White women, 16.7% and 13.6%, respectively. Women of color are disproportionately affected, encountering systemic obstacles in accessing healthcare, which is crucial for effective disease management [16, 31, 35, 77].

2.3.4 DEPRESSION

Depression, a condition marked by persistent sadness and a diminished interest in pleasurable activities, is significantly influenced by socioeconomic factors, particularly among women. Economic hardship, coupled with caregiving responsibilities, places a disproportionate burden on women, exacerbating their risk for depression. Women living below the poverty line are over twice as likely to experience depression due to the financial strain and reduced access to mental healthcare [2, 54, 96, 139, 166]. Moreover, the intersectionality of gender, income, and race further complicates this landscape. For example, despite reporting similar rates of depression as their White counterparts, African American women often experience more chronic, persistent forms of the condition [76, 103, 178, 180, 186]. Women of color, for instance, face additional layers of stress and discrimination that not only increase their risk for depression but also impact the severity and duration of depressive episodes, highlighting the need for more culturally competent care.

2.3.5 AL

AL, the cumulative "wear and tear" on the body from chronic stress, serves as a crucial biomarker for the health impacts of socioeconomic adversity, particularly among women facing the dual challenges of low income and racial discrimination [48, 64, 71, 93, 171, 175, 199]. This measure reveals the physiological consequences of constant exposure to stress, offering insight into the deep-seated health disparities that pervade income inequality and systemic racism. Research indicates that elevated AL indices are significantly more prevalent among low-income women and women of color, underscoring the physiological toll of navigating life's adversities [14, 48, 64, 71, 93, 102, 122, 152, 171, 177, 185]. For example, studies have shown that African American women exhibit higher AL scores compared to their White counterparts, reflecting the added stress of racial discrimination on top of socioeconomic challenges [11, 93, 103, 152, 185]. These disparities are not just numbers; they translate into tangible health outcomes, with higher AL associated with increased risks for chronic conditions such as hypertension, diabetes, and cardiovascular diseases [24, 55, 71, 115, 148, 171].

2.4 IMPACT OF RACIAL AND GENDER DISCRIMINATION ON ECONOMIC AND HEALTH OUTCOMES

Addressing income and health disparities demands interventions that center the SDOH framework. Through a detailed exploration, it becomes evident that the intersectionality of race and gender plays a significant role in exacerbating health disparities, with women of color facing the most severe consequences. This study not only highlights the direct correlation between income inequality and adverse health conditions but also underscores the necessity of addressing these disparities through a lens that considers the compounded effects of SES, race, and gender. The evidence presented herein lays a critical foundation for understanding the broader narrative of health inequities within the context of income inequality. It points to the essential need for a historical and policy-oriented examination of the systemic factors that have contributed to the current landscape of health disparities among women. Such an examination is crucial for identifying root causes and developing comprehensive solutions beyond surface-level interventions.

2.4.1 GENDER WAGE GAP AND OCCUPATIONAL SEGREGATION

The gender wage gap, often simplified to a misleading statistic—women earning 82 cents for every dollar earned by men in 2020—masks the deeper issue of occupational segregation and its roots in historical exclusion from education and professional fields [51, 125, 141, 157, 17, 191]. This segregation has funneled women into lower paying sectors and limited their representation in higher paying, specialized fields traditionally dominated by men [27, 68, 110, 163, 164, 176]. The systemic barriers historically limiting women's career choices and growth opportunities are evident in today's labor market. For example, women's overrepresentation in sectors such as healthcare and education often places them in roles that, despite being essential, are undervalued and underpaid compared to their male counterparts in other industries [27, 68, 163, 164]. This history of occupational segregation contributes significantly to the wage gap and hinders women's economic independence and security.

2.4.2 IMPACT OF HISTORIC DISCRIMINATION

Redlining, a discriminatory practice that began in the 1930s, systematically marked neighborhoods with predominantly African American residents as high risk for lenders [1, 57]. This policy has had enduring effects on these communities' economic and health landscapes [1, 26, 57, 113]. A large body of evidence has confirmed that neighborhoods affected by redlining continue to experience higher poverty rates and lower home values, with 74% of these areas remaining low-to-moderate income today [37, 72, 80, 112, 123, 162, 188]. The health implications are stark, with residents in redlined communities facing increased exposure to environmental pollutants, contributing to higher rates of asthma, cancer, and cardiovascular diseases [47, 69, 106, 109, 117, 128, 173].

The ripple effects of redlining extend into the realm of colorism, where the preference for lighter skin within racial or ethnic groups exacerbates health disparities for women of color [94, 126]. This bias in healthcare settings leads to darker-skinned women receiving lower quality care and facing longer wait times [94, 126, 165, 190]. Research indicates that these experiences of discrimination contribute to higher rates of stress and depression among affected individuals [7, 25, 43, 139]. For instance, studies have shown that African American and Latina women, particularly those with darker skin tones, report significant mental health challenges linked to experiences of colorism, further highlighting the health impact of systemic discrimination [4, 21, 33, 94, 132].

By systematically addressing these entrenched disparities, it is possible to establish a foundation for a more equitable future in which the pervasive effects of historical injustices no longer determine health and economic outcomes.

2.4.3 LITERATURE REVIEW SUMMARY

Addressing income and health disparities necessitates interventions that delve into the socioeconomic and racial determinants of health. Through comprehensive analysis, this study illuminates how the intersectionality of race and gender significantly amplifies health disparities, particularly affecting women of color. By examining the intricate relationship between income inequality and adverse health outcomes—specifically diabetes, hypertension, depression, obesity, and AL—this research underscores the critical need to approach these disparities through a lens that integrates the compounded effects of SES, race, and gender. This approach is among the first to scrutinize these five health outcomes within the context of income inequality, specifically for women, employing the WHO's SDOH framework as a unique lens for analysis.

The utilization of the SDOH framework represents a novel contribution to the literature, offering a comprehensive perspective that enhances our understanding of health inequities in the backdrop of income inequality. This perspective highlights the direct correlation between income disparity and health conditions and emphasizes the importance of historical and policy-oriented examinations of systemic factors contributing to the current landscape of health disparities among women. Such an examination is pivotal for identifying root causes and formulating comprehensive solutions beyond surface-level interventions.

By integrating the SDOH framework, this study contributes significantly to developing policy and programmatic interventions to improve income and health outcomes for women of all backgrounds. It lays a critical foundation for understanding the broader narrative of health inequities and points toward the essential need for targeted strategies that address the multifaceted nature of these disparities. This research underscores the urgency of adopting a holistic approach to health equity that considers the interplay of income, race, and gender and paves the way for meaningful change in women's lives across the socioeconomic spectrum.

2.5 METHODS

2.5.1 STUDY DESIGN AND SETTINGS

This study is a secondary analysis of data collected by the National Health and Nutrition Examination Survey (NHANES), which is publicly available from the National Center for Health Statistics. NHANES provides national estimates of the health and nutritional status of the US population. The study utilized the SDOH framework developed by the WHO (see Figure 2.1) to guide its research.

2.5.2 DATA COLLECTION METHOD

The NHANES data has been collected every two years since 1999, with an average response rate of 73.2% between 1999 and 2016 [134, 202]. The NHANES survey employed a combination of in-person interviews, standardized physical examinations, and laboratory tests. Participants were selected from counties across the United States, representing both metropolitan and nonmetropolitan areas in all four regions. The NHANES has published comprehensive documents outlining the sample design, estimation, and analytic guidelines [6].

2.5.3 STUDY POPULATION AND SAMPLING

The analytical sample included 22,650 participants. The study population comprised 15,855 NH White women, 2718 NH Black women, 2718 Hispanic women, and 1359 women of other NH who were 20 years and older and had participated in NHANES between 1999 and 2016.

2.5.4 MEASURES

2.5.4.1 OUTCOME VARIABLES

The study focused on five common health issues among US women: (1) obesity, (2) hypertension, (3) diabetes, (4) depression, and (5) AL score as a measure of clinical stress.

2.5.4.1.1 Obesity

We created a binary variable to identify participants who were obese [if body mass index (BMI) $\geq$ 30 kg/m^2], using BMI as the indicator. BMI is derived by dividing weight in kilograms by height in meters squared (kg/m^2) [136]. As noted by NHANES, trained health technicians obtained all body measures in the body measures room at each mobile examination center [135]. It is important to mention that both high and low ends of the BMI spectrum are considered undesirable, as high BMI is a risk factor for numerous chronic diseases and associated adverse outcomes. Conversely, low BMI can be an indicator of cancer or other severe health conditions that cause weight loss.

2.5.4.1.2 Hypertension

Hypertension was measured by taking the average of three separate blood pressure measurements during one sitting in the medical examination. The blood pressure measurements were obtained using electronic cuffs that were appropriately sized and calibrated to the ambulatory standard. Hypertension was defined as an average systolic blood pressure greater than 130 mmHg and/or diastolic blood pressure greater than or equal to 80 mmHg or if the participant reported taking antihypertensive medication(s) [49, 142].

2.5.4.1.3 Diabetes

Diabetes was defined based on two criteria. First, if participants reported that a doctor had diagnosed them with diabetes. Second, if participants were taking medication for insulin or any other diabetes medications, including pills.

2.5.4.1.4 Depression

The NHANES utilized the nine-item version of the Public Health Questionnaire-9 (PHQ-9) to assess depressive symptoms. The PHQ-9 is a brief version of the Primary Care Evaluation of Mental Disorders and measures the severity of depression on a graded scale. It is a self-administered questionnaire by the patient and has been found to be reliable and valid. A score greater than 9 has an 88% sensitivity and specificity, making it suitable for clinical use. On the Diagnostic and Statistical Manual of Mental Disorders, Fourth Edition scale, scores of 5, 10, 15, or 20 represent mild, moderate, moderately severe, and severe depression, respectively [74]. The PHQ-9 is a clinically validated survey with a sensitivity and specificity of 88% [53]. Participants were asked to rate the frequency of experiencing depressive symptoms, such as restless sleep, poor appetite, and feeling lonely, over the past 2 weeks. Each item was scored on a 4-point ordinal scale for frequency (0, not at all; 1, several days; 2, more than half the days; 3, nearly every day). The total score was calculated by summing the nine items, resulting in a maximum score of 27 [101]. To run a logistic model, we created a dummy variable with a cutoff score of 10 or higher (=1 if PHQ-9 $\geq$ 10, =0 if PHQ-9 $<$ 10), and this cutoff score has been used in other studies [86, 196].

2.5.4.1.5 AL Score

To calculate the AL score, we followed the method proposed by Chyu and Upchurch (2011), which involves eight biomarkers: (1) systolic blood pressure (mmHg), (2) diastolic blood pressure (mmHg), (3) pulse rate (beats/min), (4) BMI (kg/m^2), (5) glycohemoglobin (%), (6) direct high-density lipoprotein (HDL) cholesterol (mg/dL), (7) total cholesterol (mg/dL), and (8) serum albumin (g/dL) [36]. Biomarkers with values above the 75th percentile were classified as high risk, except for HDL cholesterol and serum albumin, where values below the 25th percentile were considered high risk [62]. This approach has been widely used in numerous studies [154, 175].

2.5.4.2 MAIN INDEPENDENT VARIABLE

2.5.4.2.1 Poverty-to-Income Ratio (PIR)

We included several control variables in our analysis to account for various factors that could potentially influence the outcomes. These covariates encompassed demographic and SES, healthcare access, and health behaviors.

For demographic and SES variables, we considered age (measured in years), marital status (1 = married, 0 = unmarried, including divorced, separated, widowed, or never married), educational attainment (less than high school, high school, or general equivalency diploma, more than high school), and the PIR. PIR serves as a proxy for income and is calculated by dividing family (or individual) income by the poverty guidelines specific to each survey year. By incorporating family income, family size, and the poverty threshold, PIR provides a more reliable measure of a family's SES. For instance, if a family of four with two children under 18 years of age has an annual income of $32,000 and a poverty threshold of $31,661, the PIR would be calculated as $32,000/$31,661 = 1.01 [32]. Using this ratio, we created a categorical variable with three categories: (1) low PIR (0–1.16), (2) medium PIR (1.17–2.82), and (3) high PIR (2.83–5.00) quintiles, ranging from low to high.

To account for healthcare access, we included two sets of variables. The first was a categorical variable indicating the type of health insurance (Medicare, Medicaid, private insurance, governmental health insurance, or any other health insurance). The second was a binary variable indicating whether the respondent had a routine place for healthcare.

Additionally, we considered three health behavior variables as controls: (1) smoking (never, former, or current smoker), (2) drinking (never, former, or current drinker), and (3) engagement in vigorous or moderate physical activities. The NHANES defined rigorous activities as engaging in at least 60 minutes of physical activity per day [133]. All these variables were self-reported responses from the participants.

2.5.4.3 STATISTICAL ANALYSIS

The aim of this study was to examine the relationship between selected health outcomes and PIR among women aged 20 years and older. To address this objective, we conducted three sets of analyses.

First, descriptive analyses were conducted to compare selected health outcomes among low-, medium-, and high-PIR groups. Demographic variables, SES indicators, access to healthcare, health insurance status, and health behavior variables were also compared between these PIR levels. Independent *t*-tests and chi-square tests were utilized for comparing variables across PIR groups.

Second, to assess the association between obesity and race, we performed two sets of weighted modified Poisson regression analyses. These models were adjusted for race, age, marital status, education, PIR category, type of health insurance, having a routine place for healthcare, smoking status, drinking status, engagement in vigorous or moderate physical activities, and year dummies.

Given that the prevalence of obesity in our sample exceeded 10%, the weighted modified Poisson regression analysis was the most appropriate model choice [120, 177, 203]. Prevalence ratios (PRs) and 95% confidence intervals (CIs) were reported as effect measures [120, 177, 203].

All models were controlled for year dummies; age; access to healthcare (including health insurance and having a routine place for healthcare); and health behavior variables such as smoking status, drinking status, and engagement in vigorous or moderate physical activities.

Weighted analyses were conducted using the NHANES individual-level sampling weights for the year 1999–2016 [134]. Statistical significance was set at $p < 0.05$, and all tests were two-sided. All statistical analyses were performed using Stata statistical software, version 15.

In the second set of analyses, we utilized the Lorenz curve to examine the distribution of income inequality (as represented by PIR) among individuals with obesity, hypertension, diabetes, depression (PHQ-9 score > 10) and elevated AL (AL $\geq$ 4). The Lorenz curve enables us to assess how the concentration of income inequality is distributed among this specific group.

The lowest PIR was assigned the first percentile, progressing toward the highest PIR as the final percentile. Perfect equality, where income is evenly distributed, is represented by the 45° line on the graph [86].

2.6 RESULTS

2.6.1 *DESCRIPTIVE ANALYSIS*

Table 2.1 presents the weighted means and standard deviations (SDs) for all variables included in the models. The average age of the sample was 50.0 (SD: 14) years, and most individuals were college educated (61%) and belonged to the middle class or higher, with a PIR of 3.3 (SD: 0.35). Eighty-six percent of the study population had health insurance coverage, 18% were current smokers, 67% were current drinkers, and 52% engaged in regular physical activity. Additionally, 12% of the population was NH Black, 70% was NH White, 12% were Hispanics, and 6% belonged to other NH racial/ethnic groups.

When comparing sociodemographic variables by PIR, it was observed that individuals with a low PIR had a higher likelihood of obesity (50%), hypertension (23%), diabetes (15%), depression (PHQ-9 score $\geq$ 10, 19%), depressive symptoms (34%), and elevated AL (39%) ($p < 0.001$). Furthermore, 39% of the low-PIR population were non-White compared to 18% of the high-PIR group. Less than 50% of the low-PIR population were married, and only 42% had a college degree or higher, as opposed to 79% in the high-PIR group. The insurance coverage rate among individuals with low PIR was 74%, 24% were current smokers, 57% were current drinkers, 39% were engaged in regular physical activity, and only 44% were employed. Further details can be found in Table 2.1.

2.6.2 *ESTIMATING THE ASSOCIATION BETWEEN SELECTED HEALTH OUTCOME AND PIR GROUPS*

Table 2.2 presents the results of the unadjusted modified Poisson models for each selected health outcome. Compared to the high-PIR population,

TABLE 2.1 Descriptive Analysis of Outcome and Control Variables in Women Aged 20 Years and Older (NHANES 1999–2016)

	All (n = 22,650)		**Very Low (n = 4628)**		**Low (n = 5463)**		**Medium (n = 5966)**		**High (n = 6593)**		
	Mean	**SD**	**Mean**	**SD**	**Mean**	**SD**	**Mean**	**SD**	**Mean**	**SD**	**Chi/ANOVA**
Obese	0.43	0.42	0.48	0.53	0.50	0.50	0.44	0.41	0.36	0.35	0.0000
Hypertension	0.17	0.32	0.17	0.40	0.23	0.42	0.18	0.32	0.13	0.24	0.0000
Has diabetes	0.10	0.26	0.12	0.35	0.15	0.35	0.11	0.26	0.07	0.19	0.0000
Has diabetes mellitus	0.11	0.27	0.13	0.35	0.16	0.36	0.12	0.27	0.08	0.19	0.0000
PHQ-9 score > 10	0.09	0.25	0.19	0.42	0.13	0.34	0.07	0.21	0.06	0.17	0.0000
PHQ-9 scale	3.44	3.62	5.16	5.69	4.24	4.88	3.26	3.16	2.59	2.49	
PHQ-9 category											
None	0.73	0.38	0.57	0.52	0.66	0.47	0.73	0.37	0.81	0.28	0.0000
Mild	0.18	0.33	0.23	0.45	0.21	0.41	0.20	0.33	0.13	0.24	0.0000
Moderate	0.06	0.21	0.13	0.35	0.08	0.27	0.05	0.18	0.04	0.15	0.0000
Moderate severe	0.02	0.12	0.04	0.21	0.04	0.18	0.02	0.11	0.01	0.07	0.0000
Severe	0.01	0.08	0.03	0.17	0.02	0.13	0.01	0.06	0.00	0.04	0.0000
AL score	2.67	1.07	2.95	1.64	2.98	1.42	2.94	1.28	2.67	1.08	0.0000
Elevated AL (AL > 4)	0.33	0.40	0.38	0.51	0.39	0.49	0.34	0.39	0.28	0.32	
Race/ethnicity											
Hispanics	0.12	0.28	0.26	0.46	0.18	0.39	0.10	0.24	0.06	0.17	0.0000
White NH	0.70	0.39	0.46	0.53	0.61	0.49	0.73	0.37	0.82	0.28	0.0000
Black NH	0.12	0.27	0.21	0.43	0.15	0.36	0.12	0.27	0.07	0.18	0.0000
Other NH	0.06	0.20	0.08	0.28	0.06	0.23	0.06	0.19	0.06	0.17	0.1292
Age (years)	49.82	14.34	43.49	18.56	51.76	18.48	50.65	14.67	50.58	10.41	
Female											

TABLE 2.1 *(Continued)*

	All (n = 22,650)		Very Low (n = 4628)		Low (n = 5463)		Medium (n = 5966)		High (n = 6593)		
	Mean	**SD**	**Mean**	**SD**	**Mean**	**SD**	**Mean**	**SD**	**Mean**	**SD**	**Chi/ANOVA**
Married	0.61	0.41	0.41	0.52	0.46	0.50	0.64	0.40	0.74	0.31	0.0000
Education											
<High school (HS)	0.16	0.31	0.39	0.52	0.29	0.45	0.12	0.27	0.04	0.14	0.0000
HS graduate/GED	0.23	0.36	0.24	0.45	0.29	0.45	0.28	0.37	0.17	0.27	0.0000
More than HS	0.61	0.42	0.37	0.51	0.42	0.49	0.59	0.41	0.79	0.29	0.0000
Has insurance	0.86	0.30	0.65	0.51	0.74	0.44	0.88	0.27	0.96	0.13	0.0000
Routine place	0.91	0.25	0.84	0.38	0.88	0.33	0.89	0.26	0.95	0.15	0.0000
Smoking status											
Never	0.59	0.42	0.51	0.53	0.56	0.49	0.58	0.41	0.64	0.34	0.0000
Former	0.23	0.36	0.15	0.38	0.20	0.40	0.26	0.36	0.25	0.31	0.0000
Current	0.18	0.33	0.33	0.50	0.24	0.42	0.16	0.31	0.11	0.22	0.0000
Drinking status											
Never	0.16	0.31	0.23	0.44	0.25	0.43	0.15	0.29	0.09	0.21	0.0003
Former	0.17	0.32	0.17	0.40	0.18	0.38	0.18	0.32	0.16	0.26	0.0000
Current	0.67	0.40	0.60	0.52	0.57	0.49	0.67	0.39	0.74	0.31	0.0000
Missing	0.001	0.03	0.0014	0.04	0.0004	0.02	0.0008	0.02	0.0015	0.03	0.0000
Physically active	0.52	0.42	0.38	0.51	0.39	0.49	0.50	0.41	0.64	0.34	0.0000
Employed	0.57	0.42	0.38	0.51	0.44	0.49	0.59	0.41	0.69	0.33	0.0000

ANOVA: analysis of variance; GED: General Educational Development very low-PIR, low-PIR, and middle-PIR populations had higher PRs for all selected health outcomes. For example, very low-PIR population had a higher PR for obesity (PR: 1.387, CI: 1.300–1.480), hypertension (PR: 1.278, CI: 1.143–1.429), diabetes (PR: 1.888, CI: 1.719–2.355), depression (PR: 4.030, CI: 3.358–4.836), and elevated AL (PR: 1.279, CI: 1.129–1.449).

Table 2.3 presents the results of the adjusted models for race/ethnicity, which showed a similar pattern to the unadjusted models. However, when compared to the Hispanic population, the White population had a lower PR for obesity (PR: 0.853, CI: 0.804–0.904) and diabetes (PR: 0.828, CI: 0.727–0.954). The Black population had higher PRs for all health outcomes except depression. Other racial/ethnic populations had a lower PR for obesity but a higher PR for hypertension.

Table 2.4 presents the results of the full model. As presented, age, smoking, and drinking were found to be predictors of obesity, hypertension, diabetes, depression, and elevated AL. Education was mostly protective for all selected health outcomes except for obesity, which may be explained by lower levels of physical activity or the type of jobs that require less movement.

In the regression results, we found a positive association between obesity and income inequality (measured using the PIR) among women. To further investigate this association across different races and ethnicity groups, we utilized Lorenz curves and Gini coefficients (GCs).

Figure 2.2A–D displays the Lorenz curves, which represent the GC, for the income-to-poverty ratio among women in the United States from 1999 to 2016. These curves compare the GC between obese and nonobese populations, stratified by race and ethnicity. Overall, the GC for obese women is 0.352 [standard error (SE): 0.002], while the GC for nonobese women is 0.379 (SE: 0.002), indicating that there is a statistically significant difference in income inequality between these groups ($p < 0.001$).

Figure 2.2A specifically focuses on the distribution of the income-to-poverty ratio among obese and nonobese White women. The GC for obese White women is 0.343 (SE: 0.003), while the GC for nonobese White women is 0.308 (SE: 0.005), indicating a significant difference in income inequality ($p < 0.001$). We also observed significant differences in income inequality between obese and nonobese Hispanic women (GC: 0.401 vs. 0.391, $p < 0.01$). Other racial and ethnic groups showed higher income inequality in obese individuals compared to nonobese individuals

TABLE 2.2 Basic Poisson Model on the Unadjusted Association Between PIR and Various Health Outcomes in US Women Aged 20 Years and Older (NHANES 1999–2016)

	Obese		Hypertension		Has Diabetes Mellitus		PHQ-9 Score > 10		Elevated AL	
	PR	95% CI	PR	95% CI	PR	95% CI	PR	95% CI	PR	95% CI
PIR (ref. high)										
Very low	1.387*	[1.300]–[1.480]	1.278*	[1.143]–[1.429]	1.888*	[1.618]–[2.204]	4.030*	[3.358]–[4.836]	1.279*	[1.129]–[1.449]
Low	1.367*	[1.279]–[1.460]	1.465*	[1.339]–[1.603]	2.088*	[1.808]–[2.412]	2.766*	[2.242]–[3.412]	1.292*	[1.166]–[1.433]
Middle	1.225*	[1.147]–[1.307]	1.227*	[1.119]–[1.346]	1.670*	[1.458]–[1.913]	1.578*	[1.304]–[1.909]	1.218*	[1.090]–[1.363]
N	20,449		20,449		20,116		13,262		7976	

*p < 0.001.

TABLE 2.3 Poisson Model to Show the Unadjusted Association Between PIR and Race/Ethnicity and Various Health Outcomes in US Women Aged 20 Years and Older (NHANES 1999–2016)

	Obese		Hypertension		Has Diabetes Mellitus		PHQ-9 Score > 10		Elevated AL	
	PR	95% CI	PR	95% CI	PR	95% CI	PR	95% CI	PR	95% CI
PIR (ref. high)										
Very low	1.260***	[1.178]–[1.346]	1.282***	[1.138]–[1.445]	1.694***	[1.454]–[1.973]	4.132***	[3.445]–[4.958]	1.252***	[1.104]–[1.419]
Low	1.282***	[1.200]–[1.369]	1.474***	[1.342]–[1.619]	1.957***	[1.701]–[2.252]	2.809***	[2.267]–[3.481]	1.276***	[1.151]–[1.413]
Middle	1.184***	[1.108]–[1.264]	1.223***	[1.114]–[1.342]	1.608***	[1.406]–[1.839]	1.588***	[1.311]–[1.922]	1.207**	[1.077]–[1.352]
Race/ethnicity (ref. Hispanics)										
White NH	0.853***	[0.804]–[0.904]	1.307***	[1.180]–[1.447]	0.828**	[0.724]–[0.947]	1.117	[0.954]–[1.308]	1.144*	[1.018]–[1.285]
Black NH	1.277***	[1.212]–[1.347]	1.708***	[1.541]–[1.894]	1.253**	[1.089]–[1.440]	1.106	[0.950]–[1.288]	1.556***	[1.387]–[1.745]
Other NH	0.535***	[0.458]–[0.626]	1.299**	[1.097]–[1.537]	1.174	[0.937]–[1.472]	0.936	[0.695]–[1.261]	0.94	[0.779]–[1.135]
N	20,449		20,449		20,116		13,262		7979	

*p < 0.05, **p < 0.01, ***p < 0.001.

TABLE 2.4 Poisson Model to Show the Association Between PIR and Various Health Outcomes in US Women Aged 20 Years and Older (NHANES 1999–2016)

	Obese		Hypertensive		Has Diabetes Mellitus		PHQ-9 Score > 10		Elevated AL	
	PR	**95% CI**	**PR**	**95% CI**	**PR**	**95% CI**	**PR**	**95% CI**	**PR**	**95% CI**
PIR (ref. high)										
Very low	1.282***	[1.191]–[1.380]	1.166*	[1.037]–[1.312]	1.569***	[1.307]–[1.884]	1.963***	[1.582]–[2.437]	1.259**	[1.099]–[1.442]
Low	1.253***	[1.169]–[1.343]	1.083	[0.990]–[1.184]	1.468***	[1.248]–[1.728]	1.727***	[1.375]–[2.169]	1.135*	[1.017]–[1.267]
Middle	1.155***	[1.079]–[1.236]	1.012	[0.925]–[1.107]	1.346***	[1.167]–[1.553]	1.234*	[1.018]–[1.496]	1.116	[0.989]–[1.259]
Race/ethnicity (ref. Hispanics)										
White NH	0.857***	[0.805]–[0.912]	0.946	[0.848]–[1.055]	0.573***	[0.501]–[0.654]	0.899	[0.762]–[1.060]	1.011	[0.895]–[1.142]
Black NH	1.258***	[1.189]–[1.331]	1.548***	[1.403]–[1.707]	1.078	[0.941]–[1.235]	0.897	[0.765]–[1.051]	1.480***	[1.323]–[1.656]
Other NH	0.540***	[0.458]–[0.637]	1.097	[0.921]–[1.306]	1.053	[0.859]–[1.292]	0.875	[0.659]–[1.161]	0.848	[0.700]–[1.026]
Age (years)	1.002*	[1.000]–[1.003]	1.045***	[1.042]–[1.049]	1.037***	[1.033]–[1.042]	0.992***	[0.988]–[0.996]	1.018***	[1.015]–[1.021]
Married	1.04	[0.985]–[1.098]	1.036	[0.967]–[1.109]	1.106	[0.982]–[1.245]	0.724***	[0.633]–[0.827]	1.037	[0.951]–[1.131]
Education (ref. less than HS)										
High-school graduate/GED	1.089*	[1.020]–[1.164]	1.039	[0.951]–[1.134]	0.858*	[0.744]–[0.989]	0.926	[0.783]–[1.095]	1.046	[0.938]–[1.168]
More than high school	0.972	[0.917]–[1.031]	0.934	[0.859]–[1.015]	0.819**	[0.710]–[0.946]	0.874	[0.733]–[1.042]	0.927	[0.836]–[1.027]
Has health insurance	1.045	[0.979]–[1.115]	0.932	[0.825]–[1.053]	1.081	[0.898]–[1.300]	0.954	[0.812]–[1.121]	1.019	[0.899]–[1.156]
Routine place to go for healthcare	1.165***	[1.070]–[1.268]	0.991	[0.864]–[1.136]	2.968***	[2.170]–[4.059]	1.111	[0.893]–[1.381]	1.178	[0.979]–[1.418]

TABLE 2.4 *(Continued)*

	Obese		Hypertensive		Has Diabetes Mellitus		PHQ-9 Score > 10		Elevated AL	
	PR	**95% CI**	**PR**	**95% CI**	**PR**	**95% CI**	**PR**	**95% CI**	**PR**	**95% CI**
Smoking status (ref. never)										
Former	1.117***	[1.055]–[1.183]	1.049	[0.976]–[1.128]	1.315***	[1.149]–[1.506]	1.261*	[1.009]–[1.576]	1.087	[0.984]–[1.199]
Current	0.908*	[0.844]–[0.978]	1.054	[0.954]–[1.164]	1.081	[0.905]–[1.291]	2.074***	[1.743]–[2.468]	1.101	[0.996]–[1.218]
Drinking status (ref. never)										
Former	1.143***	[1.062]–[1.229]	0.97	[0.887]–[1.061]	1.072	[0.934]–[1.231]	1.343**	[1.099]–[1.641]	1.102	[0.986]–[1.233]
Current	0.94	[0.878]–[1.006]	0.864***	[0.798]–[0.936]	0.777**	[0.661]–[0.912]	1.450***	[1.190]–[1.767]	0.858**	[0.767]–[0.959]
Missing	0.854**	[0.773]–[0.943]	1.780***	[1.583]–[2.001]	0.592***	[0.470]–[0.746]	2.886**	[1.428]–[5.834]	0.771*	[0.630]–[0.942]
Has vigorous or moderate activities	0.757***	[0.721]–[0.795]	0.938	[0.879]–[1.001]	0.799***	[0.720]–[0.887]	0.544***	[0.475]–[0.623]	0.761***	[0.701]–[0.826]
Employed	1.104***	[1.051]–[1.160]	0.994	[0.902]–[1.095]	0.914	[0.792]–[1.055]	0.566***	[0.495]–[0.648]	1.126**	[1.032]–[1.228]
N	19,496		19,496		19,176		12,624		7979	

$^{*}p < 0.05$, $^{**}p < 0.01$, $^{***}p < 0.001$.

(GC: 0.374 vs. 0.314, $p < 0.001$). Interestingly, in Black women, obese individuals experienced slightly higher income inequality compared to nonobese individuals (0.385 vs. 0.393, $p < 0.001$).

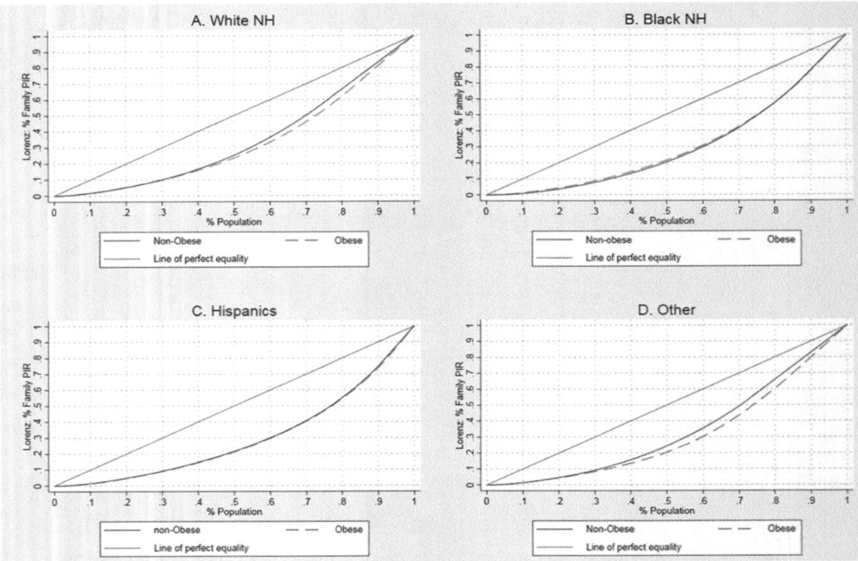

FIGURE 2.2A–D The Lorenz curves to show distribution of PIR and obesity in women aged 20 years and older between 1996 and 2016.

Source: NHANES (1996–2016).

Figure 2.3A–D examines the distribution of the income-to-poverty ratio among hypertensive and nonhypertensive women, stratified by race and ethnicity. In most racial and ethnic groups, hypertensive women experienced higher income inequality compared to nonhypertensive women. The GC for hypertensive women was 0.362 (SE: 0.001), while the GC for nonhypertensive women was 0.370 (SE: 0.001), indicating a statistically significant difference ($p < 0.05$).

As shown in Figure 2.4A–D, we explore the distribution of income among women with and without diabetes, categorized by race and ethnicity. Overall, women with diabetes experienced higher income inequality compared to women without diabetes (GC: 0.377 vs. 0.361, $p < 0.001$). However, there was considerable variation among different racial and ethnic groups, with different patterns observed across various percentiles.

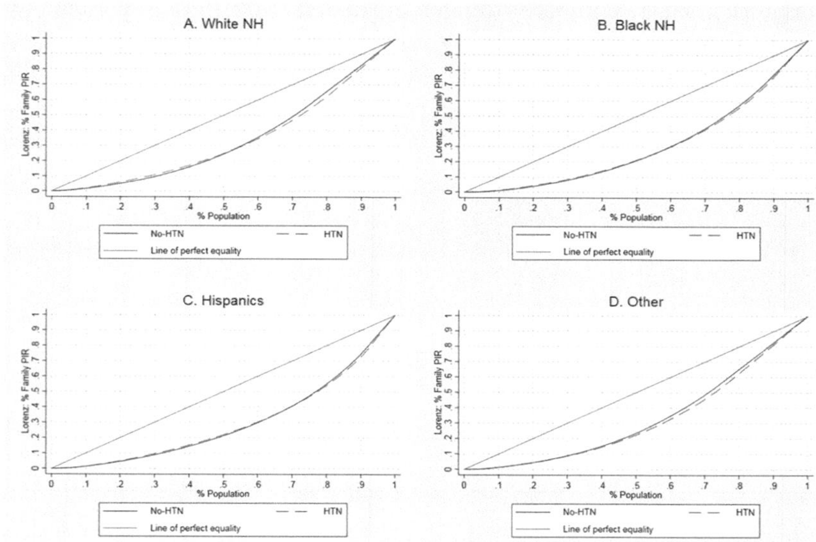

FIGURE 2.3A–D The Lorenz curves to show distribution of PIR and hypertension in women aged 20 years and older between 1996 and 2016.

Source: NHANES (1996–2016).

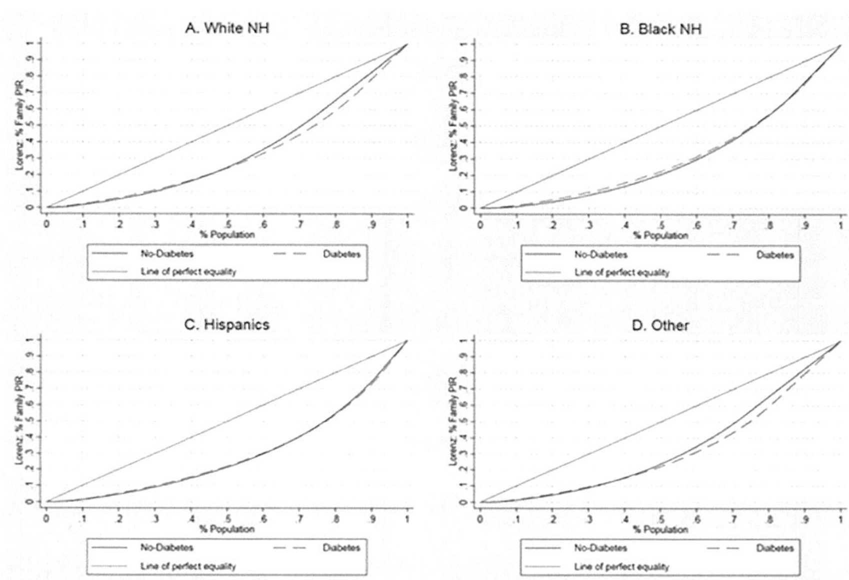

FIGURE 2.4A–D The Lorenz curves to show distribution of PIR and diabetes in women aged 20 years and older between 1996 and 2016.

Source: NHANES (1996–2016).

Figure 2.5A–D compares the income distribution among women based on their depression status (PHQ-9 score > 10). We consistently observed higher income inequality among women of different racial and ethnic backgrounds who experienced depression ($p < 0.001$). The GC for women with depression was 0.418 (SE: 0.005), while the GC for nondepressed women was 0.354 (SE: 0.002).

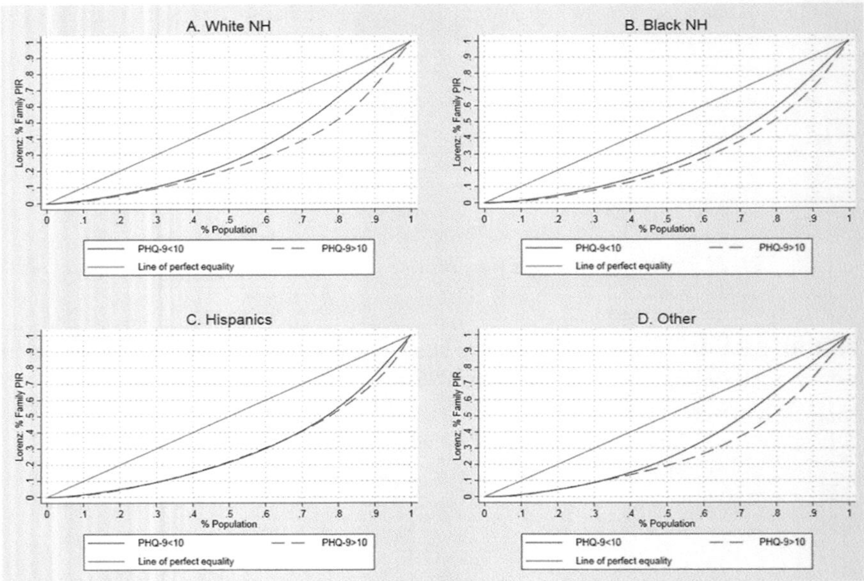

FIGURE 2.5A–D The Lorenz curves to show distribution of PIR and depression (PHQ-9 score > 10) in women aged 20 years and older between 2005 and 2016.

Source: NHANES (2005–2016).

Similarly, Figure 2.6A to D highlights the income distribution among women with elevated AL scores. We found a similar pattern of higher income inequality for women with elevated AL ($p < 0.001$). The GC for women with elevated AL was 0.373 (SE: 0.002), while the GC for women without elevated AL was 0.360 (SE: 0.002).

2.7 DISCUSSION

According to the results from a nationally representative sample of women aged 20 years and older in the NHANES data, our observations can be

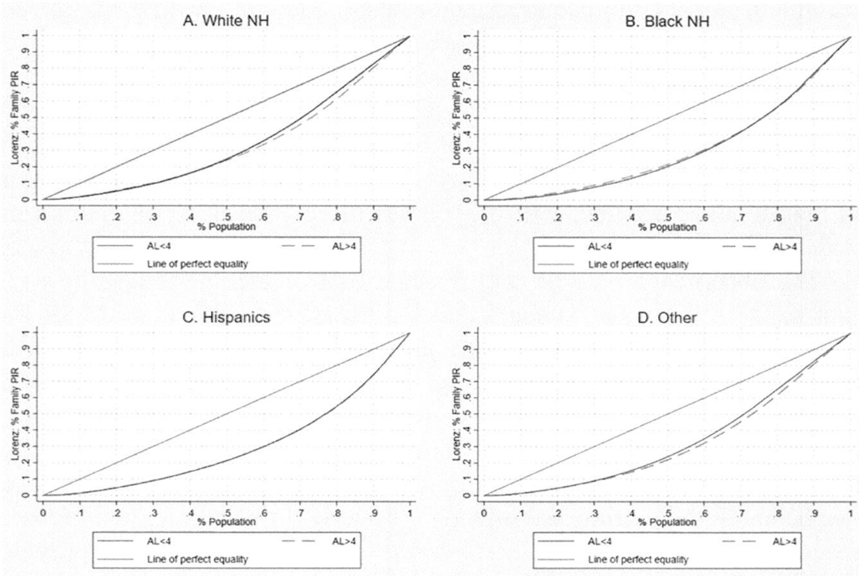

FIGURE 2.6A–D The Lorenz curves to show distribution of PIR and elevated AL in women aged 20 years and older between 2005 and 2016.

Source: NHANES (1996–2016).

summarized as follows: (1) We found consistent effects of low income as a risk factor for poor health; (2) the observed stepwise effect indicated the highest odds in the poorest group and the lowest odds in the highest-income group; (3) similar effects of income were found regardless of the domain of health (mental health and cardiometabolic risk); (4) AL may be a mechanism for some of these health differences due to income differences; and (5) the effects of income on health, across domains, persisted after controlling for race/ethnicity, demographic factors, other SES indicators, and health behaviors.

The significance of this study lies in its ability to highlight the universality of the effects of low income and inequality as a root cause of women's health disparities in the United States. In a society grappling with growing economic disparities, understanding how income inequality and income differences manifest in women's health outcomes is pivotal.

By building on existing literature on the role of income and poverty as a root cause of health inequalities [56, 90, 150, 181], our study contributes a nuanced perspective that goes beyond the conventional understanding of income inequality's impact on a single health domain. The insights gained from this study, that income is a determinant of health inequality across various domains of health, underscore the role of income as a fundamental cause of health and illness [91, 111, 184]. This observation paves the way for public and economic interventions and policy initiatives aimed at mitigating the adverse health effects of poverty and income inequalities in marginalized women, which becomes more critical in the context of widening income gaps [23].

The observed consistent and residual role of income inequality as a root cause of various women's health disparities, after controlling for other demographic, SES indicators, health behaviors, and race/ethnicity, is a compelling aspect of this study. Beyond merely identifying isolated associations, these findings underscore the systematic and pervasive influence of economic inequalities on women's mental and physical well-being across multiple domains. This aligns with a growing body of evidence emphasizing the detrimental effects of poverty, low income, and income inequality on health [73, 114, 131]. Moreover, the study's findings provide valuable insights for public health professionals, policymakers, and researchers seeking to address the broader societal determinants of health and implement strategies that promote health equity for women.

A notable finding is the stepwise increase in health risks corresponding to ascending income levels, suggesting a dose–response relationship between income and health. This means that even if we cannot close the income gap entirely, narrowing it could impact health inequalities due to income. The health difference is not only evident when the income gap is large but also at smaller degrees of income inequalities [70, 150]. This nuanced understanding of the graded impact highlights the importance of recognizing the incremental effects of income disparities across populations and society as a whole. By elucidating this dose-dependent pattern, the study adds granularity to the understanding that any level of incremental income inequality can influence women's health. Policymakers and public health practitioners can leverage these insights to tailor their economic and public interventions based on the severity of income disparities, thereby optimizing resource allocation for maximum impact.

The results of our analysis indicate that income inequality is a critical contextual risk factor for women's health disparities in the United States. It unveils the heightened health risks associated with any reduction in income, prompting a closer examination of the factors contributing to this amplified effect. Conversely, documenting stepwise improvement in health with higher income suggests that we can close the health gap as much as possible by narrowing income disparities. This view suggests that our strategies do not need to be all or nothing, and any step forward to reduce income inequality is likely to result in improved women's health and reduced health disparities. Such knowledge is hoped to guide economic and policy interventions to address specific needs in low socioeconomic contexts.

The simultaneous impact of income inequality on disparities in mental health and cardiometabolic risk, in line with the literature [13, 87, 184], accentuates the nonspecific nature of the effects of the income gap. This underscores why income is known as a root cause of health problems in the United States. In a global study, income was found to have the most significant effect across various social determinants in the United States, while in many other countries, education has been the most salient determinant of health.

Income operates through a wide range of mechanisms, serving as the lifeblood of economic systems globally. At its core, income is the financial return individuals receive for their labor, expertise, or investments. Labor income, derived from wages and salaries, represents compensation for the time and effort expended in various professions. Entrepreneurial ventures contribute to income through profits generated from business activities. Investments in financial markets, real estate, and other assets yield returns in the form of interest, dividends, and capital gains, adding to the multifaceted nature of income. Social welfare programs, government subsidies, and transfer payments further shape the income landscape, redistributing resources to address societal needs and economic inequalities. Technological advancements and globalization have introduced new avenues for income generation, such as gig economy platforms and remote work opportunities. The intricate interplay of these diverse mechanisms underscores the dynamic nature of income, influencing individual well-being, economic growth, and societal structures. Consequently, understanding the mechanism by which income affects health is essential for researchers and policymakers who wish to close the health gap due to income inequalities amid the complexities of modern economies.

Our observation of the universal effects of income on all health outcomes challenges the traditional compartmentalization of health domains and underscores the interconnectedness of mental and physical well-being. By recognizing these shared pathways, interventions can be designed holistically, addressing both mental and physical health outcomes concurrently. This integrated approach is crucial for developing effective strategies that resonate with the multifaceted nature of women's health challenges in the face of income inequality.

We also showed that income levels are linked to AL levels. This suggests that AL should be introduced as a pathway through which income inequality influences women's health [71, 160, 167]. AL, reflecting the cumulative physiological toll of stress, provides a plausible link between the social determinants of income inequality and the observed health outcomes [175, 179, 195]. By investigating mechanisms rather than merely describing disparities, the study contributes not only to theoretical frameworks but also opens avenues for targeted interventions aimed at mitigating the physiological consequences of prolonged exposure to socioeconomic disparities among women.

The robustness of the observed associations, even after meticulous control for behavioral factors, race/ethnicity, other SESs, and demographic factors, underscores the independent impact of income on women's health. This resilience against covariate adjustments strengthens the validity of the study's findings, emphasizing the need to address income inequality as a distinct determinant of population health. Policymakers and public health professionals can use this evidence to advocate for comprehensive strategies that target the root causes of health disparities, transcending traditional approaches that focus solely on individual-level risk factors.

Acknowledging the potential intersectionality of income with other social determinants of health [52, 151, 169] enriches our understanding of the complexities involved. Exploring how race/ethnicity matters in the experience of poverty for women, meaning how gender intersects and interacts with income inequality, provides a nuanced perspective on health disparities among women who have diverse backgrounds. By recognizing and addressing the complexities of intersecting multiple social identities, interventions can be tailored to account for the unique challenges faced by different subgroups of women, fostering a more inclusive and equitable approach to women's health promotion.

The practical implications of the study's findings extend to policy and intervention strategies. The identification of income inequality as a significant determinant of women's health necessitates targeted policy initiatives aimed at reducing economic disparities. Policymakers can draw on these findings to advocate for structural changes that address the root causes of income inequality, such as equitable economic policies, accessible education, and social welfare programs. Implementing interventions that specifically target women in areas characterized by high income inequality can contribute to the overall improvement of health outcomes and promote long-term societal well-being.

Although income redistribution is not a well-received and supported policy in the United States, our findings propose income redistribution policies as a tool to generate health equity in society for women. Income redistribution does not mean directly taking money from the pocket of the wealthy to the poor but providing tools and vehicles based on tax policies [129] and specific tax-exempt investments that disproportionately help the poor. Earned income tax [99], baby bonds [201], and tax relief programs [98, 170] are all among such interventions that can redistribute income indirectly and reduce the income and wealth gap. Another strategy is to increase the minimum wage to a living wage.

The robustness of the observed associations, even after controlling for various covariates, reinforces the independent and enduring nature of the impact of income inequality on women's health. These findings have important implications for policymakers, public health professionals, and advocates who must prioritize addressing societal determinants to achieve meaningful improvements in women's health. The acknowledgment of intersectionality and additional considerations calls for an inclusive approach that recognizes and addresses the unique challenges faced by different subgroups of women, fostering a more equitable and just health-care system. Moving forward, the policy implications of this study urge a reevaluation of economic and social policies to ensure they promote equitable access to resources and opportunities. Targeted interventions should prioritize areas with the highest income inequality and consider the specific needs of women in diverse socioeconomic contexts. Policymakers should advocate for structural changes that address the root causes of income inequality, thereby promoting long-term societal well-being.

While this study contributes significantly to the current understanding of the relationship between income inequality and women's health, it is not without limitations. The cross-sectional nature of the study design and potential confounding variables necessitate caution in drawing causal conclusions. Future research endeavors should adopt longitudinal approaches, delve into specific mechanisms underlying observed associations, and explore the temporal aspects of income disparities. This study lays the groundwork for a broader research agenda, highlighting the need for continued efforts to unravel the intricacies of the relationship between income inequality and women's health. In essence, this study illuminates the critical importance of addressing income inequality as a fundamental determinant of women's health. By recognizing the interconnectedness of social, economic, and health outcomes, we can chart a course toward a more equitable and healthier future for women, where opportunities and resources are distributed justly, and well-being is fostered for all.

It is crucial to underscore the potential far-reaching consequences of income inequality on women's health. By unraveling the specific pathways through which economic disparities may impact health, we hope to inform evidence-based interventions and advocate for policy changes that foster a more just and equitable healthcare landscape for women. This study, thus, emerges as a timely and imperative endeavor, aligning with a broader societal commitment to understanding and addressing the multifaceted challenges that women face in the context of evolving economic landscapes.

While this study contributes valuable insights, it is essential to acknowledge its limitations. Our study was limited to individual-level factors, and we did not investigate area-level income. We also did not collect data on wealth, neighborhoods, or zip codes. Factors such as data constraints, potential confounding variables not accounted for, and the cross-sectional nature of the study design present inherent challenges. Future research should consider longitudinal approaches, allowing for a more nuanced understanding of the dynamic relationship between income inequality and women's health. Additionally, exploring specific mechanisms underlying the observed associations and delving into the temporal aspects of income disparities could further refine our understanding. This study lays a foundation for future investigations to build upon, offering a roadmap for researchers seeking to unravel the intricacies of this multifaceted relationship.

2.8 SUMMARY

In conclusion, this study provides strong evidence of the multifaceted and detrimental role of income inequality as a root cause of health disparities among US women, revealing the consistent effect that extends across various health domains. The consistent findings underscore the urgency of addressing low income and poverty as root causes of economic disparities to promote optimal well-being among women.

The identification of a dose–response relationship and graded impact highlights the need for nuanced interventions that consider the severity of income disparities in specific communities. The comparative analysis further emphasizes the importance of understanding contextual factors that may exacerbate or mitigate the health effects associated with varying levels of income inequality. The nonspecific effects on mental health and cardiometabolic risk underscore the interconnectedness of different dimensions of health, challenging traditional compartmentalization in healthcare and advocating for holistic approaches to women's well-being. The proposed mechanism of AL adds a novel dimension to our understanding, suggesting that the physiological toll of sustained exposure to income inequality contributes to adverse health outcomes. This insight into the underlying mechanisms provides a foundation for developing targeted interventions that address the root causes of health disparities and promote resilience among women facing economic challenges.

KEYWORDS

- **poverty-to-income ratio**
- **socioeconomic**
- **obesity**
- **hypertension**
- **diabetes**
- **depression**
- **allostatic load**
- **women**

REFERENCES

1. Aaronson, D., Hartley, D., & Mazumder, B. (2021). The effects of the 1930s HOLC "redlining" maps. *American Economic Journal: Economic Policy, 13*(4), 355–392.
2. Abdalla, S. M., Shui, Y., & Galea, S. (2020). Trends in cardiovascular disease prevalence by income level in the United States. *JAMA Network Open, 3*(9), e2018150–e2018150.

3. Aburto, J. M. (2020). Dynamics of life expectancy and life span equality. *Proceedings of the National Academy of Sciences, 117*(10), 5250–5259.
4. Afzal, Z., Kamran, F., & Anjum, A. (2024). Psychosocial consequences of colorism on mental health: A systematic review. *Al-Mahdi Research Journal, 5*(3), 694–711.
5. Akarsu, M. Z. (2023). Unequal society: A detailed investigation of wage and income inequality in the United States. *Journal of the Knowledge Economy, 14*(4), 3771–3798.
6. Akinbami, L. J., Chen, T. C., Davy, O., Ogden, C. L., Fink, S., & Clark, J. (2022). National Health and Nutrition Examination Survey, 2017–March 2020 prepandemic file: Sample design, estimation, and analytic guidelines. *National Center for Health Statistics, Vital Health Stat, 2*(190), 1–36. doi: 10.15620/cdc:115434
7. Alexander, T., & Carter, M. M. (2022). Internalized racism and gendered colorism among African Americans: A study of intragroup bias, perceived discrimination, and psychological well-being. *Journal of African American Studies, 26*(2), 248–265.
8. Alsan, M., Chandra, A., & Simon, K. (2021). The great unequalizer: Initial health effects of COVID-19 in the United States. *Journal of Economic Perspectives, 35*(3), 25–46.
9. Amanat, S., et al. (2020). Exercise and type 2 diabetes. In: *Physical Exercise for Human Health* (pp. 91–105).
10. Anekwe, C. V., et al. (2020). Socioeconomics of obesity. *Current Obesity Reports, 9*, 272–279.
11. Apostolidou, E., et al. (2021). Clinical outcomes of patients with newly diagnosed acute lymphoblastic leukemia in a county hospital system. *Clinical Lymphoma Myeloma Leukemia, 21*(11), e895–e902.
12. Assari, S. (2018). Life expectancy gain due to employment status depends on race, gender, education, and their intersections. *Journal of Racial and Ethnic Health Disparities, 5*, 375–386.
13. Babones, S. J. (2008). Income inequality and population health: Correlation and causality. *Social Science & Medicine, 66*(7), 1614–1626.
14. Bai, G., et al. (2023). Trustee compensation and charity care provision in US nonprofit hospitals. *Health Affairs, 42*(4), 526–530.
15. Bak, H., & Yi, Y. (2020). When the American dream fails: The effect of perceived economic inequality on present-oriented behavior. *Psychology & Marketing, 37*(10), 1321–1341.
16. Balla, S., Gomez, S. E., & Rodriguez, F. (2020). Disparities in cardiovascular care and outcomes for women from racial/ethnic minority backgrounds. *Current Treatment Options in Cardiovascular Medicine, 22*, 1–17.
17. Balusu, P. (2022). The impact of women's representation on the gender wage gap across the United States. Available at: https://bpb-us-w2.wpmucdn.com/about.illinoisstate.edu/dist/e/34/files/2022/06/Balusu_final-2.pdf
18. Banks, N. (2020). Black women in the United States and unpaid collective work: Theorizing the community as a site of production. *The Review of Black Political Economy, 47*(4), 343–362.
19. Beccia, A. L., Jesdale, W. M., & Lapane, K. L. (2020). Associations between perceived everyday discrimination, discrimination attributions, and binge eating

among Latinas: Results from the National Latino and Asian American Study. *Annals of Epidemiology, 45*, 32–39.
20. Benusic, M., & Cheskin, L. J. (2021). Obesity prevalence in large US cities: Association with socioeconomic indicators, race/ethnicity, and physical activity. *Journal of Public Health, 43*(1), 148–154.
21. Bijou, C., & Colen, C. G. (2022). Shades of health: Skin color, ethnicity, and mental health among Black Americans. *Social Science & Medicine, 313*, 115387.
22. Blau, F. D., & Kahn, L. M. (2020). The gender pay gap: Have women gone as far as they can? In: *Inequality in the United States* (pp. 345–362). Routledge.
23. Bor, J., Cohen, G. H., & Galea, S. (2017). Population health in an era of rising income inequality: USA, 1980–2015. *The Lancet, 389*(10077), 1475–1490.
24. Borrell, L. N., Rodríguez-Álvarez, E., & Dallo, F. J. (2020). Racial/ethnic inequities in the associations of allostatic load with all-cause and cardiovascular-specific mortality risk in US adults. *PLoS One, 15*(2), e0228336.
25. Brown, A. M., Landor, A. M., & Zeiders, K. H. (2023). Weathering racism and colorism: Exploring concurrent and short-term longitudinal associations between discrimination, colorism, psychosocial health, and Black and Latinx emerging adults' relationship satisfaction. *Journal of Social and Personal Relationships. 40*(10), 3244–3268. doi: 10.1177/02654075231170900
26. Burke, L. M., & Schwalbach, J. (2021). Housing redlining and its lingering effects on education opportunity. *Backgrounder. No. 3594*. Heritage Foundation.
27. Busch, F. (2020). Gender segregation, occupational sorting, and growth of wage disparities between women. *Demography, 57*(3), 1063–1088.
28. Carlson, D. L. (2021). Time availability: Assessing causal ordering in the performance of paid labor and unpaid housework. *Journal of Comparative Family Studies, 52*(2), 180–205.
29. Carlson, D. L., Petts, R. J., & Pepin, J. R. (2022). Changes in US parents' domestic labor during the early days of the COVID-19 pandemic. *Sociological Inquiry, 92*(3), 1217–1244.
30. CBO (Congressional Budget Office). (2022). Trends in the distribution of family wealth, 1989 to 2019. Available at: https://www.cbo.gov/publication/57598
31. CDC (Centers for Disease Control and Prevention). (2023). National Diabetes Statistics Report. Available at: https://www.cdc.gov/diabetes/data/statistics-report/index.html
32. Census (United States Census Bureau). (2023). How the Census Bureau measures poverty. (Page Last Revised—June 15, 2023). Available at: https://www.census.gov/topics/income-poverty/poverty/guidance/poverty-measures.html
33. Centeno, B., Bayazitli, I., Purnell, S., Bravo, D. Y., & Mello, Z. R. (2023). Colorism unveiled: Examining how skin color discrimination is associated with academic achievement, mental health, and substance use among Latinx adolescents. *Research in Human Development, 20*(3–4), 123–140.
34. Chetty, R., et al. (2017). The fading American dream: Trends in absolute income mobility since 1940. *Science, 356*(6336), 398–406.
35. Chinn, J. J., Martin, I. K., & Redmond, N. (2021). Health equity among Black women in the United States. *Journal of Women's Health, 30*(2), 212–219.

36. Chyu, L., & Upchurch, D. M. (2011). Racial and ethnic patterns of allostatic load among adult women in the United States: Findings from the National Health and Nutrition Examination Survey 1999–2004. *Journal of Women's Health, 20*(4), 575–583.
37. Cleveland, C., & Lukes, D. (2022). The lingering legacy of redlining on school funding, diversity, and performance. Available at: https://scholar.harvard.edu/sites/scholar.harvard.edu/files/chcleveland/files/cleveland_lukes_2022_the_lingering_legacy_of_redlining_2022-10.pdf
38. Colangelo, L. A., et al. (2020). Association of resting heart rate with blood pressure and incident hypertension over 30 years in Black and White adults: The CARDIA study. *Hypertension, 76*(3), 692–698.
39. Commodore-Mensah, Y., et al. (2021). Associations between social determinants and hypertension, stage 2 hypertension, and controlled blood pressure among men and women in the United States. *American Journal of Hypertension, 34*(7), 707–717.
40. Cooksey Stowers, K., et al. (2020). Racial differences in perceived food swamp and food desert exposure and disparities in self-reported dietary habits. *International Journal of Environmental Research and Public Health, 17*(19), 7143.
41. Cooper, A. J., et al. (2021). Sex/gender differences in obesity prevalence, comorbidities, and treatment. *Current Obesity Reports*, *10*(4), 458–466.
42. Cubbin, C., et al. (2020). Longitudinal measures of neighborhood poverty and income inequality are associated with adverse birth outcomes in Texas. *Social Science & Medicine, 245*, 112665.
43. Cuevas, A. G., et al. (2021). Skin tone, discrimination, and allostatic load in middle-aged and older Puerto Ricans. *Psychosomatic Medicine, 83*(7), 805–812.
44. Darvas, Z. (2021). The unequal inequality impact of the COVID-19 pandemic. *Bruegel*. Available at: https://www.jstor.org/stable/resrep32250
45. Davis, B. A. (2020). Discrimination: A social determinant of health inequities. *Health Affairs Forefront*. Available at: https://www.healthaffairs.org/content/forefront/discrimination-social-determinant-health-inequities
46. Delevry, D., Ho, A., & Le, Q. A. (2021). Association between processes of diabetes care and health care utilization in patients with diabetes: Evidence from a nationally representative US sample. *Journal of Diabetes, 13*(1), 78–88.
47. Deo, S. V., et al. (2023). Association between historical neighborhood redlining and cardiovascular outcomes among US veterans with atherosclerotic cardiovascular diseases. *JAMA Network Open, 6*(7), e2322727.
48. Doan, S. N. (2021). Allostatic load: Developmental and conceptual considerations in a multi-system physiological indicator of chronic stress exposure. *Developmental Psychobiology, 63*(5), 825–836.
49. Egan, B. M., Zhao, Y., & Axon, R. N. (2010). US trends in prevalence, awareness, treatment, and control of hypertension, 1988–2008. *JAMA, 303*(20), 2043–2050.
50. England, P., Levine, A., & Mishel, E. (2020). Progress toward gender equality in the United States has slowed or stalled. *Proceedings of the National Academy of Sciences, 117*(13), 6990–6997.
51. Erkmen, C. P., et al. (2024). The cost of being a woman in academic cardiothoracic surgery: Joint collaboration of The Society of Thoracic Surgeons Workforces on

Diversity, Equity, and Inclusion and Cardiothoracic Surgery Practice Models. *The Annals of Thoracic Surgery, 117*(1), 59–67.
52. Etherington, C. (2015). Race, gender, and the resources that matter: An investigation of intersectionality and health. *Women & Health, 55*(7), 754–777.
53. Ettman, C. K., et al. (2020). Prevalence of depression symptoms in US adults before and during the COVID-19 pandemic. *JAMA Network Open, 3*(9), e2019686.
54. Ettman, C. K., Cohen, G. H., & Galea, S. (2020). Is wealth associated with depressive symptoms in the United States? *Annals of Epidemiology, 43*, 25–31.
55. Felix, A. S., et al. (2023). The modifying role of resilience on allostatic load and cardiovascular disease risk in the Jackson Heart Study. *Journal of Racial and Ethnic Health Disparities, 10*(5), 2124–2135.
56. Fiscella, K., & Franks, P. (2000). Individual income, income inequality, health, and mortality: What are the relationships? *Health Services Research, 35*(1 Pt 2), 307.
57. Fishback, P., et al. (2022). New evidence on redlining by federal housing programs in the 1930s. *Journal of Urban Economics, 141*, 103462.
58. Fogli, A., & Guerrieri, V. (2019). The end of the American dream? Inequality and segregation in US cities (No. w26143). *National Bureau of Economic Research.*
59. Gabriel, A., et al. (2021). Evaluating depressive symptoms among low-socioeconomic-status African American women aged 40 to 75 years with uncontrolled hypertension: A secondary analysis of a randomized clinical trial. *JAMA Psychiatry, 78*(4), 426–432.
60. Gamarel, K. E., et al. (2022). Stigma experienced by transgender women of color in their dating and romantic relationships: Implications for gender-based violence prevention programs. *Journal of Interpersonal Violence, 37*(9–10), NP8161–NP8189.
61. Garcia, R. (2022). Social determinants of health. In: *A Population Health Approach to Health Disparities for Nurses: Care of Vulnerable Populations.*
62. Gaskin, D. J., et al. (2021). Decomposing race and ethnic differences in CVD risk factors for mid-life women. *Journal of Racial and Ethnic Health Disparities, 8*, 174–185.
63. Gauthier, G. R., et al. (2021). Exacerbating inequalities: Social networks, racial/ethnic disparities, and the COVID-19 pandemic in the United States. *The Journals of Gerontology: Series B, 76*(3), e88–e92.
64. Gilmore, D. R., et al. (2022). Investigating racial differences in allostatic load by educational attainment among non-Hispanic Black and White men. *International Journal of Environmental Research and Public Health, 19*(9), 5486.
65. Glover, L. M., et al. (2020). Life course socioeconomic status and hypertension in African American adults: The Jackson Heart Study. *American Journal of Hypertension, 33*(1), 84–91.
66. Goldstein, S. P., et al. (2023). Applying a social determinants of health framework to guide digital innovations that reduce disparities in chronic disease. *Psychosomatic Medicine, 85*(7), 659–669.
67. Gooding, H. C., Walls, C. E., & Richmond, T. K. (2012). Food insecurity and increased BMI in young adult women. *Obesity, 20*(9), 1896–1901.
68. Gradín, C. (2020). Segregation of women into low-paying occupations in the United States. *Applied Economics, 52*(17), 1905–1920.
69. Graetz, N., & Esposito, M. (2023). Historical redlining and contemporary racial disparities in neighborhood life expectancy. *Social Forces, 102*(1), 1–22.

70. Gravelle, H., Wildman, J., & Sutton, M. (2002). Income, income inequality and health: What can we learn from aggregate data? *Social Science & Medicine, 54*(4), 577–589.
71. Guidi, J., et al. (2020). Allostatic load and its impact on health: A systematic review. *Psychotherapy and Psychosomatics, 90*(1), 11–27.
72. Guo-Brennan, M., & Guo-Brennan, M. (2020). Good schools for good development: Race, class, and housing. In: *Community Engagement for Better Schools: Guaranteeing Accountability, Representativeness and Equality* (pp. 57–74).
73. Guo, H., et al. (2022). Study on the impact of income gap on health level of rural residents in China. *International Journal of Environmental Research and Public Health, 19*(13), 7590.
74. Hammen, C. (2018). Risk factors for depression: An autobiographical review. *Annual Review of Clinical Psychology, 14*, 1–28.
75. Hardy, S. T., et al. (2021). Racial and ethnic differences in blood pressure among US adults, 1999–2018. *Hypertension, 78*(6), 1730–1741.
76. Hargrove, T. W., et al. (2020). Race/ethnicity, gender, and trajectories of depressive symptoms across early-and mid-life among the Add Health cohort. *Journal of Racial and Ethnic Health Disparities, 7*, 619–629.
77. Haw, J. S., et al. (2021). Diabetes complications in racial and ethnic minority populations in the USA. *Current Diabetes Reports, 21*, 1–8.
78. He, J., et al. (2021). Trends in cardiovascular risk factors in US adults by race and ethnicity and socioeconomic status, 1999–2018. *JAMA, 326*(13), 1286–1298.
79. Hess, C., Ahmed, T., & Hayes, J. (2020). Providing unpaid household and care work in the United States: Uncovering inequality. *Institute for Women's Policy Research, 26*(4).
80. Hicks, P. M., et al. (2023). Seeing red: Associations between historical redlining and present-day visual impairment and blindness. *Ophthalmology, 130*(4), 404–412.
81. Hill-Briggs, F., et al. (2021). Social determinants of health and diabetes: A scientific review. *Diabetes Care, 44*(1), 258.
82. Hoffmann, F., Lee, D. S., & Lemieux, T. (2020). Growing income inequality in the United States and other advanced economies. *Journal of Economic Perspectives, 34*(4), 52–78.
83. Holt-Lunstad, J. (2022). Social connection as a public health issue: The evidence and a systemic framework for prioritizing the "social" in social determinants of health. *Annual Review of Public Health, 43*, 193–213.
84. Huang, J. H., et al. (2020). Neighborhood characteristics associated with park use and park-based physical activity among children in low-income diverse neighborhoods in New York City.
85. Hubmer, J., Krusell, P., & Smith, A. A. Jr. (2021). Sources of US wealth inequality: Past, present, and future. *NBER Macroeconomics Annual, 35*(1), 391–455.
86. Jann, B. (2016). Estimating Lorenz and concentration curves. *The Stata Journal, 16*(4), 837–866.
87. Judge, K., Mulligan, J.-A., & Benzeval, M. (1998). Income inequality and population health. *Social Science & Medicine, 46*(4–5), 567–579.
88. Kantamneni, N. (2020). The impact of the COVID-19 pandemic on marginalized populations in the United States: A research agenda. *Journal of Vocational Behavior, 119*, 103439.

89. Karatas, S., Yesim, T., & Beysel, S. (2021). Impact of lockdown COVID-19 on metabolic control in type 2 diabetes mellitus and healthy people. *Primary Care Diabetes, 15*(3), 424–427.
90. Kawachi, I. (2000). Income inequality and health. *Social Epidemiology, 76*, 94.
91. Kawachi, I., & Kennedy, B. P. (1999). Income inequality and health: Pathways and mechanisms. *Health Services Research, 34*(1 Pt 2), 215.
92. Kelley, H., Galbraith, Q., & Strong, J. (2020). Working moms: Motherhood penalty or motherhood return? *The Journal of Academic Librarianship, 46*(1), 102075.
93. Kerr, P., et al. (2020). Allostatic load and women's brain health: A systematic review. *Frontiers in Neuroendocrinology, 59*, 100858.
94. Keyes, L., Small, E., & Nikolova, S. (2020). The complex relationship between colorism and poor health outcomes with African Americans: A systematic review. *Analyses of Social Issues and Public Policy, 20*(1), 676–697.
95. Kidd, J. D., et al. (2021). Understanding the impact of the COVID-19 pandemic on the mental health of transgender and gender nonbinary individuals engaged in a longitudinal cohort study. *Journal of Homosexuality, 68*(4), 592–611.
96. Klawetter, S., et al. (2020). Perinatal depression in low-income women: A literature review and innovative screening approach. *Current Psychiatry Reports, 22*, 1–8.
97. Klein, S., et al. (2022). Why does obesity cause diabetes? *Cell Metabolism, 34*(1), 11–20.
98. Komro, K. A., et al. (2020). Anti-poverty policy and health: Attributes and diffusion of state earned income tax credits across US states from 1980 to 2020. *PLoS One, 15*(11), e0242514.
99. Komro, K. A., et al. (2019). Effects of state-level earned income tax credit laws on birth outcomes by race and ethnicity. *Health Equity, 3*(1), 61–67.
100. Kraft, M. A., & Simon, N. S. (2020). Teachers' experiences working from home during the COVID-19 pandemic. Upbeat. Downloaded July 7, 2020.
101. Kroenke, K., Spitzer, R. L., & Williams, J. B. W. (2001). The PHQ-9: Validity of a brief depression severity measure. *Journal of General Internal Medicine, 16*(9), 606–613.
102. Langellier, B. A., et al. (2021). Allostatic load among U.S.- and foreign-born Whites, Blacks, and Latinx. *American Journal of Preventive Medicine, 60*(2), 159–168.
103. Lara-Cinisomo, S., Akinbode, T. D., & Wood J. (2020). A systematic review of somatic symptoms in women with depression or depressive symptoms: Do race or ethnicity matter? *Journal of Women's Health, 29*(10), 1273–1282.
104. Leak-Johnson, T., Yan, F., & Daniels, P. (2021). What the Jackson Heart Study has taught us about diabetes and cardiovascular disease in the African American community: A 20-year appreciation. *Current Diabetes Reports, 21*, 1–10.
105. Lee, C., Park, S., & Boylan, J. M. (2021). Cardiovascular health at the intersection of race and gender: Identifying life-course processes to reduce health disparities. *The Journals of Gerontology: Series B, 76*(6), 1127–1139.
106. Lee, E. K., et al. (2022). Health outcomes in redlined versus non-redlined neighborhoods: A systematic review and meta-analysis. *Social Science & Medicine, 294*, 114696.
107. Liao, T. F. (2021). Income inequality, social comparison, and happiness in the United States. *Socius, 7*, 2378023120985648.

108. Liddell, J. L., et al. (2021). She's the center of my life, the one that keeps my heart open: Roles and expectations of Native American women. *Affilia, 36*(3), 357–375.
109. Linde, S., et al. (2023). Historic residential redlining and present-day social determinants of health, home evictions, and food insecurity within U.S. neighborhoods. *Journal of General Internal Medicine*, *38*(15), 3321–3328.
110. Lordan, G., & Pischke, J.-S. (2022). Does Rosie like riveting? Male and female occupational choices. *Economica, 89*(353), 110–130.
111. Lorgelly, P. K., & Lindley, J. (2008). What is the relationship between income inequality and health? Evidence from the BHPS. *Health Economics, 17*(2), 249–265.
112. Lukes, D., & Christopher Cleveland. (2021). The lingering legacy of redlining on school funding, diversity, and performance. *EdWorkingPaper No. 21-363*. Annenberg Institute for School Reform at Brown University.
113. Lynch, E. E., et al. (2021). The legacy of structural racism: Associations between historic redlining, current mortgage lending, and health. *SSM-Population Health, 14*, 100793.
114. Lynch, J., et al. (2004). Is income inequality a determinant of population health? Part 1: A systematic review. *The Milbank Quarterly, 82*(1), 5–99.
115. Macit, S. M., & Acar-Tek, N. (2020). Evaluation of nutritional status and allostatic load in adult patients with type 2 diabetes. *Canadian Journal of Diabetes, 44*(2), 156–161.
116. Mahajan, Shiwani, et al. (2021). Trends in differences in health status and healthcare access and affordability by race and ethnicity in the United States, 1999–2018. *JAMA, 326*(7), 637–648.
117. Maliniak, M. L., et al. (2023). Census tracts are not neighborhoods: Addressing spatial misalignment in studies examining the impact of historical redlining on present-day health outcomes. *Epidemiology, 34*(6), 817–826.
118. Manrique-Acevedo, C., et al. (2020). Obesity and cardiovascular disease in women. *International Journal of Obesity, 44*(6), 1210–1226.
119. Mathieu-Bolh, N. (2022). The elusive link between income and obesity. *Journal of Economic Surveys, 36*(4), 935–968.
120. McNutt, L.-A., et al. (2003). Estimating the relative risk in cohort studies and clinical trials of common outcomes. *American Journal of Epidemiology, 157*(10), 940–943.
121. Meara, K., Pastore, F., & Webster, A. (2020). The gender pay gap in the USA: A matching study. *Journal of Population Economics, 33*, 271–305.
122. Miller, H. N., et al. (2021). The impact of discrimination on allostatic load in adults: An integrative review of literature. *Journal of Psychosomatic Research, 146*, 110434.
123. Mitchell, B., & Franco, J. (2018). HOLC "redlining" maps: The persistent structure of segregation and economic inequality. Available at: https://ncrc.org/wp-content/uploads/dlm_uploads/2018/02/NCRC-Research-HOLC-10.pdf.
124. Mongelli, F., Georgakopoulos, P., & Pato, M. T. (2020). Challenges and opportunities to meet the mental health needs of underserved and disenfranchised populations in the United States. *Focus, 18*(1), 16–24.
125. Mongero, L. B., Rosenthal, T. M., & Walczak, A. B. (2022). A survey of women in the perfusion workforce: 2021. *The Journal of ExtraCorporeal Technology, 54*(1), 29.

126. Monk Jr., E. P. (2021). Colorism and physical health: Evidence from a national survey. *Journal of Health and Social Behavior, 62*(1), 37–52.
127. Moseson, Heidi, et al. (2020). The imperative for transgender and gender nonbinary inclusion: Beyond women's health. *Obstetrics and Gynecology, 135*(5), 1059.
128. Mujahid, M. S., et al. (2021). Historical redlining and cardiovascular health: The multi-ethnic study of atherosclerosis. *Proceedings of the National Academy of Sciences, 118*(51), e2110986118.
129. Mulenga, A., & Ataguba, J. E. (2017). Assessing income redistributive effect of health financing in Zambia. *Social Science & Medicine, 189*, 1–10.
130. Murshed, S. M. (2022). Consequences of the COVID-19 pandemic for economic inequalities. In: *Covid-19 and International Development* (pp. 59–70). Springer.
131. National Academies of Sciences, Engineering, and Medicine, & Committee on Population. (2015). *The Growing Gap in Life Expectancy by Income: Implications for Federal Programs and Policy Responses*. National Academies Press. https://nap.nationalacademies.org/catalog/19015/the-growing-gap-in-life-expectancy-by-income-implications-for
132. Nguyen, M. (2022). *Colorism: The Psychological Effects of Skin Color Discrimination Among Ethnic/racial Minority Women* (Doctoral dissertation, Adler University).
133. NHANES. (2016). Impact of work and recreational physical activity on prediabetes condition among U.S. adults. *International Journal of Environmental Research and Public Health, 18*(4), 1378.
134. NHANES (National Health and Nutrition Examination Survey). (2018). *Analytic guidelines, 2011–2014 and 2015–2016*. Available at: https://wwwn.cdc.gov/nchs/data/nhanes/2011-2012/analyticguidelines/analytic_guidelines_11_16.pdf
135. NHANES (National Health and Nutrition Examination Survey). (2021). *National Health and Nutrition Examination Survey 1999–2000 data documentation, codebook, and frequencies*. Available at: https://wwwn.cdc.gov/Nchs/Nhanes/1999-2000/BMX.htm#BMIWT
136. National Institutes of Health, National Heart, Lung, and Blood Institute. (2020). *Assessing Your Weight and Health Risk*. Available at: https://www.nhlbi.nih.gov/health/educational/lose_wt/risk.htm
137. National Institutes of Health. (2021). *Overweight & Obesity Statistics*. Available at: https://www.niddk.nih.gov/health-information/health-statistics/overweight-obesity#:~:text=Nearly%202%20in%205%20non,(43.7%25)%2C%20have%20obesity.
138. Ogden, C. L., et al. (2020). Trends in obesity prevalence by race and Hispanic origin—1999–2000 to 2017–2018. *JAMA, 324*(12), 1208–1210.
139. Oh, S., Salas-Wright, C. P., & Vaughn, M. G. (2018). Trends in depression among low-income mothers in the United States, 2005–2015. *Journal of Affective Disorders, 235*, 72–75.
140. Okoro, O. N., et al. (2020). Access to health care for low-income African American women: Lived experiences and expectations. *Journal of Health Care for the Poor and Underserved, 31*(2), 939–957.
141. Okoro, O. N., Hillman, L. A., & Cernasev, A. (2022). Intersectional invisibility experiences of low-income African American women in healthcare encounters. *Ethnicity & Health, 27*(6), 1290–1309.

142. Olives, C., et al. (2013). Prevalence, awareness, treatment, and control of hypertension in United States counties, 2001–2009. *PLoS One, 8*(4), e60308.
143. Oncescu, J., & Loewen, M. (2020). Community recreation provisions that support low-income families' access to recreation. *Leisure/Loisir, 44*(2), 279–302.
144. World Health Organization. (2010). *A Conceptual Framework for Action on the Social Determinants of Health: Debates, Policy, and Practice.*
145. Ostchega, Y., et al. (2022). Differences in hypertension prevalence and hypertension control by urbanization among adults in the United States, 2013–2018. *American Journal of Hypertension, 35*(1), 31–41.
146. Pailhé, A., Solaz, A., & Stanfors, M. (2021). The great convergence: Gender and unpaid work in Europe and the United States. *Population and Development Review, 47*(1), 181–217.
147. Park, J. (2021). Who is hardest hit by a pandemic? Racial disparities in COVID-19 hardship in the U.S. *International Journal of Urban Sciences, 25*(2), 149–177.
148. Parker, H. W., et al. (2022). Allostatic load and mortality: A systematic review and meta-analysis. *American Journal of Preventive Medicine, 63*(1), 131–140.
149. Perry, B. L., Aronson, B., & Pescosolido, B. A. (2021). Pandemic precarity: COVID-19 is exposing and exacerbating inequalities in the American heartland. *Proceedings of the National Academy of Sciences, 118*(8), e2020685118.
150. Pickett, K. E., & Wilkinson, R. G. (2015). Income inequality and health: A causal review. *Social Science & Medicine, 128*, 316–326.
151. Ragin, C. C., & Fiss, P. C. (2017). *Intersectional Inequality: Race, Class, Test Scores, and Poverty*. University of Chicago Press.
152. Richardson, L. J., Goodwin, A. N., & Hummer, R. A. (2021). Social status differences in allostatic load among young adults in the United States. *SSM-Population Health, 15*, 100771.
153. Rieger, A., et al. (2022). The impact of the COVID-19 pandemic on gender-based violence in the United States: Framework and policy recommendations. *Psychological Trauma: Theory, Research, Practice, and Policy, 14*(3), 471.
154. Rogers, C. R., et al. (2022). Investigation of differences in allostatic load among Black men by level of educational attainment: High school graduates experience the highest levels of stress. *International Journal of Environmental Research and Public Health, 19*(6), 3580.
155. Rollston, R., & Galea, S. (2020). *COVID-19 and the Social Determinants of Health.* SAGE Publications.
156. Rosengren, A. (2021). Obesity and cardiovascular health: The size of the problem. *European Heart Journal, 42*(34), 3404–3406.
157. Savage, M. (2020). Money talks: Using prior salary as an affirmative defense in equal pay claims. *Utah Law Review, 289*.
158. Scaptura, M. N., & Boyle, K. M. (2020). Masculinity threat, "Incel" traits, and violent fantasies among heterosexual men in the United States. *Feminist Criminology, 15*(3), 278–298.
159. Schmalor, A., & Heine, S. J. (2022). The construct of subjective economic inequality. *Social Psychological and Personality Science, 13*(1), 210–219.

160. Schulz, A. J., et al. (2012). Associations between socioeconomic status and allostatic load: Effects of neighborhood poverty and tests of mediating pathways. *American Journal of Public Health, 102*(9), 1706–1714.
161. Scott, J., et al. (2020). Understanding social determinants of cardiometabolic disease risk in rural women. *Journal of Community Health, 45*, 1–9.
162. Sedivy, S. (2023). Systematic barriers to success: The impact of redlining on modern educational outcomes in Omaha public schools.
163. Shrestha, B. K., et al. (2020). Employment and wage distribution investigation in the construction industry by gender. *Journal of Management in Engineering, 36*(4), 06020001.
164. Siltanen, J. (2021). *Locating Gender: Occupational Segregation, Wages and Domestic Responsibilities*. Routledge.
165. Slaughter-Acey, J. C., et al. (2019). Skin tone matters: Racial microaggressions and delayed prenatal care. *American Journal of Preventive Medicine, 57*(3), 321–329.
166. Smith, M. V., & Mazure, C. M. (2021). Mental health and wealth: Depression, gender, poverty, and parenting. *Annual Review of Clinical Psychology, 17*, 181–205.
167. Solís, C. B., et al. (2016). Mediating pathways between parental socio-economic position and allostatic load in mid-life: Findings from the 1958 British birth cohort. *Social Science & Medicine, 165*, 19–27.
168. Spencer, L. H., et al. (2020). A scoping review of how income affects accessing local green space to engage in outdoor physical activity to improve well-being: Implications for post-COVID-19. *International Journal of Environmental Research and Public Health, 17*(24), 9313.
169. Strompolis, M., et al. (2019). The intersectionality of adverse childhood experiences, race/ethnicity, and income: Implications for policy. *Journal of Prevention & Intervention in the Community, 47*(4), 310–324.
170. Strully, K. W., Rehkopf, D. H., & Xuan, Z. (2010). Effects of prenatal poverty on infant health: State earned income tax credits and birth weight. *American Sociological Review, 75*(4), 534–562.
171. Suvarna, B., et al. (2020). Health risk behaviors and allostatic load: A systematic review. *Neuroscience & Biobehavioral Reviews, 108*, 694–711.
172. Sweeney, B. N. (2020). Gender-based violence and rape culture. In: *Companion to Women's and Gender Studies*, (pp. 285–302).
173. Swope, C. B., Hernández, D., & Cushing, L. J. (2022). The relationship of historical redlining with present-day neighborhood environmental and health outcomes: A scoping review and conceptual model. *Journal of Urban Health, 99*(6), 959–983.
174. Szewczyk, J., & Crowder-Meyer, M. (2020). Community income inequality and the economic gap in participation. *Political Behavior*, 1–26.
175. Tavares, C. D., et al. (2022). Allostatic load, income, and race among Black and White men in the United States. *American Journal of Men's Health, 16*(2): 15579883221092290.
176. Tesfai, R., & Thomas, K. J. A. (2020). Dimensions of inequality: Black immigrants' occupational segregation in the United States. *Sociology of Race and Ethnicity, 6*(1), 1–21.
177. Thorpe Jr, R. J., et al. (2017). Association between discrimination and obesity in African-American men. *Biodemography and Social Biology, 63*(3), 253–261.

178. Tobin, C. S. T. (2021). Distinguishing distress from disorder: Black-white patterns in the determinants of and links between depressive symptoms and major depression. *Journal of Affective Disorders, 279*, 510–517.
179. Tyrell, F. A., Rogosch, F. A., & Cicchetti, D. (2023). Profiles of risk, allostatic load, and mental health in low-income children. *Clinical Psychological Science, 12*(4), 586–606. doi: 21677026231183012.
180. Vyas, C. M., et al. (2020). Association of race and ethnicity with late-life depression severity, symptom burden, and care. *JAMA Network Open, 3*(3), e201606–e201606.
181. Wagstaff, A., & Van Doorslaer, E. (2000). Income inequality and health: What does the literature tell us? *Annual Review of Public Health, 21*(1), 543–567.
182. Wang, L., et al. (2021). Trends in prevalence of diabetes and control of risk factors in diabetes among US adults, 1999–2018. *JAMA, 326*(8), 704–716.
183. WHO. (2010). *A Conceptual Framework for Action on the Social Determinants of Health*. Available at: https://www.who.int/publications/i/item/9789241500852.
184. Wilkinson, R. G., & Pickett, K. E. (2006). Income inequality and population health: A review and explanation of the evidence. *Social Science & Medicine, 62*(7), 1768–1784.
185. Williams, B. M., et al. (2022). Examining educational attainment and allostatic load in non-Hispanic Black women. *BMC Women's Health, 22*(1), 75.
186. Williams, S. L., et al. (2020). A critical deconstructed quantitative analysis: Sexual and gender minority stress through an intersectional lens. *Journal of Social Issues, 76*(4), 859–879.
187. Williams, T. G., et al. (2020). Parks and safety: A comparative study of green space access and inequity in five US cities. *Landscape and Urban Planning, 201*, 103841.
188. Wilson, B. (2020). Urban heat management and the legacy of redlining. *Journal of the American Planning Association, 86*(4), 443–457.
189. Wondmkun, Y. T. (2020). Obesity, insulin resistance, and type 2 diabetes: Associations and therapeutic implications. *Diabetes, Metabolic Syndrome and Obesity, 13*, 3611–3616.
190. Wright, H. A. (2021). *A Phenomenological Examination of Colorism Among African American Women*. Hampton University: VA 23669, United States.
191. Yassine, B. B., Rojewski, J. W., & Ransom, M. M. (2022). Gender inequity in the public health workforce. *Journal of Public Health Management and Practice, 28*(2), E390–E396.
192. Yearby, R. (2020). Structural racism and health disparities: Reconfiguring the social determinants of health framework to include the root cause. *Journal of Law, Medicine & Ethics, 48*(3), 518–526.
193. Yip, T., et al. (2021). Rendered invisible: Are Asian Americans a model or a marginalized minority? *American Psychologist, 76*(4), 575.
194. Yu, Q., et al. (2021). Racial residential segregation and economic disparity jointly exacerbate COVID-19 fatality in large American cities. *Annals of the New York Academy of Sciences, 1494*(1), 18–30.
195. Yuan, D., et al. (2023). Associations of socioeconomic factors and unhealthy lifestyles with allostatic load: A meta-analysis. *International Journal of Behavioral Medicine*, 1–15.

196. Zare, H., Fugal, A., Azadi, M., & Gaskin, D. J. (2022). How income inequality and race concentrate depression in low-income women in the US, 2005–2016. *Healthcare, 10*, 8–1424.
197. Zare, H., Gaskin, D. J., & Thorpe Jr, R. J. (2021). Income inequality and obesity among US adults 1999–2016: Does sex matter? *International Journal of Environmental Research and Public Health, 18*(13), 7079.
198. Zare, H., et al. (2021). How income inequality and race/ethnicity drive obesity in US adults: 1999–2016. *Healthcare, 9*, 11–1442.
199. Zare, H., et al. (2023). Allostatic load in the US general population: Race and educational intersection. *Public Health in Practice, 6*, 100425.
200. Zatterale, F., et al. (2020). Chronic adipose tissue inflammation linking obesity to insulin resistance and type 2 diabetes. *Frontiers in Physiology, 10*, 1607.
201. Zewde, N. (2020). Universal baby bonds reduce Black-white wealth inequality, progressively raise net worth of all young adults. *The Review of Black Political Economy, 47*(1), 3–19.
202. Zipf, G., et al. (2013). National health and nutrition examination survey: Plan and operations, 1999–2010. *National Center for Health Statistics. Vital Health Stat, 1*(56). Retrieved June 25, 2019, from: https://www.cdc.gov/nchs/data/series/sr_01/sr01_056.pdf.
203. Zou, G. (2004). A modified Poisson regression approach to prospective studies with binary data. *American Journal of Epidemiology, 159*(7), 702–706.

CHAPTER 3

Impact of Social Challenges on Female Health Issues

RUKSHANA IRANI,[1] AYAN CHATTERJEE,[2*] and ARPAN RAY[3]

*Corresponding author

ABSTRACT

The objective of this chapter is to identify and assess important topics pertaining to women's health, social, cultural, and economic well-being. In India, both men and women have nearly the same life expectancy at birth. However, after birth, women's health faces adverse conditions due to numerous social challenges. Women's health issues are multifaceted, influenced by individual characteristics and broader dimensions such as sociocultural, economic, and physical environments. Malnutrition, social dynamics, poor sanitation, unequal access to housing, livelihood, education, and cultural and economic advancement are among the most common issues facing the contemporary human ecological system. By recognizing the significance of female health in contemporary society, the study aims to emphasize the intricate interplay between various social determinants. This comprehensive review on female health challenges includes reproductive health, contraception access, mental health, and various conditions such as endometriosis and breast cancer. Various factors, including discrimination, cultural beliefs, taboos, gender roles, healthcare access, and political influences, have also been discussed. This review concludes that a holistic approach to female health issues requires research, decisive social and political intervention, and proactive measures.

Holistic Approaches for Women's Sustainable Health, Volume 2: Advancements, Socioeconomic Impacts, and Innovative Strategies. Junaid Ahmad Malik, Anamika Chauhan, and Megh R. Goyal (Eds)

DOI: 10.1201/9781779641656-4

3.1 INTRODUCTION

The status of women in society has always been ignored, despite their significant contributions to development. The active and impactful participation of women in the liberation movement was quite evident but not well recognized. Our deeply rooted culture and religious ideologies further hamper their access to social, economic, political status, etc. Rethinking and reconstruction of societal norms are needed to attain gender equality [67]. A feminist perspective that can embrace both equality and differences with open hands can only pave the way toward real women's empowerment [20]. Historical patterns indicate a gap in the attention given to women's health requirements in medical research [70]. In 1985, the Public Health Service Task Force on Women's Health Issues emphasized how important it was to get women's health research underway. In 1985, the Public Health Service Task Force on Women's Health Issues [70] issued a report stating that women's health had received insufficient attention, which had an impact on the caliber of health information that was available to them. It had an impact on the medical services the women provided [25, 26].

3.1.1 IMPORTANCE OF UNDERSTANDING SOCIAL IMPACT

Social factors affect our understanding of women's health [70]. Not studying or conducting clinical trials on women in medical research, the persistent existence of social taboos surrounding menstruation and menopause indicates the substantial impact of society on the lives of women [66].

In many societies, women are only known for their reproductive roles. It hinders their access to broader aspects of health, and, thus, their overall well-being gets hampered. Women face physical, emotional, and sexual violence, which also adversely affects their health outcomes. These issues need to be properly dealt with to achieve equitable health goals. The disparities in the health of men and women remain, as there is a difference in their biological and physiological attributes. Due to systemic prejudice, women and girls suffer significant health issues. Women live in an atmosphere where they are disadvantaged due to the unequal power relations between men and women. Social standards limit these women's access to work and educational possibilities, which has an additional impact on them [67].

3.1.2 RELEVANCE TO FEMALE HEALTH ISSUES

Women are more susceptible to several health problems that require immediate attention. The prevalence of breast cancer and cervical cancer among women in low- and middle-income countries is comparatively high, and this problem is made worse by a lack of effective screening tools and preventive measures. Reproduction and fertility disorders account for one-third of women's health issues in the 15–44 years of age range. Violence, mental health challenges, and the burden of noncommunicable diseases further aggravate women's health. Adolescent girls and teenagers also remain unaffected by the health issues linked with sex and reproduction, with many giving birth to babies every year. Older women also face problems regarding pensions and healthcare facilities. Despite advances in maternal care strategies, maternal mortality due to pregnancy-related complications still exists significantly. Young women suffer from human immunodeficiency virus (HIV) infections, and risks such as tuberculosis also increase in them [7].

3.2 OBJECTIVES OF THIS REVIEW

The review set out to investigate the ways that society influences women's health. Analysis has been done on socioeconomic factors, cultural norms, access restrictions to healthcare, and government regulations pertaining to women's health. In this review, the importance of further studies on women's health has also been stressed.

3.3 IDENTIFYING GAPS AND EMERGING TRENDS

The way that gender-specific scientific research is seen has evolved globally. It is well known how important it is to research how gender and sex traits affect health outcomes [21]. Prioritizing the health of women can help achieve the fourth and fifth goals of the Millennium Development Program [68]. Society has long disregarded women's healthcare in the name of traditions and customs. But due to recent developments in science, technology, and education, there is a greater awareness of what women need for a better society [68].

- **Sex-based differences in health outcomes**: Studies show that women are more likely than men to experience certain health issues. A new strategy had to be created due to the physiological and biological variations between the sexes.
- **Personalized care through technology**: Nowadays, women have become aware of their health issues and are using devices, "digital healthcare apps," for monitoring their own health. This step toward trying to gain control over their health and well-being can also be considered a small step toward women's empowerment. Expansion of healthcare services such as telemedicine, personalized care, and improved medical technology has contributed to the improved health outcomes of women.
- **Destigmatization of women's health issues**: Women's health issues such as menstruation, sexual wellness, fertility issues, and menopause, which were earlier taboos, are openly discussed nowadays. As a result, women are also coming forward to share their problems and, thus, getting appropriate treatments and solutions to their problems. This change in the attitude of society can address women's health challenges in a more comprehensive manner.
- **Embracing holistic approaches**: Women are acknowledging the significance of various dimensions of health such as physical, mental, and emotional well-being. Contemporary women are trying to understand and appreciate the importance of a balanced diet, sleep, gut health, mental health, etc., and they are trying to adopt holistic approaches in terms of health.
- **Continued advocacy efforts**: Even though there has been a lot of progress in the field of women's healthcare, advocacy work is still necessary to close ongoing disparities. Stakeholders can ensure that the women receive personalized care by advocating policies that prioritize women's health [22].

In conclusion, we can say that health outcomes for women can only be improved by identifying the gaps and emerging trends in women's healthcare. Continued research, education, and collaboration are vital for the upgradation of women's healthcare and promotion of gender equity in healthcare delivery system. Healthcare system can fulfill the requirements of women, applying technology for the personalized care of women, understanding the sex-based health problems, advocating policies that favor women's health, and embracing a holistic way of living.

3.4 SOCIAL DETERMINANTS OF FEMALE HEALTH

Women's health is intricately connected to social determinants [68], including socioeconomic status and cultural norms. It is important to acknowledge and address these factors in order to achieve better and comprehensive outcomes in female health.

3.4.1 SOCIOECONOMIC FACTORS

A thorough investigation into the complicated and multifaceted topic of how socioeconomic variables affect women's health was conducted in recent years. The research indicated that socioeconomic position (SEP) is a key determinant of the outcomes of women's health throughout the life cycle. Poorer health outcomes were reported in women belonging to low SEP and education levels in comparison to the women having higher levels of SEP. Limited access to healthcare, nutrition, and increased exposure to environmental hazards are the contributing factors. SEP influences all the key stages of a woman's life, that is, childhood, adolescence, and adulthood. During childhood, low SEP can lead to inadequate access to nutrition and healthcare that impacts long-term health outcomes. In adolescence, low SEP can increase the chances of poor mental health.

SEP has an impact on women's health during all major life periods but particularly in infancy, adolescence, and adulthood. For instance, poor SEP throughout childhood might lead to limited access to wholesome diets and medical services, which can have a lasting impact on women's health outcomes. Income and education are the factors that shape women's health outcomes in their adulthood. Studies reported that the occurrence of metabolic syndrome was more common in women with low SEP than in women who belong to higher income levels.

Aspects such as having children and the makeup of the household were also found to be crucial in the study on the effect of SEP on women's health. Studies have indicated that improving women's health outcomes may involve addressing socioeconomic status differences. By raising women's income and educational attainment, it is possible to mitigate the unequal distribution of work and violence against them, hence lessening the negative effects of SEP on women's health. Furthermore, the relationship between socioeconomic status and women's health is a complex issue that calls for a multipronged strategy. The health outcomes of women across the life cycle can be improved by addressing the underlying causes of socioeconomic inequality [48]. Even though women generally outlive men in most nations, they still must deal with a number of issues that include greater rates of comorbidities, worse mental health, and greater disability. By 2030, there will likely be less of a global edge in female life expectancy [32]. The benefit of a longer life expectancy for females may be diminishing due to socioeconomic inequality [33].

Nonmedical factors that significantly affect health outcomes are included in the social determinants of health (SDH). These are related to the conditions under which people are born, grow, develop, work, reside, and age. Policies, developmental goals, the state of the economy, societal norms, and political systems all have an impact on these variables [68]. We observe unjust and preventable health disparities between and within nations because SDH controls the health of its citizens in a society. There is a social gradient in health, meaning that lower SEPs are linked to worse health, regardless of earning levels. Education, work circumstances, income, housing, food security, early childhood situations, and access to high-quality health services are important determinants. Studies reveal that SDH can influence health outcomes more than lifestyle choices and healthcare combined, which account for 30–55% of health outcomes. Furthermore, the population's health outcomes are greatly influenced by sectors other than health. Effective SDH management can improve health and lessen long-term health disparities, necessitating cooperative action from all societal sectors [69].

An urgent effort aimed at fostering a healthy society is needed, as women's health is a fundamental requirement for both family and societal well-being.

In the field of policymaking, it is imperative to prioritize women's education in addition to addressing the objective of decreasing economic inequality. Important steps include supporting women's access to higher education and the workforce while also recognizing and honoring their responsibilities as mothers and wives. To enhance the health of women in lower socioeconomic and educational strata, policymakers must consider the complex interactions between SDH and health status [4, 68].

Ved et al. revealed a significant gender gap in India's labor, health, and education, highlighting the need to change economic policies to advance gender equality [59, 67].

The substantial effects of joblessness and unstable employment on healthcare, as noted by Matilla-Santander et al., underscore the need for a stable legislative framework [39].

In India, women comprise over 50% of the populace. The growing number of women enrolled in graduate and undergraduate science programs is one sign of the nation's social progress. Interestingly, women comprise 15% of all research and development workers in India and account for over 35% of PhD recipients in the sciences [18].

To encourage more women to pursue jobs in Science, Technology, Engineering, and Mathematics disciplines, the Indian government has launched numerous programs. "Beti Bachao, Beti Padhao [19]" (save the daughter, educate the daughter) is one such amazing project that India's Prime Minister Narendra Modi unveiled on January 22, 2015 [23]. To address the dropping child sex ratio, this program is a part of the government's larger goals to promote women's rights and prosperity in the country. Mahila E-Haat, a website that promotes businesses owned by women, nongovernmental organizations, and self-help groups, was another initiative that was started in 2016 [30].

In addition, the government launched "Mahila Shakti Kendra" in 2017 with the goal of giving rural women access to healthcare, media literacy, education, job opportunities, and nutrition programs [15].

3.4.2 CULTURAL AND SOCIETAL NORMS

Cultural factors can significantly affect various aspects of healthcare and its outcome. Health-seeking behaviors and mental health outcomes of women are affected by cultural practices. For instance, the practice of following certain inhibitions during the menstrual period can act as a barrier to access to maternal healthcare, resulting in a greater likelihood of births at home without the assistance of medically trained nurses. Cultural beliefs and practices also increase the occurrence of postpartum depression [5].

In poor nations, where formal institutions and organizations are either nonexistent or scarce, people frequently rely on community relationships and facilities to acquire essential services such as healthcare. People follow the social norms that are prevalent in these contexts [31].

The cultural norms and practices surrounding childbirth, postpartum confinement, and the ritualistic cleansing of new mothers and infants within the community influence women's use of healthcare services and health outcomes. Knowing how cultural influences affect women's health can help reduce barriers to accessing healthcare. Together with addressing the unique health requirements of women that are influenced by cultural norms, policymakers and healthcare professionals can create interventions and policies to support equal access to healthcare for women.

- **Reproductive rights and behaviors:** In patriarchal societies, the cultural norms make women unable to exercise their reproductive rights. This affects women's access to reproductive healthcare services, including antenatal care, childbirth, and postnatal care.
- **Decision-making dynamics:** Cultural norms and gender roles prevalent in a society influence the decision-making processes within the family, especially regarding the utilization of health-care services.
- **Maternal health:** Culture affects the adoption and utilization of healthcare facilities and, thus, exerts a substantial impact on maternal health.
- **Autonomy and empowerment:** Women's status, autonomy, and empowerment are dependent upon the cultural norms prevalent in that area.
- **Gender inequality and marginalization:** Gender inequality and marginalization of women lead to their lowered status and higher levels of dependency. These are also controlled by the existing cultural norms in society [1, 67].

3.5 HISTORICAL PERSPECTIVES

The health issues of women have varied throughout history and across different cultures and societies. Midwifery and childbirth were the key health issues of women in the past. In ancient Egypt, the wall inscriptions depicted aspects of assisted childbirth, but in ancient Greece, midwifery was done according to law. Childbirth was considered a female disease in the 16th century. The introduction of modern contraception in the 1960s was extremely important, particularly in the low-income countries [47]. The 1960s saw the rise of the women's health movement, which called for parity in medical research and treatment. An important turning point was the Boston Women's Health Book Collective's release of "Our Bodies, Ourselves" in the early 1970s. To promote the participation of women in clinical trials financed by the National Institutes of Health (NIH), the Public Health Service Task Force on Women's Health Issues was established in 1983. In 1984, the National Black Women's Health Project—now called the Black Women's Health Imperative—started focusing on the health of African American women. In 1986, the NIH enacted a policy allowing women and minorities to participate in clinical research. Initiatives on maternal morbidity and opioid use disorder were financed by the Office of Research on Women's Health, which also expanded the definition of "women's health." In 2002, specialist research labs on sexual differences were established, and in 2006, the human papillomavirus (HPV) vaccination was released. By initiating research on the causative variables and interventions that supported and encouraged women in biomedical careers in 2008, the Working Group on Women in Biomedical Careers was founded in 2007 [23].

3.5.1 EVOLUTION OF WOMEN'S HEALTH ISSUES

The Women's Health Movement started in the 1960s–1970s to augment healthcare facilities for women. It gained political relevance in the 1980s and 1990s. Core concepts included diversity in the health needs of females, empowerment, and researching gender disparities in terms of health. Feminist perspectives emphasized the sociopolitical setting. Women's health can be described as sustaining wellness and preventing sickness. Women's health centers provide comprehensive treatment with a special emphasis on accessibility and professional support. Collaboration among the stakeholders is crucial for achieving success [24].

3.5.2 CHANGES OVER TIME

The recognition of the need to concentrate on women's health has advanced significantly over the past 30 years, resulting in improvements in a variety of areas related to women's well-being. These developments were largely sparked by the Public Health Service Task Force on Women's Health Issues Report, which was released in 1985. The following are few significant shifts in women's health over time:

- **Drug safety and effectiveness**: Data on the safety and efficacy of medications and medical devices by age, ethnicity, and sex must be reported by manufacturers, according to a rule published by the US Food and Drug Administration.
- **Health disparities**: Although there has been an overall improvement in health, not all women have benefited equally. The rates of the major causes of death have decreased for women from various racial/ethnic minority groups, but there are still significant health disparities, especially for underprivileged groups such as disabled, low-income, rural, immigrant, lesbian, bisexual, and transgender women.
- **HIV transmission**: Before antiretroviral medication was developed, mothers who were HIV positive had a 25–30% chance of passing the infection to their unborn children. Antiretroviral therapy used by HIV-positive women during pregnancy can reduce the risk of HIV transmission to fetuses by less than 2%.
- **Inclusion in clinical research**: To better understand how drugs, surgeries, and illnesses affect women differently from men, the NIH implemented a policy encouraging the participation of more women in clinical research.
- **Rates of breastfeeding**: In 1984, it was estimated that 60% of mothers breastfed their children; however, in the modern era, 77% of mothers begin nursing their children as soon as they are born, and 49% of mothers continue for up to 6 months after the baby is born.
- **Teen birth rate**: For every 1000 teenage girls, there were 51 adolescent pregnancies in 1985. The rate is currently 29.4 per 1000 teenage girls, partly due to the development of more dependable and potent forms of birth control.

Even with these improvements, there are still issues that need attention. Nearly half of pregnancies in the United States were found to be unplanned, and the likelihood of death from pregnancy-related complications has more than doubled since 1987. In addition, women's long-term and grave health repercussions have worsened due to the rise in obesity and sedentary lifestyles in the United States.

In conclusion, we may state that during the previous 30 years, there have been notable advancements in women's health. However, to guarantee the well-being of every woman, it is essential to consistently address the remaining issues and health inequalities in women's health [36].

3.5.3 MILESTONES IN WOMEN'S HEALTH

Maternal and child health, including family planning, became recognized as an essential part of primary healthcare at conferences such as the Safe Motherhood Initiative in Nairobi (1987) and the International Conference on Population and Development in Cairo (1994). The Cairo focus on reproductive health, emphasizing women's right to optimal physical and mental well-being, was welcomed by the Beijing World Conference on Women (1995). Priorities for women's health now differ throughout the world based on socioeconomic and cultural variables. Seventy-four percent of HIV cases in sub-Saharan Africa were discovered in young females. Every day, more than 10,000 babies and 1600 mothers lose their lives due to avoidable pregnancy problems.

Every year, almost 14 million teenage females give birth, with more than 90% of them occurring in underdeveloped nations. Moreover, 100 million females are predicted to get married before turning 18 years, mostly in underdeveloped countries. Pregnancy-related malaria interventions are not available to more than 5% of women. In total, 15%–71% of women worldwide experience abuse in romantic relationships. Over 750,000 people die from breast and cervical cancers annually, most of which occur in underdeveloped nations, underscoring the importance of preventative measures and healthcare access [47].

The achievements that have improved women's health and well-being over time are included in the category of milestones in female health. The following significant anniversaries are given as follows:

- **Access to education and information (late 19th to early 20th century):** The access of women to education has increased. Education has played a key role in empowering them with knowledge about hygiene and health [58].
- **Contraception and family planning (1960):** Approval of the first oral contraceptive pill gave women a dependable method of contraception and greater control over family planning [17].
- **Reproductive rights (1973)**: The Supreme Court of the United States gave a decision in *Roe v. Wade*, legalized abortion, and established reproductive rights for women [3].
- **Breast cancer awareness (1985)**: The recognition of Breast Cancer Awareness Month and greater attention on breast cancer research, screening, and early detection [42].
- **Cervical cancer screening (1950s)**: Development of the Pap smear, a screening test for cervical cancer that can help in early detection and prevention [50].
- **Hormone replacement therapy (1942)**: Usage of estrogen therapy for menopausal symptoms. Further research has led to a comprehensive understanding of the risks and benefits related to hormone replacement therapy [16].
- **Maternal health services (20th century)**: An improvement in maternal healthcare facilities has taken place. Development of safer childbirth practices, prenatal care, and interventions to reduce maternal mortality are the key milestones [27].
- **Research on women's health (late 20th century):** Research on women's health has helped to develop an understanding of gender-specific health issues, which in turn assisted in the development of gender-appropriate treatments [26].
- **Vaccination programs (ongoing)**: Vaccination programs for diseases such as HPV have been implemented, which have helped to prevent cervical cancer in women to a greater extent [29].
- **Mental health awareness (ongoing)**: Awareness of people on mental health issues specific to women has improved. Measures have been taken to manage conditions such as postpartum depression and eating disorders [8].

- **Osteoporosis management (late 20th century):** Osteoporosis is a condition that affects bone density and mainly affects postmenopausal women. Understanding this condition has led to better management of osteoporosis [51].
- **Increased access to healthcare (ongoing)**: Regular checkups, screenings, and preventive services for women's health have improved [52].

It is important to understand that despite significant progress, challenges and disparities still exist, and continuous efforts are required to address them effectively.

3.5.4 SHIFTING SOCIETAL ATTITUDES TOWARD FEMALE HEALTH

- **Historical perspectives:** Earlier women were not given sufficient attention [20].
- **Movement for women's rights:** First-wave feminism focused on women's health and access to healthcare services [10].
- **Education and empowerment of women:** Improvement in education levels empowered women to make the right decisions for themselves and their health [53].
- **Reproductive rights and access to contraception:** Feminist movements in the 1960s and 1970s highlighted reproductive rights and contraception access [6].
- **Advocacy for maternal health:** Maternal health became a top priority with the aim of reducing maternal mortality [28].
- **Holistic approach to women's health**: Women's health is not only confined to reproductive issues, but a holistic approach to women's health is also adopted [43].
- **Research on gender-specific health issues:** The gender differences in health and gender-specific medical approaches were taken into consideration [59].
- **Mental health awareness:** Mental health challenges specific to women were acknowledged [22].

- **Global initiatives and women's health equity:** Efforts have been taken to address gender disparities in health [70].
- Many challenges today need continued advocacy and education for improving women's health.

3.5.5 POLITICAL AND SOCIETAL RESPONSES TO FEMALE HEALTH ISSUES

Many developing countries struggle to offer adequate healthcare facilities, particularly for women and children. Policies focusing on poverty eradication, income redistribution, reproductive rights, and social and political participation of women are essential for reducing suffering and illness. Investing in female education and addressing socioeconomic factors are crucial for improving overall health and well-being [55]. Political and societal responses to female health concerns widely vary. In some places, governments have implemented policies for improving women's access to healthcare services, education, and resources. Issues such as maternal mortality, reproductive rights, and gender-based violence have also been addressed [14].

3.6 FEMALE HEALTH ISSUES: A COMPREHENSIVE REVIEW

1. **Reproductive health**: Women between the ages of 15 and 44 years have numerous issues with their sexual and reproductive health. Approximately one-third of their total health problems are related to these. Unsafe sex practices are quite dangerous in underdeveloped nations, especially for women and girls. Therefore, it is imperative to guarantee that women have access to contraception.
2. **Maternal health**: In recent years, there have been notable breakthroughs in the treatment of pregnancy and childbirth, but these advancements are not the same elsewhere in the world. Due to problems associated with pregnancy and childbirth, around 300,000 women lost their lives in 2013. Many of these deaths may have been avoided if family planning and healthcare had been widely available.

3. **Cancer**: To combat these two common malignancies among women, early detection in the case of breast and cervical cancer is essential. Every year, around 500,000 women worldwide pass away from various cancers. Unfortunately, due to a lack of screening, preventive, and treatment options, the bulk of these deaths take place in low- and middle-income nations.
4. **HIV**: After 30 years of the acquired immunodeficiency syndrome epidemic, new HIV infections disproportionately impact young women. Due to their susceptibility, they are also more likely to have tuberculosis, which is a major cause of death for women in low-income nations between the ages of 20 and 59 years. It is necessary to take precautions against other behaviors and the spread of the virus through sexual contact.
5. **Sexually transmitted infections (STIs)**: Preventing and controlling STIs such as chlamydia, gonorrhea, and syphilis is extremely important, along with HIV and HPV infections, which are the most prevalent STIs throughout the world. Improved prevention and treatment strategies are required. Untreated syphilis can contribute to over 200,000 stillbirths and early fetal deaths on a yearly basis, with an additional 90,000 newborn deaths.
6. **Violence against women**: Whether it comes from a partner or someone else, women are abused physically and sexually. Currently, one in three women under 50 years has been the victim of physical or sexual abuse, which can have both short-term and long-term effects on their health and happiness. To react proactively, health professionals must pay closer attention to cases of violence.
7. **Mental health**: Studies reveal that women are more prone to experience depression and somatic complaints, which are physiological symptoms that are not explained by physical means. Suicide is the primary cause of death for women under the age of 60 years, and depression is the most prevalent mental health problem among women. Women who are aware of mental health issues can feel more empowered [35].
8. **Noncommunicable diseases**: In 2012, noncommunicable diseases claimed the lives of over 4.7 million women before they turned 70

years. Most of these deaths occurred in low- and middle-income countries. The causes of these deaths include obesity, substance addiction, alcoholism, tobacco usage, and road accidents. In order to promote lifespan and well-being, it is imperative that girls and women are encouraged to embrace healthy habits from an early age.

9. **Young age:** Young teenage girls face a variety of sexual and reproductive health issues, including early pregnancy, STIs, and HIV. Every year, about 13 million girls under the age of 20 years become mothers. Complications linked to pregnancies and child-birth are the primary causes of mortality in these young mothers. In addition, a lot of pregnant adolescent girls experience the repercussions of unsafe abortion procedures.
10. **Old age:** As older women have spent more time doing household chores in their lives, they may have lesser retirement benefits and access to healthcare facilities compared to men [63].
11. **Endometriosis**: 10% of women worldwide (190 million) have endometriosis [69], which can cause excruciating pain during menstruation, sex, and bowel movements in addition to bloating, nausea, pelvic pain, exhaustion, and infertility. The identification and treatment of these issues are insufficient in low- and middle-income nations [64, 69].
12. **Contraception access:** In developing countries, 214 million women do not use contraception due to limited access, fear of side effects, cultural/religious opposition, and gender-based barriers. These challenges can be tackled by putting in comprehensive efforts to improve access and dismantle cultural barriers [13].
13. **Postpartum depression (PPD) and anxiety:** Approximately one in seven women is affected by PPD, which significantly affects their ability to resume normal functioning than the shorter-lived baby blues. Insufficient social support; experiences of domestic violence, including sexual, physical, and verbal abuse from a spouse; and smoking during pregnancy increase the risk of developing PPD manifold [35].

14. **Eating disorders and psychological well-being:** Adolescent girls and adult women are the primary victims of eating disorders, which pose a serious risk to their physical and mental health. Assessments for these diseases are often disregarded by healthcare professionals, despite the potentially dangerous outcomes. The common eating disorders, such as bulimia nervosa, binge eating disorder, and anorexia nervosa, are distinguished by unique diagnostic features, mental comorbidity, and medical problems [65].

3.7 SOCIAL AND CULTURAL DETERMINANTS IN FEMALE HEALTH ISSUES

- **Discrimination:** In many societies, women face discrimination rooted in cultural practices and social norms. Patriarchal societies in underdeveloped societies exhibit heightened gender biases, which pose many challenges to women. Examples include practices such as Chhaupadi in Nepal, female genital mutilation (FGM), child marriage, domestic violence, and honor killings. These harsh practices lead to severe physical and mental health consequences. In fact, many legal practices deny women rights to property, inheritance, and decision-making [56].
- **Cultural beliefs and practices:** Cultural norms and attitudes are similar to barriers that have traditionally stood in the way of women's health, especially reproductive health. These include sati, patriarchy, antiquated methods of contraception and abortion, preference for sons, pregnancy, childbirth taboos, and dowry killings [37]. The health of women and children is negatively impacted by factors such as FGM; preference for sons; inferior status of women in society; and customs around marriage, pregnancy, childbirth, and nutrition. Furthermore, substantial consequences arise for the social and economic advancement of women and society from acts of violence against women and girl children, including but not limited to rape, FGM, dowry-related violence, incest, wife beating, female feticide, female infanticide, trafficking, and prostitution. These practices and their effects on women's health are discussed as follows:

1. **FGM:** In this practice, the external female genitalia is partially or completely removed. This causes tremendous pain, bleeding, infections, and long-term complications such as urinary and reproductive problems and can even lead to death.
2. **Male preference:** The preference for male children over female children is a very common practice in many households. As a result, female children are neglected and suffer more from malnutrition, infanticide, etc.
3. **Inferior social status of women:** Women are always subjected to discrimination and subordination in society. It is the cause of their limited access to education, employment, and healthcare.
4. **Practices related to marriage:** The practices such as child marriage, forced marriage, and dowry-related violence lead to early pregnancy, maternal mortality, and physical and emotional abuse.
5. **Practices related to pregnancy and childbirth:** Harmful traditional childbirth practices, such as unhygienic delivery conditions and the use of harmful substances during pregnancy, can result in infections, maternal and infant mortality, and long-term health problems [45].

- **Cultural taboos:** Some examples of cultural taboos that can affect women's health are given as follows:

1. **Menstruation taboos:** Menstruation is taboo in many cultures, which restricts women's activities and their access to menstrual hygiene supplies. If proper hygiene precautions are not taken, this may have an impact on women's mental and physical health as well as cause health issues [57].
2. **Breastfeeding taboos:** Cultural beliefs about breastfeeding discourage women from breastfeeding their infants [46]. This can result in malnourishment in infants and also increase the risk of complications in the mother [12].

3. **Childbirth taboos:** Access to prenatal care, birth techniques, and postpartum support for women may be impacted by cultural norms surrounding labor and parturition. Seeking medical attention during childbirth is taboo in some cultures, which increases the risk of mother and newborn mortality many times [54].
4. **Sexual taboos:** Cultural taboos surrounding sexuality and reproductive health may restrict women from accessing proper contraception facilities. These taboos prevent them from seeking treatment for STIs or discussing sexual health openly. This leads to unintended pregnancies, unsafe abortions, and increased susceptibility to sexual violence [34].
5. **Dietary taboos:** Cultural practices regarding food and nutrition during pregnancy and breastfeeding may result in dietary restrictions for women, which result in nutritional deficiencies and poor maternal and infant health outcomes [49].
6. **Genital cutting taboos:** In certain cultural traditions, certain practices, such FGM/cutting (FGM/C), have a long history. FGM/C is still practiced in many communities despite the grave health risks to women involved because of cultural views regarding marriageability and purity [40].

- Gender roles and expectations for women vary across different cultures and societies, but some common examples include:
  1. **Appearance and beauty standards**: Women are often objectified and subjected to social pressure to meet ideals of beauty, such as being young, slender, and appealing. This may exacerbate eating disorders, problems with body image, and low self-esteem in females [9].
  2. **Career limitations:** Despite advances in gender equality [67], women continue to face challenges in obtaining leadership positions in male-dominated industries. Gender stereotypes discourage women from pursuing certain careers and, thus, limit their opportunities in the workplace [11].
- **Domestic responsibilities:** Women's primary responsibility is the household chores, childcare, and caring for the family members.

This causes "double burden" for working women who struggle a lot to balance their responsibilities toward both family and profession [61].

1. **Emotional labor:** Societies expect women to perform emotional labor, such as giving support and empathy. It can be emotionally exhausting for women. Women are forced to prioritize the needs of others over their own [38].
2. **Reproductive roles:** Women are thought to bear the primary responsibility for reproduction and family planning. It leads to societal pressure to marry and have children. The women who do not marry or have children are treated differently in society [2].
3. **Sexual expectations:** Cultural norms make women play some specific roles and behaviors. They are expected to adhere to virginity, modesty, and sexual availability. These expectations lead to objectification and gender-based violence toward women [44].
4. **Submissiveness and compliance**: Women have historically been viewed as meek, accommodating, and submissive in all situations. This restricts women's independence and self-assurance in several spheres of life, such as partnerships and decision-making [62].

3.8 HEALTHCARE ACCESS AND POLICIES

3.8.1 BARRIERS TO HEALTHCARE ACCESS

Cultural considerations restrict women's access to the socioeconomic resources necessary to maintain their health and well-being in many nations [41]. These complex barriers to healthcare access might be influenced by a range of sociocultural influences. Some of these obstacles are explained by the article "Socio-Cultural Factors of Gender Roles in Women's Healthcare Utilization in Southwest Nigeria." The following are some of the main obstacles that this study found:

- **Cultural beliefs and practices:** Cultural beliefs influence women's perceptions of health and sickness. They prefer using traditional methods rather than reaching advanced healthcare facilities.
- **Financial constraints:** Women are not economically independent and, thus, financial barriers make them unable to afford transportation to healthcare facilities and costs of the services.
- **Geographical accessibility:** Rural or remote areas lack adequate infrastructure of healthcare. Long distances to healthcare facilities, poor road transport, and limited networking can act as colossal hurdles for obtaining healthcare.
- **Limited education:** Ignorance due to lower levels of education in women affects their understanding of the importance of healthcare services. This causes underutilization of services and poorer health outcomes.
- **Sociocultural norms:** Societal and cultural norms restrict women's autonomy in decision-making regarding healthcare. In many cultures, women are expected to seek permission from male members of the family before accessing healthcare services that result in delay or avoidance of necessary and prompt care.

These barriers need to be handled carefully and require a multifaceted approach. Interventions should be incorporated to improve women's healthcare access, which involve community engagement, economic empowerment, and education of women. Moreover, healthcare policies should be designed with a deep understanding of the sociocultural context [59, 60].

3.8.2 GOVERNMENT POLICIES AND WOMEN'S HEALTH

The Sustainable Development Goals (SDGs) can only be accomplished by guaranteeing women's equality in the public and private spheres, according to the United Nations. They must be given equitable access to education, healthcare, and career opportunities to feel empowered. The United Nations established SDG-5 to advance gender equality [67] and to abolish forced and early marriages, sexual exploitation, trafficking,

FGM, and other kinds of violence against women. It is necessary to inspire women to participate in political and economic decision-making. They ought to be empowered to obtain financial resources and reproductive healthcare treatments on their own [61–65].

3.9 STRATEGIES FOR FUTURE RESEARCH AND INTERVENTION

From a public health aspect, it is important to invest in early education for everyone, with a special focus on girls. This investment plays a vital role in determining lifelong health outcomes of women. Education, for both formal achievements and health literacy, should be taken care of, as it also plays a pivotal role in enhancing socioeconomic position and, thus, serves as a strong predictor of future employment and income. Education fosters the acquisition of knowledge and skills that increase women's self-assurance, competence, and openness to receiving health education. It is necessary to acknowledge the diversity within the female population as well as that of men. Research in this area should, in theory, examine how different SEP characteristics interact with gender. Adolescent girls and women who fall within the reproductive age range ought to get education and empowerment through various policies and programs, enabling them to access resources and proactively manage their health [41].

3.10 SUMMARY

Women's health outcomes are governed by complex interactions among social, cultural, and political factors. Comprehending the socioeconomic determinants of female health is crucial in addressing societal inequities and executing efficacious intervention tactics. The significance of acknowledging historical viewpoints, significant achievements in women's health, and comprehending shifting societal perceptions on women's health has been emphasized by this review. This overview has covered the main concerns related to female health, mental health, infectious diseases, cancer, and reproductive health.

Government policies and the obstacles to accessing healthcare have been critically examined. To improve women's health and status, the assessment stressed the need for equitable healthcare and legislative reform. Furthermore, to enhance women's health outcomes, future research and intervention tactics should reduce information gaps, encourage new trends, and apply evidence-based practices. Improving women's health and creating a society where everyone may prosper requires cooperation between healthcare professionals, legislators, researchers, and community partners.

KEYWORDS

- **cultural**
- **female**
- **gender**
- **health**
- **malnutrition**
- **social**
- **taboos**
- **women**

REFERENCES

1. Addai, I. (2000). Determinants of use of maternal child health services in rural Ghana. *Journal of Biosocial Science*, 32, 1–15.
2. Azuh, D., Fayomi, O., & Ajayi, L. (2015). Socio-cultural factors of gender roles in women's healthcare utilization in Southwest Nigeria. *Open Journal of Social Sciences*, 3, 105–117.
3. Baheiraei, A., Bakouei, F., Mohammadi, E., Montazeri, A., & Hosseni, M. (2015). The social determinants of health in association with women's health status of reproductive age: A population-based study. *Iran Journal Public Health*, *44*(1), 119–29.
4. Blaydes, L. & Platas, M. R. (2020). Religion, family structure, and the perpetuation of female genital cutting in Egypt. *Journal of Demographic Economics*, *86*, 305–328.
5. Blehar, M. C. (2003). Public health context of women's mental health research. *The Psychiatric Clinics of North America*, *26*(3), 781–799. doi: 10.1016/s0193-953x(03)00039-x.
6. Britannica, The Editors of Encyclopaedia. "Roe v. Wade". *Encyclopedia Britannica*; (accessed on 31 Jan. 2024).
7. Burkett, E. (2024). Women's rights movement. *Encyclopedia Britannica*.

8. Bustreo, F. (2015). *Ten Top Issues for Women's Health*. World Health Organization. http://www.who. int/life-course/news/commentaries/2015-intl-womens-day/en.
9. Chakrabarti, S., & Chakrabarti, A. (2018). Food taboos in pregnancy and early lactation among women living in a rural area of West Bengal. *Journal of Family Medicine and Primary Care*, *8*(1), 86–90.
10. Chandra, P. S., Varghese, M., & Supraja, T. (2016). Women's mental health. *International Encyclopedia of Public Health*, *2*, 434–443.
11. Christianson, M., Teiler, Å., & Eriksson, C. (2021). A woman's honor tumbles down on all of us in the family, but a man's honor is only his: Young women's experiences of patriarchal chastity norms. *International Journal of Qualitative Studies on Health and Well-Being*, *16*(1), e1862480.
12. Ciciolla, L., & Luthar, S. S. (2019). Invisible household labor and ramifications for adjustment: Mothers as captains of households. *Sex Roles*, *81*(7–8), 467–486.
13. Cleland, J., Conde-Agudelo, A., Peterson, H., Ross, J., & Tsui, A. (2012). Contraception and health. *Lancet*, *380*(9837), 149–156.
14. Council of Europe (coe.int). (n.d.). Feminism and women's rights movements – Gender matters.
15. Davidson, P. M., McGrath, S. J., Meleis, A. I., Stern, P., DiGiacomo, M., Dharmendra, T., Campbell, J. C., Hochleitner, Messias, D. K., Brown, H., Teitelman, A., Sindhu, S., Reesman, K., Richter, S., Sommers, M. S., Schaeffer, D., Stringer, M., Sampselle, C., Anderson, D., & Covan, E. K. (2011). The Health of women and girls determines the health and well-being of our modern world: A white paper from the International Council on Women's Health Issues. *Health Care for Women International*, *32*(10), 870–875.
16. Dutta, K. (2018). Women entrepreneurs in rural India: Challenges and opportunities. *International Journal of Molecular Sciences*, *6,* 215–220.
17. Fait, T. (2019). Menopause hormone therapy: Latest developments and clinical practice. *Drugs Context*, *2*, e212551.
18. Gailits, N., Mathias, K., Nouvet, E., Pillai, P., & Schwartz, L. (2019). Women's freedom of movement and participation in psychosocial support groups: Qualitative study in northern India. *BMC Public Health*, *19*(1), 725–730.
19. Garg, K. C., & Kumar, S. (2014). Scientometric profile of Indian scientific output in life sciences with a focus on the contributions of women scientists. *Scientometrics, 98*, 1771–1783.
20. Gauffenic, A. (1985). Le statut social de la femme. Pour un nouvel ordre mondial (The social status of women. For a new world order). *Tiers Monde*, *26*(102), 273–281.
21. Goldin, C., & Katz, L. F. (2002). The power of the pill: Oral contraceptives and women's career and marriage decisions. *Journal of Political Economy, 110*(4), 730–770.
22. Göttgens, I., & Oertelt-Prigione, S. (2023). Editorial: Emerging trends in global women's health—sex and gender differences in disease. *Frontiers in Global Women's Health*, *4*, 1304382.
23. Gupta, R., Nimesh, R., Singal, G. L., Bhalla, P., & Prinja, S. (2018). Effectiveness of India's national programme to save the girl child: Experience of Beti Bachao Beti Padao (B3P) programme from Haryana State. *Health Policy Plan, 33*, 870–876.

24. GYN Surgical Solutions. (2023). Emerging trends in women's healthcare, online. Hologic (gynsurgicalsolutions.com)
25. HHS (US Department of Health and Human Services). (1985). *Women's health: Report of the Public Health Service Task Force on Women's Health Issues. Public Health Reports, 100*(1), 73–106.
26. Institute of Medicine (US). (2003). Improving birth outcomes within health care systems. In: *Improving Birth Outcomes: Meeting the Challenge in the Developing World.* National Academies Press (US): New York.
27. Institute of Medicine (US). (2010). *Women's Health Research: Progress, Pitfalls, and Promise*. National Academies Press: New York.
28. Jat, T. R., Deo, P. R., & Goicolea, I. (2013). The emergence of maternal health as a political priority in Madhya Pradesh- India: A qualitative study. *BMC Pregnancy Childbirth, 13*, 181–185.
29. Kaarthigeyan, K. (2012). Cervical cancer in India and HPV vaccination. *Indian Journal of Medical and Paediatric Oncology*, *33*(1), 7–12.
30. Kapur, R., & Narayan, S. (2020). Women empowerment in India: More needs to be done. *ISAS Insights, 628*, 1–5.
31. Khang, Y. H., Bahk, J., Lim, D., Kang, H. Y., Lim, H. K., Kim, Y. Y., & Park, J. H. (2019). Trends in inequality in life expectancy at birth between 2004 and 2017 and projections for 2030 in Korea: Multiyear cross-sectional differences by income from national health insurance data. *BMJ Open, 9*(7), e030683.
32. Konduru, D., & Kundargi, R. G. (2019). A brief analysis of food practices and food taboos on women health in Andhra Pradesh, India. *International Journal of Community Medicine and Public Health*, *6*(12), 5088–5094.
33. Kontis, V., Bennett, J. E., Mathers, C. D., Li, G., Foreman, K., & Ezzati, M. (2017). Future life expectancy in 35 industrialized countries: Projections with a Bayesian model ensemble. *Lancet, 389*(10076), 1323–1335.
34. Kumar, R., & Maity, B. (2022). Cultural norms and women's health: Implications of the practice of menstrual restrictions in Nepal. *World Development Perspectives*, *2022,* 1–38.
35. Lakkis, N. A., & Mahmassani, D. M. (2015). Screening instruments for depression in primary care: A concise review for clinicians. *Postgraduate Medicine*, *127*(1), 99–106.
36. Lee, N. C. (2015). Progress in women's health, 1985–2015. *Public Health Reports*, *130*(2), 121–122.
37. Macklin, R. (2006). Global inequalities and human rights in women's sexual and reproductive health. *Gaceta Médica de México*, *2006*(Suppl 2), 5–11.
38. Matilla-Santander, N., Martín-Sánchez, J. C., González-Marrón, A., Cartanyà-Hueso, À., Lidón-Moyano, C., & Martínez-Sánchez, J. M. (2020). Precarious employment, unemployment and their association with health-related outcomes in 35 European countries: A cross-sectional study. *Critical Public Health, 31*, 404–415.
39. McCreary, D. R., & Rhodes, N. (2001). On the gender-typed nature of dominant and submissive acts. *Sex Roles*, *44*(5–6), 339–350.
40. McDaniel, S. A. (1988). Women's roles and reproduction: The changing picture in Canada in the 1980s. *Atlantis, 14*(1), 1–12.

41. Mujeed, S., Li, S., Jabeen, M., Nassani, A. A., Askar, S. E., & Zaman, K. (2021). Technowomen: Women's autonomy and its impact on environmental quality. *Sustainability*, *13*(4), 1611–1615.
42. Napoli, M. (2002). Holistic health care for native women: An integrated model. *American Journal of Public Health*, *92*(10), 1573–1575.
43. Nishimura, Y., & Acoba, J. D. (2022). Impact of breast cancer awareness month on public interest in the United States between 2012 and 2021: Google trends analysis. *Cancers (Basel)*, *14*(10), e2534.
44. O'Neil, A., Russell, J. D., Thompson, K., & Martinson, M. L., & Peters, S. A. (2020). The impact of socioeconomic position (SEP) on women's health over the lifetime. *Maturitas*, *140*, 1–7.
45. Office of the United Nations High Commissioner for Human Rights. Fact sheet no. 23: Harmful traditional practices affecting the health of women and children.
46. Osman, H., El Zein, L., & Wick, L. (2009). Cultural beliefs that may discourage breastfeeding among Lebanese women: A qualitative analysis. *International Breastfeed Journal*, *2*(4), 12–18.
47. Razavi, S. (2007). *The Political and Social Economy of Care in a Development Context, Conceptual Issues, Research Questions and Policy Options* (p. 50). Gender and Development Programme, UNSRID: Geneva.
48. Rushwan, H. (2008). Milestones in women's health. *International Journal of Gynecology & Obstetrics*, *101*(1), 1–2.
49. Russell, J. D., Thompson, K., Martinson, M. L., & Peters, A. E. (2020). The impact of socioeconomic position (SEP) on women's health over the lifetime. *Maturitas*, *140*, 1–7
50. Safaei, J. (2009). Democracy and women's health. *Mens Sana Monographs*, *7*(1), 20–36.
51. Safaei, J. (2012). Democracy, human rights and women's health. *Mens Sana Monographs*, *10*(1), 134–142.
52. Safaeian, M., & Solomon, D. (2007). Cervical cancer prevention - cervical screening: Science in evolution. *Obstetrics and Gynecology Clinics of North America*, *34*(4), 739–741.
53. Shanks, G., Sharma, D., & Mishra, V. (2019). Prevention and treatment of osteoporosis in women. *Obstetrics, Gynaecology & Reproductive Medicine*, *29*(7), 201–206.
54. Sharma, S., Teijlingen, E. V., & Hundley, V. (2016). Dirty and 40 days in the wilderness: Eliciting childbirth and postnatal cultural practices and beliefs in Nepal. *BMC Pregnancy Childbirth*, *16*, 147–151.
55. Singh, S., Sinha, K. L. & Agrawal, V. P. (2018). Empowering women through higher education. *International Journal for Environmental Rehabilitation and Conservation*, *9*(2), 17–22.
56. Stolp, H., & Fox, J. (2015). Increasing receipt of women's preventive services. *Journal of Women's Health*, *24*(11), 875–881.
57. Unesco.org. (2016). *Institute for Lifelong Learning (UIL)'s Annual Reports)*.
58. USA for UNFPA. (n.d.). Left in the dark: How does period taboos put women and girls at risk? https://www.usaforunfpa.org/left-in-the-dark-how-period-taboos-put-women-and-girls-at-risk/.

59. Ved, R., Scott, K., Gupta, G., Ummer, O., Singh, S., & Srivastava, A. (2019). How are gender inequalities facing India's one million ASHAs being addressed? Policy origins and adaptations for the world's largest all-female community health worker programme. *Human Resources for Health, 17*, 1–15.
60. Verma, A., & Mulani, M. (2018). Challenges and issues of working woman in 21st century. *International Journal of Research in all Subjects in Multi Languages (National Conf. On 21st Century: Changing Trends in the Role of Women-Impact on Various Fields)*, *6*(3), 1–5.
61. Vlassoff, C. (2007). Gender differences in determinants and consequences of health and illness. *Journal of Health, Population, and Nutrition*, *25*(1), 47–61.
62. Voges, M. M., Giabbiconi, C., Schöne, B., Waldorf, M., Hartmann, A. S., & Vocks, S. (2019). Gender differences in body evaluation - do men show more self-serving double standards than women? *Frontiers in Psychology*, *10*, e437146.
63. Wilfley, D. E., & Grilo, C. M. (1994). Eating disorders: A women's health problem in primary care. *Nurse Practitioner Forum*, *5*(1), 34–45.
64. Short, S. E., & Zacher, M. (2022). Women's health: Population patterns and social determinants. *Annual Review of Sociology*, *48*(1), 277–298.
65. World Bank (International Economics Department. (2008). *World Development Indicators*. World Bank Publications: Development Data Group: Washington – DC. https://hdl.handle.net/10986/11855
66. World Health Organization (who.int). (2000). Ten top issues for women's health, online.
67. World Health Organization (who.int). (2021). The future we expect: Women's health and gender equality, online.
68. World Health Organization (who.int). (2022). Social determinants of health, online.
69. World Health Organization (who.int). (2023). Endometriosis, online.
70. World Health Organization (who.int). (n.d.). Women's health, online.

CHAPTER 4

Impact of Marital Relations on Women's Health

DIPALI SAXENA* and SHWETA KESWANI

*Corresponding author

ABSTRACT

A holistic approach to women's health takes seriously not just the physical but also the mental, emotional, and spiritual aspects of well-being. This concept argues that all these areas are interconnected and can influence one another. Marital functioning has a strong and powerful impact on women's strength. Adverse extents of marital operational have unintended impacts on well-being consequences through unhappiness and health habits, and direct effects on circulatory, hormone, and other biological mechanisms, according to studies conducted over the last decade, particularly women's marital interaction studies. This chapter focuses on the road that leads from the marriage connection to various areas of women's health. It is important to recognize that the impact of marital relations on women's health is complex and multifaceted, and individual experiences may vary widely. Different factors have a significant influence on women health, like on mental health, physical health, emotional health, and so on. To facilitate convey a comprehensive overview of recent research on the relationship between marriage and women's health, we brought together recent literature from a variety of fields, including community health, behavioral sciences, and the field of medicine. Marital distress and poor quality of life often go together in the lives of women, which also affects women's health. Additionally,

Holistic Approaches for Women's Sustainable Health, Volume 2: Advancements, Socioeconomic Impacts, and Innovative Strategies. Junaid Ahmad Malik, Anamika Chauhan, and Megh R. Goyal (Eds)

DOI: 10.1201/9781779641656-5

seeking support from healthcare providers, counselors, or support groups can be beneficial for women facing challenges in their marital relationships that affect their health and well-being.

4.1 INTRODUCTION

Women represent over 50% of the world's population, but their unemployment rates are substantially lower than men's. However, current trends indicate a steady increase in the percentage of women in the workforce. Modernization, social development, and education among women have enabled some women to enter formerly unthinkable professions. Work-life balance is, however, more critical today than ever before, and Indian organizations are recognizing it. Women are entering the workforce in a society where "most of the household responsibilities and pressure of bringing up the children have been placed on them." The author investigates variations in marital relations as a constructive trend toward increased liberty for spouses. Because the couples' expressive, spiritual, rational, and substantial requirements take precedence above mere permanence, as defined by traditional marriages [16]. Some sociologists today debate the conventional role of marriage and family in species preservation.

Globalization, women joining professions and gaining economic autonomy, and the disappearance of the social shame attached to divorced persons all contribute to adjustments in the conventional definition of marriage. The situation requires a long period of commitment and consideration prior to marriage. As a result, dating, courting, and the duration of engagement, when treated honestly, play a critical part in the accomplishment or failure of any wedding. The longer a pair knows one another before marrying, the better their marriage will be. The situation is a well-known truth that brief association, fast marriage, and misery in marriage or divorce go hand in hand; those who had been acquainted for three years or more prior to marriage found gladness in marriage.

The association between marriage and healthiness is complicated. Marital significance can have a significant impact on health outcomes as well as affect them. Healthy people may have a higher chance of becoming and staying married if they are seen as more suitable marriage partners due to their physical attractiveness, earning potential, mental well-being, level of self-sufficiency, or likelihood of longevity. Researchers in the social sciences refer to these phenomena as the "selection" of healthy individuals for marriage. If this is the only explanation for the relationship between marriage and health, then marriage does not benefit health. Instead, the observed health inequalities between wedded and unwedded people are the result of healthier people being further liable to get married.

Alternatively, there could be an actual causal relationship between marriage and improved health. Marriage may improve health outcomes in several ways. It may result in two earnings and economies of scale, which will improve economic well-being. Having more income may enhance health outcomes by increasing access to healthcare or reducing stress. Furthermore, a spouse can help monitor and encourage healthy behaviors (such as good eating habits and frequent exercise) while discouraging harmful ones. Marriage can also provide an emotionally rewarding, personal relationship that meets the desire for social connection, which can have an impact on both physical and mental health. Most investigations believe that the link between marriage and health is a result of both the selection of healthier individuals into marriage and the actual health benefits derived from marriage.

To build upon the comprehensive reviews highlighting the adverse health impacts of marital conflict [15], it is essential to recognize both the positive and negative dimensions of marital dynamics. This includes examining the health-related advantages and risks associated with spousal support, along with understanding gender-based variations in how marital interactions influence physiological processes and health outcomes. Marital strain can result in health issues such as sleep disturbances and metabolic alterations that increase susceptibility to obesity, metabolic syndrome, and diabetes.

This chapter provides an overview of the myriad factors shaping women's health, alongside theories and models elucidating the connection between marriage and well-being. Various elements exert substantial influence on women's health, encompassing mental, physical, and emotional dimensions. We synthesized recent literature from diverse fields such as public health, social sciences, and medical science to offer a comprehensive insight into contemporary research on the interplay between marriage and women's health.

4.2 MARRIAGE AND ITS TYPES

Marriage presents a multifaceted dynamic within the contemporary landscape of constant change. Individuals enter matrimony for a multitude of reasons. Beyond the primal considerations of sex and sexual attraction, motives such as love, financial stability, companionship, security, emotional fulfillment, relief from loneliness or dissatisfaction at home, shared interests, and aspirations for children play pivotal roles in shaping the decision to wed. Certain psychologists delve into the concept of homogamy in marriage, positing that individuals naturally gravitate toward partners who align with their desires and preferences. Modern shifts in values and social consciousness have an impact on traditional understandings of marriage and family.

Marriage is defined as a socially sanctioned union for sexual companionship, commencing with a formal declaration and aiming for lifelong commitment. It is established through a clear marital contract delineating the reciprocal rights and responsibilities of both partners and any future offspring. These definitions underscore essential aspects of matrimony, encompassing the integration of individuals into society, commitment and public acknowledgment, the expectation of permanence, procreation, and the mutual rights and duties shared by spouses. Beyond mere sexual attraction, biological unity, and social integration, marriage represents a profound commitment, involving complete devotion to one another and the acceptance of responsibilities that contribute to mutual welfare.

In traditional contexts, marriage and family life are built upon five distinct types of relationships between men and women. These encompass promiscuity, group marriage, polyandry, polygamy, and monogamy. Promiscuity involves unrestricted sexual encounters devoid of regulations concerning age, marital status, or familial ties. Group marriage entails multiple men marrying multiple women without specific pairings between individuals. Polyandry occurs when one woman is married to multiple men, while polygamy refers to one man marrying multiple women. Monogamy, the prevailing marital model across cultures today, denotes a one-to-one partnership between spouses. Because humans are bisexual by nature, the complementing male–female partnership benefits both parties. Although there seems to be a growing trend among a small fraction of the population toward single living, single parenting, and same-sex marriages, this does not undermine marriage's foundations.

4.3 STATUS OF MARRIAGES IN THE 21ST CENTURY

Humans have always experienced some type of official marital dissolution. Since the mid-19th century, when industrialization began, the likelihood of a marriage ending in divorce (or annulment) has been less than 10%. In 1974, divorce became the most prevalent endpoint of marriage. By 1985, the divorce rate had consistently risen to more than 55%. It has soared around 50% in the previous 20 years. The ongoing research is influencing marriage dynamics in the 21st century, owing to significant demographic and cultural shifts, including decreased marriage rates, increased instances of cohabitation, the legalization of same-sex marriage, and changes in the age at which individuals marry.

The cultural evolution of marriage has transitioned from a formal institution primarily focused on family and economic stability to a pursuit of love and companionship, and more recently, in the late 20th century, to a means of individual choice and self-fulfillment. The increasing acceptance of premarital cohabitation has normalized unmarried couples living together, a dynamic phenomenon with significant implications for subsequent marriage and children. Exploring the reasons behind cohabitation, the contrast between traditional and egalitarian gender roles, and the consequences of cohabitation before marriage enables us to identify protective measures and anticipate the impact of this evolving relationship structure. Many researchers argue that individuals choose to cohabit for reasons such as financial and sexual convenience, as well as to demonstrate heightened commitment—a transitional stage between dating and marriage.

Nevertheless, the absence of standardized vocabulary or terminology (such as husband, wife, and fiancé) suggests that cohabitation before marriage has not been fully institutionalized. While many people believe that cohabitation will enhance future marriages, research indicates that couples who live together before marriage experience higher divorce rates and shorter durations of marriage. The primary factors contributing to the lack of reinforcement of future marriages through cohabitation include unconventional perspectives (such as egalitarian beliefs and role division), deficiencies in problem-solving and communication abilities, and a lack of self-awareness and awareness of one's partner.

Living together without marriage is often a spontaneous occurrence for many individuals, rather than a deliberate choice, as it gradually evolves over time. Some researchers suggest that contemporary marriages are under strain due to societal and cultural shifts, leading to a sense of "suffocation" [4]. Marriage is now expected to fulfill lofty objectives such as happiness and personal fulfillment, yet constraints stemming from modern economic and societal realities hinder couples from dedicating the necessary time and effort to nurture their marriage to meet these expectations.

4.4 MARITAL RELATIONS AND HEALTH

Health is a complex notion that incorporates a wide range of indicators, including behavioral, physical, and emotional results. There is a significant correlation between marriage and health, with married individuals experiencing lower rates of morbidity and mortality across various health risks such as cancer, heart attacks, and surgical procedures. However, the extent of these effects varies depending on gender, potentially influenced by the differing social positions of men and women.

An extensive empirical study has focused on the correlation among ""better" or "worse" marriages and "sickness and health" through the last half-century. Marriage has undergone significant sociodemographic transformations over time, including a decline in marriage rates, an increase in the age at which individuals marry, a surge in divorce rates during the 1960s and 1970s, and a rise in cohabitation and same-sex marriage [8]. While most research on the relationship between marital status and health has centered on heterosexual couples, there is a need for further exploration into the health implications of same-sex marriage. Both the mere act of being married and the quality of one's marriage have been associated with a broad spectrum of health outcomes. Researchers have delved into the social-cognitive, emotional, behavioral, and biological mechanisms that underlie these connections.

Marital quality for men as well as women is a multidimensional concept, encompassing both subjective and objective factors such as satisfaction, happiness, adjustment, love and affection, understanding, communication, disputes, shared participation in activities, and so on. Married quality refers to "satisfaction, happiness, adjustment, and other related dimensions and evaluations of the marital relationship" [7]. In recent times, researchers have directed their attention toward the importance of marital quality in relation to physical health. The findings of this research consistently indicate that positive aspects of marriage, such as marital satisfaction and enjoyment, contribute positively to physical well-being, while negative marital dynamics, such as conflicts, can have detrimental effects. However, much of this research has predominantly focused on the correlation between marital quality and physical health in younger individuals rather than older adults.

Marital well-being influences health outcomes both indirectly through effects on depression and health habits, and directly *via* circulatory, hormonal, immunologic, neurosensory, and other physical mechanisms. High marriage quality has been associated with lower vulnerability to depression, self-rated health, fewer physical problems, and subjective well-being and happiness. Based on an extensive literature review, most studies examining the link between marital quality and health focused on samples with mean ages in the late 30s and early 40s. However, some exceptions were noted, particularly in studies involving couples managing a spouse's chronic illness. Nonetheless, marital quality is likely to serve as a significant asset for the physical health of older individuals, even in the absence of chronic stressors like caregiving for an unwell spouse.

This study explores the associations between marital quality and physical well-being in a probability-based sample of middle-aged and older adults. A strong marital bond is associated with improved health outcomes, including higher self-rated health, fewer physical ailments, and reduced depression. Moreover, marital quality and status also yield benefits for maternal health.

4.5 STATUS OF WOMEN HEALTH

The status of women's health after marriage can vary significantly depending on various factors such as the quality of the marital relationship, access to healthcare, socioeconomic status, cultural norms, and individual circumstances. In some cases, marriage may positively impact women's health by providing emotional support, access to healthcare resources through their spouse's insurance, and opportunities for a healthier lifestyle through shared responsibilities and mutual encouragement. However, in other instances, marriage may exacerbate existing health issues or introduce new challenges, particularly in cases of marital conflict, domestic violence, or disparities in decision-making power within the relationship. Additionally, societal expectations around gender roles and responsibilities may place undue stress on married women, impacting their mental and physical well-being. Overall, the status of women's health after marriage is complex and multifaceted, influenced by a wide range of factors that require careful consideration and support from various stakeholders, including healthcare providers, policymakers, and community organizations.

Marital conflict or satisfaction has a more pronounced impact on women's health compared to men's, resulting in unhappy married women experiencing similar health outcomes to single women. Studies conducted in laboratories indicate that women exhibit stronger reactions to marital discord than men. Research published in the September 2023 issue of Health Psychology, a publication of the American Psychological Association, suggests that women in fulfilling marriages enjoy better health outcomes than their unmarried counterparts or those in unsatisfactory marriages.

Every type of marriage carries inherent physical, sexual, and emotional risks for women. Women encounter physical dangers such as domestic violence perpetrated by family members and spouses. Sexual risks emerge when women decline sexual advances from their husbands or are coerced into engaging in unwanted sexual activities. Unfavorable aspects of marriage contribute to heightened stress levels among women [11]. Stress typically manifests in physical symptoms, a phenomenon known as somatization, where individuals express psychological distress, stress stemming from underlying life challenges, and health issues through bodily complaints. This development of somatization prompts these women to seek medical attention for culturally accepted and nonstigmatized health concerns.

Until recently, numerous women's health concerns were largely disregarded in medical research, with women historically being underrepresented in clinical trials. Previous studies in women's health primarily focused on issues related to fertility and reproduction, while research on other illnesses predominantly centered on men. Presently, the diagnosis and treatment of most women are based on strategies that have proven effective for men. However, the efforts of women's health advocates and the recognition of disparities in medical research have prompted a more comprehensive research agenda. This emerging research aims to uncover both the similarities and differences in health-related matters between men and women.

Women often encounter fragmentation within the healthcare system when seeking reproductive healthcare and other medical services. Additionally, women tend to visit healthcare providers more frequently than men. Women demonstrate a keen interest in, and understanding of healthcare matters. However, the availability of reliable healthcare information has been limited. National studies suggest that women may express lower satisfaction levels with the information provided by their healthcare providers compared to men, as well as with the level of communication they receive from their physicians. Moreover, numerous studies indicate that healthcare professionals treat women differently from men. In contrast to men, healthcare providers may conduct fewer comprehensive evaluations for similar complaints, downplay their symptoms, offer fewer interventions for identical diagnoses, prescribe certain medications more frequently, or provide less detailed explanations in response to their inquiries.

4.5.1 DETERMINANTS OF WOMEN'S HEALTH

Women's health is influenced by a myriad of determinants that encompass various aspects of their lives. Socioeconomic status stands as a fundamental determinant, with income, education, and employment status profoundly impacting access to healthcare, nutrition, and other essential resources. Access to healthcare services plays a critical role, encompassing preventive care, reproductive health services, and treatment for chronic and acute conditions. Social and cultural factors, including societal norms, cultural practices, and gender roles, shape women's health behaviors, decision-making autonomy, and exposure to discrimination and violence. Reproductive health is a significant determinant, with access to family planning services, maternal healthcare, and safe childbirth directly impacting women's well-being. Lifestyle factors such as diet, physical activity, substance use, and stress management also play a crucial role in determining women's health outcomes. Environmental factors, including exposure to pollutants and unsafe living conditions, can have adverse effects, particularly during pregnancy and infancy. Understanding and addressing these determinants are essential for promoting women's health equity and addressing disparities in health outcomes.

Economic hardship, geographic setting, societal marginalization stemming from caste, gender, sexual orientation, and disability all exert notable influences on women's health, alongside elements like employment, housing, environmental conditions, and educational opportunities. While some of these challenges impact the general populace, women often experience them uniquely due to their marginalized social status. It is essential to recognize the disproportionate impact on women and their resultant health outcomes. Taking a comprehensive approach to women's health entails understanding it within the broader context of their social circumstances and personal encounters, rather than limiting analysis to biomedical perspectives.

The health status of women in India is characterized by a complex interplay of various factors, including socioeconomic disparities, cultural norms, access to healthcare, and gender-based discrimination. While progress has been made in certain areas, significant challenges persist, contributing to disparities in health outcomes between men and women. One of the key issues affecting women's health in India is maternal health. Despite improvements in recent years, maternal mortality rates remain high, particularly in rural and marginalized communities. Access to quality maternal healthcare services, including antenatal care, skilled birth attendance, and postnatal care, continues to be limited in many parts of the country.

Reproductive health is another area of concern, with challenges ranging from limited access to family planning services and contraceptives to high rates of teenage pregnancies and unsafe abortions. Women in India also face a high burden of reproductive tract infections, including sexually transmitted infections. Nutrition and food security are significant determinants of women's health, with a large proportion of women and girls experiencing malnutrition and micronutrient deficiencies. Gender disparities in access to food, healthcare, education, and employment contribute to these challenges.

Violence against women, including domestic violence, sexual assault, and dowry-related violence, remains a pervasive issue in India, impacting women's physical and mental health. Stigma and cultural barriers often prevent women from seeking help or accessing support services. Additionally, women in India often face barriers to education and employment opportunities, limiting their economic independence and access to healthcare services. Social norms and practices, such as early marriage and son preference, further exacerbate gender disparities in health outcomes.

While efforts have been made to address these challenges through various government programs and initiatives, sustained action is needed to improve the health status of women in India. This includes investing in comprehensive maternal and reproductive healthcare services, addressing gender-based violence, promoting gender equality and women's empowerment, and addressing the social determinants of health.

4.5.2 *WOMEN'S HEALTH IN THE GLOBAL CONTEXT*

In the global context, women's health is influenced by a wide range of factors that vary across different regions and countries. While progress has been made in certain areas, significant challenges remain, affecting the health and well-being of women worldwide. Globally, women's health primarily focuses on obstetric and gynecologic issues, including family planning, pregnancy, childbirth, sexually transmitted infections, gynecologic conditions and cancers, menopause, and infectious and noncommunicable diseases (NCDs). Women and girls in these regions encounter diseases and health outcomes that may not be prevalent in developed nations. Maternal mortality, obstetric fistulas, female genital mutilation, HIV/AIDS, malaria during pregnancy, and cervical cancer are significantly more common in resource-poor settings, where access to many clinical and diagnostic resources is limited.

Women with disadvantaged socioeconomic backgrounds face the greatest risk, irrespective of age or location. Healthcare providers should be alerted to women with low education levels, minority backgrounds, and migrant status, as they are most likely to seek medical attention late, with undiagnosed conditions, and experience treatment complications. Addressing these concerns is imperative for global health efforts worldwide. Multiple risk factors leading to these health issues often coexist within the same woman. Reflecting the evolving landscape of women's health challenges, particularly in low- and middle-income countries, the World Health Organization has stressed the need to broaden the women's health agenda beyond reproductive health and adopt a life-course approach.

Women, especially those from middle- or low-income countries, are more prone to experiencing depression, anxiety, and other mental health issues. Over the past three decades, the number of women affected by mental health problems resulting in disability or death has remained consistent worldwide. Mental health issues can impact women across all stages of life, affecting not only the individual but also their families and communities. Vulnerability, societal stigma, and limited resources, particularly in resource-constrained settings, exacerbate this burden.

Addressing the health needs of women globally requires a comprehensive approach that addresses the social, economic, and political factors that shape women's health outcomes. This includes investing in healthcare systems that are accessible, affordable, and gender-responsive, promoting gender equality and women's empowerment, and addressing the underlying determinants of health, such as poverty, discrimination, and violence.

4.5.3 MILLENNIUM DEVELOPMENT GOALS

The millennium development goals (MDGs) were a set of eight international development targets established by the United Nations in 2000, aimed at addressing poverty, hunger, disease, gender inequality, and other global challenges by the year 2015. While the MDGs did not explicitly focus on married women's health, several of the goals indirectly influenced the well-being of women within marital relationships.

For instance, Goal 3 of the MDGs aimed to promote gender equality and empower women. Achieving this goal involved targets such as eliminating gender disparities in primary and secondary education and increasing the proportion of women in wage employment. Gender equality is closely linked to women's health within marital relationships, as it can influence women's decision-making power regarding their own health, access to healthcare services, and exposure to risks such as domestic violence.

Additionally, Goal 5 of the MDGs focused on improving maternal health, aiming to reduce maternal mortality and achieve universal access to reproductive healthcare. This goal directly addressed the health needs of women during pregnancy and childbirth, including those within marital relationships. Access to maternal healthcare services can significantly impact the health outcomes of both women and their children, contributing to improved overall well-being within families.

While the MDGs did not specifically target marital women's health as a standalone issue, progress toward achieving goals related to gender equality and maternal health can have significant implications for the health and well-being of women within marital relationships. The subsequent sustainable development goals (SDGs), adopted in 2015, continue to prioritize gender equality and women's health, furthering the global commitment to addressing the health needs of all women, including those within marital unions.

4.6 MODELS AND THEORIES: HOW MARITAL RELATIONS AFFECT HEALTH

The correlation between marital satisfaction and health is a component of a broader array of studies that consistently highlight strong correlations between interpersonal connections and physical well-being. Two primary categories of models have been suggested to elucidate the mechanisms by which social support impacts physical health.

4.6.1 MODELS TO EXPLAIN HOW MARITAL RELATIONS ARE AFFECTED BY A PHYSICAL CONDITION

Various theoretical models outline the pathways through which marital relationships impact physical health. These models include:

- **Health behavior model**: Marital relationships can influence health behaviors such as diet, exercise, and substance use. Spouses may encourage or discourage healthy behaviors, leading to differences in physical health outcomes.
- **Psychophysiological model**: This model posits that marital quality affects physiological processes such as hormone levels, immune function, and cardiovascular activity, which in turn influence physical health.
- **Social support model**: This model suggests that marital relationships provide emotional, instrumental, and informational support, which buffers against stress and promotes better physical health outcomes.
- **Socioeconomic status model**: Marital relationships often intersect with socioeconomic status, with higher-quality marriages associated with greater economic resources and social support networks.

Socioeconomic status, in turn, impacts access to healthcare, living conditions, and other determinants of physical health.

- **Stress and coping model**: According to this model, marital quality influences an individual's ability to cope with stress. High-quality marriages provide support and resources that help individuals effectively manage stressors, thereby mitigating the adverse effects of stress on physical health.

According to Cohen [3], main-effect models and elevated levels of social connectivity will foster health benefits, irrespective of an individual's stress levels. Enhanced involvement within one's social circle provides individuals with a sense of belonging, significance, and autonomy, as well as a perceived feeling of safety and belongingness, and a mechanism for incentivizing health-supporting actions or penalizing health-compromising behaviors, all of which contribute to well-being.

As per the stress-buffering model, the adverse impacts of stress stemming from external sources (e.g., workplace stressors) are alleviated by robust social support networks, which can directly alleviate stress-inducing situations (e.g., intervening on behalf of a friend) or by reducing stress perceptions. In both models, close interpersonal connections, such as marriage, are expected to have a significant influence in furnishing social support.

4.6.2 THEORIES TO EXPLAIN HOW MARITAL RELATIONS AFFECT HEALTH

Married individuals tend to possess a confidant, someone dependable with whom they can converse, compared to those without intimate partners. While marriage does not assure emotional support, it enhances the likelihood of its presence. Emotional support mitigates psychological distress, such as depression and anxiety, thereby fostering overall well-being. The absence of standardized measures for emotional support leaves intriguing theoretical questions unresolved. Women both offer and receive more emotional aid than men. Generally, a household consisting of two women would boast the highest emotional support levels of any partnership, followed by a married couple of opposite genders; conversely, a household of two men would experience the lowest support levels among partnerships.

The primary theoretical rationales for the health benefits of marriage are emotional and economic support. Cohabitating couples theoretically fall between married pairs and single individuals in terms of health advantages. Additional potential contributing factors include a healthy lifestyle, household composition, division of labor, and decision-making within the household, sexual relationships, or legal standing. Adjusting for explanatory variables or mediators aims to diminish the connection to zero, statistically "explaining" why unions influence health. When researchers possess a robust theory with reliable measures of theoretical factors (as opposed to crude, dichotomized measures with low reliability), they aim to account for the association by reducing it to zero. This approach serves as the theoretical antithesis to minimizing a connection to insignificance due to spurious associations caused by selection bias.

According to explanatory theories, the correlation between marital quality and health is part of a broader realm of research that consistently illustrates strong connections between social bonds and physical well-being. A recent meta-analysis of 148 studies discovered that individuals with robust social connections had a 50% greater likelihood of survival [5]. Indeed, social support has been deemed one of the most extensively documented psychological factors influencing physical health outcomes.

The escalating prevalence of nonmarital cohabitation in developed countries may confound existing hypotheses elucidating marriage's health advantages. Nonetheless, research on cohabitation and its effects on health and well-being is still nascent. The prevailing belief is that cohabitation provides greater well-being benefits than being single but fewer economic, psychological, and health advantages compared to marriage [9]. However, "cohabiting" encompasses a diverse array of circumstances regarding reasons for cohabitation (e.g., as a precursor to eventual marriage or not), and sociodemographic factors and selection effects associated with cohabitation (described later when discussing marital status) modify the association. Indeed, the consequences of cohabitation on mortality diverge from those of marriage based on ethnicity, socioeconomic status, age, gender, and their interactions. Moreover, evidence on the relationship between relationship quality and health outcomes, the focal point of this research, and whether it differs between married and cohabiting individuals, remains scarce. Nonetheless, we assert that in committed partnerships (married or otherwise), relationship quality should correlate with physical well-being.

4.7 FACTORS AFFECTING WOMEN'S HEALTH

Several factors influencing the health of married women have been identified in research. These encompass the quality of the marital relationship, including communication, emotional support, and conflict resolution, which significantly impacts various health outcomes for women. Stressful marital experiences, such as conflict or dissatisfaction, contribute to psychological distress, affecting both mental and physical health. Social support, particularly from spouses and broader social networks, serves as a buffer against stress and fosters better health outcomes. Economic factors within the marital relationship, such as financial strain or disparities in income, can affect access to healthcare and overall well-being. Gender dynamics, including power dynamics and decision-making autonomy, also influence women's health behaviors and outcomes within marriages. Some factors are listed below:

4.7.1 MARITAL RELATIONSHIPS AND PHYSICAL HEALTH OF A FEMALE

Marital relationships play a significant role in influencing a woman's physical health. Research suggests that the quality of the marital relationship, including aspects such as communication, emotional support, and conflict resolution, can have direct implications for a woman's physical well-being. Positive marital interactions and emotional support have been linked to better cardiovascular health, immune function, and overall longevity. Conversely, marital conflict, dissatisfaction, and lack of support can contribute to increased stress levels, which may manifest in physical symptoms such as headaches, gastrointestinal issues, and compromised immune function.

Moreover, the presence of supportive marital relationships can encourage healthier lifestyle behaviors, such as regular exercise, balanced nutrition, and avoidance of harmful substances like tobacco and alcohol, all of which contribute to better physical health outcomes for women. Additionally, marital relationships can influence healthcare-seeking behaviors and adherence to medical recommendations, further impacting a woman's ability to manage and prevent health conditions. Overall, the quality of marital relationships plays a crucial role in shaping a woman's physical health and well-being. Researchers have identified a positive impact of marriage on women's physical health, shown through reduced rates of certain health conditions and illnesses. Recent studies suggest a possible link between marriage and a reduced risk of cardiovascular disease for women, though no similar effect has been observed for men. Marriage may influence physical health through enhanced access to and utilization of healthcare, with studies indicating that being married often allows individuals to access health insurance through a spouse's policy. This access increases the likelihood of having insurance coverage and decreases the chance of losing it after major life events like job loss—a benefit particularly significant for women. Research also shows that marriage is associated with shorter hospital stays, fewer doctor visits, and lower rates of nursing home admissions. Some findings even suggest that married individuals may use preventive services, such as cancer screenings, more frequently.

These healthcare advantages are linked to lower healthcare costs for married individuals, particularly older adults. For instance, the decreased risk of nursing home admission and shorter hospital stays associated with marriage contribute to lower overall costs. Notably, marriage's effect on reducing healthcare costs appears to be independent of its influence on physical health, as married individuals often receive informal care from their spouses, leading to fewer extended hospital stays and nursing home admissions. This cost-saving effect is especially pronounced for men, as wives are more likely to provide at-home care. Although some researchers have used statistical methods to explore these outcomes, the strongest evidence for marriage's positive impact on longevity comes from the consistent findings across numerous studies rather than the results of any single investigation.

Factors in marital relations that can affect the physical health of women are:

- **Healthcare**: Married men and women are also more likely to maintain health insurance. Furthermore, married people use hospitals and health facilities less frequently than others, are discharged from hospitals earlier on average than unmarried people, and spend half the time in hospitals as single people. Married people are also less likely to be admitted to a nursing home after leaving the hospital.

- **Lifestyle**: A lower proportion of married women than widowed, divorced or separated, never married, or cohabiting people had only "fair to poor health." Married women report greater health than divorced, separated, widowed, or never-married women. Married people smoke and binge drink less frequently than cohabitees. Women who marry consume less alcohol, whereas married males who divorce consume more alcohol and smoke cigarettes. Married young individuals are less likely to be alcoholics than those who are not in a romantic relationship.
- **Longevity**: Married women have shown lower mortality rates, with reduced risks of death from accidents, diseases, self-inflicted harm, and suicide. Compared to their married counterparts, divorced or separated individuals face an 83% higher risk of suicide, those who have never married have a 48% higher risk, and bereaved individuals have a 41% higher risk. Additionally, longevity tends to increase with the duration of marriage, as people married longer have lower mortality rates than those who are single. Numerous studies report a strong association between marriage and extended life expectancy, though current research has some limitations. Many studies primarily offer basic comparisons between married and unmarried groups, which may not account for the possibility that healthier individuals are more likely to marry. The most reliable studies on marriage and health tend to focus on health indicators just before and after marriage. However, because longevity is assessed at life's end, observing the direct impact of marital changes on lifespan remains challenging.
- **Severe illness**: Married individuals have shown higher survival rates across various stages of cancer progression compared to those who are unmarried. Married people tend to respond better to cancer treatments, with outcomes comparable to those of individuals 10 years younger. For instance, married men with prostate cancer have longer life expectancies, while unmarried women with breast cancer are more likely to be diagnosed at a later stage and face higher three-year morbidity rates specific to breast cancer. Additionally, after adjusting for age, married individuals have a lower mortality risk from conditions like liver cirrhosis, lung cancer, tuberculosis, and diabetes than those

who are never married, divorced, or widowed. The likelihood of survival following a heart attack is also higher for married people. Furthermore, individuals who are always unmarried or widowed show a greater likelihood of experiencing a stroke compared to their married counterparts.

- **STDs and pregnancy**: Married women provide superior prenatal care and consistently avoid dangerous substances than unattached mothers. Married women are less likely to have low birth weight children than mothers who are permanently cohabiting or have a romantic involvement with their baby's father. Married women have much fewer abortions than unmarried women. Marriage might impact health by influencing behaviors such as alcohol use, drug usage, cigarette smoking, food, and exercise. Recent study reveals that marriage has a major impact on both men's and women's health behaviors, but the evidence is mixed. Marriage is related with healthier behaviors in certain circumstances, but less healthy behaviors in others. Marriage is frequently shown in studies to lower excessive drinking and overall alcohol intake, and the effects are identical for young men and young women. In contrast to studies on alcohol and drug use, research on the influence of marriage on weight and physical activity suggests that marriage may have a detrimental impact on healthy behaviors and promote a more sedentary lifestyle. Several robust studies suggest that marriage leads to modest weight increases for both men and women—usually averaging less than five pounds. Additional study implementing longitudinal data is additionally required to investigate the impacts of marriage on physical activity in order to evaluate whether the association observed in cross-sectional analysis persists when more rigorous estimating approaches are utilized.

4.7.2 MARITAL RELATIONSHIPS AND HER MENTAL HEALTH

Marital relationships exert a profound influence on a woman's mental health. The quality of the marital bond, characterized by factors like communication, emotional support, and conflict resolution, significantly impacts a woman's psychological well-being. Positive marital interactions and emotional support contribute to greater resilience against stress, lower levels of anxiety and depression, and enhanced overall psychological functioning. Furthermore, the presence of a supportive marital relationship can serve as a protective factor against mental health challenges, providing a sense of security, stability, and belongingness. The ability to confide in a spouse and receive empathy and understanding can foster emotional resilience and help women cope effectively with life stressors.

However, it is essential to recognize that negative marital experiences, such as conflict, criticism, or emotional neglect, can have detrimental effects on a woman's mental health, leading to feelings of loneliness, despair, and low self-worth. These negative interactions within the marital relationship can contribute to the development or exacerbation of mental health disorders. Overall, the quality of marital relationships plays a pivotal role in shaping a woman's mental health outcomes, highlighting the importance of nurturing healthy and supportive partnerships for psychological well-being.

Mental health issues for women are rarely discussed. Approximately 15% of women suffer from mental problems, compared to 11% of men. Between the late 1960s and 1990s, psychiatric studies conducted in rural/urban, north/south Indian communities found that 1.3% of women were diagnosed with severe mental disorder and about 10–11% of women were diagnosed with common mental disorder (CMD). Gynecological morbidity is strongly associated with CMD. Premenstrual discomfort is reported by approximately 12–15% of women. Postpartum depression is a common reason why many women require treatment. Women's mental health is impacted by their daily survival. The pressure of their livelihoods, the various tasks that they must fulfill both within and outside the home, can create immense stress and worry. Increased poverty, discrimination, and violence all have an impact on mental health. Globalization has had a significant detrimental influence on mental health, resulting in increased unemployment, poverty, a lack of access to resources and treatment, an overburden of work, violence, and the mere battle to survive. Suicide attempts have been found to be higher among women.

CMD is a term used to describe emotional symptoms that are common in community and primary care settings and indicate a breakdown in normal functioning, but are frequently overlooked. These clinical and subclinical symptoms disrupt an individual's daily routine and general functioning, significantly affecting everyday living [11]. CMD typically appears as a combination of mild to moderate depression, anxiety, and unexplained physical symptoms. These diseases are classed under ICD-10 as "neurotic," "stress-related and somatoform disorders," and "mood disorders." CMD is typically characterized by physical manifestations rather than odd behavior or personality abnormalities. Common CMD complaints include insomnia, fatigue, anxiousness, depressive symptoms, feelings of hopelessness, irritability, forgetfulness, difficulties concentrating, and other nonspecific symptoms that might result in functional impairment. The influencing factors of mental health that affect women's health are listed below:

- **Anxiety and stress**: Stress and anxiety disorders are the most prevalent mental illnesses among Indian women. Women are more likely than men to encounter these mental health disorders, although they are less likely to receive treatment. Disadvantaged socioeconomic standing, mental illness stigma, and the belief that depression and anxiety are not serious disorders all lead to a failure to seek treatment. Furthermore, there is a gender bias in which male primary care practitioners fail to notice emotional disorders in female patients [12]. Adults and children in married homes encounter less psychological distress than their counterparts in divorced families. Married men had lower levels of stress hormones, while married women suffered less psychological anguish. Married mothers experience more love and connection, less ambivalence, and less conflict with their spouses than cohabiting and single women do.
- **Community**: Older married couples receive more social assistance than older cohabiters, and married mothers receive more social support than single mothers. Those in intact marriages are less likely to believe that most individuals will take advantage of others. Married parents spend more on schooling and less on alcohol and smoking than cohabiting parents.
- **Depression**: Research consistently suggests that marriage is associated with lower rates of depression, though current evidence has limitations that future studies should seek to address. The most comprehensive research often examines the impact of marriage and marital changes by assessing depressive symptoms immediately before and after these transitions, helping to control

for differences between those who marry and those who do not. However, this approach may introduce additional sources of bias, the effects of which are unclear. Generally, married individuals report lower levels of depression compared to those who are cohabiting. Married mothers tend to experience less depression, enjoy greater partner support, and have more stable relationships than mothers who are cohabiting. Additionally, adolescents living with married parents are less likely to experience depression than those living in stepfamilies or single-parent households, regardless of the presence of additional adults.

- **Drug and alcohol use**: Married people are more likely to stop using marijuana, thanks in part to increased self-control. Continuously married adults are less likely to say that they occasionally drink too much. Married ladies have fewer drinking problems. Adolescents from intact married homes use cocaine less frequently than those from divorced families. Teenagers from intact households are less likely to start smoking than those whose parents have never married or are divorced.
- **Happiness:** Married people are considerably more likely to report happiness than cohabiters, and those who do not cohabit before marriage report happier marriages than those who do. Married people (both those in intact marriages and those who have divorced and remarried) are the most likely to express pride in their employment. Married women with infants have the most favorable views and report creating better home conditions than single and cohabiting mothers.
- **Suicide:** Married persons are the least likely to commit suicide. Adolescents raised in divorced households are more prone to commit suicide [13].

4.7.3 MARITAL RELATIONSHIPS AND HER EMOTIONAL HEALTH

Marital relationships have a profound impact on a woman's emotional health. The quality of the marital bond, characterized by factors such as communication, trust, intimacy, and mutual support, significantly influences a woman's emotional well-being. Positive marital relationships, marked by open communication, empathy, and mutual respect, contribute to emotional stability and satisfaction. These relationships provide a sense of security, belongingness, and comfort, fostering feelings of happiness, contentment, and fulfillment. Emotional support from a spouse can serve as a buffer against life's stressors, helping women navigate challenges with greater resilience and optimism.

Conversely, negative marital experiences, such as conflict, criticism, or emotional neglect, can undermine emotional well-being. Marital discord and dissatisfaction can lead to feelings of loneliness, frustration, and sadness, contributing to emotional distress and vulnerability to mental health issues such as anxiety and depression. Moreover, the absence of emotional support within the marital relationship can exacerbate feelings of isolation and inadequacy, impacting self-esteem and overall emotional health.

Women in unsupportive or hostile marital relationships may experience heightened levels of emotional confusion, leading to decreased life satisfaction and diminished overall well-being. Married women in India are more likely to experience emotional stress than unmarried women. Research in high-income countries has demonstrated that the quality of marital relationships has a considerable impact on spouses' physical and emotional well-being [15]. The level of marital discontent has a negative impact on physical and emotional health [10]. However, research in low- and middle-income countries has only lately begun to investigate the association between marital quality and women's mental health.

Similarly, improved marital happiness protects against depression. It has also been proposed that higher and perceived discontent with marriage relates to an increased risk of CMD. Marital adjustment is described as "the state in which husband and wife have an overall feeling of happiness and satisfaction with their marriage and each other." Women's marital adjustment problems may be caused by psychological, social, and biological stress because of changing to distinct social roles and obligations in a new family, as well as caring for the family, childbirth, and maternal roles. The emotional health of women is intricately linked to the quality of their marital relationships. Nurturing positive, supportive, and emotionally fulfilling partnerships can promote emotional resilience, happiness, and overall psychological wellness for women.

Previous research on marital adjustment has revealed a variety of psychological, social, demographic, and personal aspects connected with marital adjustment and their impact on the married relationship. Living with in-laws, employment duties, gender-specific tasks, money management, childbearing and rearing, anger management, and sexual relationships are all important areas of adjustment for married couples. Although researchers have focused on these factors impacting marital adjustment, there is minimal information from India about how stress from marital adjustment affects women's emotional well-being, underlining the need for further research in this area.

4.8 MARITAL DISTRESS AND WOMEN HEALTH

Nobody has a perfect marriage, and most couples could use some support from time to time. Many locations provide pre-marital preparation and marriage enrichment programs, including the Prevention and Relationship Enhancement Program and the Relationship Enhancement Program. All couples can benefit from the specialized education provided by marriage and family therapists. To participate in marital therapy, you do not have to be in a disturbed marriage. Many people in stable marriages take this option to improve their relationship. Marital distress is indistinguishable from the normal ups and downs of marriage. People in disturbed marriages are essentially dissatisfied with their connection. Furthermore, their disappointment appears to be ongoing rather than episodic. Couples experiencing high degrees of marital misery dispute frequently; the conflict goes unsolved and becomes exhausting. Alternatively, the spouses may not argue, but rather stand apart in utter estrangement, no longer doing sweet things for one another and talking.

A marital or committed partnership includes a secure, ongoing relationship with someone who can provide both support and stress, both of which play a role in the development of cardiovascular disease. Unlike other stresses, which are typically temporary or transient, marital stress can be persistent and continuing. Ten prior research studies suggest that couples in their mid-40s experience the highest levels of marital stress, despite varying sources and intensities across life stages.

4.8.1 MARITAL DISCORD AND DEPRESSION

Distressed marriage relationships and depression are typically linked. Both syndrome depression and depressive symptoms are highly linked to marital distress. Unhappy marriages were a strong risk factor for major depressive illness in both men and women, with a 25-fold increase over untroubled marriages. The association is bidirectional: disturbed marriages worsen depressive symptoms, whereas depression promotes lower marital quality [1].

The link between marital distress and depression has significant implications for physical functioning. Depression affects various biological systems (e.g., endocrine, immunological, cardiovascular, metabolic, and neurocognitive), and these changes are sufficient to increase several health risks, including early death. Depression increases inflammation, which is one of the primary causes of poor health.

A variety of disorders and systemic diseases are characterized by increased inflammation, including cardiovascular disease, diabetes, metabolic syndrome, rheumatoid arthritis, asthma, multiple sclerosis, chronic pain, and psoriasis; each of these is associated with an increased risk of depression [16]. In addition to physiological changes, depressed people are more likely to have poorer health habits, such as a higher risk of alcohol and drug abuse, insufficient sleep and nutrition, and less exercise, all of which have negative health consequences in and of themselves.

Furthermore, depression may initiate the inflammatory response, leading to increased cytokine surges in response to stressors or infections. Depression and stress interact to increase the chance of infection, prolong infectious episodes, and slow wound healing, all of which can contribute to long-term proinflammatory cytokine production.

First, inflammation-induced mood and behavior changes appear to be more common in women than in men. For example, women respond to temporary increases in inflammation with larger sensations of loneliness and social alienation than men, which likely contributes to the 2:1 gender ratio in depressive illnesses. Furthermore, antecedent depression, somatic symptomatology, interpersonal stresses, childhood adversity, obesity, and physical inactivity are all factors that raise inflammation, and women have disproportionately higher representation than males in each of these categories.

Marital caregivers' stress has been extensively documented in dementia concerned literature. Women face more negative consequences while caring for a husband with dementia than men when they become caregivers. Although rigorous caring significantly increases health risks, the data discussed above show that even nondisabling diseases can raise the stakes. Husbands' high blood pressure and stroke history were associated with greater levels of depressive symptoms in their spouses, whereas wives' health problems were not associated with husbands' depressive symptoms.

4.8.2 MARITAL DISCORD AND SLEEP

Marital disputes also disrupt day-to-day sleep: on days when couple interactions were more unfavorable, women had poorer actigraphy-assessed sleep that night. Furthermore, marital disagreement has a contagious effect on sleep; wives reporting poorer relationship quality led to husbands sleeping worse at night [4].

The link between marital dispute and sleep has a dose-response relationship: more harmful conflict increases the probability of sleep disturbance. Divorced victims of intimate partner violence had more persistent sleep issues than unvictimized divorcees, and those who experienced continuous aggression slept even worse than those subjected to less frequent violence.

Poor sleep is linked to cardiovascular disease, cancer, obesity, diabetes, and early death. Though married people sleep better than singles on average, marital strife reduces sleep quality and quantity. Those in more stressed marriages report higher levels of insomnia than their happily married counterparts, and their sleep disturbances worsen over time. For example, unhappily married older persons' sleep issues intensified over four years [2]. Over a year, more destructive and less constructive disagreement led to decreases in actigraphy-measured sleep quality and duration.

Yang and colleagues reported that higher sleep issues led to lower marital quality four years later. Thus, the bidirectional ties between marital quarrel and sleep disturbance create a positive feedback loop in which discord-induced sleep problems intensify conflict, potentially leading to long-term marital dysfunction. Sleep deprivation, in turn, increases the production of proinflammatory cytokines and cellular inflammatory signaling, which contributes to sadness. Increased inflammation feeds back to disrupt sleep. In this approach, marital discord generates a synergistic cascade of depression, sleep disruption, and inflammation, heightening the risk for comorbidities and death. In addition to its significant inflammatory effects, poor sleep affects hunger regulation and food choice. It is not unexpected that inadequate sleep has been linked to obesity and the metabolic syndrome.

4.8.3 MARITAL PATHS TO OBESITY AND ITS COMORBIDITIES

Depression and stress have been closely linked to obesity, with research showing that depressed adults have a 58% greater likelihood of becoming obese. One major prospective study found that older adults with depression accumulated visceral fat over five years, whereas nondepressed adults showed a reduction in this type of fat. Chronic stress and stressful experiences have also been associated with weight gain, with longitudinal studies indicating that long-term stress and life events contribute to the onset of metabolic syndrome, in which central obesity is a key component. These findings carry important implications for individuals in strained marriages, given the strong connection between marital conflict and depression.

Marital distress and depression can influence neurochemistry, neurobiology, and behavior in ways that encourage metabolic changes related to obesity. For instance, both depression and marital strain can elevate cortisol levels, which increases cravings for high-calorie "comfort" foods. Additionally, cortisol elevation stimulates insulin production, leading to persistent high cortisol and insulin levels, which in turn promote visceral fat accumulation. Marital distress can also affect ghrelin, an appetite-stimulating hormone, encouraging increased food intake [6].

Recent research from our lab examined how marital conflict affects couples' metabolic responses to high-fat meals, focusing on metabolic processes crucial for weight management and fat storage. Resting energy expenditure, which accounts for 65% to 75% of daily energy expenditure, plays a vital role in maintaining energy balance and weight control. Lower resting energy expenditure raises the risk of weight gain, while elevated insulin levels stimulate appetite and contribute to visceral fat accumulation.

4.8.4 METABOLIC SYNDROME

Metabolic syndrome is categorized by the National Cholesterol Education Program standards as mild dyslipidemia, central obesity, hypertension, and insulin resistance/hyperglycemia. This cluster includes traits that are all associated with an increased risk of cardiovascular disease and diabetes. Women who reported higher marital happiness had a considerably lower chance of developing the metabolic syndrome over an 11.5-year period than women who were dissatisfied with their marriages or were unpartnered. Even after controlling for age, demographic features, and psychosocial and behavioral risk variables, women in unsatisfied marriages were more than three times more likely to develop the metabolic syndrome than those in impeccable marriages.

A cross-sectional study found that marital distress increased the risk of metabolic syndrome in women, but not men. In a four-year follow-up, the effect was stronger for women, and if husbands reported marital distress at the start, wives were more likely to develop metabolic syndrome after four years. A couples-based analysis later showed that marital quality affected metabolic syndrome only through depressive symptoms rather than directly, contrasting with earlier findings that linked marital distress to metabolic syndrome in women independently. This discrepancy may be due to differences in classification and depression measures used across studies.

Diabetes is a fast-growing chronic health issue in the USA and requires consistent management, often influenced by spousal behaviors, such as encouragement of a healthy lifestyle or shared habits. Marital conflict raises risk factors for diabetes, including metabolic syndrome and inflammation. Studies on marital quality and diabetes prevalence showed mixed results: women with increasing positive marital quality had a lower diabetes risk, while men with worsening marital quality surprisingly had better outcomes. Moreover, having a spouse with metabolic syndrome or diabetes significantly raises one's own risk by 26–30%, with a spousal history of diabetes or prediabetes doubling the risk.

Marital distress is strongly linked with depression, both in short-term and long-term studies. Individuals in distressed marriages generally have poorer responses to treatments for depression and are more likely to experience relapse. Individual treatments for depression typically do not address marital distress, resulting in less effective outcomes than couple-based interventions, which tend to improve both relationship quality and depression symptoms.

4.9 IMPLICATIONS OF PRACTICES AND POLICIES ON WOMEN'S HEALTH

The implications of practices and policies on marital women's health are significant and multifaceted. Access to healthcare, reproductive health services, mental health support, and domestic violence prevention are crucial factors that can impact the well-being of marital women. Policies promoting gender equality, empowerment, and health education are essential for addressing the unique health needs and challenges faced by married women within the context of marriage. Overall, prioritizing women's health, safety, and empowerment within marital relationships is crucial for promoting better health outcomes and creating healthier marital dynamics.

4.9.1 CURRENT POLICIES AND PRACTICES ON WOMEN'S HEALTH

The Global Strategy for Women's, Children's, and Adolescents' Health (2016–2030) is an ambitious plan aimed at ending preventable maternal, newborn, and child deaths, including stillbirths, by 2030, while enhancing their health and safety. This strategy seeks to prioritize these groups within the SDG agenda, harnessing their potential for significant positive change. It provides actionable guidance to drive progress through a multisectoral approach, effectively translating the SDG agenda into practical steps for impact. The Platform for Action emphasized the importance of gathering and assessing health data by sex. Many countries, UN agencies, and nongovernmental organizations have now committed to gender mainstreaming, which is the assessment of how every proposed policy action may have distinct repercussions for men and women, as a method for attaining gender equality.

As per the Women in Global Health Policy report 2023, women's leadership and global health to assess the pace of change at the global level, the impact of the pandemic, and inform our recommendations with country experiences from India, Kenya, and Nigeria. Women in the health workforce are demanding change and demanding the right to compete fairly for leadership roles. Current policies and practices related to marital women's health vary across different regions and countries, influenced by cultural norms, healthcare systems, and socioeconomic factors. Here are some common policies and practices that may impact marital women's health.

Policies related to healthcare access play a significant role in marital women's health. Ensuring affordable and accessible healthcare services, including reproductive health services, prenatal care, and mental health support, is essential. This may involve government-funded healthcare programs, insurance coverage for essential health services, and initiatives to improve healthcare infrastructure in underserved areas. Policies related to reproductive rights and family planning have a direct impact on married women's health. Access to contraception, safe abortion services, and comprehensive sexual education can empower women to make informed decisions about their reproductive health and prevent unintended pregnancies, thereby reducing maternal mortality and improving overall health outcomes.

Policies aimed at preventing domestic violence and intimate partner violence are crucial for protecting marital women's health and safety. This includes legal protections, support services for survivors, and public awareness campaigns to challenge societal attitudes that perpetuate violence against women. Additionally, policies may focus on promoting healthy relationship dynamics and providing resources for couples counseling and conflict resolution. Policies that support work-life balance and provide adequate maternity leave can positively impact marital women's health. Maternity leave policies that allow women to take time off work to recover from childbirth and bond with their newborns promote physical and mental well-being. Additionally, flexible work arrangements and support for childcare can help women balance their professional and caregiving responsibilities.

Policies aimed at promoting gender equality and empowering women in marital relationships can have long-term benefits for women's health. This includes initiatives to address gender-based discrimination, promote women's education and economic empowerment, and challenge traditional gender roles and stereotypes. Empowered women are better able to advocate for their own health needs, make informed decisions about their bodies, and access resources and support services.

Overall, policies and practices related to marital women's health should prioritize equity, autonomy, and empowerment, recognizing the diverse needs and experiences of women within marital relationships and addressing systemic barriers to health and well-being. By implementing comprehensive approaches that address both individual and structural factors, policymakers can promote positive health outcomes for marital women and contribute to broader efforts to achieve gender equality and social justice.

4.9.2 SUGGESTIONS FOR FUTURE RESEARCH

Research on marital relations and their effects on women's health is crucial for understanding the complex interplay between intimate relationships and well-being. Here are some potential implications for future research in this area:

- **Biopsychosocial approach**: Adopt a biopsychosocial approach to examine the pathways through which marital relations influence women's health. This involves considering biological, psychological, and social factors, including physiological responses to stress, mental health symptoms, social support networks, and access to healthcare.
- **Cultural context**: Consider the influence of cultural norms, values, and beliefs on marital relations and women's health outcomes. Comparative studies across diverse cultural contexts can provide insights into how cultural factors shape relationship dynamics, gender roles, and health behaviors within marital relationships.
- **Health disparities**: Explore how disparities in marital quality and access to resources impact women's health disparities. Investigating how factors such as income inequality, educational attainment, and neighborhood characteristics intersect with marital relations can shed light on the social determinants of health among women in different populations.
- **Intersectionality**: Investigate how intersecting identities (such as race, ethnicity, socioeconomic status, sexual orientation, and disability) intersect with marital relations to influence women's health outcomes. Recognizing the diversity of experiences within marital relationships can help researchers develop more inclusive and nuanced understandings of this topic.
- **Intervention studies**: Design and evaluate interventions aimed at improving marital relations and enhancing women's health outcomes. Interventions may focus on communication skills training, conflict resolution strategies, stress management techniques, and promoting equitable division of household labor. Assessing the effectiveness of these interventions can inform

evidence-based practices for supporting couples' relationships and women's health.

- **Life course perspective**: Take a life course perspective to understand how experiences in early life, transitions across the life span, and cumulative advantages or disadvantages influence marital relations and women's health trajectories over time. Examining critical periods of vulnerability and resilience can inform strategies for promoting healthy aging and well-being among women in marital relationships.
- **Longitudinal studies**: Conduct longitudinal studies to explore how changes in marital quality and dynamics over time impact women's health outcomes. Tracking couples' relationships and health status over an extended period can provide valuable insights into the long-term effects of marital relations on women's physical and mental well-being.
- **Technology and social media**: Examine the role of technology and social media in shaping marital relations and women's health. Research could explore how digital communication tools, social networking platforms, and online support communities impact relationship dynamics, social support networks, and access to health information among couples.

By addressing these research implications, scholars can advance our understanding of the complex connections between marital relations and women's health, ultimately informing interventions and policies aimed at improving outcomes for individuals and couples alike.

4.9.3 RECOMMENDATIONS FOR PROMOTING WOMEN'S HEALTH WITHIN THE CONTEXT OF MARITAL RELATIONS

Promoting women's health within the context of marital relations requires a multifaceted approach that addresses both individual and relational factors. By implementing the following recommendations, couples can work together to promote women's health within the context of marital relationships, fostering a supportive environment that prioritizes the well-being of both partners. Here are some recommendations:

- **Access to healthcare**: Ensure equitable access to healthcare services for women within marital relationships. This involves addressing barriers such as financial constraints, lack of transportation, and limited availability of healthcare providers. Encourage regular health check-ups, screenings, and preventive care for both partners.
- **Community resources**: Connect couples with community resources and support networks that promote women's health. This could include local health clinics, support groups, women's centers, and online forums where couples can access information, services, and peer support.
- **Couples counseling**: Offer couples counseling or relationship education programs that integrate discussions about health and well-being. These programs can provide a supportive environment for couples to address concerns related to communication, intimacy, and health behaviors. Emphasize the importance of mutual support and collaboration in maintaining both partners' health.
- **Education and awareness**: Provide education and raise awareness about women's health issues within marital relationships. This includes promoting knowledge about reproductive health, family planning, mental health, and preventive care. Empower women and their partners with accurate information to make informed decisions about their health.
- **Gender equity**: Promote gender equity within marital relationships to support women's health and well-being. Encourage shared decision-making, equal participation in household responsibilities, and mutual respect for each other's autonomy and choices. Addressing power imbalances and promoting gender equality can positively impact women's health outcomes.
- **Mental health support**: Prioritize mental health support for women within marital relationships. Offer resources for managing stress, anxiety, depression, and other mental health concerns. Normalize discussions about mental health and encourage seeking professional help when needed.

- **Physical activity and nutrition**: Encourage physical activity and healthy eating habits within the household. Engage in activities such as walking, biking, or exercising together as a couple. Plan and prepare nutritious meals together, emphasizing the importance of a balanced diet for overall health and well-being.
- **Regular check-ins**: Encourage regular check-ins between partners to discuss health-related concerns, goals, and priorities. Foster an environment where both partners feel comfortable sharing their needs and supporting each other's health and well-being.
- **Stress management**: Provide resources and support for stress management techniques within marital relationships. High levels of stress can negatively impact women's health, so promoting coping strategies such as mindfulness, relaxation techniques, and effective communication skills can help couples navigate challenges together.
- **Support for reproductive health**: Offer support for women's reproductive health needs within marital relationships. This includes access to contraception, family planning services, prenatal care, and support during pregnancy and childbirth. Encourage open communication about reproductive goals and preferences between partners.

4.10 CONCLUSIONS

The worldwide outline for females' health should be strengthened and transformed, as should a gender-disaggregated approach to health explore and strategy development. While NCDs are the most prevalent reasons for morbidity and mortality in women worldwide, they have received relatively little consideration in global health-improvement measures. Adequate means and directed efforts at the local, national, and worldwide levels are needed to enhance NCD results for women during their lives. Furthermore, to develop, assess, and provide the best healthcare interferences and policies for illness obstacles and care, gender disparities must be investigated on a regular basis in all disciplines of well-being and remedy. A life-course approach for treating NCDs, along with sex-disaggregated assets, along with utilization of healthcare data informed by a feminist perspective, has the potential to significantly boost the health of worldwide.

There is much evidence linking marital quality to health outcomes, ranging from intracellular signaling to mortality. Marital relations significantly impact women's health, influencing physical, mental, and emotional well-being. Research suggests that healthy marital relationships can contribute to positive health outcomes for women, while marital discord or negative relationship dynamics can be detrimental to their health. Positive marital relations, characterized by open communication, mutual respect, and emotional support, can provide a protective buffer against stress and promote overall well-being. Supportive partners may encourage healthy behaviors, such as regular exercise, balanced nutrition, and seeking medical care when needed. Additionally, strong social support within marriage can mitigate the negative effects of stress on women's health.

Conversely, strained or unhealthy marital relationships can contribute to various negative health outcomes for women. Chronic relationship conflict, lack of emotional support, and feelings of loneliness or isolation within marriage can increase the risk of mental health issues such as depression, anxiety, and low self-esteem. Marital stress has also been linked to physiological changes in women's bodies, including increased inflammation and immune dysfunction, which can contribute to the development or exacerbation of physical health conditions. A greater awareness of how marriage impacts health could be beneficial to facilitate conversations about the role and goals of public policy in upgrading marriage—and could give new meaning to the phrase "healthy marriage."

4.11 SUMMARY

The relationship between women's health and marital relations is complex and multifaceted. Healthy marital relationships can serve as a protective factor, promoting women's physical, mental, and emotional well-being. Supportive partners can encourage healthy behaviors, provide emotional support, and mitigate the negative effects of stress on women's health. Unhealthy marital relationships can contribute to various negative health outcomes for women, including mental health issues, physiological changes, and exacerbation of existing health conditions. Therefore, promoting healthy marital relations characterized by open communication, mutual respect, and support is essential for fostering women's health and well-being. This requires addressing issues such as relationship conflict, power imbalances, and access to resources and support services. By prioritizing the promotion of healthy marital dynamics, we can create environments that support women's health and contribute to overall family well-being.

KEYWORDS

- **distress**
- **emotional**
- **health**
- **marital**
- **marriage**
- **mental**
- **physical**
- **sleep**
- **women**

REFERENCES

1. Beach, S. R. H. (2014). The couple and family discord model of depression: Updates and future directions. In: Agnew, C. R., & South, S. C. (Eds.), *Interpersonal Relationships and Health: Social and Clinical Psychological Mechanisms*, (pp. 133–155).
2. Chen Jen, H., Waite, L., Kurina, L. M., Thisted, R. A., McClintock, M., & Lauderdale, D. S. (2015). Insomnia symptoms and actigraph-estimated sleep characteristics in a nationally representative sample of older adults. *The Journals of Gerontology Series A: Biological Sciences and Medical Sciences, 70*(2), 185–192.
3. Cohen, S. (2004). Social relationships and health. *American Psychologist*, *59*(8), 676–684.
4. Finkel, E. J., Hui, C. M., Carswell, K. L., & Larson, G. M. (2014). The suffocation of marriage: Climbing Mount Maslow without enough oxygen. *Psychological Inquiry, 25*, 1–41.
5. Hughes, E. L., & Parkes, K. R. (2007). Work hours and well-being: The roles of work-time control and work-family interference. *Work & Stress, 21*(3), 264–278.

6. Jaremka, L. M., Glaser, R., Malarkey, W. B., & Kiecolt-Glaser, J. K. (2013). Marital distress prospectively predicts poorer cellular immune function. *Psycho Neuro Endocrinology*, *38*(11), 2713–2719.
7. Joshi, O., Desai, S., & Vanneman, R. (2017). Marital quality and spousal choice: An Indian scenario. *Population Association of America*.
8. Liu, H. (2012). Marital dissolution and self-rated health: Age trajectories and birth cohort variations. *Social Science and Medicine*, *74*(7), 1107–1116.
9. Liu, R. T. (2017). The microbiome as a novel paradigm in studying stress and mental health. *American Psychologist*, *72*(7), 655–667.
10. Lorenz, F. O., Wickrama, A. S., & Conger, D. Glen, H., & Elder, Jr. (2006). The short-term and decade-long effects of divorce on women's midlife health. *Journal of Health and Social Behavior*, *47*, 111–125.
11. Maitra, S., Brault, M. A., Schensul, S. L., Schensul, J. J., Nastasi, B. K., Verma, R. K., Burleson, J. A. (2015). An approach to mental health in low-and middle-income countries: A case example from urban India. *International Journal of Mental Health, 44,* 215–230.
12. Malhotra, S., & Shah, R. (2015). Women and mental health in India: An overview. *Indian Journal of Psychiatry*, *57*, 205.
13. Maria, M., et al., (2008). Suicide and marital status in Italy. *Psychiatric Quarterly*, *79*, 275–285.
14. Prigerson, H. G., Paul, K. M., & Robert, A. R. (2000). Preliminary explorations of the harmful interactive effects of widowhood and marital harmony on health, health service use, and health care costs. *The Gerontologist*, *40*, 349–357.
15. Robles, T. F., Slatcher, R. B., Trombello, J. M., & McGinn, M. M. (2014). Marital quality and health: A meta-analytic review. *Psychological Bulletin, 140*, 140–187.
16. Slavich, G. M., Way, B. M., Eisenberger, N. I., & Taylor, S. E. (2010). Neural sensitivity to social rejection is associated with inflammatory responses to social stress. *Proceedings of the National Academy of Sciences of the United States of America, 107*, 14817–14822

CHAPTER 5

Lost Daughters: The Silent Injustice of Present Society

SANJIB KUMAR HALDAR[1*] and MEGH R. GOYAL[2]

*Corresponding author

ABSTRACT

This chapter explores the emotional journey of a daughter caught in the complexities of societal norms. Set in a seemingly progressive society, the protagonist struggles with identity and belonging, facing invisible prejudices that reflect broader systemic injustices. The narrative emphasizes the tension between personal loss and societal expectations, illustrating the impact of conformity on marginalized individuals. The daughter becomes a symbol of those whose stories are suppressed by societal norms. Through poignant storytelling, the chapter challenges readers to confront uncomfortable truths about the invisible threads of injustice that shape contemporary life. It calls for breaking the silence and dismantling the barriers that perpetuate inequality, urging action against the injustices that remain hidden beneath the surface.

5.1 INTRODUCTION

5.1.1 UNVEILING THE SILENT INJUSTICE

In the shadows of contemporary society, a silent injustice (SJ) persists, often overlooked and underexplored—the plight of lost daughters (LS). This introduction peels back the layers of this societal phenomenon,

Holistic Approaches for Women's Sustainable Health, Volume 2: Advancements, Socioeconomic Impacts, and Innovative Strategies. Junaid Ahmad Malik, Anamika Chauhan, and Megh R. Goyal (Eds)

DOI: 10.1201/9781779641656-6

shedding light on the overlooked narratives of daughters who, for various reasons, find themselves estranged or neglected. The phenomenon of lost daughters, as highlighted by Sen [10], is a pervasive issue affecting many regions globally. Sen's study underscores the widespread nature of this problem and its roots in deeply ingrained societal norms that devalue female children. These lost daughters embody a collective voice yearning to be heard, challenging the prevailing norms that contribute to their silent suffering. The exploration begins by acknowledging the existence of this silent injustice and establishing the need to delve deeper into the complexities that shroud the lives of these overlooked individuals.

The term "lost daughters" encompasses a spectrum of experiences, including abandonment, neglect, or societal dismissal, pushing these individuals to the periphery of attention and care. This introduction aims to initiate a compassionate conversation around the stories of these daughters, acknowledging the complexities that surround their experiences and the broader implications for societal well-being. By recognizing this silent injustice, we pave the way for a more empathetic understanding and collective responsibility to address the challenges faced by these daughters.

5.1.2 NAVIGATING THE COMPLEX LANDSCAPE

The second point of introduction navigates the intricate landscape that defines the experiences of lost daughters. It delves into the diverse factors contributing to their marginalization, such as societal expectations, gender biases, and economic disparities (ED). By understanding the complex interplay of these elements, we embark on a journey to unravel the nuanced stories of lost daughters and the impact of societal norms on their lives. This exploration goes beyond mere observation, aiming to dissect the roots of the silent injustice embedded in the present society. From familial dynamics to broader cultural influences, the introduction aims to provide a comprehensive understanding of the multifaceted challenges faced by lost daughters. Various responses and interventions have been proposed and implemented to address the issue of the lost daughter. Gupta (2019) explores the global intersectionality of social justice and suggests that multifaceted approaches are necessary to tackle the root causes of this issue [5]. By recognizing the intersections of gender, social expectations, and economic factors, we lay the groundwork for a holistic examination that seeks not only to identify the injustices but also to propose pathways toward a more equitable and compassionate society. Similarly, Nair [7] offers an international comparative study, demonstrating that the issue of lost daughters is not confined to any single country but is a global concern influenced by various cultural and socioeconomic factors. In essence, this introduction serves as compass-guiding readers through the uncharted territory of the silent injustice faced by lost daughters. By acknowledging the existence of this societal blind spot and delving into the complexities that define the experiences of these daughters, we set the stage for a profound exploration that seeks not only to expose the injustices but also to advocate for transformative change in our present society.

5.1.3 DISCUSSIONS

5.1.3.1 ROOTS OF MARGINALIZATION

The authors begin the discussion by excavating the roots of the marginalization faced by lost daughters within the present societal framework. It is imperative to recognize that the term "lost daughters" encompasses a spectrum of experiences, including but not limited to abandonment, neglect, and societal indifference. According to Roy, these daughters often become casualties of prevailing norms, rooted deeply in societal expectations, gender biases, and economic disparities, sociological analysis, and sociological perspectives [9].

The patriarchal underpinnings of many societies contribute significantly to the marginalization of daughters. Gender biases, perpetuated through cultural norms and familial expectations, relegate daughters to subordinate roles. This subjugation, when combined with economic factors, creates a volatile environment where daughters become susceptible to abandonment or neglect. The discussion aims to dissect these intersecting factors, shedding light on how societal structures play a pivotal role in rendering these daughters "lost" within their own communities. Beyond individual circumstances, the discussion delves into broader cultural influences that sustain the silent injustice faced by lost daughters. Societal norms that prioritize male heirs, reinforce traditional gender roles, and stigmatize deviations from established family structures (FS) contribute to the marginalization of daughters. By unraveling these intricate threads, we gain a deeper understanding of the systemic forces at play, forming the foundation for transformative interventions. Chatterjee [2] discusses patterns across different cultural contexts and advocates for culturally sensitive interventions.

5.1.3.2 TOWARD TRANSFORMATIVE EMPATHY AND ACTION

The second facet of our discussion propels us from understanding the roots of marginalization to envisioning transformative measures. Recognizing the silent injustice faced by lost daughters is the first step; the subsequent imperative is to cultivate empathy and advocate for systemic change. This section explores avenues for societal introspection and collective action to dismantle the structures perpetuating the marginalization of lost daughters. Transformative empathy involves a paradigm shift in societal attitudes toward daughters. It necessitates challenging ingrained biases and fostering inclusivity in familial and communal settings. The discussion advocates for educational initiatives to promote awareness about gender equality and the consequences of perpetuating traditional gender norms. By addressing the root causes, communities can foster an environment where daughters are valued, protected, and provided equal opportunities. Furthermore, the discussion emphasizes the role of policy interventions and legal frameworks. Meanwhile, Mishra (2011) discusses the social factors influencing the lives of lost daughters and the adequacies in legal frameworks that fail to protect them adequately [6] in safeguarding the rights of daughters. Dasgupta (2018) offers a human rights perspective, emphasizing the need for international collaboration and robust legal frameworks to protect the rights of daughters [4]. By challenging discriminatory practices and promoting gender-inclusive policies, societies can create a more equitable landscape. Grassroots movements, community engagement, and collaborative efforts are pivotal in effecting lasting change. This section aims to inspire a collective commitment to dismantling the silent injustice faced by lost daughters, fostering a society where every daughter is seen, heard, and afforded the dignity and opportunities she deserves.

This chapter delves into issues related to lost daughters focusing on case studies, their contributing factors, their consequences to create awareness among government agencies and societies, and relatives, so that this issue of lost daughters can be minimized.

5.2 FACTORS CONTRIBUTING TO ISSUE OF LOST DAUGHTERS

5.2.1 ECONOMIC FACTORS

The economic factor is a significant contributor to the silent injustice experienced by lost daughters in the present society. Economic disparities, often rooted in gender biases, create an environment where daughters face heightened vulnerability, neglect, and abandonment. In many societies, the birth of a daughter is accompanied by financial concerns, especially in regions where dowry systems persist. Families burdened by economic constraints may view daughters as financial liabilities, contributing to their marginalization. The economic devaluation of female labor further exacerbates the vulnerability of daughters, limiting their access to resources and opportunities. Economic hardship is another critical factor that exacerbates the plight of lost daughters. Patel (2015) conducts a case study on the economic factors contributing to this issue, revealing how financial pressures lead families to sell their daughters into child labor, marriage, or even trafficking [8]. Economic pressures force families into difficult choices, and in some cases, daughters become victims of neglect or abandonment due to perceived economic hardships. The silent injustice perpetuated by economic factors underscores the need for comprehensive economic reforms, addressing gender-based economic disparities, and empowering daughters through financial means. Sengupta [11] provides a comparative analysis of economic inequality and its impact on the vulnerability of daughters, highlighting the intersection of poverty and gender discrimination.

5.2.2 SOCIAL FACTORS

The social factor plays a pivotal role in unraveling the silent injustice faced by lost daughters within present society. Deeply entrenched societal norms, influenced by cultural beliefs, create an environment where daughters encounter discrimination, neglect, and abandonment from an early age. Sharma (2012) provides an anthropological perspective on the societal impacts that contribute to the phenomenon of lost daughters. Sharma's research points to patriarchal norms and gender biases that prioritize male children over female children, leading to practices such as female infanticide, neglect, and abandonment [12].

Gender stereotypes, ingrained in societal expectations, perpetuate the notion that daughters are inherently inferior or less capable than their male counterparts. Verma [14] adds a feminist exploration of these social injustices, emphasizing how patriarchal structures perpetuate the marginalization and mistreatment of daughters. Norms related to marriage, familial duties, and societal roles contribute to sidelining daughters. The prevailing cultural stigma surrounding issues such as premarital pregnancies or unconventional life choices further exacerbates the challenges faced by daughters, leading to their social exclusion or abandonment. Challenging ingrained social norms is paramount in fostering a more inclusive and equitable societal framework for daughters. Addressing the social factor involves promoting cultural shifts, dismantling gender stereotypes, and advocating for societal acceptance and support for the well-being of lost daughters.

5.2.3 POPULATION GROWTH FACTORS

The population analysis factor emerges as a crucial aspect influencing the silent injustice faced by lost daughters in the present society. Demographic dynamics, including population growth patterns, cultural preferences for male offspring, and family planning practices, contribute significantly to the challenges faced by daughters. Singh (2020) analyzes the population dynamics and the challenges, providing insights into how demographic imbalances arise from gender-based disparities. His study highlights the broader societal implications, including skewed sex ratios and the perpetuation of gender inequality [13].

In regions where cultural norms prioritize male heirs, daughters may encounter neglect or abandonment due to societal expectations regarding family lineage and population continuity. Family planning practices that favor male offspring can result in adverse consequences for daughters, who may be marginalized or undervalued within demographic considerations. Addressing the population factor involves navigating the complexities of cultural preferences, promoting gender-neutral family planning practices, and challenging demographic norms that perpetuate the silent injustice against daughters.

5.2.4 TECHNOLOGICAL FACTORS

The technological factor unveils a dual-edged impact on the silent injustice faced by lost daughters in the present society. While technological advancements (TA) bring opportunities for progress, they also contribute to new challenges and vulnerabilities for daughters. Kumar (2019) explores the role of technological advancements in increasing the vulnerability of lost daughters. His research suggests that while technology can aid in tracking and rescuing lost daughters, it also facilitates trafficking networks that exploit these girls [14].

Technological shifts can lead to gender-based disparities in access to education and employment opportunities, affecting the life trajectories of daughters. Additionally, the rise of social media and online platforms may expose daughters to cyberbullying, harassment, or online exploitation, adding new dimensions to their challenges. Addressing the technological factor requires a nuanced approach that leverages technology for the empowerment of daughters while concurrently addressing the risks and vulnerabilities associated with technological advancements. Developing policies, raising awareness, and providing digital literacy are essential components of mitigating the impact of technology on the silent injustice faced by lost daughters.

5.3 PATTERNS ACROSS INDIA

5.3.1 GEOGRAPHIC DISPARITIES

The silent injustice experienced by lost daughters' manifests are consistent patterns across India, marked by geographic disparities (GD) that exacerbate their vulnerability and marginalization. Regions with deep-rooted cultural norms and societal expectations often witness a more pronounced manifestation of this injustice. In many rural areas, daughters face heightened challenges due to prevailing cultural norms that prioritize male heirs and perpetuate gender-based discrimination. The geographic concentration of such communities intensifies the silent injustice, leading to higher instances of neglect, abandonment, or unequal treatment.

Additionally, limited access to education and healthcare facilities in certain regions amplifies the challenges faced by daughters, perpetuating a cycle of disadvantage. Understanding and addressing geographic disparities is essential for formulating targeted interventions and policies that can mitigate the silent injustice faced by lost daughters. Initiatives focusing on education, healthcare, and community engagement can contribute to breaking the patterns of inequality and creating a more equitable environment for daughters across diverse geographical contexts.

5.3.2 URBAN REALITIES

Contrary to the belief that urban settings provide more opportunities for progress, the silent injustice faced by lost daughters is also prevalent in metropolitan areas, albeit often concealed by the veneer of development. Urbanization brings its own set of challenges, with daughters navigating through complex societal dynamics that may seem progressive but carry underlying biases. In urban settings, daughters may face challenges related to education, employment, and societal expectations. Das [3] examines educational barriers faced by the lost daughters, highlighting the long-term implications for their personal development and societal participation. The fast-paced nature of metropolitan lifestyle can contribute to the erosion of traditional support systems, leaving daughters vulnerable to issues such as isolation, mental health concerns, or economic disparities. The pressure to conform to societal ideals of success and achievement may exacerbate the silent injustice, leading to a different yet equally impactful set of challenges. Recognizing the nuanced nature of the silent injustice in urban areas is crucial for developing comprehensive strategies. Urban-centric policies that address issues such as workplace discrimination, mental health support, and community engagement can play a pivotal role in dismantling the patterns of injustice faced by daughters in metropolitan settings. Analyzing the patterns of injustice faced by lost daughters across the nation unveils a complex interplay of cultural, societal, and geographic factors. Tailoring interventions to address these specific patterns is essential for creating meaningful and sustainable change, ensuring that daughters are afforded equal opportunities and protection regardless of their geographical location.

5.4 IMPACTS OF ISSUE OF LOST DAUGHTERS

5.4.1 INTERGENERATIONAL TRAUMA

The silent injustice experienced by lost daughters reverberates across generations, leaving an indelible mark on the fabric of families and communities. One of the profound impacts is inter-generational trauma, as the psychological and emotional scars inflicted on daughters often transcend their own experiences, influencing the well-being of subsequent generations. The cycle of injustice is perpetuated as daughters who have faced neglect, discrimination, or abandonment may grapple with mental health issues, low self-esteem, or a sense of inadequacy. These struggles can significantly impact their ability to provide a nurturing environment for their own children. Thus, the trauma endured by lost daughters becomes an inheritance passed down through generations, shaping the outlook and life chances of their descendants. Addressing inter-generational trauma necessitates a holistic approach that encompasses mental health support, community-based interventions, and educational initiatives. Breaking the cycle requires not only empowering lost daughters but also equipping future generations with the tools to overcome the legacy of silent injustice and build healthier, more resilient communities.

5.4.2 SOCIOECONOMIC CONSEQUENCES

The silent injustice faced by lost daughters has far-reaching socioeconomic consequences that extend beyond individual households to impact the prosperity of entire communities. The consequences of the silent injustice against daughters are profound and multifaceted. Bhattacharya (2016) conducted a psychological analysis of the impacts on family structures, noting how the loss of daughters leads to emotional and psychological trauma for families and communities [1].

Discrimination against daughters contributes to gender-based economic disparities, limiting their access to education and employment opportunities. This, in turn, hinders the overall economic growth and development of communities. The underutilization of female potential denies societies the full spectrum of talent, creativity, and innovation. The perpetuation of silent injustice against daughters stifles the socioeconomic progress of communities by impeding the contributions women could otherwise make to various sectors. Addressing these disparities requires dismantling systemic barriers, promoting gender-inclusive policies, and fostering environments where daughters can thrive academically and professionally. Recognizing the socioeconomic ramifications of the silent injustice against lost daughters is crucial for formulating comprehensive strategies aimed at community development. By breaking down barriers that limit the potential of daughters, societies can harness the collective strength and talents of their entire population, paving the way for shared prosperity and sustainable growth.

5.5 SUMMARY

In this chapter, authors delve into the multifaceted dimensions of a pervasive issue that often lurks in the shadows, such as discrimination, neglect, and injustice faced by daughters in contemporary society. This exploration unfolds across various points, each shedding light on different aspects of the silent tragedy. The introduction sets the stage by framing the overarching theme—the silent injustice that plagues the lives of daughters in our present societal landscape. It emphasizes the subtlety of this injustice, often overshadowed by louder societal narratives, yet profoundly impactful in shaping the destinies of countless daughters. The discussion section unfolds with a focus on two key points, meticulously examining the intricate web of factors contributing to the silent injustice faced by lost daughters. Economic factors, social dynamics, population pressures, and technological influences intertwine to create an environment where daughters are systematically disadvantaged. This comprehensive analysis lays bare the complexity of the issue, dispelling any notion that the silent injustice faced by daughters is a singular, isolated problem. Moving on to the examination of patterns across the nation (PAN), the narrative broadens its scope to encompass the widespread nature of this injustice. It becomes evident that the plight of lost daughters is not confined to specific regions but reverberates across diverse communities and cultural contexts (CC). This section serves to underscore the urgency of addressing the issue as a collective societal responsibility rather than relegating it to the realm of isolated incidents. The exploration then delves into the far-reaching impacts of the silent injustice, highlighting the inter-generational trauma passed down through daughters who have experienced discrimination. Additionally, the socioeconomic ramifications underscore the broader consequences that extend beyond individual households, affecting the overall prosperity of communities. This nuanced understanding of impacts emphasizes the need for holistic interventions that address both immediate and long-term repercussions. The examination of factors, patterns, and impacts sets the stage for proposing solutions to overcome the barriers faced by lost daughters. The narrative emphasizes the importance of dismantling systemic prejudices, fostering inclusive policies, and creating environments where daughters can thrive. "Lost daughters" serves as a poignant exploration of a pervasive societal issue that demands collective attention and action. By unraveling the silent injustice faced by daughters, this discourse aims to spark awareness, incite empathy, and propel society toward a path of inclusivity and justice for all its members. The narrative not only calls for acknowledgment but also urges communities to actively engage in dismantling the barriers that perpetuate the silent injustice faced by lost daughters in our present society.

ACKNOWLEDGMENTS

I would like to express my sincere gratitude to all those who contributed to the completion of this work, "Lost Daughters: The Silent Injustice of Present Society." First and foremost, I extend my heartfelt thanks to my mentors for their invaluable guidance, support, and constructive feedback throughout the research process. Their expertise has played a crucial role in shaping the direction of this study. I am deeply appreciative of the individuals who generously shared their experiences through interviews, providing invaluable insights that have enriched the depth and authenticity of this research.

KEYWORDS

- **discrimination**
- **gender disparity**
- **inequality**
- **lost daughters**
- **present society**
- **silent injustice**
- **social neglect**
- **societal awareness**

REFERENCES

1. Bhattacharya, S. (2016). Impacts of lost daughters on family structures: A psychosocial analysis (PSA). *Family Dynamics Journal*, *32*(2), 98–115.
2. Chatterjee, N. (2014). Patterns across the nation: Lost daughters in cultural contexts. *Cross-Cultural Studies*, *18*(3), 132–149.
3. Das, A. (2017). Educational barriers and lost daughters: A study in gender disparities. *Education Research Quarterly*, *28*(1), 45–63.
4. Dasgupta, B. (2018). Lost daughters: A human rights perspective. *Human Rights Quarterly*, *23*(4), 198–215.
5. Gupta, V. (2019). Lost daughters: Exploring the intersectionality of social injustice. *Journal of Intersectionality Studies*, *12*(1), 78–95.
6. Mishra, R. (2011). Social factors influencing the lives of lost daughters. *Social Justice and Equality*, *38*(4), 205–222.
7. Nair, A. (2015). Lost daughters in the global context: An international comparative study. *Global Perspectives Journal*, *31*(2), 124–141.
8. Patel, S. K. (2015). Economic factors and the plight of lost daughters: A case study. *Economic and Political Studies*, *40*(4), 267–285.
9. Roy, D. (2018). Lost daughters and the social stigma: A sociological analysis. *Sociological Perspectives*, *45*(1), 34–51.
10. Sen, A. (2010). The silent injustice: Lost daughters in contemporary society. *Gender Studies Journal*, *25*(3), 145–162.
11. Sengupta, M. (2016). Lost daughters and economic inequality: A comparative analysis. *Economic Disparities Review*, *27*(3), 160–177.
12. Sharma, R. (2012). Societal impacts on lost daughters: An anthropological perspective. *Journal of Social Anthropology*, *30*(2), 88–105.
13. Singh, P. (2020). Population faced by lost daughters. *Population Studies Review*, *35*(3), 178–195.
14. Verma, A. (2013). Lost daughters: A feminist exploration of social injustice. *Feminist Review*, *22*(4), 210–227.

CHAPTER 6

Reclaiming Female Postpartum Reproductive Health in Low- and Middle-Income Countries: A Scoping Review

EMI GRACE MARY GOWSHIKA R.

ABSTRACT

This scoping review investigates how female postpartum reproductive health is framed, assessed, and studied in low- and middle-income countries (LMICs) up to 12 months postpartum among women aged 15–49. The review included studies published between 2001 and 2021, resulting in 46 articles after narrowing an initial search of 812 papers. Of the 46 studies, five focused on positive aspects of reproductive health, 13 on negative outcomes, and 28 addressed both without specifying direction. The most common outcome assessed was the resumption of sexual activity. Studies were primarily conducted in sub-Saharan Africa (27), followed by the Middle East (10), Asia (5), Africa (3), and multi-geographical regions (1). Negative sexual health issues included uterine prolapse, vaginismus, perineal tears, dyspareunia, episiotomy, prolapse, female genital cutting, infection, obstetric fistula, postnatal pain, and loss of sexual arousal. While most studies employed quantitative methods, eight qualitative studies revealed challenges in accessing sexual health information and reluctance to seek help for postpartum reproductive issues. The review highlights a significant gap in postpartum reproductive

Holistic Approaches for Women's Sustainable Health, Volume 2: Advancements, Socioeconomic Impacts, and Innovative Strategies. Junaid Ahmad Malik, Anamika Chauhan, and Megh R. Goyal (Eds)

DOI: 10.1201/9781779641656-7

health research in LMICs, with a need for broader integration of sexual health in postpartum care.

6.1 INTRODUCTION

Female health is frequently discussed in terms of their ability to procreate, with little focus on the vast range of outcomes that are specific to females or that affect them more than other genders [20, 56]. Area of reproductive health has faced significant criticism for its perceived lack of attention on the "S" in Sexual and Reproductive Health. The criticisms focus on the underfunding of and absence of policies pertaining to female reproductive health [24, 27]. Reproductive health is defined as "the positive and respectful approach to sexual relationships, including pleasurable and safe sexual experiences, free from coercion, discrimination, or violence" and is an important aspect of sustainable development goal-5 (SDG-5) [60, 62]. Although indicators focus on sexual rights infringements, such as female genital cutting (FGC), child marriage, and sexual violence than the positive ones, like reproductive resumption of sexual activities.

Females undergo physiological and psychological changes during conception and childbirth, and a wealth of research has shown how pregnancy can affect female reproductive health. This includes the need for reproductive wellness guidance during prenatal appointments and childbirth education programs [4, 35]. Additionally, several studies on high-income countries have investigated certain outcomes related to sexual dysfunction or function throughout the postpartum phase. These investigations highlight the frequency of sexual deaths, including incontinence, dyspareunia, altered pleasure perceptions after childbirth and lack of desire, and the necessity of appropriate therapies and counseling techniques to manage them [17, 22, 28]. Furthermore, it is important to consider the psychological impacts of the postpartum period, since postnatal depression affects one in five women and can significantly affect sexual pleasure [35]. Even in high-income nations, postnatal reproductive wellness is still regionalized, underfunded, and lacks policy backing, despite the evidence supporting interventions.

Many women give birth at home or in settings unprepared for obstetric emergencies in nations with low- and middle-incomes (LMICs), which puts them at risk for immediate and long-term postpartum issues, including morbidities related to their sexual health [16, 26, 30, 37]. Important areas of focus for reproductive wellness education and counseling are prenatal and postnatal care; however, there are significant differences in the availability of these services within and between LMIC contexts [9, 13, 35]. Furthermore, significant gaps have been discovered in recent attempts to assess the coverage of excellent services [9, 13]. Maternal health services are frequently restricted to advice on the use of postpartum contraceptives to prevent short-interval pregnancies. Postnatal care, which is typically less comprehensive than antenatal services, emphasizes primarily danger indications to the neonates [6, 52]. Only few emphasize on frequency of postnatal reproductive wellness difficulties and strategies to reduce complications and encourage correct reproductive health in LMICs due to these care gaps.

Therefore, this chapter attempts to compile the body of knowledge about female reproductive well-being in the postnatal phase, with a particular emphasis on studies pertaining to sexual dysfunction and function in women residing in low- and middle-income countries. Research guidelines for practice in LMICs may be written based on these findings.

6.2 METHODOLOGY

6.2.1 PROCEDURE FOR SCOPING REVIEW

This review selected articles that delved into female reproductive health by 12 months following childbirth and were conducted among the objects aged 15–49 in LMICs. Inclusion criteria also required that these studies were published within the last two decades (from 2001 to 2021). Initially, a search on PubMed yielded 812 articles. Subsequently, the review was narrowed down to focus exclusively on studies addressing positive and negative reproductive functions, resulting in a selection of 46 articles (Figure 6.1). Five investigations focused on positive aspects of reproductive health, 13 examined degrading aspects, while 28 articles addressed positive and degrading reproductive health practices without specifying a particular direction.

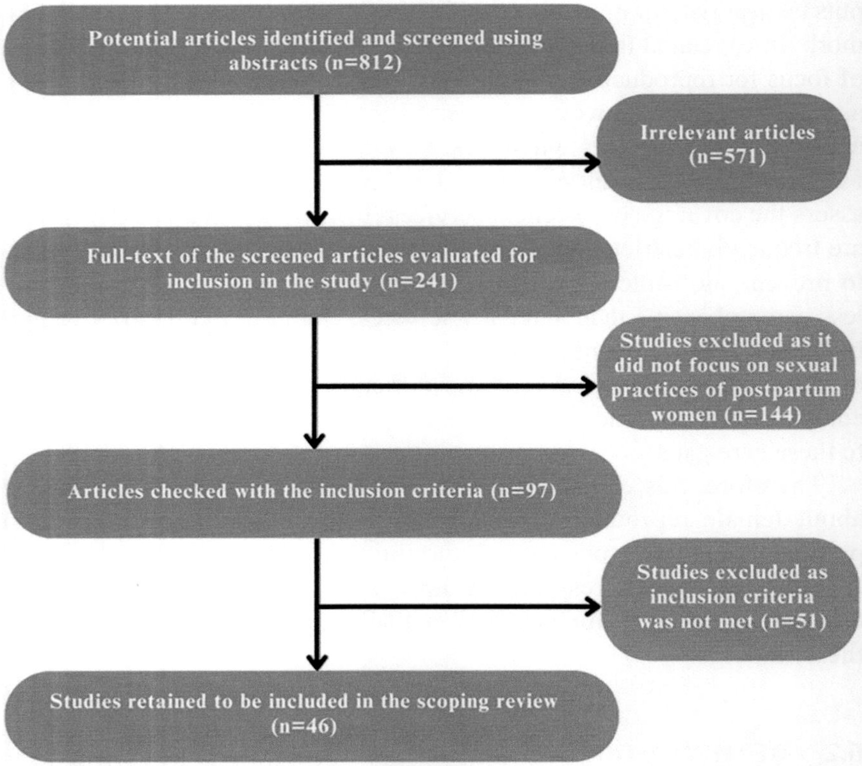

FIGURE 6.1 Quorum diagram for scoping review.

6.2.2 INCLUSION CRITERIA

- Research that was related to the sexual health of women after giving birth: (1) 1 year following birth was the definition of postpartum in this review. (2) This investigation focuses on reproductive functioning (resuming reproductive behaviors, feeling sexually fulfilled, sex satisfaction, sexual excitement, intimacy, and pleasure) and sex disorders (including dyspareunia, sexual assault, and sexual pressure) to provide a deeper insight on reproductive health and to be in accordance with World Health Organization's concept of sexual health, which includes both positive and negative experiences.
- Females of sexual age of 15–49 years were the focus of studies.

- Research undertaken in low- or low-middle-income countries, as classified by the World Bank (2021–2022).
- Investigations in English only.
- Research conducted during 2001–2021.

6.2.3 EXCLUSION CRITERIA

- Research that did not involve women less than a year post-childbirth (that is, research involving exclusively male partners or caregivers).
- Research that did not focus on sexual health, particularly sexual function or dysfunction as described above.
- Research that only focused on abstinence from sex in connection to conception and parental decision-making, as well as studies that focused on postpartum fertility, continuous or unplanned pregnancies, abortion, and negative postnatal family decisions.
- Review of the literature, case studies, study procedures, and gray literature; and investigations that were related to the viewpoints of male reproductive activity during the postnatal period.
- Investigations focusing on extremely particular targets, like only HIVpositive females.
- Studies related to complications encountered "prior or afterward," instead of "during the postpartum" period.

6.3 RESULTS

Forty-six publications met the final requirements for inclusion and exclusion (Tables 6.1–6.3). Of these 46 papers, 5 indicated good aspects of sexual health, 13 indicated negative aspects, and the rest of the 28 indicated the combination of constructive as well as destructive aspects of sexual outcomes or the absence of any direction. The most often studied result was having intercourse again after giving birth. Sub-Saharan Africa accounted for 27 of the studies, with the remaining geographic distribution occurring in the Middle East (n = 10), Asia (n = 5), and the region of North Africa (n = 3); and one study examined 17 Surveys of Demographics and Health (DHS) [15]. Eight research studies, either alone or in addition to other studies, collected the qualitative data. Most studies, including cross-sectional, prospective cohort, and clinical trial designs, were quantitative in nature.

TABLE 6.1 Investigations Related to Constructive Sexual Health Post-Childbirth

References	Study Design	Site of Study	Study Population	Key Outcomes
Anharan et al. [7]	Cross-sectional	Iran	366 women receiving postpartum care 4 months after childbirth in health centers from Mashhad	• Sexual functions of women in different feeding groups varied significantly ($p = 0.04$) • Sexual functions were highest among the exclusive breastfeeding group, followed by breastfeeding + complementary feeding, only formula feeding, and breastfeeding + formula feeding groups • These groups were found to differ in satisfaction scores and mean lubrication ($p = 0.01$)
Mirzaei et al. [43]	Cross-sectional	Iran	604 pregnant and breastfeeding, and women not pregnant and breastfeeding	• The Female Sexual Function Index (FSFI) scores were equivalent for pregnant and lactating women. • The FSFI scores for lactating women for different domains, including reproductive desire ($p < 0.001$), arousal ($p < 0.001$), pain ($p < 0.001$), and ejaculation ($p = 0.007$), were less compared to nonlactating or nonpregnant women • 37% reported sexual dysfunction among pregnant and lactating women compared to 54% in women not pregnant or breastfeeding ($p < 0.001$)
Nezhad and Goodarzi [45]	Cross-sectional	Iran	128 postpartum (6–36 weeks after childbirth) married couples- Ahvaz, Iran	• 91% felt healthy by 2 months postpartum • Sexuality was significantly related to gender, and not significantly to intimacy, sexual, and marital satisfaction • Women's self-appearance was positively connected with sexuality ($p < 0.001$) • Fatigue and intercourse were negatively related ($p < 0.001$)
Zamani et al. [63]	Clinical trial	Iran	80 postpartum females between 18 and 35, from health centers in 3–12 months after childbirth in Mashhad, Iran	• 8 weeks post-counseling for the intervention group, reproductive satisfaction was significant in the experimental group ($p = 0.03$) • Reproductive satisfaction score before and after the counseling was significant in the experimental group only ($p < 0.001$)
Zare et al. [64]	Clinical trial	Iran	79 postpartum care women after 8 weeks of childbirth from health centers in Mashhad, Iran	• At 4 and 8 weeks, pelvic floor muscles strengthened significantly in the intervention group performing pelvic floor exercises ($p < 0.001$) • In experimental ($p < 0.001$) and control ($p = 0.001$) groups, the self-efficacy scores were higher • Differences in self-efficacy scores were noticed in intervention and control groups after 8 weeks of intervention ($p = 0.001$)

TABLE 6.2 Investigations Related to Destructive Sexual Health Post-Childbirth

References	Study Design	Site of Study	Study Population	Key Outcomes
Achour et al. [1]	Prospective Cohort	Tunisia	Vaginismus infected pregnant women, followed into postpartum ($n = 20$)	• Among those who had vaginal delivery, 75% of them had their vaginismus eased • 20% were found to be disinterested in treating their vaginismus • 60% preferred motherhood to sexual life • During pregnancy, 70% felt misunderstood by their healthcare providers
Adanikin et al. [2]	Prospective Cohort	Nigeria	181 women until 6 months postpartum in Ado-Ekiti hospital	• Sexual intercourse was resumed by 27.6% within 6 weeks, 63.3% within 3 months, and 36.2% within 6 months • Dyspareunia was prevalent in 36.2% till 6 months • Dyspareunia or perineal injury was not the result of sexual intercourse
Ahmed et al. [3]	Propsective Cohort	Bangladesh	Four categories of deliveries ($n = 1037$): • Perinatal death • Uncomplicated normal vaginal birth • C-section with no complications • Severe complications during pregnancy/delivery	• The type of deliveries had a significant impact on genital infection ($p = 0.04$), perineal tear ($p < 0.001$), and uterine prolapse ($p < 0.001$) • Incidence of uterine prolapse was less likely in c-section than vaginal deliveries
Assarag et al. [12]	Cross-sectional	Morocco	All women aged between 18 to 49 in Al Massira district ($n = 1210$)	• One of the more common complaints was raised by 44% postpartum • Among those with complaints, 91% did not consult a healthcare provider • 10% reported gynecologic issues, including sexual problems, infected episiotomy, and uterine prolapse • Complaints were higher among women aged 30 and above with delivery complications

TABLE 6.2 *(Continued)*

References	Study Design	Site of Study	Study Population	Key Outcomes
Boene et al. [14]	Qualitative	Mozambique	14 women, each with and without a fistula diagnosis, aged between 16 and 49	• Among the 14 with fistula, 10 had stillbirth, 6 had first birth, 9 had c-section delivery • Most of the patients reported that their sexual activity was halted since the diagnosis of fistula
Gudu and Abdulahi [29]	Prospective Cohort	Ethiopia	Out of 1125 other, 288 nulliparous women	• FGC was believed by 90.3% to have a negative influence on labor and delivery • In 83%, an anterior episiotomy was required to aid delivery • 29% experienced perineal tearing • 39% experienced postpartum complications
Islam et al. [33]	Randomized experiment	Pakistan	Group 1: 100 patients with mediolateral episiotomy Group 2: 100 delivered without episiotomy	• Postnatal pain and dyspareunia were reported among 69% with episiotomy and 12% without episiotomy
Jambola et al. [34]	Cross-sectional	Ethiopia	509 women in their sixth week postpartum	• 20.2% resumed sexual activity within 6 weeks postpartum • 16.9% received guidance for sexual intercourse postpartum • 22.4% reported sexual problems on resuming intercourse • Problems commonly found included: • Impaired sexual desire (10.4%) • Dyspareunia (41.7%) • Vaginal tightness (6.5%) • Multivariate analysis indicated an association between the mother's secondary level education with resuming sexual activity
Lagro et al. [38]	Cross-sectional	Zambia	3 months postpartum women with a baby gestational age of>22 weeks or a weight of>500g	• 90% resumed sexual intercourse within 2 months postpartum • 31% reported vaginal discharge, 7% reported abnormal vaginal bleeding

TABLE 6.2 *(Continued)*

References	Study Design	Site of Study	Study Population	Key Outcomes
				• 90% resumed sexual intercourse within 2 months postpartum • 31% reported vaginal discharge, 7% reported abnormal vaginal bleeding • 17% indicated abnormal vaginal swab results, which tested for lower abdomen pain, infections, fever, and badly smelling discharge • Tender uterus was reported among 10% of those who underwent a vaginal swab
Nazari et al. [44]	Cross-sectional and Qualitative	Iran	Cross-sectional: 250 pregnant women in third trimester	• Qualitative themes: • Sexual needs during postpartum were avoided • Limited awareness • Incorrect beliefs • Education and reproductive health were not significant in the four groups of women ($p = 0.12$)
Oboro and Tabowel [48]	Panel study	Nigeria	122 married women from Kwale Zonal Hospitals, Delta State of Nigeria	• Sexual problems reported during 6 weeks, 3 and 6 months include the following: • Uterine tightness (33%, 21%, 11%) • Painful intercourse (55%, 34%, 19%) • Lack of muscle tone in vagina (22%, 17%, 10%) • Difficulty in ejaculation (41%, 27%, 15%) • Bleeding post sex (19%, 9%, 6%) • 37% reported diminished sexual satisfaction postpartum ($p = 0.004$) • Sexual dysfunction was increased to 47% postpartum compared to prepregnancy (21%) ($p < 0.001$) • 12% out of the 68% who needed healthcare facilities sought professional assistance for sexual dysfunction. • Only 29% discussed sexual health, 98% discussed contraceptives with professionals in clinics

TABLE 6.2 *(Continued)*

References	Study Design	Site of Study	Study Population	Key Outcomes
Surkan et al. [58]	Prospective Cohort	Bangladesh	Married females aged 13 to 44 in Gaibandha and Rangpur with singletons ($n = 39{,}434$)	• Reproductive tract infection ($p < 0.001$) and uterine prolapse ($p < 0.001$) at 3 months postpartum escalated the risk of poor mental health symptoms at 6 months postpartum
White [61]	Qualitative	Cambodia	11 FGDs with 88 women and 20 birth attendants from Khmer	• Resuming sex very soon after childbirth triggered pain, bleeding, and weakness • Dry skin, insomnia, and back stiffness were commonly reported

TABLE 6.3 Investigations Related to Constructive and Destructive Sexual Health Post-Childbirth ($n = 28$)

References	Study Design	Site of Study	Study Population	Key Outcomes
Alum et al. [5]	Cross-sectional	Uganda	374 women within 6 months postpartum in teaching hospitals	• Within 6 weeks of childbirth, 21.6% resumed sexual activities • Higher income, never used contraceptives, low parity, and spouses with high education levels were associated with women resorting to earlier sexual practices postpartum
Anzaku et al. [8]	Cross-sectional	Nigeria	14 weeks postpartum women at teaching hospital in Jos, Nigeria ($n = 340$)	• 77.9% of genital injuries were healed • 29.9% had vaginal lacerations • 19.7% had episiotomies • By this time, 67.6% resumed sexual activities • Reasons for not indulging in sexual activities by this time included: • Disinterest (5.5%) • Spouse not available (38.2%) • To prevent pregnancy (16.4%) • Cultural reasons (3.6%) • Unwell (12.7%)

TABLE 6.3 *(Continued)*

References	Study Design	Site of Study	Study Population	Key Outcomes
				• Advised by a healthcare professional (1.8%) • 5.6% pursued medical advice for sexual problems • 22.2% experienced sexual problems • Through multivariate regression analysis, those who underwent vaginal childbirth were prone to many reproductive issues ($p = 0.01$)
Asadi et al. [11]	Qualitative	Iran	23 postpartum women and their healthcare providers	• Postpartum women reported the following reasons for not resuming sexual activities: • Less sexually attractive than before • Uneasiness due to loosened vaginal muscles • Decreased self-confidence • Dyspareunia • Burning or dryness leading to less sexual desire
Borda et al. [15]	Cross-sectional	Involved 17 DHS countries	15 out of 17 countries included all women, and the other 2 only married women	• The least sexual activity was reported during 0–2.9 months postpartum by all women from each country • The majority of women from 13 countries reported sexual activities by 3–5.9 months • Women not exclusively breastfeeding among 10 countries reported resuming sexual activity resumption than actively breastfeeding women • With the return of menses, sexual activity was resumed by women in 16 countries
Dadabhai et al. [18]	Prospective Cohort	Malawi	460 HIV-uninfected and 418 HIV-infected postpartum women	• Both groups reported resorting to sexual activities in almost 6% after 6 weeks postpartum and 82% at 12 months post childbirth • Marital status was directly associated with early sexual activity resumption in both groups

TABLE 6.3 *(Continued)*

References	Study Design	Site of Study	Study Population	Key Outcomes
Desgrees-du-Lou and Brou [19]	Qualitative	Cote d'Ivoire	Parents of weaned children under age 5, men (n = 10), women (n = 23)	• The pointers noted for abstinence from sexual activities until complete weaning were as follows: • Taboos of breastfeeding issues • Until menses resumed for the woman • Risk of pregnancy • Desire of their partner • Risks of STIs and/or HIV
Ezebialu and Eke [21]	Cross-sectional	Nigeria	860 postpartum mothers at the first postnatal clinic visit	• Vaginal intercourse was resumed by 29.7% at their first clinical visit • Those not resumed sexual activity had a significant association with place of residence (p = 0.001), return of menses (p = 0.004), mode of childbirth (p = 0.039), minimal/ no education (p = 0.009), marital status (0.002), and age extremes (p = 0.007) • Sexual activity resumption was strongly related to menses and absence of HIV ($p < 0.001$) • Reasons for abstinence included: • Lack of interest (9.1%) • Avoiding pregnancy (64.5%) • Fear of pain (2.5%) • Unavailability of partner (14.9%) • No reason (11.6%) • Full physical recovery (39.5%)
Gadisa et al. [23]	Cross-sectional	Ethiopia	14 weeks postpartum, women were selected randomly (n = 330)	• 14% started intercourse <4 weeks • 53.9% started intercourse <6 weeks postpartum • On the spouse's request, 77% resumed sex • Early sex resumption was associated with low income, sexual activity during pregnancy, monogamous marriage, using a contraceptive and having a c-section delivery.

TABLE 6.3 *(Continued)*

References	Study Design	Site of Study	Study Population	Key Outcomes
Glynn et al. [25]	Cross-sectional	Multicountry (Cameroon, Zambia, Kenya)	6 antenatal clinics: Yaounde, Cameroon (n = 1532) Kisumu, Kenya (n = 1480) Ndola, Zambia (n = 1021)	• Abstinence from sexual activity >6 months postpartum was reported in more than half of them from Yaounde, 13% in Ndola, and 17% in Kisumu • Abstinence greater than 12 months revealed by 8% in Kisumu, 23% in Yaounde, and 4% in Ndola • In Yaounde, postpartum abstinence was associated with HIV and amenorrhea • In Ndola, postpartum abstinence was associated with HIV, but not in Kisumu
Iliyasu et al. [31]	Cross-sectional	Nigeria	Postpartum mothers with children under 5 years (n = 300)	• 6–11 months postpartum, 76.7% women resumed sex • Returning to sexual practices was influenced by: • Healing of perineal wounds (77.3%) • Drainage of lochia (66%) • Stimulate lactation (81.3%) • Stamina of mother (92.7%) • Ritual practices were not believed by educated women ($p < 0.01$), which included: • Confinement = 40 days (12.3%) • Hot ritual baths (86%) • Eating spicy foods (85.3%) • Those with medical complaints resorted to traditional remedies (66%) and modern medicines (25%). • 9% did not use any medication
Iliyasu et al. [32]	Cross-sectional	Nigeria	Mothers attending postnatal clinics (n = 317)	• Episiotomies were done on 52.1%, perineal tears were experienced by 25% and vaginal lacerations by 70.8% • Postpartum abstinence was followed between 4 and 28 weeks, after which 66.9% resorted to sexual practices • Reasons for abstinence included: • Lack of interest (2.9%)

TABLE 6.3 *(Continued)*

References	Study Design	Site of Study	Study Population	Key Outcomes
				• Avoiding pregnancy (13.3%) • Infant being very young (81%) • Divorced/widowed (2.9%) • Dyspareunia (32.5%) • Vaginal dryness/soreness (15.6%) • Diminished sexual desire (31.6%) • Vaginal discharge (6.1%) • Vaginal looseness (15.6%) • Reasons for indulgence included: • Own desire (14.6%) • Partner's desire (67.5%) • Strong significant associations for resuming sex were found in cohabiting with husband ($p = 0.001$), infant's age 1–6 months ($p = 0.02$) and >6 months ($p = 0.001$), vaginal delivery ($p = 0.05$), not resumed menses ($p = 0.003$), having 5 or more living children ($p = 0.03$)
Kinuthia et al. [36]	Prospective Cohort	Kenya	HIV-uninfected pregnant women ($n = 1252$)	• Resumption of early sex 2–36 weeks post childbirth was related to: • Partner's age • Being married • History of anal sex • Primary education and beyond • C-section delivery • Unknown HIV status of partner
Lundberg and Trieu [39]	Cross-sectional and Qualitative	Vietnam	Vietnamese postpartum women ($n = 115$)	• 3–4 months post childbirth, sexual activity was avoided • Reasons for avoiding sexual activity included: • Impact on health • Improper perineal healing

TABLE 6.3 *(Continued)*

References	Study Design	Site of Study	Study Population	Key Outcomes
				• Uterine prolapse issues • Risk of pregnancy • Disinterest in sex • Caring for infants
Maamri et al. [40]	Cross-sectional	Tunisia	6 months postpartum women (n = 100)	• Postpartum abstinence from sexual activities lasted for 21 months • Sexual activity was resumed by women who underwent instrumental vaginal delivery 6 months postpartum (p = 0.01) • Reasons for abstinence included: • Fear of pregnancy (13%) • Lack of desire (37%) • Fear of pain (32%) • Physiological changes (31%) • Reduced sexual satisfaction (33%) • Dyspareunia (14%)
Mbekenga et al. [41]	Qualitative	Tanzania	2 RCH clinics, Tanzania (n = 10)	• Reasons provided for abstinence from sexual activities included: • Absence of information to treat episiotomy wounds • No proper health education in clinics • Until cessation of breastfeeding for 4 years • Infant developmental problems
Mekonnen [42]	Cross-sectional	Ethiopia	Postpartum women within 12 months in Gondar city, Northwest Ethiopia (n = 634)	• Vaginal delivery without episiotomy (61.4%), with episiotomy (11.8%), and instrumental forceps (6.5%); the others had c-section delivery • Before 6 weeks postpartum, 26.9% resumed sex • 69.2% reported no issues during sexual activities • Early resumption of sex was associated, through multivariable logistic regression analysis with:

TABLE 6.3 *(Continued)*

References	Study Design	Site of Study	Study Population	Key Outcomes
				• Partner demand • Low parity • Using family planning • In postnatal care • Urban residence
Nkwabong et al. [46]	Retrospective Cohort	Camerron	6 weeks postpartum women between November 2013 to December 2013 (n = 120)	• 79.1% resumed sexual activities • Vaginal and uncomplicated deliveries increased the number of women starting sexual activities before 6 weeks postpartum compared to c-section deliveries ($p < 0.001$) • Perineal trauma was more prevalent among those who had an episiotomy ($p < 0.001$)
Nolens et al. [47]	Prospective Cohort	Uganda	Childbirth through SSCs in Mulago National Referral Hospital, Kampala, Uganda	• 90.7% had a known perineal discomfort: • 34% had an intact perineum • 35.9% had an episiotomy • 0.8% had third-degree tear • 29.8% had second-degree tear • Vacuum extraction during labor vs. C-section had reduced pain post 6 weeks ($p < 0.001$) and 6 months ($p = 0.05$) • Women who had vacuum extraction (40%) vs. C-section (28.3%) resumed sex at 6 weeks postpartum ($p = 0.01$)
Odar et al. [49]	Cross-sectional	Uganda	3–6 months postpartum women at Mugalo Hospital immunization clinics (n = 216)	• 87.2% episiotomies healed, and 12.8% were infected • 66.4% resumed sexual intercourse after 3 months • Reasons for sexual activity resumption included: • Husband's demands (46%) • Cultural demands (10%)

TABLE 6.3 *(Continued)*

References	Study Design	Site of Study	Study Population	Key Outcomes
				• Convenience (37%) • Reasons for abstinence from sex included: • Health advice (37%) • Not well (18%) • Husband's demands (23%) • Not interested (22%) • Dyspareunia (62.5%) • Vaginal bleeding (15.6%) • Vaginal discharge (18.8%) • Tears and injuries (3.1%) • Older women were found to sought professional help during medical problems ($p = 0.01$)
Osinde et al. [50]	Cross-sectional	Uganda	Women from postpartum hospital ($n = 131$)	• Within 6 weeks postpartum, 58% resumed sexual activities • Early resort to sex was significantly associated with the education level of the husbands' ($p = 0.05$) • Reasons for delay in resuming sexual activities included: • Fear of pregnancy • Unhealed wounds • Geographic separation from spouses
Rezaei et al. [51]	Cross-sectional	Iran	Women from 10 urban health centers ($n = 380$)	• Sexual dysfunction was reported in 76.3% • Lack of sexual desire was reported by 79% • Sexual dysfunction was most likely found in women who exclusively breastfed, as reported by a multivariate regression analysis ($p = 0.01$)

TABLE 6.3 *(Continued)*

References	Study Design	Site of Study	Study Population	Key Outcomes
Shabangu and Madiba [53]	Qualitative	Eswatini	Purposive selection of 15 postpartum women from a health facility	• Most of them resumed sexual intercourse after their infant turned 6 months old • Women were not allowed to live with their husbands postpartum, leading to delayed sexual activities • A major disadvantage included the increase in HIV among men, as they were not prevented from having sexual activities with other women
Sheikhi et al. [54]	Randomized controlled trial	Iran	3–5 days postpartum women with low-grade perineal tears (n = 94)	• 96% had an episiotomy and 4% had perineal tears • After counseling, SFI score escalated from 12.7 to 17.4 ($p < 0.001$) • Difference was observed in the intervention group after counseling, which included: • Arousal ($p = 0.009$) • Desire ($p = 0.001$) • Orgasm ($p = 0.001$) • Lubrication ($p = 0.001$) • Dyspareunia ($p = 0.003$)
Shirvani et al. [55]	Cross-sectional	Iran	3–12 months postpartum women from January to July 2008 (n = 490)	• Postpartum sexual abstinence was noticed for 57.17 ± 27.95 days • Beyond 45 days, 52.9% were following abstinence • Reasons for abstinence included: • Avoiding pregnancy (2.5%) • Fear of pain (8.6%) • Bleeding (0.6%) • Tiredness (2.2%) • Reduced sexual desire (40%) • Sexual function was positively correlated with: • Postpartum duration ($r = 0.17$) • Marriage duration ($r = –0.08$)

TABLE 6.3 *(Continued)*

References	Study Design	Site of Study	Study Population	Key Outcomes
Sule-Odu et al. [57]	Prospective Cohort	Nigeria	Breastfed one baby for >= 6 months and have delivered singleton babies (n = 371)	• 84.6% abstained from sexual practices after 1 month postpartum • Abstinence was associated with age, social status, and feeding pattern
Ugwu et al. [59]	Prospective Cohort	Nigeria	Intervention group-C-section delivery (n = 50) Control group-vaginal delivery (n = 50)	• 25% of women who had vaginal delivery experienced perineal tearing • 6 weeks postpartum, 74.4% c-section women resumed sex vs. 52.1% vaginal delivery women • The mean scores were higher for c-section women related to pain, satisfaction, and orgasm ($p < 0.05$)
Zulu [65]	Mixed method	Malawi	Rural areas: south (n = 273), north (n = 288), central (n = 550)	• Reasons for abstinence included: • Contaminate breast milk • Male partner's ill-health • Postpartum bleeding • Most of them resumed sexual activities between 3 and 6 months postpartum

6.3.1 CONSTRUCTIVE SEXUAL HEALTH

Libido, fulfillment, enjoyment, orgasm, pelvic floor power, reproductive confidence, female sexual function, and intimacy were the outcomes of five studies [7, 43, 45, 63, 64] that looked at favorable sexual wellness during the postpartum period (Table 6.1). Interestingly, all five studies were carried out within Iran, mostly in the framework of interventions or with the use of control groups. It was discovered how a program of strengthening the pelvic floor muscles affected both sexual self-efficacy and pelvic floor strength, and it was discovered that the intervention group significantly outperformed the control group in both measures [64]. Participants in the intervention group reported higher levels of sexual satisfaction, according to the evaluation of the efficacy of sexual health counseling [63]. Two other studies, with varying degrees of success, looked at the relationship between newborn feeding patterns and sexual function [7, 43]. Furthermore, the study on intimacy and sexuality in relationships revealed that a high degree of intimacy could operate as a constructive factor against the detrimental aspects of low sexual pleasure on general satisfaction in marriage [45].

6.3.2 DESTRUCTIVE SEXUAL HEALTH

Vaginismus, dyspareunia, a caesarean, perineal tears, rupture, infection, fistula during delivery, cutting of female genitalia, after childbirth pain, prolapse of uterus, force to return to intercourse, reproductive assault, and loss of sexual arousal were among the detrimental sexual health outcomes that were observed in thirteen studies (Table 6.2).

One of the most researched adverse effects on postpartum women's sexual health was dyspareunia, or painful sex. In Nigeria [2], more than one-third of women experienced dyspareunia six months after giving birth. Dyspareunia was among the most often reported sexual illnesses in Ethiopia; one in five women complained of it when they resumed sexual activity after giving birth [34]. When dyspareunia and episiotomy were compared in Pakistan [33], patients with the procedure had a higher prevalence of dyspareunia (69% vs. 12%). Furthermore, dyspareunia at three months following delivery was more common among females who had experienced trauma or indicated prenatal dyspareunia. In Nigeria, it was observed that the painful sexual activity reduced the time following delivery, with roughly 55% of females complaining about uncomfortable sex at 2 months following delivery and reducing to <20% at six months after childbirth [48].

If forceful or compelled intimacy is examined, resumption of sex was also included in the bad consequences related to sexual health. Although the duration of postpartum sexual abstinence varied depending on cultural circumstances, it was generally observed in all settings, yet not every woman who returned to intercourse did so voluntarily. In Ethiopia, specifically, half of the females who started sex under 6 weeks after giving birth claimed to have been under pressure from their husbands to do so. Even though our search turned up just three qualitative studies that focused specifically on poor sexual wellness, these studies were useful in clarifying cultural perceptions and anxieties about postpartum sexual health [61]. Women in Mozambique who had fistulas reported no intercourse since the condition began. One of the women said her spouse had taken advantage of her "handicap" to get a second wife [14].

Most women experienced reproductive health complications after delivery across studies and settings, but there was no evidence of help-seeking or intervention engagement. Women in Tunisia reported experiencing vaginismus symptoms after giving birth, yet 60% of them did not think that having sex was more important than being a mother. Additionally, no woman finished a pelvic-floor training program or sought out sexologist treatment [1]. Furthermore, according to several research studies, women felt uneasy talking to healthcare practitioners about sexual health-related issues or that they were ill-prepared to address them. In Nigeria, just 29% of women in the research reported having conversations on sexual health, even though 98% of them said they had received counseling on contraception [48]. Similarly, Iranian women perceived that medical professionals frequently disregarded their postpartum needs related to sexual health [44].

A cross-sectional analysis of unusual discharge from the vagina in Zambian women, genital tearing and complications after childbirth associated with FGC in the nation of Ethiopia, and urinary tearing as well as genital rupture in Bangladesh were among the other findings. RTIs were also linked to prolapse of the uterus and postpartum depression [3, 29, 38, 58].

6.3.3 NEUTRAL SEXUAL HEALTH

Table 6.3 ($n = 28$) summarizes studies that evaluated women's health after childbirth from a neutral standpoint or that looked at positive as well as negative effects relating to sexual health. Notably, bulk of research in this category focuses on the frequency or correlates with resuming sex; little attention is paid to the advantages or disadvantages of scheduling sex during the postpartum phase. Resuming sex was linked to a woman's menstrual cycle returning, according to a multicountry DHS investigation; qualitative evidence from Malawi and Cote d'Ivoire supported this practice [15, 19, 65].

Resuming sexual activity was correlated with their husbands' expectations or requirements in terms of sex [8, 32, 40, 53]. The demand placed on women to restart sex was illustrated in a qualitative study conducted in Cote d'Ivoire. Although some women thought polygynous weddings were helpful in permitting extended periods of abstinence, others showed concerns associated with STI risks [19]. According to a Kenyan study, having forced intercourse in the previous month was linked to higher chances of having sex again [36].

Few studies examined the relationship between cultural behaviors and women's sexual health, regardless of when sex is resumed. Women in Nigeria engage in a variety of postpartum behaviors, such as hot ceremonial baths, lying on warm beds, and eating foods during periods of postpartum abstinence [31]. Significant regional heterogeneity in cultural customs still existed in Malawi; however, postnatal abstinence was described as necessary for the healing of the mom, partner, and child, and early resumption was associated with several health issues [65].

Notably, women reported in the qualitative data that they felt less attractive to men and that their desire and sexual health were affected by their lower self-esteem; on the other hand, their partner's approval of altered bodies helped them feel less anxious about having sex [11]. Some women said nothing more than the fact that they were too exhausted to have sex [39].

In research pertaining to both positive and bad sexual health, women also reported having trouble talking to medical professionals about sex or asking for help [8]. Less than a third of postpartum women in a Nigerian study requested guidance for the reproductive illnesses; common excuses for not seeking health care included feeling self-conscious, thinking the issue would go away on by itself, traditions and customs, and lacking a female doctor to consult [32]. Women in Tanzania reported receiving excessive health education all at once during prenatal care, and they believed that some of this knowledge ought to be dispersed throughout the course of postnatal visits [41]. Women in Uganda said that they were unaware of when to restart having relations and how to manage the related health and safety concerns since health providers' advice was inconsistent at the time of discharge [49].

6.4 DISCUSSION

Only 5 of the 46 research articles indicated sexual health in LMICs during the postpartum period, with most of the investigations focusing on good sexual health. Instead, postpartum morbidities or delivery problems (episiotomies, fistula, and prolapse) were typically used to frame discussions about sexual health. Furthermore, most of the research was done in sub-Saharan Africa; although there were about three times as many articles from this region as there were from other regions, many of these investigations only looked at the incidence or predictors of sexual resuming. Overall, compared to higher-income nations, the research on female reproductive health after delivery within LMICs is still quite small. This underscores the need to investigate a broader spectrum of reproductive health consequences, especially those pertaining to good sexual health.

This review makes it abundantly evident that postpartum women in LMICs require more information on sexual health. Previous research from throughout the world has brought attention to the dearth of information on good sexual wellness, which is impacted by people's access to sexuality education, which includes information on dangers and weaknesses, access to sexual wellness treatment, and the creation of environments that are supportive of constructive reproductive health [60]. This chapter revealed that females who witnessed reproductive health problems during the postpartum phase were reluctant to seek medical attention. This was due to their feelings of embarrassment as well as their perception that medical professionals lacked the necessary training to address problems pertaining to women's sexual health. Furthermore, a lot of women resorted to cultural customs that were mostly upheld by family members because they were unsure of the ideal time for a safe resumption of sex. To enable women to resume sex when they believe it is appropriate for them and their relationships, postnatal care services must incorporate sexual health education, including advice on seeking treatment for any potential sexual health morbidities. Furthermore, normalizing sexual health problems helps lessen women's feelings of shame and stigma, especially during the period when their bodies are going through significant physical and hormonal changes. Given delays in the resumption of sexual activity and the recognition of associated dysfunctions, expanding the reach of postpartum care services well into the postpartum period and providing specific instructions for healthcare professionals on how to incorporate information on sexual health into postpartum protocols are imperative.

While maternal healthcare facilities are growing quickly in LMICs, focus is now also being placed on evaluating the quality of these services in addition to ensuring their availability. However, sexual health counseling is not currently included in quality of services assessments, and most of them have only paid passing attention to the substance of prenatal services rather than the quality of postnatal care [10]. The research and practice field lacks a firm understanding of when and in what manner sexual health is addressed in the absence of data to assess the reception and subject matter of sexual counseling and health education as part of prenatal and/or postnatal care services [9]. Considering the significant influence these data will have on developing clinical practice guidelines, future research must aim to close this data gap. The meticulous implementation of the scoping protocol, the use of library resources in the development and revision of the method of search, and the study's emphasis on a neglected subject that encompasses both beneficial and detrimental sexual health outcomes are its main strengths. Nevertheless, there are some limitations to this research. Many research studies on sexual wellness in postpartum times with small sample sizes or scant metrics are included in this scoping review chapter.

Because most of the included research articles remained cross-sectional in nature, inferences about the temporal relationships were constrained. Furthermore, some studies were excluded from the current scoping review because it was impossible to determine whether the results were unique to the first-year postpartum because the inclusion criteria for those studies did not specify the timing within the postpartum period. Because so many publications met our final criteria, methodological rigor was not evaluated as a component of this evaluation. Finally, as our search technique did not specifically look at women's sexual health in connection to conception and contraception, it is possible that some papers that looked more widely at women's sexual wellbeing in the period following delivery were overlooked.

6.5 SUMMARY

There is a need to further look at sexual health issues beyond the post-partum period and to investigate obstacles that prevent women with sexual health morbidities from getting care. It is necessary to investigate positive women's sexual health further, including any variables that might support positive sexual health throughout the postpartum phase. In the end, women's sexual health may be prioritized among global development priorities, like the SDGs, and the breadth of their health needs can be fully met, regardless of the situation, by expanding the set of indicators related to positive sexual health.

KEYWORDS

- **dyspareunia**
- **episiotomy**
- **negative sexual health positive sexual health**
- **postpartum**
- **sexual activity**

REFERENCES

1. Achour, R. (2019). Vaginismus and pregnancy: Epidemiological profile and management difficulties. *Psychological Research and Behavior Management*, *12*, 137–143.
2. Adanikin, A. I. (2015). Resumption of intercourse after childbirth in southwest Nigeria. *European Journal of Contraception and Reproductive Health Care*, *20*(4), 241–248.
3. Ahmed, F. A. (2012). Occurrence and determinants of postpartum maternal morbidities and disabilities among women in Bangladesh, MATLAB. *Journal of Health and Population Nutrition*, *30*(2), 143–158.

4. Allen, L. & Fountain, L. (2007). Addressing sexuality and pregnancy in childbirth education classes. *The Journal of Perinatal Education*, *16*(1), 32–36.
5. Alum, A. C. (2015). Factors associated with early resumption of sexual intercourse among postnatal women in Uganda. *Reproductive Health*, *12*(1), 1–15.
6. Amouzou, A. (2017). Measuring postnatal care contacts for mothers and newborns: An analysis of data from the MICS and DHS surveys. *Journal of Global Health*, *7*, 2–10.
7. Anharan, Z. K. (2015). Postpartum sexual function in women and infant feeding methods. *Journal of Pakistan Medical Association*, *65*(3), 1–7.
8. Anzaku, A. & Mikah, S. (2014). Postpartum resumption of sexual activity, sexual morbidity and use of modern contraceptives among Nigerian women. *Annals of Medicine and Health and Scientific Research*, *4(*2), 210–216.
9. Arroyave, L. (2021). Inequalities in antenatal care coverage and quality: An analysis from 63 low and middle-income countries using the ANC content-qualified coverage indicator. *International Journal of Equity Health*, *20*(102), 1–10.
10. Arroyave, L., Ghada, E. & Barros, A. J. D. (2021). A new content-qualified antenatal care coverage indicator: Development and validation of a score using national health surveys in low- and middle-income countries. *Journal of Global Health*, *11*, e04008.
11. Asadi, M., Noroozi, M. & Alavi, M. (2021). Exploring the experiences related to postpartum changes: Perspectives of mothers and healthcare providers in Iran. *BMC Pregnancy and Childbirth*, *21*(7), 1–31.
12. Assarag, B. (2013). Maternal postpartum morbidity in Marrakech: What do women feel what doctors diagnose? *BMC Pregnancy and Childbirth*, *13*, 1–16.
13. Benova, L. (2018). Not just a number: Examining coverage and content of antenatal care in low-income and middle-income countries. *BMJ Global Health*, *3*(e000779), 1–11.
14. Boene, H. (2020). Obsteric fistula in southern Mozambique: Qualitative study on women's experiences of care pregnancy, delivery and post-partum. *Reproductive Health*, *17*(1), 1–24.
15. Borda, M. R., Winfrey, W. & McKaig, C. (2010). Return to sexual activity and modern family planning use in the extended postpartum period: Analysis of findings from seventeen countries. *African Journal of Reproductive Health*, *14*, 72–79.
16. Campbell, O. M., & Graham, W. J. (2006). Strategies for reducing maternal mortality: Getting on with what works. *The Lancet*, *368*(9543), 1284–1299.
17. Cattani, L., De Maeyer, L., Verbakel, J. Y., Bosteels, J., & Deprest, J. (2022). Predictors for sexual dysfunction in the first year postpartum: A systematic review and meta-analysis. *BJOG*, *129*(7), 1017–1028.
18. Dadabhai, S. (2020). Resumption of postpartum sexual activity and menses among HIV- infected women on lifelong antiretroviral treatment compared to HIV-uninfected women in Africa. *International Journal of Gynaecology and Obstetrics*, *149*(2), 211–218.
19. Desgrees-Du-Lou, A. & Brou, H. (2005). Resumption of sexual relations following childbirth: Norms, practices and reproductive health issues in Abidjan. *Cote d'Ivoire Reproductive Health Matters*, *13*(25), 155–163.
20. Editorial, L. (2007). Women: More than mothers. *Lancet, 370*, e1283.

21. Ezebialu, I. U. & Eke, A. C. (2012). Resumption of vaginal intercourse in the early postpartum period: Determinants and considerations for child spacing in a Nigerian population. *Journal of Obstetrics and Gynaecology (Lahore), 32*(4), 353–356.
22. Fan, D. (2017). Sexual dysfunction and mode of delivery in Chinese primiparous women: Systematic review and meta-analysis. *BMC Pregnancy and Childbirth, 17*(1), 408–415.
23. Gadisa, T. B. (2021). Early resumption of postpartum sexual intercourse and its associated risk factors among married postpartum women who visited public hospitals of Jimma zone, Southwest Ethiopia: A cross-sectional study. *PLoS One, 16,* 1–8.
24. Gilby, L. (2021). Global health without sexual and reproductive health and rights? Analysis of United Nations documents and country statements, 2014–2019. *BMJ Global Health, 6*(3), 1–10.
25. Glynn, J. R. (2001). Research letters: Is long postpartum sexual abstinence a risk factor for HIV? *AIDS, 15*(8), 1059–1061.
26. Gon, G. (2018). The frequency of maternal morbidity: Systematic review of systematic reviews. *International Journal of Obstetrics and Gynaecology, 141*(1), 20–38.
27. Gruskin, S. (2019). Sexual health, sexual rights and sexual pleasure: Meaningfully engaging the perfect triangle. *Sexual and Reproductive Health Matter, 27*(1), 29–40.
28. Grussu, P., Vicini, B. & Quatraro, R. M. (2021). Sexuality in the perinatal period: A systematic review of reviews and recommendations for practice. *Sexual & Reproductive Healthcare, 30,* e100668.
29. Gudu, W. & Abdulahi, M. (2017). Labor, delivery and postpartum complications in nulliparous women with female genital mutilation admitted to Karamara hospital. *Ethiopian Medical Journal, 55*(1), 11–17.
30. Hardee, K., Gay, J. & Blanc, A. K. (2012). Maternal morbidity: Neglected dimension of safe motherhood in the developing world. *Global Public Health, 7*(6), 603–617.
31. Iliyasu, Z., Kabir, M., Galadanci, H. S., Abubakar, I. S., Salihu, H. M., & Aliyu, M. H. (2006). Postpartum beliefs and practices in Danbare village, Northern Nigeria. *Journal of Obstetrics and Gynaecology, 26*(3), 211–215.
32. Iliyasu, Z. (2018). Correlates of postpartum sexual activity and contraceptive use in Kano Northern Nigeria. *African Journal of Reproductive Health, 22*(1), 103–112.
33. Islam, A. (2013). Morbidity for episiotomy. *Journal of Pakistan Medical Association, 63*(6), 696–701.
34. Jambola, E. T. (2020). Early resumption of sexual intercourse and its associated factors among postpartum women in western Ethiopia: Cross-sectional study. *International Journal of Womens' Health, 12,* 381–391.
35. Johnson, C. E. (2011). Sexual health during pregnancy and the postpartum (CME). *The Journal of Sexual Medicine, 8*(5), 1267–1284.
36. Kinuthia, J. (2017). Sexual behavior and vaginal practices during pregnancy and postpartum: Implications for HIV prevention strategies. *Journal of Acquired Immune Deficiency Syndrome, 74*(2), 142–149.
37. Koblinsky, M. (2012). Maternal morbidity and disability and their consequences: Neglected agenda in maternal health. *Journal of Health and Population Nutrition, 30*(2), 124–130.

38. Lagro, M. (2003). Postpartum health among rural Zambian women. *African Journal of Reproductive Health, 7*(3), 41–48.
39. Lundberg, P. C. & Thu, T. T. N. (2011). Vietnamese women's cultural beliefs and practices related to the postpartum period. *Midwifery*, *27*(5), 731–736.
40. Maamri, A. (2019). Sexuality during the postpartum period: Study of a population of Tunisian women. *Tunis Medicine*, *97*(5), 704–710.
41. Mbekenga, C. K. (2011). Joy, struggle and support: Postpartum experiences of first-time mothers in a Tanzanian suburb. *Women Birthing*, *24*(1), 24–31.
42. Mekonnen, B. D. (2020). Factors associated with early resumption of sexual intercourse among women during extended postpartum period in Northwest Ethiopia: Cross-sectional study. *Contraception and Reproductive Medicine*, *5*(1), 1–8.
43. Mirzaei, N. (2021). Sexual function, mental health, and quality of life under strain of COVID-19 pandemic in Iranian pregnant and lactating women: Comparative cross-sectional study. *Health and Quality of Life Outcomes*, *19*(66), 1–8.
44. Nazari, S. (2021). Postpartum care promotion based on maternal education needs: Mixed study. *Journal of Education and Health Promotion*, *10*(July), 1–6.
45. Nezhad, M. Z. & Goodarzi, A. M. (2011). Sexuality, intimacy, and marital satisfaction in Iranian first-time parents. *Journal of Sex & Marital Therapy*, *37*(2), 77–88.
46. Nkwabong, E., Ilue, E. E. & Nana, N. T. (2019). Factors associated with the resumption of sexual intercourse before the scheduled six-week postpartum visit. *Tropical Doctrine*, *49*(4), 260–264.
47. Nolens, B. (2018). Birthing experience and quality of life after vacuum delivery and second-stage caesarean section: Prospective cohort study in Uganda. *Tropical Medicine in International Health*, *23*(8), 914–922.
48. Oboro, V. & Tabowei, T. (2002). Sexual function after childbirth in Nigerian women. *International Journal of Gynaecology and Obstetrics*, *78*(3), 249–250.
49. Odar, E., Wandabwa, J. & Kiondo, P. (2003). Sexual practices of women within six months of childbirth in Mulago hospital, Uganda. *African Health Sciences, 3*(3), 117–123.
50. Osinde, M. O., Kaye, D. K. & Kakire, O. (2012). Influence of HIV infection on women's resumption of sexual intercourse and use of contraception in the postpartum period in rural Uganda. *International Journal of Gynaecology and Obstetrics*, *116*(2), 170–171.
51. Rezaei, N. (2017). Postpartum sexual functioning and its predicting factors among Iranian women. *Malays Journal of Medical Sciences*, *24*(1), 94–103.
52. Sacks, E. & Langlois, E. V. (2016). Postnatal care: Increasing coverage, equity, and quality. *Lancet Global Health, 4*, e442–e443.
53. Shabangu, Z. & Madiba, S. (2019). The role of culture in maintaining post-partum sexual abstinence of Swazi women. *International Journal of Environmental Research and Public Health*, *16*(14), 1–18.
54. Sheikhi, Z. P., Navidian, A. & Rigi, M. (2020). Effect of sexual health education on sexual function and resumption of sexual intercourse after childbirth in primiparous women. *Journal of Education and Health Promotion, 9,* 1–6.
55. Shirvani, M. A., Nesami, M. B. & Bavand, M. (2010). Maternal sexuality after childbirth among Iranian women. *Pakistan Journal of Biological Sciences*, *13*(8), 385–389.

56. Strobino, D. M., Grason, H. & Minkovitz, C. (2002). Charting a course for the future of women's health in the United States: Concepts, findings and recommendations. *Social Science and Medicine*, *54*(5), 839–848.
57. Sule-Odu, A. O. (2008). Postpartum sexual abstinence and breastfeeding pattern in Sagamu, Nigeria. *African Journal of Reproductive Health*, *12*(1), 96–100.
58. Surkan, P. J. (2017). Risk of depressive symptoms associated with morbidity in postpartum women in rural Bangladesh. *Maternal and Child Health Journal*, *21*(10), 1890–1900.
59. Ugwu, E. O., Dim, C. C. & Eleje, G. U. (2021). Effects of mode of delivery on sexual functions of parturient in Nigeria: Prospective cohort study. *International Uro-gynaecologic Journal*, *32*(7), 1925–1933.
60. UNFPA. (2020). *Measuring SDG Target 5.6: Ensure Universal Access to Sexual and Reproductive Health and Reproductive Rights* (Publication 3067, p. 38, online). UNFPA: New York.
61. White, P. M. (2004). Heat, balance, humors, and ghosts: Postpartum in Cambodia. *Health Care Women International*, *25*(2), 179–194.
62. World Health Organization (WHO). (2006). *Defining Sexual Health—Report on a Technical Consultation on Sexual Health* (p. 30, online), 21–31 January 2002. Sexual health document series. WHO: Geneva (<DHS layout17.indd (paho.org)>).
63. DSH layout17.indd (paho.org) DSH layout17.indd (paho.org)
64. Zamani, M. (2019). The effect of sexual health counselling on women's sexual satisfaction in postpartum period: Randomized clinical trial. *International Journal of Reproductive Biomedicine*, *17*(1), 41–50.
65. Zare, Z. (2015). The effect of pelvic floor muscle exercises on sexual quality of life and marital satisfaction in primiparous women after childbirth. *Iran Journal of Obstetrics and Gynaecology*, *20*(3), 347–353.
66. Zulu, E. M. (2001). Ethnic variations in observance and rationale for postpartum sexual abstinence in Malawi. *Demography*, *38*(4), 467–470.

PART II

PSYCHOLOGICAL AND EMOTIONAL WELL-BEING

CHAPTER 7

Impact of Mental Health and Psychological Stress on Women's Heart Health

AMAL ABDELLAOUI

ABSTRACT

The psychological stress on the woman life leads to a risk factor for the coronary heart disease (CHD). This chapter deals with mental disorders and psychological stress on potential risks for women who are changing gender roles and lacking attention to epidemiology and etiology of female heart health. Literature documents the link between psychological stress and women coronary diseases. Generally, the vulnerability to mental disorders (depression and anxiety) is higher for women at all stages of their lives. Females with clinical depression could have an occurrence of cardiovascular disease twice than those without any depression. This chapter investigates the neurobiology mechanisms of mental disorders in women and the links between them and the CHD risk. Besides, this review presents different psychological disorders (such as depression, anxiety, etc.) and their effect on CHD in women; and several treatments for psychological disorders like medications and psychotherapies.

7.1 INTRODUCTION

During the last two decades, it has been confirmed that psychological disorders (such as anxiety and depression) are not related to the mind

Holistic Approaches for Women's Sustainable Health, Volume 2: Advancements, Socioeconomic Impacts, and Innovative Strategies. Junaid Ahmad Malik, Anamika Chauhan, and Megh R. Goyal (Eds)

DOI: 10.1201/9781779641656-9

but they are physical and effective illness like any other body illness. Consequently, these disorders can affect the whole body, including the cardiovascular system [1, 9, 23]. Several studies have demonstrated the connection between psychological health and cardiovascular disease (CVD). However, there is no effective illustration that psychological malady is a contributor to cardiovascular disorder for patients with coronary malady, myo-cardinal infraction, and heart breakdown [10, 15].

Psychological or mental disorders are terms employed to describe several symptoms of an individual's daily life that are not ordinary. An individual with a psychological disorder can exhibit symptoms such as anxiety, depression, confused emotions, hallucination, and anger. Different life situations may lead to losing a job, bereavement, stress, sleep deficiency, assault, drug/alcohol consumption, or accidents [10].

Sometimes, it is not easy for doctors and patients to ascribe a fundamental role of psychological well-being due to symptoms overlap of CVD such as chest tightness, palpitations, and breath shortness [1].

Several treatments have been suggested to prevent the coronary heart diseases (CHDs); however, the mental disorder remains the important source of disability and even mortality in females [12]. In terms of clinical course and pathophysiology, there is a difference concerning adult females and males. In case of women, CHD manifests late in life compared to man with slight connection of coronary arteries toward atherosclerotic plaques. However, women have similarly the same CHD morbidity and mortality as men, even atherosclerotic plaque protection [24]. These gender differences in pathophysiology, especially the breakdown of little coronary arteries to dilate during stress (microvascular coronary disease) and an inequality concerning vasoconstricting and vasodilating substances of endothelium regulation, could be significant in myocardial ischemia etiology than the plaque problem [8]. The American Heart Association (AHA) stated that young women with CHD have elevated mental issues associated with high CHD risk, as depression and anxiety, and post-traumatic stress disorder (PTSD) [27]. Ultimately, the studies have recommended a deep function of psychological and emotional issues on cardiovascular health in women, although research investigations are significantly limited in this domain [10].

The current chapter aims to target the impact of different psychological disorders on the cardiovascular health of women and ways to remedy these issues. Therefore, the first part of the chapter investigates the neurobiological mechanisms of mental disorders in women and the relation between the neurobiological system and psychological health. The second part describes the different mental disorders (such as depression, anger, anxiety, social relationship, and others) and their effect on the coronary health of women. Finally, different treatments (such as medication and psychotherapies) for psychological disorders have been discussed.

7.2 NEUROBIOLOGY SYSTEM AND MENTAL DISORDERS IN WOMEN

7.2.1 NEUROBIOLOGY OF MENTAL DISORDERS IN WOMEN

Mental disorders (also known as psychiatric disorders) are referred to a large range of conditions affecting a person's daily life, especially feeling, thinking, mood, or behavior. Consequently, these disorders affect considerably interpersonal relationships and whole well-being.

The mental disorders can affect women as men, but certain mental conditions could be more present or prevalent differently in women. Among the most known mental disorders, are: depression, eating disorders, anxiety disorders, PTSD, bipolar disorder, borderline personality disorder (BPD), obsessive-compulsive disorder (OCD), and perinatal mood disorders [10]. This chapter, especially, delves into the impact of depression, anxiety, and stress issues on coronary heart health (CHD) in women.

In early life of women, the mental illness like the stress and trauma, can have lasting impacts on neurobiological and cognitive functions that in return affect the physical health and can lead to CVD [25]. On other hand, the physical and emotional abuse can also have long-term effects on women [5]. For instance, the childhood sexual abuse can generate PTSD in women adulthood. Generally, the psychological disorders occur twice as common in women life as in men [10]. In terms of neurobiology, these disorders have similarly the same aspects with an overlap of symptoms, especially sharing a common augmented risk for CVD [6]. Generally, phycological trauma leads to PTSD with symptoms, such as emotional numbing or withdrawal, elimination of trauma reminders, negative distorted thoughts, poor concentration and memory, sleep disturbances, nightmares, and so on [10]. As a result, these symptoms are expression of stress-based modification in both the brain and neurobiology system [3]. PTSD causes a perturbation of the neurohormonal systems (hypothalamic–pituitary–adrenal [HPA] axis, cortisol, and norepinephrine system) that play a serious role in the stress reaction. In some studies, it has been found that brain areas involved in fear, memory, and learning response (amygdala, prefrontal cortex, and hippocampus), are affected in women with PTSD [6]. Compared to women, normal men show an important cortisol response for challenges achievement and women show an important cortisol response to social rejection [19].

Another common mental illness in early life of women is the depression that is characterized by losing interest in things or a depressed mood that lasts at least for two weeks. Among the depression symptoms, there is loss of appetite, crying spells, reduced sleep, agitation, poor concentration, restlessness, energy lost, guilt, feelings of hopelessness and worthlessness, and sometimes suicide thoughts [10]. Anxiety disorders include generalized anxiety disorder (GAD), OCD, phobic disorder, and panic disorder [10].

7.2.2 NEUROBIOLOGY MECHANISMS OF MENTAL DISORDERS

Neurobiologically, the norepinephrine system and the HPA axis play a serious role in the stress response. Under threatening circumstances, the HPA has the role to regulate the metabolic modification in response to stressor to ensure the survival of the person [10]. Corticotropin releasing factor is liberated from paraventricular nucleus of hypothalamus, and it plays the role of fear-related behavior stimulator as well as activating the noradrenergic neurotransmitter system [2]. Besides, the norepinephrine system like brain fire alarm, increases the alertness and fear levels and stimulates the respiratory and cardiovascular systems and responses to stress [10]. Stress impacts several brain zones, such as the medial prefrontal cortex, amygdala, and hippocampus [17]. The early stress in life of individuals is related to the long-run sensitization of the HPA axis [14]. The medial prefrontal cortex, significantly sensitive to stress, is especially implied in the relation between CVD and stress as illustrated in Figure 7.1 [14]. The alteration of the medial prefrontal cortex functioning impacts outputs from this zone that has the role of regulating the psychological reactions to stress in the periphery with risk of cardiovascular implications [10]. Compared to men, the studies suggest that the psychological disorders (e.g. social rejection) cause significant cortisol response in women while men could be more sensitive to stress linked to achievement issues [10].

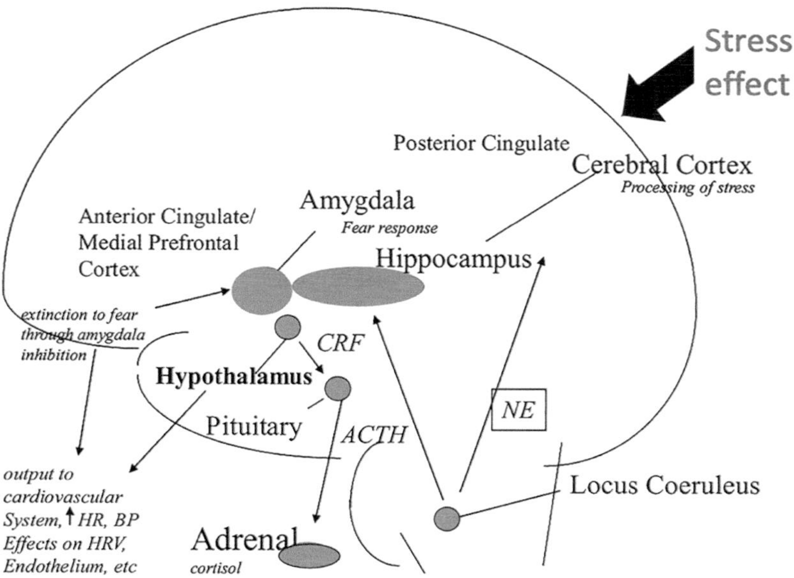

FIGURE 7.1 Illustration of neurobiology of functioning of coronary function and stress effects.

7.3 PSYCHOLOGICAL DISORDERS AND CARDIOVASCULAR SYSTEM IN WOMAN LIFE

7.3.1 EFFECT OF DEPRESSION ON THE CARDIOVASCULAR SYSTEM

7.3.1.1 DEPRESSION AND CVD

Depression affects women more than men and is considered as a reliable interpreter of incident and recurrent CHD in women life [1]. For both females and males, the depression corporal symptoms, like the fatigue, could be narrowly linked to clinical CHD symptoms and indicating an early CHD [9, 10]. One research study concluded that more strict depression symptoms were related to augmented risk of cardiovascular death due to a dose response connection [9].

The relationship among anxiety, depression and CHD is bidirectional, which means that anxiety and depression can enhance the risk of CVD development, and the CVD can lead to an increase of the risk of depression/anxiety development [1]. Moreover, the depression can enhance the myocardial infraction development risk, unexpected death, stroke, and atrial fibrillation in patients with angina [21].

Consequently, AHA endorses that depression, diabetes, hyperlipidemia, smoking, and hypertension need to be acknowledged as a main risk factor for CHD [1]. It is about 80% enhanced risk of worsening CHD development [1]. Besides, the AHA has inferred that depression can stimulate the beginning and danger of cardiovascular risk issues of diabetes, hypertension, and high levels of low-density lipoprotein as well as can accelerate the atherosclerosis [1]. Ultimately, depression increases the risk of having an unhealthy lifestyle (e.g., smoking, salt, diet higher in calories and saturated fat, and decreases in exercise) and medication compliance [1, 10]. A good lifestyle and healthy compliance with treatments cannot be undervalued. Effects of depression on heart disease can be summarized as follow [1]:

- Augment the atherosclerosis rate.
- Increase the cortisol levels leading to augmented blood glucose levels and pressure of blood.
- Increase the inflammation and the risk of coronary artery occlusion.
- Increase the other hormones leading to an increase of the rate of resting heart and a significant elevation in heart rate with exertion.
- Increase the platelets activity, leading to an accumulating and creating a plug into an artery, and an obstacle of the blood flow.

7.3.1.2 PREVENTION OF DEPRESSION AND ITS SYMPTOMS

To prevent depression and its effects on cardiovascular system, some treatments (the medication, the mindful meditation, and the exercise) can be adopted depending on the person and depression stage [1].

- **Medications:** Several medications are available, such as [1] (1) selective serotonin reuptake inhibitors (SSRIs) and serotonin–norepinephrine reuptake inhibitors (SNRIs) approved by principal care or psychiatrist, (2) therapy treatment with a social worker or psychologist, and (3) cognitive behavioral therapy (CBT) that is helpful for stress, anxiety, and depression with sorrow reaction, but this technique is not supportive in case of major depression.

- **Exercise:** Doing aerobic exercise with light or moderate intensity (e.g., 30 min/day), walking on treadmill, Brisk walking, cycling, jogging, playing sports, climbing stairs, and swimming.

- **Breathing exercise**: Like yoga, pranayama, slow breathing in 10–15 min sessions daily with breathing rate of 6 breaths/minute.
- **Mindful meditation**: A meditation practice of almost 10 min/day with an experienced sitting eye closed, and cross-legged on a chair or cushion with the back at straight position. During meditation, the whole attention is focused on the abdomen movement when breathing in and out. Only focusing on putting the awareness of the breath that is going in and out of the nostrils [1].

7.3.1.3 ANXIETY AND CVD

Another psychological disorder that has a risk for CVD is anxiety. General anxiety (stress and anger) has been revealed to anticipate CVDs [17]. Continuing stressful stimuli (such as caregiver strain, work stress, marital stress, low socioeconomic status, and low social support) have been associated to an elevated risk of coronary artery disease and other contrary cardiac actions as well as emotional stressors [18]. The effect may be gradual with further anxiety episodes, stress, and anger connected with an increased risk of CVDs as well as overlapping signs with chest pain, despite normal effect of coronary arteries and heart pounding [17]. Anxiety disorders can result in the liberation of the adrenaline hormone leading to a temporary increase in the blood pressure [1]. Consequently, it leads to arteries contraction that may result in myocardial infraction inducing cardiac anomalies in individuals' life with or without structural coronary disease [1]. Recurrent temporary growths in blood pressure can cause disruption of the plaques and myocardial infraction. For the patients with weakened aorta (e.g., survivors of an aortic dissection), may generate an aortic dissection or failure [1].

The most common relationship between anxiety disorders and exposure to psychological trauma is PTSD and depression, especially in childhood [10]. This allows to infer that the nexus between anxiety disorders and coronary disease risk in women is less strong than for PTSD and depression.

7.3.1.3.1 Anxiety Mechanisms

There exist several mechanisms associating emotional factors, stress with high CHD risk in women (Figure 7.2). Lifestyle and behavioral factors are highly linked to stress-based psychopathology and CD risk [2]. PTSD, depression, and childhood trauma are related to unhealthful behaviors like sedentary routine, smoking, poor adherence to medication, and preventive solutions [7, 26]. For instance, childhood sexual abuse is linked to obesity in their adulthood life, noticeable even after obesity control behavior. The alteration of systems of neurohormonal stress response due to recurrent stress is plausible mechanisms illustrating the linkage between CHD and stress. It has been stated that repeated activation of the sympathetic and parasympathetic nervous systems removal with stress cause long-run dysregulation of these two systems by elevating the blood pressure, plasma glucose, heart rate, dyslipidemia, and insulin resistance [10]. The stress-induced norepinephrine liberation triggers the transcription issue NF-kB in starting the inflammatory cascade and circulating monocytes with long-lasting abnormalities in immune system [10].

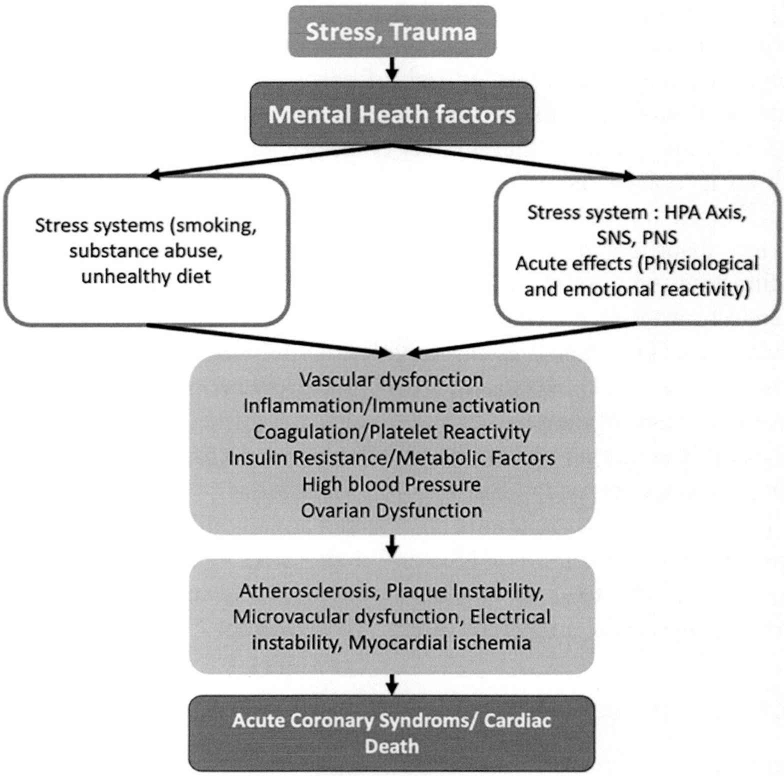

FIGURE 7.2 Illustration of associated mechanisms between behavioral and emotional factors to CHD in women.

PTSD and depression have also been also linked to evidence immune dysregulation and high levels of inflammatory biomarkers [16, 22]. Research studies indicate that some psychological factors such as depression may have some shared genetic pathways with coronary diseases [10]. Depression and coronary disease can be like a different phenotypic expression of the identical genetic substrate, especially in women [10, 27]. For women, the mutual genetic factors could generate depression-CVD in all age-based groups. In contrast, for men, these factors are only in younger age groups [10]. The depression heritability has been assessed as 42% in women compared with 29% in case of men [10]. Besides, the epigenetic mechanisms could be included due to DNA methylation in case of several psychological disorders like depression and PTSD as well as it has an effect in the pathophysiology CVD [10]. Also, epigenetics can lead to changes in gene expression affecting different phenotypes like mental health and CVD [10].

In daily life, the psychological factors could enhance the CHD risk via acute effects like prompting severe coronary syndromes, inducing silent ischemia or even intensifying cardiovascular responsiveness. For instance, a depressive mood may induce ischemia in CHD's patients and ruptures of anger can induce severe MI [13]. Daily-life emotional reactivity, depression, and anxiety are linked to myocardial ischemia during mental stress [4].

To overcome the stress effect, diverse approaches for treatment should be fitted. Generally, the most psychological involvements or drug treatment have exhibited a lower value for CHD's results improvement, especially for women [10].

7.3.1.3.2 Anxiety Treatment

Efficient treatments for anxiety and overstated stress can enhance long-run cardiovascular health and can successfully improve the life quality [9]. Generally, it is highly recommended for patients with mental health to discuss frequently with their doctors especially because mental illness usually is undiagnosed.

Anxiety treatments include medications and nonmedications (CBT, yoga, slow breathing exercise, mindfulness meditation, exercise, etc.). For example, a moderate intensity aerobic exercise for 30 min can reduce the myocardial infraction risk and death owing to CHD [23].

Mindfulness's objective is to be conscious of the present moment without any judgment and focusing only on the breath in the body. The most important part of this practice is that the person can return his attention at any moment to this anchor and focus on his breath and just letting its attention be. The individual state improvement can be observed after a few weeks, especially if the mindful meditation is practiced long term and facilitated by an expert. It helps to reduce stress and emotional response, lowering blood pressure, smoking cessation, and overall can enhance the daily life quality [23].

7.3.1.4 EFFECTS OF OTHER NEGATIVE PSYCHOLOGICAL FACTORS ON CHD

- **Hostility:** Another psychology disorders generating negative emotions include hostile behaviors, attitudes and emotions. Hostility is a component of certain psychological disorders or personality trait but not typically a mental illness. It refers to pattern of aggressive behaviors or anger and feelings toward others. Individuals with high hostility level may express anger fast and have difficulty managing and regulating their emotions. Some studies of CHD in women showed that adverse behavior scores anticipated considerably risk for upcoming coronary disease [10, 23]. Other studies focused on the nexus between adversity-based concepts and CHD in women, in which results illustrated those cynical behaviors like doubt of others enhanced risk of death but not CHD incident, especially among Afro-American women [23]. These studies reported higher scores for men for mean hostile behaviors or angry emotions. The anger experiences are less strongly related to CHD in women compared to men.
- **Anger suppression**: The frequency or intensity of anger emotion and hostility and associated emotions could be also linked to CHD risk in women. In a study, it was stated that self-silencing like keeping feelings during conflicts with spouse without sharing, was linked to a four-fold enhanced CHD risk in women [3]. In another study, women hospitalized for a severe CHD, elimination of angry emotions was considerably linked to risk of a cardiac death [10].

- **Social relationship**: An empirical attention has been noticed because of social relationship, network diversity, and other's support as phycological factors associated to CHD in women. Some studies reported that large size of social network and being married were each linked to reduced mortality risk [23]. Another study investigated the link between the CHD and social relationship in women and men distinctly with mixed outcomes. The results illustrated that noticed social care was not linked to CHD for both women and men. However, it was illustrated that the presence of a partner can reduce the CHD risk for men and not for women, as well as a considerable relationship was noticed for women between low social support and loneliness CHD risk incident [3, 20]. Besides, stress associated to family responsibilities and interpersonal relationship, has received more awareness relatively to CHD in women but could be less meaningful in men's CHD [9]. The incident CHD risk increases with increased hours spent with children or grandchildren caring as well as hours spent in disabled or ill spouse caring [9]. Ultimately, based on the changes in the presence, frequency, and value of social relationship, it has been concluded that the kindhearted social support is more essential for women's CHD. Further data reported that psychological stress related to relational fields could be more significant for women than stress related work [9].
- **Eating disorder** is a complex psychological condition distinguished by abnormal eating habits, and behaviors impacting individual's well-being. It includes bulimia nervosa, binge-eating, and anorexia nervosa disorder [9]. Bulimia nervosa includes binge eating episodes followed by vomiting, fasting, or excessive exercise as a compensatory behavior. Electrolyte imbalance linked to bulimia nervosa generates dangerous irregular heart rhythms (arrhythmias) that can lead to cardiac arrest. For binge-eating disorder includes persistent episodes of consumption of considerable quantity of food without any compensatory attitude [9]. In anorexia nervosa, there is often an exhibition of intense fear of weight gaining, leading to excessive exercise, distorted body image and severe calorie restriction and causing the heart muscle and reduction of cardiac volume and mass. Generally, these disorders can generate profound effects on cardiovascular

health of women and emotional disorders such as anxiety and social withdrawal [9]. Moreover, eating disorder can be challenged by chronic stress of daily life contributing to an overactive sympathetic nervous system, increasing the cortisol and adrenaline levels and raising blood pressure and heart rate. Repeatedly, persistent stress contributes to the development of hypertension and enhances risk of CHD [9].

7.4 TREATMENT OF PSYCHOLOGICAL DISORDERS ON CHD IN WOMEN

Psychological health and cardiovascular health are complex issues, and their concerns should be discussed with doctors and healthcare professionals. This section presented some employed treatments to reduce effects of psychological disorders and consequently reduction of their effects on the cardiovascular health of women. Generally, the medication treatment depends on individual patient characteristics, specific diagnosis and potential side effects. For a comprehensive treatment plan, it is recommended to use the medications in conjunction with psychotherapy [10].

7.4.1 PSYCHOLOGICAL DISORDERS: MEDICATIONS [1, 11]

- **Antianxiety medication**: The benzodiazepine family (e.g., Xanax, Valium, Ativan, etc.) that acts on the central nervous system to induce a calming effect. However, it is typically employed for short-term relief of severe anxiety symptoms. An alternative of benzodiazepine family with a lower risk of dependency, is buspirone that is used for GAD.
- **Antidepressants** include three categories that are SNRIs, SSRIs, and Tricyclic antidepressants (TCAs): (1) SSRIs aim to improve the serotonin levels in the brain leading to relieve depression and anxiety symptoms. This category includes escitalopram, fluoxetine, sertraline; (2) SNRIs affect both serotonin and norepinephrine levels and provide a relief for depression and certain anxiety disorders; (3) TCAs include the amitriptyline and imipramine classes. They affect serotonin and norepinephrine levels. However, they are less commonly prescribed because of more side effects.

- **Mood stabilizers** like lithium and anticonvulsants that are used for bipolar disorder to stabilize the mood and prevent episodes of depression.
- **Antipsychotic medications** include typical antipsychotics (e.g., haloperidol and chlorpromazine) that treat psychosis symptoms but may have side effects, and atypical antipsychotics (e.g., risperidone, quetiapine, and olanzapine) that are often employed to treat a large range of psychiatric syndromes with some side effects.
- **Attention-deficit/hyperactivity disorder (ADHD) medications** include stimulants methylphenidate (Ritalin and amphetamine/dextro-amphetamine) that are employed to manage symptoms of ADHD.

7.4.2 PSYCHOTHERAPY TREATMENT

Psychotherapy approach includes a variety of therapeutic interventions employed to manage specific needs of individuals having mental issues. Some common therapeutic treatments [1, 10] are:

- **Talk therapy** (known also by psychotherapy) contains three main therapies: (1) CBT: it is effective of different disorders like anxiety, depression, and eating disorders. This therapy emphasizes identification and modifications of the negative thoughts and bad behaviors generating mental issues; (2) dialectical behavior therapy combines CBT techniques with mindfulness and acceptance techniques to manage intense emotions. This therapy is particularly helpful in the case of BPD; and (3) interpersonal therapy: basically, employed to treat depression with a focus on improving interpersonal relationship and communication skills.
- **Behavioral therapy** includes three therapies: (1) applied behavior analysis: it focuses on changing behaviors via systematic interventions and positive reinforcement. This therapy is employed for individuals with autism spectrum disorders; (2) exposure therapy: it exposes gradually individuals to feared situations or objects to reduce their anxiety responses. This therapy is commonly used to treat anxiety disorders; (3) behavioral activation: based on CBT technique, the behavioral activation focuses on increasing

individuals' engagement in positive activities to enhance their mood and reduce their depression symptoms.

- **Mindfulness-based approaches** include two main classes: (1) mindfulness-based stress reduction: usually employed for chronic pain, depression, and anxiety. This technique reduces stress and improves overall well-being; (2) mindfulness-based cognitive therapy: gathers mindfulness approaches related to cognitive-behavioral approaches to prevent the recurrence of depressive episodes.

7.5 SUMMARY

Psychological disorders, such as depression, stress, and anxiety, can have a significant influence on cardiovascular health in women. These psychological conditions may act as independent risk factors or interact with other lifestyle elements to lead to developing CHD. Healthcare professionals should take a multidisciplinary approach, involving mental and cardiovascular health specialists, to assess and treat women with mental disorders.

In this chapter, the neurobiology mechanisms of mental/psychological disorders and their relationship with coronary disease in women have been investigated. Besides, several psychological disorders such as depression, anxiety, stress, social relationship, and so on have been detailed to identify their effects of CHD in women. Ultimately, different ways of psychological disorders treatment have been presented to remedy and prevent these disorders and restrict their impact on CHD risk on women.

KEYWORDS

- **cardiovascular disease**
- **coronary health disease**
- **medication**
- **psychological disorder**
- **psychotherapy**
- **female heart health**

REFERENCES

1. Andre-Petersson, L., Engstrom, G., Hedblad, B., Janzon, L., & Rosvall, M. (2007). Social support at work and the risk of myocardial infarction and stroke in women and men. *Social Science & Medicine, 64,* 830–841.
2. Arborelius, L., Owens, M. J., Plotsky, P. M., & Nemeroff, C. B. (1999). The role of corticotropin-releasing factor in depression and anxiety disorders. *The Journal of Endocrinology, 160,* 1–12.
3. Boyle, S. H., Samad, Z., Becker, R. C., Williams, R., Kuhn, C., Ortel, T. L., Kuchibhatla, M., Prybol, K., Rogers, J., O'Connor, C., Velazquez, E. J., & Jiang, W. (2013). Depressive symptoms and mental stress-induced myocardial ischemia in patients with coronary heart disease. *Psychosomatic Medicine, 75*(9), 822–831.
4. Bremner, J. D. (2002). *Does Stress Damage the Brain? Understanding Trauma-related Disorders from a Mind-Body Perspective.* W.W. Norton: New York.
5. Bremner, J. D., & Vaccarino, V. (2015). Neurobiology of early life stress in women. In: *Psychosocial Stress and Cardiovascular Disease in Women: Concepts, Findings, Future Perspectives* (pp. 161–168). Springer International Publishing: Cham.
6. Breslau, N., Davis, G. C., & Schultz, L. R. (2003). Posttraumatic stress disorder and the incidence of nicotine, alcohol, and other drug disorders in persons who have experienced trauma. *Archives of General Psychiatry, 60*(3), 289–294.
7. Bugiardini, R., & Merz, C. N. B. (2005). Angina with normal coronary arteries: A changing philosophy. *JAMA, 293*(4), 477–484.
8. Chaddha, A, Robinson, E. A., Kline-Rogers, E., Alexandris-Souphis, T., & Rubenfire, M. (2016). Mental health and cardiovascular disease. *The American Journal of Medicine, 129*(11), 1145–1148. doi: 10.1016/j.amjmed.2016.05.018.
9. Chaput, L. A., Adams, S. H., Simon, J. A., Blumenthal, R. S., Vittinghoff, E., Lin, F., Loh, E., & Matthews, K. A. (2002). Hostility predicts recurrent events among postmenopausal women with coronary heart disease. *American Journal of Epidemiology, 156*(12), 1092–1099. doi: 10.1093/aje/kwf158.
10. Kyoung-Im, C. (2016). Women, stress and heart health: Mindfulness-based stress reduction and cardiovascular disease. *Kosin Medical Journal, 31*(2), 103–112.
11. Mallik, S., Spertus, J. A., Reid, K. J., Krumholz, H. M., Rumsfeld, J. S., Weintraub, W. S., Agarwal, P., Santra, M., Bidyasar, S., Lichtman, J. H., & Wenger, N. K., Vaccarino, V. (2006). Depressive symptoms after acute myocardial infarction: Evidence for highest rates in younger women. *Archives of Internal Medicine, 166*(8), 876–883.
12. Mehta, L. S., Beckie, T. M., DeVon, H. A., Grines, C. L., Krumholz, H. M., Johnson, M. N., & Wenger, N. K. (2016). Acute myocardial infarction in women: A scientific statement from the American Heart Association. *Circulation, 133*(9), 916–947.
13. Mostofsky, E., Maclure, M., Tofler, G. H., Muller, J. E., & Mittleman, M. A. (2013). Relation of outbursts of anger and risk of acute myocardial infarction. *The American Journal of Cardiology, 112*(3), 343–348.
14. Pani, L., Porcella, A., & Gessa, G. L. (2000). The role of stress in the pathophysiology of the dopaminergic system. *Molecular Psychiatry, 5,* 14–21.

15. Pepine, C. J. (2004). Ischemic heart disease in women: Facts and wishful thinking. *Journal of the American College of Cardiology*, *43*(10), 1727–1730.
16. Plantinga, L., Bremner, J. D., Miller, A. H., Jones, D. P., Veledar, E., Goldberg, J., & Vaccarino, V. (2013). Association between posttraumatic stress disorder and inflammation: A twin study. *Brain, Behavior, and Immunity, 30*, 125–132.
17. Riba, M., Wulsin, L., & Rubenfire, M. (2011). *Psychiatry and Heart Disease: The Mind, Brain, and Heart.* Wiley-Blackwell: Hoboken, NJ, USA.
18. Rozanski, A., Blumenthal, J. A., Davidson, K. W., Saab, P. G., & Kubzansky, L. (2005). Epidemiology, pathophysiology, and management of psychosocial risk factors in cardiac practice: Emerging field of behavioral cardiology. *Journal of the American College of Cardiology*, *45*(5), 637–651.
19. Stroud, L. R., Salovey, P., & Epel, E. S. (2002). Sex differences in stress responses: Social rejection versus achievement stress. *Biological Psychiatry, 52*(4), 318–327.
20. Thomas, A. J., Kalaria, R. N., & O'Brien, J. (2004). Depression and vascular disease: What is the relationship? *Journal of Affective Disorders*, *79*(1–3), 81–95.
21. Thurston, R. C., & Kubzansky, L. D. (2009). Women, loneliness, and incident coronary heart disease. *Psychosomatic Medicine*, *71*(8), 836–842.
22. Uddin, M., Aiello, A. E., Wildman, D. E., Koenen, K. C., Pawelec, G., de Los Santos, R., Goldmann, E., & Galea, S. (2010). Epigenetic and immune function profiles associated with posttraumatic stress disorder. *Proceedings of the National Academy of Sciences of the United States of America, 7*(20), 9470–9475.
23. Vaccarino, V. (2010). Ischemic heart disease in women: Many questions, few facts. *Circulation Cardiovascular Quality and Outcomes, 3,* 111–115.
24. Vaccarino, V., Badimon, L., Corti, R., de Wit, C., Dorobantu, M., Manfrini, O., Koller, A., Pries, A., Cenko, E., & Bugiardini, R. (2013). Presentation, management, and outcomes of ischemic heart disease in women. *Nature Reviews Cardiology, 10*(9), 508–518.
25. Vaccarino, V., & Bremner, J. D. (2015). Sex-specific differences in acute myocardial infarction. *Gender Differences in the Pathogenesis and Management of Heart Disease*, *2015,* 191–213.
26. Whooley, M. A., De Jonge, P., Vittinghoff, E., Otte, C., Moos, R., Carney, R. M., & Browner, W. S. (2008). Depressive symptoms, health behaviors, and risk of cardiovascular events in patients with coronary heart disease. *JAMA*, *300*(20), 2379–2388.
27. Xu, H., Beltrame, J. F., & Krumholz, H. M. (2015). Sex differences in perceived stress and early recovery in young and middle-aged patients with acute myocardial infarction. *Circulation, 131*(7), 614–623.

CHAPTER 8

Stress Management Intervention for Breast Cancer Survivors

MUZAMIL JAN,[1] MOHD YOUNUS ZAROO,[2] and SIMPLE SHARMA[3*]

*Corresponding author

ABSTRACT

Breast cancer arises from mutations in breast cells, leading to tumor growth, typically in the ducts or lobules. Risk factors include age, genetic mutations, reproductive history, dense breast tissue, and a personal or family history of cancer. The main symptom is a lump in the breast or under the armpit. Early detection through clinical breast exams, ultrasounds, magnetic resonance imaging, biopsies, and mammograms is essential. Breast cancer accounts for over 23% of all global cancers in women. Treatment is personalized and may include surgery, chemotherapy, hormonal therapy, biological therapy, and radiation. Complementary therapies like massage and acupuncture can also be integrated. Emotional challenges are common, and factors such as education, support, and financial stability impact quality of life. Awareness of normal breast changes is crucial for early detection. Addressing psychosocial well-being through interventions across various settings can significantly enhance long-term care and support for breast cancer patients.

8.1 INTRODUCTION

The breasts are located at the front (anterior) and sides (lateral) of the chest area (thorax). The breasts reach from the top of the sternum to the

Holistic Approaches for Women's Sustainable Health, Volume 2: Advancements, Socioeconomic Impacts, and Innovative Strategies. Junaid Ahmad Malik, Anamika Chauhan, and Megh R. Goyal (Eds)

DOI: 10.1201/9781779641656-10

midaxillary line laterally, and from the second rib to the bottom of the sixth rib cartilage superiorly. Along the lower border of the pectoralis major muscle, the axillary tail is formed by the superior lateral section of the mammary gland as it spreads toward the axilla. The form and size of a woman's breasts are determined by genetic factors, racial background, dietary habits, age, history of childbirth, and menopausal stage. The form of breasts can vary, ranging from spherical, cone-shaped, variably drooping, pear-shaped, to narrow and flattened. A normal breast is 10–12 cm in diameter and 5–7 cm thick, giving it a conical shape. Typically, the upper outer quadrant area has the largest portion of breast tissue. This upper outer quadrant is more commonly affected by both breast cancer and benign (noncancerous) breast conditions [8].

8.1.1 BREAST CANCER

Cancer occurs when cells experience uncontrolled proliferation. Breast cancer is a cancerous tumor that develops in the breast tissue. The disease can appear as either unilateral or bilateral breast enlargement. Generally, breast cancer is more commonly diagnosed in women aged 50 or over; however, it can also impact males and younger women [16]. Most breast lumps are benign, meaning they are noncancerous and do not metastasize beyond the breast. However, some nonmalignant tumors may raise a woman's risk of breast cancer. Breast lumps may be caused by a variety of illnesses, including cancer. However, the majority of lumps are caused by benign illnesses such as fibrocystic breast disease and cysts. Fibrocystic breast disease produces noncancerous alterations in the breast tissue, resulting in lumpiness, discomfort, and pain. Breast cysts are small sacs filled with fluid that can develop in the breast [17]. Breast cancer arises from the mutation of breast cells, leading to the development of malignant tumors as a result of uncontrolled growth. Alternative treatment options include surgical tumor excision and therapies aimed at eliminating cancer cells. Breast cancer is a common kind of cancer that primarily affects women. Cancer can develop in several regions of the breast, including the milk-producing tubes known as invasive ductal carcinoma and the fatty tissue called invasive lobular carcinoma [22]. A small number of malignancies, such as sarcomas and lymphomas, can arise in breast tissues but are not classed as breast cancer. Breast cancer can metastasize via the circulatory or lymphatic system, allowing cancerous cells to infiltrate different areas of the body. The lymphatic system is a complex network of lymph nodes, blood vessels, and organs that facilitates the movement of lymph fluid throughout the body. Breast cancer cells can invade lymphatic vessels and grow within lymph nodes [27].

- The majority of lymphatic arteries in the breast flow into [1].
- Axillary lymph nodes are beneath the arm, whereas internal mammary nodes are around the breastbone.
- Lymph nodes near the collarbone, including supraclavicular and infraclavicular.

8.1.2 IMPORTANCE OF ADDRESSING BREAST CANCER

The detection of cancer cells in lymph nodes indicates an elevated probability of their metastasis, or dissemination, to other organs through the lymphatic system. However, metastases do not necessarily accompany lymph node cancer in all women, and even women without lymph node cancer may get them in the future [35]. Many people dread receiving a diagnosis of any sickness, particularly cancer, and having to endure surgery. However, surgery for breast cancer raises extra problems. Breast cancer is distressing not just because it is potentially fatal, but also because it exposes women to the possibility of losing a bodily part that is sexualized and highly prized in many cultures [23]. This chapter will synthesize current information, including empirical data as well as theoretical and methodological contributions from numerous studies on the social, emotional, and psychological condition of women with breast cancer [18].

8.2 RISK FACTORS FOR BREAST CANCER

Studies suggest that several factors influence an individual's probability of acquiring breast cancer. The primary risk factors are being female and being over the age of 50, with the preponderance of cases occurring in women in this age range. Some women get breast cancer in the absence of any known risk factors, and having a risk factor does not guarantee that a woman will be diagnosed with the illness. Although certain women may be at risk for getting breast cancer, it is generally considered to be a rare illness among them [36]. Age advancement, genetic mutations, reproductive record, dense breast tissue, personal history of breast cancer or specific benign breast conditions, family history of breast or ovarian cancer, prior radiation therapy, and exposure to certain medications are all recognized as intrinsic risk factors for breast cancer. These factors cannot be changed. Modifiable risk factors encompass insufficient physical activity, postmenopausal obesity or overweight, hormone therapy, a history of pregnancy, and excessive alcohol use [37].

8.2.1 SYMPTOMS AND INDICATIONS OF BREAST CANCER

The presence of a lump is not universally observed in individuals with breast cancer, and the symptoms might differ depending on the specific kind of cancer [39]. Common manifestations of this disorder include the presence of a tumor in the breast or chest wall region, bleeding or discharge from the nipple, breast pain, inflammation or swelling in one breast, and the nipple being pushed inward or retracted [38]. While these symptoms do not necessarily indicate breast cancer, any new breast changes should be evaluated. Early detection is crucial for treatment options [28]. A painless breast lump [40] is often the first sign, though many lumps are detected through routine mammograms. Most women do not exhibit any obvious symptoms when they are diagnosed. Early-stage breast cancers [42] are seldom detectable without imaging such as mammograms [41]. Common early warning signals include [9]:

1. Visible alterations in the skin, such as swelling, inflammation, or noticeable differences in the appearance of one or both breasts
2. Alterations in breast size or morphology
3. Alterations in the look of the nipple
4. Excretion of substances other than breast milk
5. Mastalgia
6. Presence of palpable masses or lymph nodes in or around the breast.

8.3 BREAST CANCER SCREENING

Breast cancer screening entails detecting cancer before symptoms occur [43]. Women should be informed about screening choices, benefits, and risks so that they may make an informed decision with their healthcare practitioner about whether or not to be tested [44].

8.3.1 CLINICAL BREAST EXAMINATION

A doctor or nurse physically palpates the breasts to discover abnormalities during a clinical breast examination (CBE). It should be done yearly during routine check-ups. The healthcare provider carefully feels the breasts, underarms, and collar bone area, both visually and by touch, while the woman is sitting and lying down [29].

Knowing how one's breasts generally appear and feel might help one recognize signs such as lumps, soreness, or size changes, all of which should be reported to a doctor. Breast self-exams do not lower breast cancer mortality [2].

8.3.2 BREAST ULTRASOUND

Breast ultrasounds (BUSGs) utilize sound waves to generate sonograms, which are images of the inside of the breasts. While not a standard screening test, it can be useful in assessing breast tumors, particularly those that are not detectable on mammograms and in cases with thick breast tissue. Ultrasound can differentiate between fluid-filled cysts and solid masses that may require further testing. It can also guide biopsy needles into suspicious areas [19]. An ultrasound probe is moved over the skin, sending and receiving sound waves that create images on a computer screen. Some pressure may be felt, but it should not be painful [45].

8.3.3 BREAST MAGNETIC RESONANCE IMAGING

Breast magnetic resonance imaging (MRI) generates comprehensive cross-sectional pictures of the breast by using a powerful magnetic field, radio waves, and computers. It does not utilize radiation [24].

8.3.4 BIOPSY

A breast biopsy is a medical technique that entails extracting a small sample of breast tissue to ascertain the presence of malignant cells inside the tissue for diagnostic purposes. It is the best way to evaluate a suspicious lump or area. Potential side effects include breast appearance changes, bruising, swelling, soreness, and infection at the biopsy site [30].

8.3.5 MAMMOGRAM

A mammogram is a diagnostic technique that uses X-rays to identify breast cancer in its early stages, before the manifestation of any symptoms, when it is most amenable to treatment. Mammograms conducted regularly decrease the likelihood of death from breast cancer. During the operation, the breast is compressed between two plates to immobilize it and ensure it remains flat, while X-ray pictures are captured from various angles. Some pressure is felt, but it should not be painful. Though all breasts are unique, any concerning areas on the mammogram may require further evaluation [46].

8.4 PREVALENCE OF BREAST CANCER

Timely identification of breast cancer is essential for efficiently controlling the illness. The possibility of finding a cure for breast cancer exists when the disease is detected in its initial stage and treated well. Nevertheless, in cases when the diagnosis is made at a later stage, the opportunity for curative treatment is sometimes no longer available, therefore requiring the implementation of palliative care to alleviate the suffering of both patients and their families [47].

8.4.1 PREVALENCE OF BREAST CANCER AT THE INTERNATIONAL LEVEL

Among the female population, breast cancer is the most widespread form of cancer, representing around 23% of all documented occurrences worldwide. By 2030, it is estimated that there will be a worldwide total of 2 million instances of breast cancer, with developing nations playing a substantial role in the overall impact. This is an algorithmically generated forecast. Breast cancer is the most prevalent kind of cancer that impacts women in both developed and developing nations. Breast cancer is the predominant kind of cancer. There has been a steady rise in the prevalence of this phenomenon in nations with incomes categorized as low to moderate in recent years. This phenomenon may be ascribed to a multitude of variables, such as a rise in life expectancy, urbanization, and the adoption of Western habits. The majority of fatalities, amounting to 269,000, are ascribed to countries with low and moderate incomes. A significant number of women in these nations receive a diagnosis of breast cancer at an advanced stage because of a lack of knowledge about early detection procedures and restricted availability of healthcare services (WHO 2003) [10]. Within the female population of the United Kingdom, breast cancer is the leading cause of death attributed to cancer. Breast cancer is the most common and often encountered kind of cancer. Approximately 11% of females will receive a diagnosis of breast cancer at some point in their lifetime. Approximately 41,000 new instances of breast cancer are projected to be detected in women during the current year. On the other hand, the mortality rate for breast cancer in the entire population is around 42 deaths per 100,000 women each year. Despite these statistics, women are reaping the benefits of the progress made in the identification and treatment of breast cancer. This is supported by the findings that mortality rates in the United Kingdom are declining at a more rapid pace in comparison to all other nations. Despite the prevalence of breast cancer, a substantial proportion of women can have fulfilling lives following their diagnosis with the illness. It is projected that the current number of women in the United Kingdom who have been diagnosed with breast cancer and are still alive today will surpass 170,000 over the course of the next decade. Breast cancer incidence shows substantial variation across different countries, with the greatest rates seen among women living in industrialized Western nations and the lowest rates recorded among women in Eastern countries [31]. It is now believed that the development of breast cancer is influenced by a mix of environmental and genetic variables that contribute to the occurrence of the illness. Japan has a markedly lower prevalence of breast cancer in comparison to the United Kingdom, the United States, and Australia, despite these nations sharing similar levels of economic prosperity. This suggests that the economic conditions of a nation have little effect on the occurrence of breast cancer in that particular country. When an individual relocates from an area with a low occurrence of breast cancer to one with a high occurrence, there is a discernible rise in the frequency of this ailment [48]. The International Agency for Research on Cancer is collaborating with population-based cancer registries in Algeria, China, Costa Rica, Cuba, India, the Philippines, and Thailand to examine cancer survival rates in economically disadvantaged countries. The results of this study are then contrasted with the data collected from the surveillance, epidemiology, and end result (SEER) program of the National Cancer Institute in the United States, as well as the EUROCARE survival study conducted in European countries. These findings indicate that there are significant disparities in patient survival rates across nations that lack sufficient financial resources. The 5-year relative survival rate for breast cancer in women under the age of 75 in developing nations ranged from 43 to 63%. In contrast to the United States, the survival rates throughout the time periods of 1967 to 1973, 1974 to 1986, and 1986 to 1991 were 65, 76, and 82%, respectively. Tumors that impact the large intestine, breast, and cervix show significant differences in survival rates, with a higher likelihood of surviving if they are detected and treated early. To reduce cancer mortality rates in impoverished countries, it is essential to identify the specific components of cancer control, such as primary prevention, early detection measures, and therapy, that are most likely to be successful [3, 55]. The early detection and prevention of illnesses can be achieved with the implementation of breast self-examination (BSE) to identify breast lumps. While breast cancer can affect people from all demographic groups, its epidemiology shows substantial diversity. The occurrence, length, and death rates of breast cancer differ, giving rise to multiple concerns about the cause, detection, and treatment choices for the illness [20].

8.4.2 PREVALENCE OF BREAST CANCER AT THE NATIONAL LEVEL

Breast cancer is the most prevalent kind of cancer among women in India. Among women, breast cancer is the most prevalent type of cancer. In India, a woman is diagnosed with breast cancer every four minutes, and every eight minutes, a woman dies directly from the illness. Furthermore, there is a noticeable increase in the incidence of breast cancer among women in India. It is estimated that roughly 70,218 women in India lost their lives as a direct consequence of breast cancer in the year 2012, making India the nation with the largest number of deaths that can be ascribed to the ailment. In India, the majority of the population is comprised of young people, and it is anticipated that the incidence of breast cancer among females will increase in the country. This is because young people make up the majority of the population. An increasing number of women in India, aged between 30 and 50, are being diagnosed with breast cancer, and this trend is expected to persist in the coming years. Breast cancer is a condition that specifically impacts women. Breast cancer is the leading cause of death among women worldwide in relation to any type of cancer. This holds true irrespective of the nature of the illness. Poorer nations experience a significantly higher rate of breast cancer. India experiences an annual incidence of about 0.8 million new instances of cancer, resulting in the death of over 0.5 million individuals. It is estimated that the annual incidence of cancer in India exceeds 2.5 million individuals. Based on the Twenty-Year Report of the Population-Based Cancer Registries 2004–2006, released by the National Cancer Registry Programme (NCRP), Indian Council of Medical Research, the occurrence of breast cancer in India ranged from 23 to 32 cases per 100,000 women. This information was obtained from the data collected over two years. The Indian Cancer Registry was used to acquire this information. The investigation leading to the discovery of this significant knowledge was conducted by a business called the Indian Council of Medical Research. The NCRP is responsible for overseeing a nationwide network of cancer registries [36]. This obligation arises from the partnership it has established with the Indian Council of Medical Research.

According to a 1999–2000 National Cancer Registry report, the major sites of cancer among women in six Indian cities are:

- In Bangalore, breast cancer is the leading cancer site (22.1%), followed by cervix (18.7%), together constituting over 40% of total cancers.
- In Barshi (Maharashtra), it is cervix (43.24%), followed by breast cancer (12.2%).
- In Bhopal, breast cancer (24.4%) is followed by cervix (21.4%).
- According to the Chennai Registry, the first cancer site is the cervix (25.2%), and breast cancer is second (22.5%).
- In Delhi, breast cancer is first (25.1%), and cervix is second (16.4%).
- In Mumbai, breast cancer is the leading (25.7%), and cervix is second (14.3%) (NCRP 2013).

India has a different incidence of breast cancer than Western nations in several ways, most notably in terms of age at beginning and stage of diagnosis. Compared to instances in Western nations, most cases of breast cancer in India happen 10 years sooner, mostly in the premenopausal stage. Early breast cancer comprises 60–70% of all reported cases of breast cancer at different cancer institutes in India. In contrast, early breast cancer accounts for sixty to seventy percent of occurrences in industrialized nations. Most patients in India seek medical attention when their condition has advanced, resulting in low survival and high death rates. Over 70% of patients seek therapy at an advanced stage [32].

8.5 TREATMENT FOR BREAST CANCER

The management of breast cancer may vary depending on the kind of cancer and the degree of its metastasis. People with breast cancer usually need many treatments, and physicians from various specializations commonly work together to treat breast cancer. Surgeons conduct surgeries, medical oncologists provide medications, and radiation oncologists use radiation to treat cancer. The doctor can discuss the risks, advantages, and side effects of each therapy choice. Sometimes, people seek a "second opinion" from another cancer doctor to help choose the most suitable treatment. The treatment of breast cancer includes the following [4].

8.5.1 BREAST SURGERY

A procedure in which surgeons remove cancer.

8.5.2 CHEMOTHERAPY

A treatment that involves the utilization of specialist drugs to reduce or eliminate cancer cells. It is possible to administer the drugs either orally, intravenously, or both.

8.5.3 TREATMENT WITH HORMONES

Because of this, cancer cells are unable to get the hormones that are necessary for their proliferation.

8.5.4 BIOLOGICAL TREATMENT

This works with the immune system to help kill cancer cells or deal with the bad effects of other cancer medicines.

8.5.5 RADIATION THERAPY

The elimination of cancer cells is accomplished by the utilization of high-energy rays, which are analogous to X-rays.

8.5.6 ALTERNATIVE AND COMPLEMENTARY MEDICINE FOR PATIENTS

Some examples of complementary and alternative medical techniques include massage therapy, acupuncture, tai chi, consumption of green tea, and the use of vitamins and herbal supplements. Additional modalities encompass acupuncture and massage therapy.

8.6 PSYCHOLOGICAL EXPERIENCES OF BREAST CANCER SURVIVORS

A considerable amount of research has investigated the psychosocial dimensions of breast cancer. To fully understand how women cope with the loss of their breasts, it is necessary to consider the broader context of their marital and social life. As breasts are part of female identity and define its aesthetic importance, the disease and surgery of the organ have social ramifications, as women live in a society where the female body is objectified and aestheticized. Theories about body image hold that society plays an important role in shaping one's body image. Thus, physical changes to the female body also have consequent social implications [49]. Each woman's experience of breast cancer is shaped by societal constructs, and the illness may profoundly influence a woman's perception of her own identity. Clinical explanations and treatment side effects fail to capture the actual psycho-social experience of breast cancer, necessitating an examination of the "patient's experience" of sickness within her social setting [11]. Breast cancer patients' quality of life is affected by their level of education, the help they get from their spouse, their job, and their ability to pay their bills. Women with unmarried children, nodal and/or metastatic cancer, and those who are presently getting active treatment had a much worse quality of life. The cancer diagnosis in the family brings a social stigma that may impair the children's marriage chances. The number of unmarried children has a big impact on breast cancer survivors' mental well-being. The loss of a personal impression of good health, combined with the dread of dying from cancer, forces women to seek support and knowledge both internally and outside. Bonding with other women with breast cancer resulted in an extension of self-boundaries, which provided comfort, a desire to change life goals, and a greater appreciation for helpful individuals and life itself [33]. Positive thinking, a sense of purpose in life, and strong family support all contribute to treatment completion and survival. Timely health-seeking behavior, appropriate general medicine, and emotional support from friends and family members were found to be critical elements in efficient coping.

Spirituality exerted a significant influence on people's coping methods. Sexually active women are more prone to encountering difficulties with their body image. The challenges encompass hair loss due to chemotherapy, apprehensions regarding weight fluctuations, deteriorating mental well-being, diminished self-confidence, and struggles in comprehending one's partner's emotions. These issues are also linked to mastectomy and likely reconstruction. Experiencing vaginal dryness, experiencing diminished mental well-being, being married, having a partner who struggles to comprehend one's thoughts, and facing more challenges with body image are all factors linked to a higher likelihood of experiencing sexual issues. The severity of these sexual problems was considerably different across different ethnic groups [50]. Breast cancer survivors report sexual disturbance and a complete loss of sexual desire. They see themselves as having lost their femininity, physical beauty, and attractiveness. Women experience "survivor loneliness" after undergoing breast cancer therapy. Some women are reported to be more susceptible to psychological disturbance. Loneliness is an important aspect of breast cancer survival. Mastectomy dramatically improved sexual functioning and satisfaction compared to breast conservation. Assessing perceived social support among breast cancer patients might help determine who will benefit from social sharing. Interventions might assist the social network and surroundings in responding to the socio-emotional features of breast cancer patients as they go through the disease. Women are more apprehensive about their breast cancer diagnoses. Women who undergo screening for excessive worry may be able to find those breast cancer patients who are most likely to suffer from excruciating pain as a result of their disease. Women establish their own coping mechanisms for treatment-related discomfort and side effects. Breast cancer patients with effective pain management methods have decreased levels of worry, tiredness, and sadness [12]. Therefore, using pain management techniques may enhance fatigue and alleviate psychological anguish in females diagnosed with breast cancer. The purpose of this study is to evaluate the link between protective buffering, psychological distress, and relationship satisfaction from the perspective of couples who are coping with breast cancer. Breast cancer survivors credit their cancer to God's will. Regardless, they are actively involved in their medical care. These findings can help researchers create a paradigm for creating culturally sensitive health treatments [5, 54]. Identifying stress predictors among caregivers may aid in stress prevention efforts for this population. After receiving a breast cancer diagnosis, both patients and partners endure substantial distress. Partners are as likely to feel unsupported by their patients and sad. There is an urgent need to address the enormous anguish experienced by both patients and spouses as a result of a lack of assistance. All cancer centers must offer psychosocial therapy that focus on the spouses of breast cancer patients in order to address their emotional needs. Surgeons and treatment facilities should educate patients about breast cancer therapy's pros and cons. This is especially crucial for women belonging to racial/ethnic minority groups who have received a breast cancer diagnosis. Breast cancer survivors have a moderate comprehension of clinical studies. As a result, it is critical for patients to be well-informed, to have their worries regarding involvement alleviated, and to understand the advantages of participation [21].

8.7 RAISING BREAST CANCER PREVENTION AND DETECTION AWARENESS

Breast cancer is a prevalent malignancy that affects people globally and is a significant global public health concern. The increased focus on breast cancer awareness, public scrutiny, and advancements in breast imaging has collectively led to enhanced identification and examination of the illness. It is important for every woman to have a clear understanding of the normal appearance and texture of her breasts in order to be able to identify any alterations. Breast Cancer Awareness Month is observed every October and holds special significance globally, especially in India. In a country where breast cancer is becoming more prevalent, Breast Cancer Awareness

Month plays a crucial role in educating, empowering, and inspiring action. This campaign serves as a beacon of hope and knowledge, encouraging women in India and around the world to take charge of their breast health. By raising awareness, dispelling myths, and fostering a culture of proactive health management, we can help ensure the timely detection of breast cancer, leading to effective treatment and significant improvements in survival rates. It is essential to continuously promote awareness, support early detection, and provide assistance to those affected by breast cancer [46]. This initiative holds immense significance for several reasons.

8.7.1 RISING INCIDENCE

Among Indian women, breast cancer has emerged as the predominant form of cancer, surpassing cervical cancer in terms of prevalence. India is witnessing an alarming pattern concerning breast cancer. In 2016, there were around 118,000 reported cases of breast cancer among individuals of Indian descent. According to the most recent data, India represented 13.5% of all breast cancer cases worldwide and accounted for 10.6% of the total breast cancer-related fatalities. Among women in India, breast cancer has emerged as the most prevalent form of cancer, surpassing cervical cancer. India has a significantly higher incidence of breast cancer. In 2016, a total of 118,000 individuals from India were diagnosed with breast cancer. According to the most recent data, India accounts for 13.5% of the global breast cancer incidences and 10.6% of all breast cancer-related fatalities. Gaining knowledge about individual risk factors, such as familial background, genetic predisposition, and lifestyle decisions, might enable women to actively take measures to safeguard their breast health. The numbers are concerning, highlighting the urgent need for increased awareness [25].

8.7.2 EARLY DETECTION

Around 60% of breast cancer cases in Indian women are diagnosed at advanced stages (Stage III or IV), resulting in worse survival rates. A recent study conducted in Mumbai found that doing clinical breast exams every two years in women aged 50 and older led to a notable 30% reduction in mortality attributable to breast cancer. Performing regular BSEs, undergoing clinical breast exams, and receiving mammography screenings can assist in the timely identification and management of breast cancer. Raising awareness about early detection can save lives. Here is the information paraphrased, with references, headings, and subheadings kept as they were.

8.7.3 STIGMA AND MYTHS

There are widespread myths in Indian society, especially in rural areas, regarding the contagiousness of cancer and the belief that a cancer diagnosis could damage the family's reputation. A study found that many women believed breast issues were the result or reflection of poor character, leading them to hide symptoms. This awareness month seeks to debunk myths, reduce stigma, and promote open discussions [13].

Women should adhere to recommended screening guidelines, such as mammograms and clinical breast exams, as advised by healthcare professionals. Every woman needs to learn how to perform BSEs regularly and report any unusual changes to a healthcare provider promptly. Reducing alcohol consumption, staying physically active, maintaining a healthy weight, and avoiding hormone replacement therapy can all help lower the risk of breast cancer. Additionally, advocating for better access to healthcare, particularly in underserved areas, is crucial to ensure that all women have the opportunity for early detection and treatment [51].

8.8 STRESS MANAGEMENT

Emotional suppression (the attempt to restrict the expression of unpleasant emotions) has been a major focus in psychosocial studies on cancer patients. This concept is increasingly recognized as a significant psychological component that influences psychosocial adjustment in breast cancer patients, and it may modulate health outcomes. Over the last three decades, much of the research on psychosocial risk factors in cancer has focused on the behavior patterns implicated in cancer initiation and prognosis. Emotional suppression is a crucial factor in coping with patients' psychological adjustment throughout cancer diagnosis and treatment. Individuals who are afflicted with life-threatening diseases, such as breast cancer, are likely to feel emotional distress; however, the degree of difficulty that they experience might vary from patient to patient [6].

8.8.1 INTERVENTION APPROACH TO BREAST CANCER SURVIVORS

An intervention is a set of plans aimed at changing behavior or improving health among people as a whole. Intervention techniques are adaptable to meet individuals' needs and offer them better solutions to problems. There are different types of intervention programs, for example, psycho-education, skill training, and counseling. Multiple strategy interventions are usually the most effective in eliciting desires and long-term change. Interventions can have different settings, including workplaces, communities, healthcare departments, insurance organizations, and homes [14, 53].

8.8.2 EFFORTS TO PREVENT THE OCCURRENCE OF BREAST CANCER

Breast cancer is a major issue for women, but with proper education and preventative measures, the chances can be reduced. Considerations that may help women stay healthy and prevent breast cancer to a considerable extent include: regular exercise and obesity prevention, avoiding obesity, maintaining a healthy weight, maintaining a BMI between 20 and 24, timely marriage and childbearing, having children at the right age, avoiding late childbirths and breastfeeding, avoiding pills containing estrogen, avoiding long-term hormone therapy, avoiding hormone replacement therapy, getting adequate sleep, avoiding junk food, a high-protein diet, an antioxidant-rich, low-calorie, and low-fat diet, drinking little or no alcohol, and avoiding smoking [34].

8.8.3 BREAST SELF-AWARENESS

An examination of the breasts that a woman can do on her own is called a breast self-exam for breast awareness. Although most breast changes observed during a self-examination for breast awareness are harmless, some modifications may suggest a more severe problem, such as breast cancer. Healthcare practitioners emphasize the need for women to become familiar with their own breasts to promptly identify any deviations from the usual and promptly report them [52]. The following actions must be taken to be ready for a BSE for breast awareness:

1. Seek a medical professional for clarification. It may be beneficial for a woman to go over the procedure and instructions with her doctor before starting her BSEs for breast awareness.
2. If a woman is menstruation, she ought to schedule her period for when her breasts are the least sensitive. Every month, throughout her menstrual cycle, her hormone levels fluctuate, resulting in alterations to her breast tissue. When her period starts, the swelling starts to go down. The week following the end of her menstrual cycle is often the ideal time to do a self-examination for breast awareness.
3. Begin with a visual examination of breasts:
   a. Position your arms alongside your body and face a mirror while being shirtless (for males) or braless (for females). To visually inspect the breasts, perform the following steps.
   b. Direct your gaze straight ahead and examine your face for any signs of dimpling, puckering, or changes in symmetry, size, or shape.
   c. Determine whether the nipples are inverted or retracted.
   d. Examine breasts by pressing your own hands on your hips.
   e. Examine breasts while raising your own arms upward and pressing your palms together.
   f. Raise the breasts to check for symmetry in the ridges running down the bottom.

8.8.4 BREAST SELF-EXAMINATION

Typical techniques for carrying out the breast exam's manual portion include:

- **Lying on one side:** Select a level surface, such as a bed, on which to rest your back. Breast tissue spreads out while you are lying down, which makes it thinner and more tactile.
- **In the bathtub:** To make your fingertips slide over your skin more smoothly, lather soap on your breasts and fingers.

Some general guidelines to bear in mind when inspecting breasts are as follows:

- **Make use of your own finger pads:** During the exam, it is recommended to utilize the pads of your three middle fingers instead of their tips. If a woman is experiencing difficulty in feeling with her fingertips, she might consider using a more delicate part of her hand, such as her palm or the dorsal side of her fingers.
- **Utilize a range of different pressure levels:** Applying varying degrees of pressure on all of the breast tissue allows one to experience varied levels of depth within the breast. This is the principle behind the breast sensitivity technique. Applying light pressure will allow you to feel the tissue that is next to the skin, applying moderate pressure will allow you to penetrate farther, and applying hard pressure will allow you to feel the tissue that is close to the chest and the ribs. Before moving on to the next spot, you should always be sure that you have applied each pressure level.
- **Allow adequate time:** Exercise patience. The thorough examination of the breasts may need a few minutes.
- **Reproduce a sequence of actions or elements consistently:** To achieve a comprehensive examination of the whole breast, adopt a meticulous technique. Take into account the clock face positioned above the chest or the individual slices of pie. Commence from the clavicle and go downward toward the nipple. Subsequently, proceed to relocate the fingers to the subsequent region.

8.8.5 SELF-EVALUATION AWARENESS

Know what is normal and seek medical attention if your breasts change. If the following symptoms are seen [7], a doctor should be contacted promptly.

- Breast lumps, knots, or thickening
- Breast enlargement, redness, warmth, or darkening of the breasts
- Variations in the look or sensation of the breasts, such as thickening or a more pronounced fullness
- On the breast skin, dimples, puckers, bulges, or ridges may be present

- Pulling in of the nipple or other breast regions is one of the symptoms of a nipple infection. Other symptoms include abrupt discharge. Nipple infections can cause itching, scaling, or a rash on the nipple
- Nipple inversion, redness, warmth, swelling, itching, scales, blisters, or rashes, and bloody nipple discharge
- A firm lump or knot around the armpit
- Nipple inversion with a persistent ache

8.9 EARLY DETECTION OF BREAST CANCER VIA SCREENING

Prompt identification and thorough evaluation of breast cancer are crucial for the health and welfare of women. Screening tests help expedite the prompt detection of breast cancer, when the likelihood of survival is highest [26].

8.9.1 GET SCREENED

- Consult a healthcare practitioner to determine whether screening tests are appropriate for high-risk women.
- Women who have a moderate risk of developing breast cancer should get an annual mammography beginning at the age of 40.
- Additionally, CBEs should be conducted every three years starting at the age of 20, and then annually beyond the age of 40 [15].

8.10 CONCLUSION

Breast cancer has an impact on women in terms of their psychological, social, and emotional adaptation. The disruption in family, social communication, increase in anger, anxiety, low self-esteem, financial worry, and fear of death was observed among breast cancer survivors. Breast cancer puts immense pressure on patients themselves as well as on their partners and their family members. Breast cancer survivors are facing problems psycho-socially as well as emotionally. Although many breast cancer survivors have gotten rid of the disease, they still have a negative impact of it, be it on their emotional wellness, their mental stability, or even their sexuality. Illiteracy plays a vital role in keeping these survivors from lagging. Their little knowledge about early detection of breast cancer is one of the several causes that led to the onset of this illness in their bodies. Had they been educated about breast self-examination and other examinations, treatments, and surgeries, they would not have had to suffer through various stages. This disease has led these survivors to devalue themselves due to body disfigurement. Although the relation between the family members, relatives, and friends has improved, self-esteem levels are visibly low among the survivors. Emotional suppression is an important aspect in dealing with patients' psychological adjustment after they have been diagnosed and treated for cancer. Patients with life-threatening conditions, such as breast cancer, undergo emotional distress; however, the depth of the unhappiness varies per patient.

KEYWORDS

- **causes**
- **diagnosis**
- **treatment**
- **psychosocial impact**
- **awareness**
- **knowledge**

REFERENCES

1. Al-Dubai, S. A., Qureshi, A. M., Saif-Ali, R., Ganasegeran, K., Alwan, M. R., & Hadi, J. I. (2011). Awareness and knowledge of breast cancer and mammography among a group of Malaysian women in Shah Alam. *Asian Pacific Journal of Cancer Prevention*, *12*(10), 2531–2538.
2. Amin, T. T., Al Mulhim, A. R., & Al Meqihwi, A. (2009). Breast cancer knowledge, risk factors, and screening among adult Saudi women in a primary health care setting. *Asian Pacific Journal of Cancer Prevention*, *10*(1), 133–138.
3. Anderson, K. N., Schwab, R. B., & Martinez, M. E. (2014). Reproductive risk factors and breast cancer subtypes: A review of the literature. *Breast Cancer Research and Treatment*, *144*, 1–10.

4. Akashi-Tanaka, S., Fukutomi, T., Nanasawa, T., Matsuo, K., Hasegawa, T., & Tsuda, H. (2000). Treatment of noninvasive carcinoma: Fifteen-year results at the National Cancer Center Hospital in Tokyo. *Breast Cancer*, *7*, 341–344.
5. Bevers, T., El-Serag, H., Hanash, S., Thrift, A. P., Tsai, K., Maresso, K. C., & Hawk, E. (2020). Screening and early detection. In: *Abeloff's Clinical Oncology* (pp. 375–398). Elsevier.
6. Bray, F., Ferlay, J., Soerjomataram, I., Siegel, R. L., Torre, L. A., & Jemal, A. (2018). Global cancer statistics 2018: GLOBOCAN estimates of incidence and mortality worldwide for 36 cancers in 185 countries. *CA: A Cancer Journal for Clinicians*, *68*(6), 394–424.
7. Brinton, L. A., Figueroa, J. D., Awuah, B., Yarney, J., Wiafe, S., Wood, S. N., & Clegg-Lamptey, J. N. (2014). Breast cancer in Sub-Saharan Africa: Opportunities for prevention. *Breast Cancer Research and Treatment*, *144*, 467–478.
8. Brinton, L. A., Bernstein, L., & Colditz, G. A. (1998). Summary of the workshop: Workshop on physical activity and breast cancer, November 13-14, 1997. *Cancer: Interdisciplinary International Journal of the American Cancer Society*, *83*(S3 3), 595–599.
9. Cady, B., Steele Jr, G. D., Morrow, M., Gardner, B., Smith, B. L., Lee, N. C., & Winchester, D. P. (1998). Evaluation of common breast problems: Guidance for primary care providers. *CA: A Cancer Journal for Clinicians*, *48*(1), 49–63.
10. Chlebowski, R. T., Hendrix, S. L., Langer, R. D., Stefanick, M. L., Gass, M., Lane, D., & WHI Investigators. (2003). Influence of estrogen plus progestin on breast cancer and mammography in healthy postmenopausal women: The Women's Health Initiative Randomized Trial. *JAMA*, *289*(24), 3243–3253.
11. Chlebowski, R. T. (2013). Nutrition and physical activity influence on breast cancer incidence and outcome. *The Breast*, *22*, S30–S37.
12. Clegg-Lamptey, J., Dakubo, J., & Attobra, Y. (2009). During treatment in Ghana? A pilot study. *Ghana Medical Journal*, *43*(3).
13. Cobleigh, M. A., Vogel, C. L., Tripathy, D., Robert, N. J., Scholl, S., Fehrenbacher, L., & Slamon, D. J. (1999). Multinational study of the efficacy and safety of humanized anti-HER2 monoclonal antibody in women who have HER2-overexpressing metastatic breast cancer that has progressed after chemotherapy for metastatic disease. *Journal of Clinical Oncology*, *17*(9), 2639–2639.
14. Doaa, G. M., Eman, S. A. A., & Nadia, M. T. (2015). Effect of a breast-self-examination (BSE) educational intervention among female university students. *American Journal of Nursing Science*, *4*(4), 159–165.
15. Dupont, W. D., Page, D. L., Parl, F. F., Vnencak-Jones, C. L., Plummer Jr, W. D., Rados, M. S., & Schuyler, P. A. (1994). Long-term risk of breast cancer in women with fibroadenoma. *New England Journal of Medicine*, *331*(1), 10–15.
16. Dupont, W. D., & Page, D. L. (1985). Risk factors for breast cancer in women with proliferative breast disease. *New England Journal of Medicine*, *312*(3), 146–151.
17. Early Breast Cancer Trialists' Collaborative Group. (2011). Effect of radiotherapy after breast-conserving surgery on 10-year recurrence and 15-year breast cancer death: Meta-analysis of individual patient data for 10 801 women in 17 randomised trials. *The Lancet*, *378*(9804), 1707–1716.

18. Fisher, B., Costantino, J. P., Wickerham, D. L., Redmond, C. K., Kavanah, M., Cronin, W. M., & Bowel Project Investigators. (1998). Tamoxifen for prevention of breast cancer: Report of the National Surgical Adjuvant Breast and Bowel Project P-1 Study. *JNCI: Journal of the National Cancer Institute*, *90*(18), 1371–1388.
19. Fisher, B., Dignam, J., Wolmark, N., Wickerham, D. L., Fisher, E. R., Mamounas, E., & Oishi, R. H. (1999). Tamoxifen in treatment of intraductal breast cancer: National Surgical Adjuvant Breast and Bowel Project B-24 randomised controlled trial. *The Lancet*, *353*(9169), 1993–2000.
20. Finne, P. (2000). *Development and Validation of Methods for Detection of Prostate Cancer,* (Doctoral dissertation, Helsingin yliopisto).
21. Gann, P. H., & Morrow, M. (2003). Combined hormone therapy and breast cancer: A single-edged sword. *JAMA*, *289*(24), 3304–3306.
22. Grady, D. (2002). A 60-year-old woman trying to discontinue hormone replacement therapy. *JAMA*, *287*(16), 2130–2137.
23. Grunfeld, E., Gray, A., Mant, D., Yudkin, P., Adewuyi-Dalton, R., Coyle, D., & Vessey, M. (1999). Follow-up of breast cancer in primary care vs specialist care: Results of an economic evaluation. *British Journal of Cancer*, *79*(7), 1227–1233.
24. Grunfeld, E., Mant, D., Yudkin, P., Adewuyi-Dalton, R., Cole, D., Stewart, J., & Vessey, M. (1996). Routine follow up of breast cancer in primary care: Randomised trial. *BMJ*, *313*(7058), 665–669.
25. Haber, D. (2002). Prophylactic oophorectomy to reduce the risk of ovarian and breast cancer in carriers of BRCA mutations. *New England Journal of Medicine*, *346*(21), 1660–1662.
26. Hadi, M. A., Hassali, M. A., Shafie, A. A., & Awaisu, A. (2010). Evaluation of breast cancer awareness among female university students in Malaysia. *Pharmacy Practice*, *8(*1), 29.
27. Harford, J. B. (2011). Breast-cancer early detection in low-income and middle-income countries: Do what you can versus one size fits all. *The Lancet Oncology*, *12*(3), 306–312.
28. Hoskins, K. F., Stopfer, J. E., Calzone, K. A., Merajver, S. D., Rebbeck, T. R., Garber, J. E., & Weber, B. L. (1995). Assessment and counseling for women with a family history of breast cancer: A guide for clinicians. *JAMA*, *273*(7), 577–585.
29. Huang, Z., Hankisen, S., Colditz, G., et al. (1997). Dual effects of weight and weight gain on breast cancer risk. *JAMA*, *278*, 1407.
30. John, E. M., & Kelsey, J. L. (1993). Radiation and other environmental exposures and breast cancer. *Epidemiologic Reviews*, *15*(1), 157–162.
31. Lee, K., Kruper, L., Dieli-Conwright, C. M., & Mortimer, J. E. (2019). The impact of obesity on breast cancer diagnosis and treatment. *Current Oncology Reports*, *21*, 1–6.
32. Lee-Feldstein, A., Anton-Culver, H., & Feldstein, P. J. (1994). Treatment differences and other prognostic factors related to breast cancer survival: Delivery systems and medical outcomes. *JAMA*, *271*(15), 1163–1168.
33. Lemlem, S. B., Sinishaw, W., Hailu, M., Abebe, M., & Aregay, A. (2013). Assessment of knowledge of breast cancer and screening methods among nurses in university hospitals in Addis Ababa, Ethiopia, 2011. *International Scholarly Research Notices*, *2013*(1), 470981.

34. Li, C. I., Malone, K. E., Porter, P. L., Weiss, N. S., Tang, M. T. C., Cushing-Haugen, K. L., & Daling, J. R. (2003). Relationship between long durations and different regimens of hormone therapy and risk of breast cancer. *JAMA*, *289*(24), 3254–3263.
35. Malone, K. E., Daling, J. R., Thompson, J. D., O'Brien, C. A., Francisco, L. V., & Ostrander, E. A. (1998). BRCA1 mutations and breast cancer in the general population: Analyses in women before age 35 years and in women before age 45 years with first-degree family history. *JAMA*, *279*(12), 922–929.
36. Moore, M., & Kinne, D. (1995). Clinical Highlights from the National Cancer Data Base, 1999. *CA: A Cancer Journal for Clinicians*, *49*(3), 145–158.
37. Mouridsen, H., Gershavovich, M., & Sun, Y. (2001). Superior efficacy of letrozole (Femeray) versus tamoxifen as first-line therapy for postmenopausal women with advanced breast cancer: Results of a phase III study of the International Letrozole Breast Cancer Group. *Journal of Clinical Oncology*, *19*, 2596.
38. Nabholtz, J. M., Buzdar, A., Pollak, M., Harwin, W., Burton, G., Mangalik, A., & Von Euler, M. (2000). Anastrozole is superior to tamoxifen as first-line therapy for advanced breast cancer in postmenopausal women: Results of a North American multicenter randomized trial. *Journal of Clinical Oncology*, *18*(22), 3758–3767.
39. Naku Ghartey Jnr, F., Anyanful, A., Eliason, S., Mohammed Adamu, S., & Debrah, S. (2016). Pattern of breast cancer distribution in Ghana: A survey to enhance early detection, diagnosis, and treatment. *International Journal of Breast Cancer*, *2016*(1), 3645308.
40. Obrist, M., Osei-Bonsu, E., Awuah, B., Watanabe-Galloway, S., Merajver, S. D., Schmid, K., & Soliman, A. S. (2014). Factors related to incomplete treatment of breast cancer in Kumasi, Ghana. *The Breast*, *23*(6), 821–828.
41. Oladimeji, K. E., Tsoka-Gwegweni, J. M., Igbodekwe, F. C., Twomey, M., Akolo, C., Balarabe, H. S., & Oladimeji, O. (2015). Knowledge and beliefs of breast self-examination and breast cancer among market women in Ibadan, South West, Nigeria. *PloS One*, *10*(11), e0140904.
42. Pietras, R. J., Fendly, B. M., Chazin, V. R., Pegram, M. D., Howell, S. B., & Slamon, D. J. (1994). Antibody to HER-2/neu receptor blocks DNA repair after cisplatin in human breast and ovarian cancer cells. *Oncogene*, *9*(7), 1829–1838.
43. Pike, M. C., Spicer, D. V., Dahmoush, L., & Press, M. F. (1993). Estrogens, progestogens, normal breast cell proliferation, and breast cancer risk. *Epidemiologic Reviews*, *15*(1), 17–35.
44. Potischman, N., Swanson, C. A., Siiteri, P., & Hoover, R. N. (1996). Reversal of relation between body mass and endogenous estrogen concentrations with menopausal status. *JNCI: Journal of the National Cancer Institute*, *88*(11), 756–758.
45. Rossouw, J. E., Anderson, G. L., Prentice, R. L., LaCroix, A. Z., Kooperberg, C., Stefanick, M. L., & Writing Group for the Women's Health Initiative Investigators. (2002). Risks and benefits of estrogen plus progestin in healthy postmenopausal women: Principal results From the Women's Health Initiative randomized controlled trial. *JAMA*, *288*(3), 321–333.
46. Sambanje, M. N., & Mafuvadze, B. (2012). Breast cancer knowledge and awareness among university students in Angola. *Pan African Medical Journal*, *11*(1), 70.
47. Scherber, S., Soliman, A. S., Awuah, B., Osei-Bonsu, E., Adjei, E., Abantanga, F., & Merajver, S. D. (2014). Characterizing breast cancer treatment pathways in

Kumasi, Ghana, from onset of symptoms to final outcome: Outlook towards cancer control. *Breast Disease*, *34*(4), 139–149.

48. Singletary, K. W., & Gapstur, S. M. (2001). Alcohol and breast cancer: Review of epidemiologic and experimental evidence and potential mechanisms. *JAMA*, *286*(17), 2143–2151.
49. Smith, H. O., Kammerer-Doak, D. N., Barbo, D. M., & Sarto, G. E. (1996). Hormone replacement therapy in the menopause: A pro opinion. *CA: A Cancer Journal for Clinicians*, *46*(6), 343–363.
50. Thune, I., Brenn, T., Lund, E., & Gaard, M. (1998). Tamoxifen for early breast cancer: An overview of the randomised trials. *Lancet (London, England)*, *351*(9114), 1451–1467.
51. Vogel, C. L., Cobleigh, M. A., Tripathy, D., Gutheil, J. C., Harris, L. N., Fehrenbacher, L., & Press, M. (2002). Efficacy and safety of trastuzumab as a single agent in first-line treatment of HER2-overexpressing metastatic breast cancer. *Journal of Clinical Oncology*, *20*(3), 719–726.
52. Winchester, D. J., Menck, H. R., & Winchester, D. P. (1997). The National Cancer Data Base report on the results of a large nonrandomized comparison of breast preservation and modified radical mastectomy. *Cancer: Interdisciplinary International Journal of the American Cancer Society*, *80*(1), 162–167.
53. Woods, E. R., Helvie, M. A., Ikeda, D. M., Mandell, S. H., Chapel, K. L., & Adler, D. D. (1992). Solitary breast papilloma: Comparison of mammographic, galactographic, and pathologic findings. *AJR. American Journal of Roentgenology*, *159*(3), 487–491.
54. Osei-Afriyie, S., Addae, A. K., Oppong, S., Amu, H., Ampofo, E., & Osei, E. (2021). Breast cancer awareness, risk factors and screening practices among future health professionals in Ghana: A cross-sectional study. *PLoS One*, *16*(6), e0253373.
55. Amoako, Y. A., Awuah, B., Larsen-Reindorf, R., Awittor, F. K., Kyem, G., Ofori-Boadu, K., et al. (2019). Malignant tumours in urban Ghana: Evidence from the city of Kumasi. *BMC Cancer*, *19*, 1–12.

CHAPTER 9

Social and Professional Support for Psychological and Mental Disorders: Improvement of Female Health

ASOKE KUMAR SAHA, CHINMOY KUMAR MONDAL, ROPAK ROY, HAMIDA ZINAT, and AFRIMA PARVEN

*Corresponding author

ABSTRACT

The state of one's mental health is a crucial component of their overall well-being, influencing every aspect of life. Specifically, women encounter distinct obstacles that can increase their vulnerability to psychological issues and mental disorders. This chapter explores how social and professional support critically contributes to the improvement of women's mental health, ultimately leading to enhanced overall well-being. Women encounter a range of stressors, including societal expectations, family and career pressures, and biological factors like hormonal fluctuations. These stressors can significantly affect their mental health, making it essential to address the issue comprehensively.

9.1 INTRODUCTION

The intricate interplay between mental health and overall well-being is a fundamental aspect of human existence. The prevalence of psychological issues, ranging from everyday stress to severe disorders, underscores the need for robust support systems [4, 5].

Holistic Approaches for Women's Sustainable Health, Volume 2: Advancements, Socioeconomic Impacts, and Innovative Strategies. Junaid Ahmad Malik, Anamika Chauhan, and Megh R. Goyal (Eds)

DOI: 10.1201/9781779641656-11

This chapter explores the significance of social and professional support in addressing psychological issues, emphasizing their roles, benefits, challenges, and the evolving and dynamic landscape of mental healthcare.

9.2 THE IMPORTANCE OF SOCIAL SUPPORT

Studies have consistently shown that social support networks play a pivotal role in promoting mental health among women. Friends, family, and community support systems offer a crucial safety net, providing emotional reassurance, companionship, and practical assistance when needed. Professional support, including mental health services, therapy, and counseling, complements social support by offering evidence-based interventions for psychological and mental disorders. It enables women to access the specialized care they may require addressing their unique challenges. Women grappling with posttraumatic stress disorder, eating disorders, anxiety disorders, or depression may significantly benefit from professional assistance. Various therapeutic approaches, including the application of cognitive behavioral therapy (CBT), the use of prescribed medications, and the incorporation of mindfulness techniques, have been effective in enhancing the mental well-being of women. Women, particularly those belonging to marginalized communities, frequently encounter obstacles when trying to access mental health services. Tackling these challenges, which encompass societal stigma, financial limitations, and inadequate awareness, is crucial to ensuring that every woman can access the necessary support. Public health campaigns and educational initiatives can help destigmatize mental health issues and encourage women to seek professional assistance when required.

- **Definition of social support:** Social support encompasses the assistance individuals receive from their social networks, including family, friends, colleagues, and community connections. In the context of mental disorders, social support plays a pivotal role in alleviating symptoms, fostering resilience, and promoting overall well-being.
- **Types of social support:** Social support revolves around (1) emotional support (i.e., providing empathy and care to help cope with emotions), (2) instrumental support (i.e., offering tangible aid or help with practical tasks), (3) informational support (i.e.,

providing guidance, advice, or information to solve problems, and (4) appraisal support (offering feedback or evaluation to understand situations better) from one's social network. It can take in many forms, from familial and friendly bonds to connections within peer groups and the broader community. Together, these four support systems form a comprehensive framework of support.

- **Impact on mental health:** Research has shown a positive relationship between strong social support and mental health [10]. Supportive relationships can lead to decreased stress, enhanced self-esteem, and a feeling of inclusion, thereby nurturing resilience in the face of psychological difficulties.
- **Challenges in social support:** Despite its benefits, social support encounters challenges such as stigma, misunderstanding, and the potential for strained relationships. It is imperative to address these challenges to maximize the beneficial effects of social support on mental well-being.

9.3 IMPORTANCE OF PROFESSIONAL SUPPORT

- **Definition of professional support:** Professional support entails interventions led by trained mental health professionals. Such professionals employ evidence-based strategies to address psychological issues to diagnose, treat, and support individuals with mental disorders; and include psychologists, psychiatrists, therapists, and counselors [8].
- **Role of professional support:** Professional support provides specialized expertise, diagnostics, and treatment options, which significantly improve the mental health landscape. It is crucial for individuals needing personalized interventions that go beyond what social support can provide.
- **Accessibility and challenges in professional support:** Access to professional support remains a global challenge, driven by socioeconomic status, systematic issues within the healthcare infrastructure and geographical, cultural differences, and other factors. Additionally, the stigma surrounding mental disorders may deter individuals from seeking professional help, highlighting the need for destigmatization efforts.

9.3.1 INTEGRATION OF SOCIAL AND PROFESSIONAL SUPPORT

- **Holistic approach to mental health:** Integrating social and professional support creates a comprehensive approach to mental healthcare. Collaboration between informal support networks and mental health professionals can bridge gaps and offer a more holistic framework.
- **Community-based programs:** Community-based mental health programs, combining peer support groups with professional guidance, have emerged as successful models. These initiatives leverage the strengths of both social and professional support to create inclusive and accessible services.

9.4 ROLE OF TECHNOLOGICAL ADVANCEMENTS ON FEMALE MENTAL HEALTH

Moreover, incorporating mental health services within primary healthcare facilities can enhance availability and diminish the social disapproval linked to seeking help. Cooperation among healthcare professionals, local groups, and social services is vital in establishing a nurturing atmosphere for women's mental well-being. In professional settings, establishing an environment that promotes mental health and support is crucial. Women who balance their professional careers alongside family responsibilities frequently face a heightened risk of experiencing burnout and developing stress-related disorders. Employers can implement policies that promote work-life balance, provide mental health resources, and destigmatize conversations around mental health. These measures can contribute to a more mentally resilient female workforce. Social and professional support must also consider the intersectionality of women's identities. Women of color as well as those with disabilities frequently encounter unique challenges and experiences that require specialized approaches to support and care. Inclusive and culturally competent services are vital to ensuring that the mental health needs of all women are met. In conclusion, social and professional support systems are integral in improving women's mental health. Identifying and addressing the distinct stressors and obstacles experienced by women, providing accessible and destigmatized mental health services, and fostering supportive environments in both personal and professional contexts are essential steps toward enhancing the overall well-being of women. By prioritizing women's mental health, we can foster a society that is more inclusive, mentally healthy, and beneficial not only for women but for the entirety of society.

- **Online communities and resources:** Online communities and resources offer women a platform to access information, exchange experiences, and receive support. Websites, forums, and apps dedicated to women's mental health create virtual spaces where women can connect and find support and advice, all accessible conveniently in their personal spaces.
- **Telehealth and online support:** Technological advancements have revolutionized mental healthcare, offering online counseling, therapy apps, and telehealth services. Telehealth services, online therapy platforms, and mental health apps provide convenient and accessible support, overcoming geographical and logistical barriers [1]. These platforms provide convenient options for seeking professional guidance and connecting with peer support networks, overcoming geographical barriers.
- **Challenges and ethical considerations:** While technology enhances access to support, it also introduces issues related to confidentiality, data integrity, and security, and the risks for a depersonalized therapeutic experience. Locating a perfect equilibrium between technological innovations and ethical concerns is essential for technology to effectively integrate into mental healthcare.

9.5 WORKPLACE SUPPORT FOR FEMALE MENTAL HEALTH

- **Corporate responsibility:** Recognizing the influence of mental health on productivity and the well-being of employees, many organizations are adopting workplace mental health programs. These initiatives may include employee assistance programs, mental health days, and awareness campaigns to create a supportive and stigma-free work environment. By enacting policies that promote work-life balance, offering mental health leave days, and cultivating a supportive organizational culture, organizations contribute significantly to establishing an environment, where women experience a sense of worth and encouragement [5].

- **Reducing stigma in the workplace:** Workplace environments can contribute to or alleviate mental health stigma. Organizations can play an instrumental role in diminishing the stigma surrounding mental health disorders by fostering open communication, promoting a supportive culture, and providing resources. This foundational support is crucial in motivating individuals to pursue professional support. This includes on-site childcare facilities, flexible work arrangements, and awareness programs to reduce stigma associated with postpartum mental health issues.

9.6 CULTURAL COMPETENCE IN SUPPORT SYSTEMS

- **Understanding diverse perspectives:** Cultural competence is imperative in both social and professional support systems. Recognizing and respecting diverse cultural backgrounds ensures that support services are inclusive and effective for individuals from a range of social backgrounds, ethnicities, and religions.
- **Cultural challenges in professional support:** Mental health professionals must be equipped with cultural competence to navigate the nuances of diverse populations. Understanding cultural perceptions of mental health, stigma, and help-seeking behavior is pivotal for providing effective support.

9.7 MENTAL DISORDERS: A COMPREHENSIVE EXPLORATION

The intricate relationship between mental disorders and social and professional support systems is a critical aspect of mental healthcare. Mental disorders, such as anxiety, depression, and more severe conditions like schizophrenia, bring about significant challenges to individuals' well-being. This essay delves into the broad landscape of social and professional support for mental disorders, highlighting their roles, impact, challenges, and the evolving paradigms in mental healthcare.

9.7.1 ROLE OF SOCIAL SUPPORT IN MENTAL DISORDERS

Extensive research demonstrates the positive correlation between robust social support and better outcomes for individuals with mental disorders. Strong social networks contribute to reduced symptom severity, enhanced treatment adherence, and improved quality of life for those grappling with mental health challenges.

Despite its potential benefits, social support encounters challenges in the context of mental disorders. Stigma, lack of understanding, and communication barriers may hinder the effectiveness of social support networks. Addressing these challenges is crucial for optimizing the supportive role of family, friends, and communities.

- **Importance of social networks:** Social support from family, friends, and communities plays a pivotal role in women's mental health. Strong social networks contribute to resilience, stress reduction, and a sense of belonging, acting as protective factors against psychological and mental disorders.
- **Women's peer support groups:** Women-specific peer support groups provide a safe space for shared experiences, nurturing a sense of camaraderie, empathy and understanding. These groups address issues such as body image, motherhood, and relationships, establishing a supportive environment for women as they navigate their mental well-being.
- **Role of family and community:** Families and communities are essential components of a woman's support system. Understanding, empathy, and open communication within these networks contribute to an environment that encourages seeking help and reduces the stigma associated with mental health issues.
- **Challenges in social support for women:** Despite its benefits, social support for women's mental health encounters challenges, including societal stigma, gender norms, and cultural expectations. Efforts to destigmatize mental health discussions and promote inclusivity are essential for optimizing the positive impact of social support.

9.7.2 ROLE OF PROFESSIONAL SUPPORT FOR FEMALE MENTAL DISORDERS

Mental health professionals play diverse roles in the management of mental disorders, ranging from diagnostic assessments and psychotherapy to medication management and crisis intervention. Their expertise is particularly crucial for severe and persistent mental illnesses that may require specialized care.

- **Specialized care for women:** Mental health professionals, including psychologists, therapists, and gynecologists, play a crucial role in providing specialized care for women. Tailoring interventions to address women-specific issues, such as reproductive health concerns and life transitions, contributes to more effective treatment.
- **Therapeutic approaches:** Psychotherapy and counseling offer women a safe space to explore and address mental health challenges. CBT, Dialectical Behavior Therapy, and Trauma-Informed Care are particularly beneficial in addressing the diverse needs of women facing psychological and mental disorders.
- **Role of women's health practitioners:** Gynecologists and obstetricians are well-positioned to integrate mental health screenings into routine women's health visits. Recognizing the interconnectedness of physical and mental well-being, these practitioners contribute to early identification and intervention for mental health challenges.
- **Access to women-centric mental health services:** Providing mental health services that are finely tuned to the distinct needs of women is critical. This encompasses services for reproductive health, postpartum mental healthcare, and trauma-informed approaches that consider the distinct challenges encountered by women throughout their lives.

9.7.3 INTEGRATION OF SOCIAL AND PROFESSIONAL SUPPORT SYSTEMS: HOLISTIC APPROACH

- **Comprehensive approach to mental healthcare:** To effectively manage mental health, it is crucial to integrate social and professional support systems. Collaboration between informal support networks and mental health professionals can address the multifaceted nature of mental disorders, combining emotional support with evidence-based interventions.
- **Community-based programs:** Community-based mental health programs that integrate peer support groups with professional guidance have demonstrated success. These initiatives leverage

the strengths of both social and professional support to create inclusive and accessible services for individuals with varying degrees of mental health challenges.

- **Collaboration between social and professional support:** The integration of social and professional support creates a holistic approach to women's mental health. Collaborative efforts between informal support networks and mental health professionals address the complexity of women's experiences, combining emotional support with evidence-based interventions [7].
- **Educational campaigns:** Public awareness campaigns fulfill a crucial function in mitigating the stigma surrounding mental health concerns among women. These campaigns effectively educate communities, families, and individuals about the commonality and manageability of mental disorders, thereby fostering a supportive environment that encourages seeking assistance [3].

9.7.4 CULTURAL COMPETENCE IN MENTAL HEALTH SUPPORT SYSTEMS

The symbiotic relationship between social and professional support is essential for nurturing mental well-being. Recognizing the significance of informal as well as formal support systems, addressing challenges, and embracing technological advancements enable workplaces, communities, and individuals to promote a mental healthcare approach that is both comprehensive and efficient. By fostering a culture of understanding, empathy, and collaboration, society can create a robust framework that supports individuals on their journey toward mental well-being.

- **Understanding diverse perspectives:** Cultural competence is essential in both social and professional support systems for mental disorders. Recognizing and respecting diverse cultural backgrounds ensures that support services are inclusive and tailored to the unique needs of individuals from a range of ethnicities, religions, and social backgrounds.
- **Cultural challenges in professional support:** Mental health professionals must be equipped with cultural competence to navigate the complexities of diverse populations. Understanding cultural perceptions of mental health, stigma, women's roles,

reproductive health, and help-seeking behavior is pivotal for providing effective and culturally sensitive support to individuals with mental disorders [6].

- **Understanding cultural nuances:** Cultural competence is crucial in both social and professional support systems for women's mental health. Recognizing and respecting diverse cultural backgrounds ensures that support services are inclusive and sensitive to the unique challenges faced by women from a range of ethnicities, religions, and social settings.

Comprehensive support for individuals with mental disorders requires a synergistic approach that embraces both social and professional dimensions. Recognizing the critical roles of informal support networks and mental health professionals, addressing accessibility challenges, leveraging technological innovations, and promoting cultural competence contribute to a more effective and inclusive mental healthcare system. By nurturing a collaborative and empathetic environment, society can play a pivotal role in supporting individuals on their journey toward mental well-being in the face of mental disorders.

The complex interplay between psychological and mental health issues poses unique challenges for women, necessitating a multifaceted approach to support their well-being. This essay explores the diverse facets of social and professional support systems and their impact on enhancing women's mental health. By analyzing the obstacles encountered by women, the influence of social and professional support, and the significance of a comprehensive approach, we can gain deeper insights into addressing the intricate mental health needs of women [2, 9].

9.8 SUMMARY

The enhancement of women's mental health requires a comprehensive and tailored approach that embraces both social and professional dimensions. Recognizing the unique challenges faced by women, addressing stigma, leveraging technology, and promoting cultural competence contribute to a more effective and inclusive mental healthcare systems. By fostering collaborative efforts between informal support networks, mental health professionals, workplaces, and technological innovations, society can create an environment that supports women on their path to mental well-being.

KEYWORDS

- **social and professional support**
- **psychological**
- **mental disorders**
- **women's health**

REFERENCES

1. Becker, M. H. (1974). The Health Belief Model and personal health behavior. *Health Education Monographs, 2*(4), 324–508.
2. Cohen, S., & Wills, T. A. (1985). Stress, social support, and the buffering hypothesis. *Psychological Bulletin, 98*(2), 310–357.
3. Hankin, B. L., Abramson, L. Y., Moffitt, T. E., Silva, P. A., McGee, R., & Angell, K. E. (1998). Development of depression from preadolescence to young adulthood: Emerging gender differences in a 10-year longitudinal study. *Journal of Abnormal Psychology, 107*(1), 128–140.
4. Kessler, R. C., & McLeod, J. D. (1984). Sex differences in vulnerability to undesirable life events. *American Sociological Review, 49*(5), 620–631.
5. Mojtabai, R., Olfson, M., & Mechanic, D. (2002). Perceived need and help-seeking in adults with mood, anxiety, or substance use disorders. *Archives of General Psychiatry, 59*(1), 77–84.
6. Satcher, D. (2001). *Mental Health: A Report of the Surgeon General.* U.S. Department of Health and Human Services.
7. Uchino, B. N. (2004). *Social Support and Physical Health: Understanding the Health Consequences of Relationships.* Yale University Press.
8. Wang, P. S., Berglund, P., & Kessler, R. C. (2003). Patterns and correlates of contacting clergy for mental disorders in the United States. *Health Services Research, 38*(2), 647–673.
9. World Health Organization. (2013). *Mental Health Action Plan 2013–2020* (p. 45; 9789241506021). World Health Organization: Geneva.
10. Zineldin, M. (2021). Neurological and psychological determinants of depression, anxiety, and life quality. *International Journal of Preventive Medicine, 12*, 95–99. doi: 10.4103/ijpvm.IJPVM_237_19

CHAPTER 10

Holistic Approach to Menopause and Menstruation Issues in Females

JAYMALA KUMAWAT,* VRUSHALI NEVE, YOGITA SHINDE, ARCHANA SHAHA, and DIPALI TALELE

*Corresponding author

ABSTRACT

A female's reproductive journey is impacted by menopause transition and the regular monthly cycle, which influences her physical, emotional, and social well-being. Research studies recommend a holistic approach for effective control of menopausal and menstruation-related issues by accounting for social, intellectual, and biological factors. The organic details draw attention to the complex hormonal changes that are the essence of menstruation and menopause. To create efficient treatment programs, it is imperative to comprehend these physiological processes. The study also examines newer studies on diet, hormone therapy, and lifestyle modifications to improve overall health and manage symptoms during those phases. This approach acknowledges the substantial influence that hormone fluctuations have by accounting for mental clarity, emotional balance, and intellectual fitness. Techniques to support emotional fitness are covered along with stress management, cognitive-behavioral therapy, and mindfulness exercises. The sociocultural issues also highlight the methods in which women's experiences with menopause and menstruation are shaped by healthcare systems, cultural norms, and societal attitudes. A thorough plan should address social taboos, offer inclusive, compassionate healthcare, and encourage education on those subjects.

Holistic Approaches for Women's Sustainable Health, Volume 2: Advancements, Socioeconomic Impacts, and Innovative Strategies. Junaid Ahmad Malik, Anamika Chauhan, and Megh R. Goyal (Eds)

DOI: 10.1201/9781779641656-12

This review chapter provides an overview of current research findings, clinical procedures, and community-based treatments for menopause and menstruation-related issues.

10.1 INTRODUCTION

10.1.1 SIGNIFICANCE OF MENOPAUSE AND MENSURATION

A woman's menopause, which marks the end of her reproductive years, is a significant life turning point. It generally occurs between the ages of 45 and 55, with an average age of around 51. The term "menopause" refers to the natural reduction in reproductive hormones that causes the menstrual cycle to stop for a period of 12 consecutive months [1].

The physical and psychological effects of menopause on women's health are what make it significant. The physical symptoms associated with menopause are mood swings, hot flashes, vaginal dryness, nocturnal sweats, and reduced sex desire [2]. These symptoms may significantly affect a woman's quality of life and necessitate medical treatment. An increased risk of osteoporosis, cardiovascular disease, and other disorders in women is one of the long-term health implications of menopause. Certain tumors are seen postmenopausally. Thus, to lower their chance of developing these disorders, women should take care of their health both during and after menopause [1].

Menopause is frequently seen as a taboo topic in our society, and many women feel alone or ashamed when they talk about their experiences. This may result in a lack of sympathy and empathy for menopausal women, which may worsen their mental and emotional health. The menopause, in general, is a major life shift that has an impact on women socially, emotionally, and physiologically. It is critical that women get menopause education, knowledge, and support so that they can move through this time of life with ease and confidence [1].

10.1.2 RATIONALE FOR A COMPREHENSIVE APPROACH TO MENOPAUSE

Because menopause and menstrual health are such complex problems with such wide-ranging effects on women's lives; therefore, a thorough approach to these issues is essential. The following main justifications for a thorough approach are necessary [2].

- **Menopause** is a complicated time duration due to the intricate interactions between hormonal, physical, and psychological changes. A detailed knowledge of these developments and their implications for women's health is made possible by a holistic approach.
- **Menopausal experiences** might differ greatly from one woman to the next. Numerous variables, including lifestyle, genetics, and medical history, might affect the timing and intensity of menopausal symptoms. A comprehensive strategy considers these unique variations. Long-term health effects (such as osteoporosis, cardiovascular disease, and several types of cancers) are among the disorders for which menopause is linked to an elevated risk [2].
- **A thorough approach** enables the investigation of these long-term health impacts as well as treatments and prevention techniques.
- **Considerations for quality of life**: The quality of life for women can be greatly impacted by menopausal symptoms. An all-encompassing strategy looks at approaches to better manage symptoms and promote general health.
- **Social and cultural issues**: Several social and cultural issues, such as views on aging and menopause, access to healthcare, and cultural preconceptions on women's health, have an impact on menopause. A thorough approach considers these elements and how they affect the experiences of women [2].
- **Interdisciplinary perspectives**: Medicine, psychology, sociology, anthropology, and other disciplines can all contribute to our understanding of the interdisciplinary themes of menopause and menstrual health. These viewpoints are integrated in a comprehensive method to offer a thorough knowledge of tissue [1].

This review chapter examines research studies on diet, hormone therapy (HT), and lifestyle modifications, and a holistic approach to improve overall health and manage symptoms associated with menopause and menstruation.

10.2 METRICS OF THE BODY

10.2.1 EFFECTS OF HORMONE FLUCTUATIONS

Hormone fluctuations affect many facets of women's physiology and health, and they are crucial to menopause and menstrual health. The following are the main hormones at play and their effects:

- **Estrogen**: Throughout the menstrual cycle, estrogen levels vary, and they decrease during menopause. Menstrual cycle regulation, bone density maintenance, and cardiovascular health are all aided by estrogen. A reduction in estrogen is associated with symptoms of menopause (such as hot flashes, nocturnal sweats, mood swings, and dry vagina).
- **Progesterone**: During the menstrual cycle, progesterone levels fluctuate and peak during the luteal phase. When a pregnancy develops, progesterone plays a role in both preparing the uterus and sustaining the pregnancy. Progesterone levels drop during menopause, which may be a factor in irregular menstrual periods and other symptoms [3].
- **Follicle-stimulating hormones** (FSH): As the ovaries lose their sensitivity to progesterone and estrogen during menopause, FSH levels rise. Menstrual cycle discontinuation and the start of menopausal symptoms are linked to elevated FSH levels [3].
- **Luteinizing hormone** (LH): Due to alterations in ovarian function, LH levels also rise after menopause. LH plays a role in the development of ovarian follicles and the control of the menstrual cycle.
- **Testosterone** affects muscle mass, libido, and bone health in women; however, it is present in modest amounts. Menopause may cause a drop in testosterone levels, which may have an impact on energy and sexual drive [2].

10.2.2 MENOPAUSE AND MENSTRUAL PHYSIOLOGICAL METHODS

Examining the biological changes and processes that take place in the body during these phases is a key component of physiological methods for researching menopause and menstrual health. These techniques can offer insightful information about the changes that take place in terms of hormones, physiology, and metabolism, as well as the implications for women's health. The following are several important physiological techniques [3]:

- **Hormone testing** measures the concentrations of important hormones in the blood or saliva, including progesterone, estrogen, FSH, and LH. This can be used to evaluate menopause or the stage of the menstrual cycle, as well as ovarian function and hormone balance.
- **Ultrasound imaging** can be used to view the uterus and ovaries, evaluate the development of follicles, and identify any anomalies. During the menstrual cycle, transvaginal ultrasonography is frequently used to measure endometrial thickness and ovarian follicles [3].
- **Bone density testing:** Because osteoporosis is a prevalent issue during and after menopause owing to hormonal changes, bone health may be assessed, and problems can be identified by bone density testing, such as dual-energy X-ray absorptiometry scans.
- **Cardiovascular assessment:** Cardiovascular exams can be used to determine a person's risk of cardiovascular disease, which rises after menopause. These evaluations may include blood pressure monitoring, cholesterol profiling, and other procedures [2].
- **Metabolic testing** includes lipid profiles and glucose tolerance tests. This can evaluate metabolic health and the likelihood of diseases like metabolic syndrome and diabetes, which can be impacted by menopausal hormone fluctuations.
- **Menstrual cycle monitoring:** By using tools like calendar tracking or applications to track the cycles, women can gain valuable information about the length, regularity, and irregularities of menstrual cycles [3].

10.2.3 TECHNIQUES FOR MANAGING HORMONE SHIFTS

- **Changes in one's lifestyle** can help better control hormone fluctuations and improve general health. Regular exercise can aid with hormone regulation, stress reduction, and mood enhancement. It is crucial to get enough sleep because menopause-related sleep disruptions might throw off the hormone balance. Additionally, hormone balance and general health can be enhanced by stress management practices like yoga, meditation, or mindfulness [3].

- **Dietary changes:** Eating a healthy, balanced diet (rich in fruits, vegetables, whole grains, and lean meats) helps to improve hormone balance and overall health (Figure 10.1). Certain foods contain phytoestrogens or omega-3 fatty acids, which may help to reduce menopausal symptoms. Examples of these foods are fatty fish, flaxseeds, and soy products. Reducing alcohol, caffeine, and spicy foods—all of which can cause hot flashes—might be advantageous as well [2].

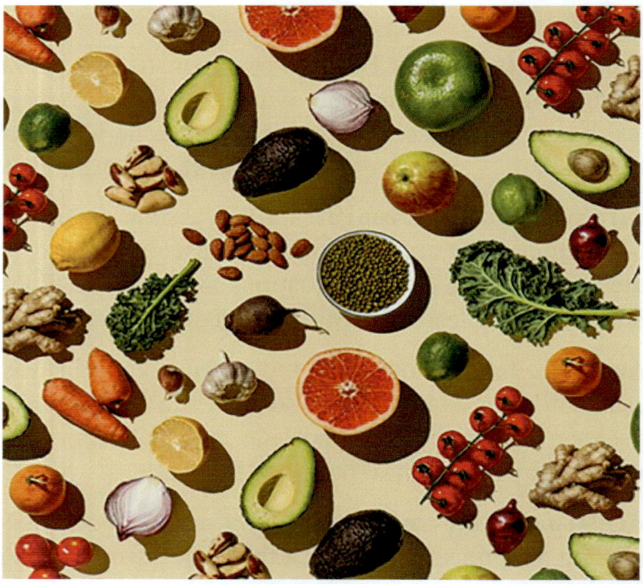

FIGURE 10.1 Dietary changes for management of menopause phase in females.

Source: DownToEarth. https://www.downtoearth.org.in/food/fibre-is-your-body-s-natural-guide-to-weight-management-90382

- **The use of hormones [6]:** During menopause, hormone changes are commonly managed using HT. In HT, hormones that the body can no longer generate in sufficient levels are replaced by taking either estrogen alone, or, in the case of women with uteruses, estrogen coupled with progesterone. Hot flashes, nocturnal sweats, mood swings, and vaginal dryness are all menopausal symptoms that can be alleviated with HT. There are hazards associated with HT; therefore, it is crucial to consider the advantages and disadvantages with a healthcare professional [2, 6].

- **Alternative therapies:** Acupuncture, herbal supplements (such as black cohosh and evening primrose oil), and bioidentical hormone treatment are some of the alternative therapies that some women find helpful in relieving menopausal symptoms. These treatments are not controlled in the same way as traditional treatments; therefore, it is crucial to speak with a medical professional first before attempting them [3].
- **Frequent health checkups:** Throughout the menopause, regular health checkups are crucial for tracking hormone levels, bone density, and general wellness. Medical professionals can provide advice on how to control menopausal symptoms and lower the chance of developing long-term health issues [3].

10.3 A MENTAL PERSPECTIVE

10.3.1 THE EFFECT OF HORMONE FLUCTUATIONS ON COGNITIVE FITNESS

Menopausal hormone swings can significantly affect memory, focus, and general cognitive function, among other aspects of cognitive fitness. Hormone changes can impact cognitive fitness in the following important ways:

- **Memory and estrogen:** Estrogen is essential for brain activity, which includes forming and retrieving memories. Certain women may have memory issues during menopause, when their estrogen levels drop, making it harder for them to recall specifics or names. This phenomenon is commonly known as "menopausal brain fog."
- **Cognitive function:** In addition to affecting executive function, attention, and processing speed, estrogen also affects other facets of cognitive function. During menopause, some women may experience changes in their ability to concentrate or do multitask.

- **Mood and cognitive health:** Changes in hormone levels can also have an impact on mood, which can therefore influence cognitive health. Mood swings, such as elevated anxiety or anger, can impact general well-being and cognitive performance.
- **Brain structure and function:** Estrogen contributes to the upkeep of brain networks and individual brain cells. Cognitive decline may be exacerbated by changes in brain structure and function brought on by declining estrogen levels during menopause [3].
- **Menopause and Alzheimer's disease:** According to research studies, menopause's hormonal changes may raise one's chance of getting Alzheimer's later in life. To fully comprehend the connection between menopause, hormone fluctuations, and the risk of Alzheimer's disease, further research is necessary.

It is crucial to consider that not all women undergo cognitive changes throughout menopause, and that individual differences in the severity of these changes might occur. Elements like menopause-related cognitive decline may also be influenced by lifestyle choices, genetics, and general health [4].

10.3.2 EMOTIONAL STABILITY AND MENTAL HEALTH

- **Mood swings:** Hormonal changes brought on by menopause can cause mood swings such as melancholy, anxiety, and irritability. These mood swings can affect relationships and daily life, and they can be difficult to control.
- **Depression and anxiety:** During menopause, some women may be more susceptible to experiencing depression and anxiety. Hormone fluctuations can impact the brain's neurotransmitters, including serotonin, which are involved in mood regulation.
- **Stress response:** Women are more vulnerable to stress and its negative impacts on mental health since hormonal fluctuations can also influence the body's stress response. Mood disorders and other mental health problems can be exacerbated by prolonged stress.
- **Menopausal symptoms** like hot flashes and night sweats can cause sleep disturbances, which can make you tired and irritable. Insufficient sleep can affect mental health and mood as well.

- **One's feeling of self-worth and body image** might be affected by menopausal changes, such as weight gain or changes in body shape. Hormonal shifts in addition to these changes may exacerbate emotional instability.
- **Coping mechanisms:** To handle the emotional and mental health difficulties associated with menopause, women may need to learn new coping mechanisms (such as asking friends, family, or mental health experts for assistance) as well as practicing stress-reduction strategies like mindfulness or relaxation exercises [4].

10.3.3 TECHNIQUES FOR PRESERVING EMOTIONAL BALANCE

The following methods that support resilience and mental health can be used to maintain emotional balance throughout menopause and monthly fluctuations.

- **Techniques for cognitive behavioral therapy (CBT):** CBT is a popular treatment strategy that can assist women in coping with the emotional difficulties associated with menopause. The primary objective of CBT techniques is to identify and modify maladaptive thinking and behavior patterns. This can lessen stress, anxiety, and depressive symptoms in women and help them create more effective coping mechanisms [4].
- **Techniques for mindfulness:** Women who practice mindfulness techniques such as yoga, meditation, and deep breathing exercises might benefit from increased awareness of their thoughts and feelings. These techniques can ease tension, encourage relaxation, and enhance general emotional health. Women who practice mindfulness might also grow to be more accepting and compassionate toward themselves and their menopausal experiences.
- **Stress management techniques:** During menopause, maintaining emotional equilibrium requires effective stress management. Women who practice progressive muscle relaxation, journaling, and guided imagery can experience a decrease in stress and an increase in their capacity to handle day-to-day difficulties. It is also critical that women give self-care activities that encourage enjoyment and relaxation top priority.

- **Assistance networks:** Having a solid support system in place can help women through menopause by offering them both practical and emotional support. This can include those who can provide understanding, support, and direction, such as friends, family, support groups, or mental health experts.
- **Choosing a healthier lifestyle:** Emotional well-being during menopause can be enhanced by regular exercise, a healthy diet, adequate sleep, and abstaining from alcohol and tobacco. These lifestyle selections can be beneficial.
- Women should take care of their *physical well-being*, which helps to support their emotional well-being. Women can improve their emotional resilience and balance during menopause and other monthly changes by adopting these practices into their daily life [2–4].

10.4 SOCIETAL AND CULTURAL RELATIONSHIPS

10.4.1 EDUCATING WOMEN ABOUT THE MENOPAUSE AND MENSTRUATION

Promoting health literacy and enabling women to effectively manage their reproductive health depend on educating them about menopause and menstruation, and explain the concept of menopause, including its average age of onset, the function of hormones, and the possible emotional and physical changes that may take place. The following are some essential elements that ought to be covered in an education section:

- **Menopause symptoms:** List the typical signs and symptoms of menopause, including mood swings, altered menstrual cycles, hot flashes, vaginal dryness, and night sweats. Describe how different women will have varying degrees of symptoms [5].
- Talk about the *long-term health hazards* that come with going through menopause, including osteoporosis, cardiovascular disease, and some types of cancer. Stress the value of maintaining regular health examinations and screenings.
- **Managing menopause:** Educate women about lifestyle modifications that can help them manage the symptoms of menopause

and lower their chance of developing related health issues. These modifications include nutrition, exercise, and stress management. Talk about the function of HT and other available therapies [4].

- **Understanding menstruation**: Inform women on the phases, typical duration, and functions of hormones like progesterone and estrogen during the menstrual cycle.
- **Menstrual hygiene:** Disseminate knowledge regarding menstrual hygiene habits, such as using sanitary items and disposing of them properly. Dispute frequent misunderstandings and beliefs regarding the menstrual cycle.
- **Period disorders:** Discuss the causes and treatments of common menstruation problems, such as amenorrhea (absence of periods), dysmenorrhea (painful periods), and menorrhagia (heavy periods) [5].
- **Reproductive health:** Stress the value of routine gynecological examinations and cancer and other problems with reproductive health. Women should be encouraged to talk to a healthcare provider about any worries or changes in their menstrual cycle [3].
- **Cultural and social attitudes:** Discuss taboos and stigmas related to menopause and menstruation, as well as cultural and societal attitudes in general. Encourage candid discussions about these subjects to foster support and understanding [5].

10.4.2 SOCIAL ATTITUDES AND CULTURAL NORMS

Diverse countries and cultures have rather distinct social views and cultural conventions around menopause and menstruation. Women's experiences and views of menopause and menstruation can be greatly influenced by these attitudes and standards. The following are some prevalent cultural norms and societal attitudes around these subjects:

- **Taboos and stigmas:** Menstruation is associated with taboos and stigmas in certain cultures, which causes shame and secrecy surrounding the subject. Open discussion of menstruation may make women feel awkward or ashamed, which may limit their access to resources and assistance [4].

- **Menopause as a sign of aging:** Menopause is frequently regarded as a normal aspect of aging and is even linked to wisdom and maturity in certain cultures. Menopause, however, could be seen more unfavorably in other cultures, with women perceived of being "old" or "past their prime" [4].
- **Effect on gender roles:** Gender norms and expectations may be impacted by menstruation and menopause. Certain cultural norms may dictate that women should perform roles or exhibit behaviors during their menstrual cycle or menopause. This may have an impact on how women view themselves and are seen by others [2].
- **Cultural traditions and beliefs:** Throughout history, many societies have developed unique traditions and beliefs around the menstrual cycle and the menopause. For instance, menarche, or the start of the menstrual cycle, and menopause are observed with rituals or ceremonies in certain societies. These practices can differ greatly and impact women's experiences in both positive and negative ways [3].
- **Access to healthcare:** Women's access to menstrual and menopausal healthcare can also be impacted by cultural norms and attitudes. Ladies in certain cultures have beliefs that prevent women from getting medical attention for menstruation abnormalities or menopausal symptoms, or they may not be aware of the therapies that are available [4].
- **Education and awareness:** A society's degree of education and awareness regarding menstruation and menopause can be influenced by cultural attitudes and customs. There may be extensive educational programs and candid conversations regarding these subjects in certain cultures, but there may be little information available in others [5].
- **Economic and social status:** Menstruation and menopause-related attitudes and conventions can be influenced by socioeconomic circumstances. During various periods of life, women's access to healthcare, education, and assistance can be influenced by their social and economic standing [5].

10.4.3 HOW DO HEALTHCARE SYSTEMS FUNCTION?

The menstrual cycle and menopause experiences of women can be significantly impacted by the way healthcare systems operate. The following are some crucial elements of healthcare systems:

- **Compassion and inclusivity:** When it comes to women's health, particularly menopause and menstruation, healthcare systems ought to work toward being both compassionate and inclusive. This entails giving women from different backgrounds courteous, nonjudgmental care that is attentive to their needs [4].
- **Patient-centered treatment:** Medical professionals should adopt a patient-centered strategy that respects and involves women in making decisions regarding their treatment [5].
- **Cultural sensitivity:** Medical professionals working with women should be cognizant of and considerate of their cultural customs and beliefs, particularly those surrounding menopause and menstruation [5].
- **Accessibility:** Regardless of their location, social position, or any other factors that may affect their ability to get care, all women should have equitable access to healthcare services.
- **Information:** Accurate and current information regarding menopause and menstruation is largely provided by healthcare systems. This contains details on signs and symptoms, available treatments, and precautions [4].
- **Education and awareness:** Through community outreach, educational materials, and public health campaigns, healthcare institutions should raise public knowledge and understanding of menopause and menstruation [5].
- **Support services:** Counseling, support groups, and access to specialized treatment are just a few of the support services that healthcare systems ought to provide to women going through menopause or other menstrual diseases [4, 5].

10.5 COLLABORATIVE RESEARCH AND PRACTICE

10.5.1 COMBINING PSYCHOLOGICAL, NATURAL, AND SOCIAL COMPONENTS

In menopause and menstruation study and practice, integrating psychological, natural, and social components can result in a more holistic and comprehensive knowledge and approach to women's health. These elements can be mixed in the following ways:

- **Psychological:** Understanding the emotional and mental components of menopause and menstruation is part of the psychological component. This can involve management and changes that affect mood, looking into coping mechanisms for symptom management, and dealing with mental health conditions including anxiety and depression [6].
- **Research:** Carry out studies on mood swings, stress reduction strategies, and psychological therapies to investigate the psychological impacts of menopause and menstruation [2].
- **Practice:** To help women overcome emotional challenges associated with menstruation and menopause, incorporate psychological treatments such as CBT and mindfulness-based stress reduction into therapeutic practice [3].
- **Natural component** focuses on the biological mechanisms underlying menopause and menstruation, as well as natural therapies for these conditions. This can involve investigating natural alternatives to hormone replacement treatment as well as the effects of diet, exercise, and herbal supplements on symptoms [4].
- **Research:** Examine the efficaciousness of lifestyle modifications and natural therapies in the management of menstrual problems and menopausal symptoms.
- **Practice:** Include natural methods in treatment regimens for women pursuing complementary or alternative therapies, such as acupuncture, herbal supplements, and dietary adjustments.
- **Social component**: The social component considers the cultural and sociological elements that shape women's menstrual and

menopausal experiences. This can involve researching societal perceptions and customs, dealing with stigma and taboos, and encouraging knowledge and consciousness.[5]

- **Research**: Examine how socioeconomic determinants, such as cultural norms, access to healthcare, and social support systems, affect how women experience menopause and menstruation [1].
- **Practice**: Create initiatives and therapies that address socioeconomic factors that influence health, such as poverty, discrimination, and limited access to education, to improve women's health outcomes throughout menopause and menstruation [6].

10.5.2 ADOPTING A THOROUGH APPROACH

Menopause and menstruation experiences can be greatly impacted by encouraging women to live healthier lifestyles. The following are some essential strategies for implementing a comprehensive plan to encourage healthy lifestyles:

- **Nutrition and diet:** Women should be urged to have a diet rich in whole grains, fruits, vegetables, lean meats, and other nutrients that is balanced and healthful. Eating a healthy diet can help control weight, reduce the risk of chronic diseases, and enhance overall health throughout menstruation and menopause.
- **Encourage frequent physical activity** as a component of a healthy lifestyle: Exercise supports bone health, lowers stress, elevates mood, and helps manage weight—all of which are crucial during menopause and menstruation.
- Women should be encouraged to use **stress-reduction methods** like deep breathing, yoga, meditation, mindfulness [1], and workouts. Controlling stress can enhance general well-being and lessen the effects of menopausal symptoms.
- **Healthy sleep habits:** Emphasize the value of getting adequate rest and following appropriate sleeping procedures. Inadequate sleep has a negative impact on general health and exacerbates menopausal symptoms.

- **Avoiding hazardous substances**: Advise women to abstain from smoking, binge drinking, and using other dangerous substances. These drugs raise the chance of developing chronic illnesses and aggravate menopausal symptoms [3].
- **Frequent health check-ups:** Encourage women to make appointments with their healthcare providers for routine health check-ups. Throughout menopause and menstruation, routine examinations can support the monitoring of hormone levels, bone density, and general health.
- **Education and awareness**: Disseminate knowledge about menstruation and the menopause, including symptoms, available treatments, and lifestyle choices that may have an impact on a woman's health during these times [5].

10.6 COLLABORATIVE AND INTERDISCIPLINARY RESEARCH

10.6.1 ENDORSING INTEGRATIVE MEDICINE

Supporting the use of integrative medicine in menopausal and menstrual research can lead to a more comprehensive approach to women's health. Integrative medicine integrates complementary and alternative therapies with standard medical care to address the mental, emotional, and spiritual aspects of health. Several research applications for integrated medicine include the following:

- **Combining conventional and alternative therapies:** Research in integrative medicine can investigate the efficacy of combining traditional therapies, like HT, with complementary therapies, like acupuncture or herbal supplements, to treat menstrual disorders and menopausal symptoms [2].
- **Mind-body techniques:** Studies can explore how menstrual health and menopausal symptoms are affected by mind-body techniques like yoga, meditation, and mindfulness. These techniques can lessen tension, elevate mood, and encourage general health and wellness [1].
- **Nutrition and lifestyle interventions**: Research on integrative medicine might concentrate on how diet, exercise, stress reduction,

and other lifestyle choices affect menopause and menstruation. The general health and hormonal balance can be supported by these approaches [3].

- **Herbal and botanical medications:** Studies can assess the safety and effectiveness of using herbal and botanical medications to treat menstrual problems and menopausal symptoms. For some women, these natural remedies might be an alternative to traditional medical care [4].
- **Collaboration among disciplines:** Integrative medicine promotes cooperation between many specialties, such as psychology, naturopathy, acupuncture, conventional medicine, and nutrition. Multidisciplinary research can enhance patient outcomes and offer a more thorough understanding of women's health challenges [5].
- **Putting the patient first:** Integrative medicine strongly emphasizes treating each patient as an individual with their own needs and preferences in mind. This approach is known as patient-centered care. Research might investigate how this approach can improve menstruation and menopausal symptoms and outcomes for patients [6].

10.6.2 WOMEN'S HEALTH RESEARCH AND DESTINY MANDATES

Recognizing the significance of comprehending women's health requirements and advocating for practices and policies that assist women's health and well-being are prerequisites for incorporating women's health research into future mandates. Here are some crucial things to remember:

- **Research financing:** Menstruation and menopause studies, as well as other studies related to women's health, should receive priority financing under current requirements. This could advance our knowledge of women's health challenges and result in the creation of interventions and treatments that work better [2].
- **Policy development:** The formulation of laws pertaining to women's health may be influenced by destiny mandates. The specific requirements of women should be taken into consideration by policies, which should support reproductive health, encourage healthy lifestyles, and provide access to healthcare [3].

- **Healthcare access:** Destiny mandates ought to endeavor to guarantee that ladies possess the ability to obtain all-inclusive healthcare treatments, encompassing screenings, preventive care, as well as remedies for menstruation problems and menopausal symptoms.
- **Education and awareness**: Destiny mandates have the potential to increase knowledge and understanding of women's health issues, such as the significance of routine checkups, early illness identification, and self-care techniques [4].
- **Cultural sensitivity:** Cultural considerations that may have an impact on women's health and well-being should be included in policy directives. This entails dispelling myths and taboos related to menopause and menstruation as well as advocating for medical procedures that are culturally aware [6].
- **Collaborative research:** Research projects involving a variety of fields and stakeholders may be encouraged by specific directives. This may result in a deeper comprehension of the problems with women's health and creative solutions [6].

10.7 SUMMARY

When treating menopause and menstrual problems in women, a holistic approach considers the social, emotional, physical, and cultural facets of women's health. This method acknowledges that a range of issues affect women's health and that they need all-encompassing treatment. The essential elements of a holistic approach include: (1) Physical health: Using a combination of traditional and alternative therapy, physical health needs are met, including menopause symptoms like hot flashes, night sweats, and menstruation abnormalities; (2) Emotional well-being: promoting emotional well-being by using mindfulness exercises, psychotherapy, and stress-reduction strategies to address mood swings and enhance general mental health; (3) Social support: Assisting women in navigating menopause and menstruation by offering social support networks and resources, such as education and awareness campaigns. Understanding and addressing cultural beliefs is known as cultural sensitivity and menstrual habits to guarantee that care is inclusive and sensitive to cultural differences; (4)

Comprehensive treatment: Providing women with comprehensive and individualized treatment by integrating several facets of care, such as lifestyle interventions, mind-body therapies, and nutrition; (5) Research and education: In order to better understand and treat menopause and menstruation, women's health research and education are encouraged.

KEYWORDS

- **holistic approach**
- **menopause**
- **menstruation**
- **women's health**

REFERENCES

1. Grady, D., Hill, S., & Bush, T. (1998). Random investigation looking at the impact of estrogen and progestin on postmenopausal women's secondary prevention of coronary heart disease. *Heart Health is the Focus of the Heart and Estrogen/ Progestin Alternative Research Institute (HERS), 280*(7), 605–613.
2. Grodstein, F., Stampfer, M. J., & Colditz, G. A. (1997). Death and hormone therapy administered after menopause. *The New England Journal of Medicine, 336*(25), 1769–1775.
3. Maturitas-Hoffmann, M., Hammar, M., Lindh-Astrand, L., Kjellgren, K. I., & Brynhildsen, J. (1996). Long-term postmenopausal estrogen therapy is associated with a decreased mortality rate. *Obstetrics and Gynecology*, *87*(1), 6–12.
4. Rossouw, J. E., Anderson, G. L., & Prentice, R. L. (2002). Major outcomes of progestin plus estrogen in healthy postmenopausal girls: Benefits and risks from the randomized controlled trial of the Ladies' Fitness Initiative. *JAMA, 288*(3), 321–333.
5. Takeshi, A., Takumi, Y., & Seiichiro, F. (1999). The menopause in an aging population. In: *The Menopause in Millennium* (p. 107). The Parthenon Publishing Institution: New York.
6. Wardle, P. G. (1997). Managed care of hormone replacement therapy in menopause. *Current Opinion Obstetrics and Gynecology*, *9*(4), 270–277.
7. Damman, C. (2023). *Fibre is Your Body's Natural Guide to Weight Management.* University of Washington.

CHAPTER 11

Role of NGOs, Nonprofit, and Community Organizations in Empowering Female Health

PRIYA GOGIA, INDRESH KUMAR,* SHIKHA MALIK, and PRACHI SINHA

*Corresponding author

ABSTRACT

The female health concerns often remain overlooked due to pervasive gender inequality that limits their access to education, economic opportunities, social freedoms, and healthcare services. Women frequently lack autonomy in healthcare decisions and family planning, and societal biases exacerbate their health challenges. Numerous nongovernmental organizations (NGOs) work globally to improve women's health by offering reproductive health services, advocating for women's rights, and addressing gender-based violence. Research indicates that NGOs play a crucial role in bridging healthcare gaps, though their effectiveness is often constrained by government inefficiencies. Self-help groups (SHGs) are community-based organizations that promote mutual support and empowerment among women. Studies reveal that SHGs can positively impact women's health by raising awareness and increasing community participation. Civil societies play a pivotal role in advocating for women's health and rights, influencing policy changes, and providing support services. Addressing women's health requires a multifaceted approach involving NGOs, SHGs, and civil societies. These organizations complement governmental efforts, providing essential services, advocating for

Holistic Approaches for Women's Sustainable Health, Volume 2: Advancements, Socioeconomic Impacts, and Innovative Strategies. Junaid Ahmad Malik, Anamika Chauhan, and Megh R. Goyal (Eds)

DOI: 10.1201/9781779641656-13

policy changes, and empowering women. Collaborative strategies and systematic involvement of these organizations are essential for improving women's health globally.

11.1 INTRODUCTION

11.1.1 SCENARIO OF WOMEN'S HEALTH

According to the United Nations (UN), although nearly half (49.6%) of the global population consists of women, their health concerns are often overlooked in numerous countries [34]. Throughout much of the world, women have not received the social rights commensurate with those granted to men, resulting in gender inequality that has undermined their access to education, economic opportunities, social freedoms, and healthcare services. In various regions, women lack the autonomy to travel independently, rely on others for healthcare decisions, and have limited involvement in family planning. Societal preference for boys has led to a rise in female feticide and infanticide, perpetuating lifelong neglect of women's hygiene and nutritional needs [3].

The reports from the UN and the World Bank revealed that a significant portion of the global population is affected by poverty, and 767 million women and children are experiencing significant challenges [33, 35]. This poverty directly impacts their access to essential healthcare services [21]. A 2020 study published in the Health Care Women International Journal highlighted that women, who contribute two-thirds of the world's working hours, receive only 10% of the total global income [33]. It is important to note that this data do not include women engaged in domestic work.

Despite constituting a significant portion of the global population and making substantial contributions to development, women have not received adequate healthcare services that they deserve. Women and men differ behaviorally and physiologically, indicating that a one-size-fits-all approach is insufficient across various social contexts [21]. Understanding women's health issues is crucial as their well-being significantly influences the health of future generations. It is crucial to focus on women's health, considering the distinct challenges they encounter that differ from those faced by men.

11.1.2 HEALTH-RELATED PROBLEMS THAT AFFECT WOMEN

Women have distinct health requirements distinct from those of men, experiencing a range of biological stages, such as menstruation, pregnancy, childbirth, and menopause, that present unique challenges. Recognizing common health issues affecting women, leading organizations like the WHO have advocated for special attention to be given to these concerns [33, 36]. Key issues concerning women's health in India encompass cancer, inadequate nutrition, noncommunicable diseases, mental health, human immunodeficiency virus (HIV)/acquired immunodeficiency syndrome (AIDS), sexually transmitted diseases, and violence against women [12].

Women face the highest risk of developing breast and cervical cancers. Annually, approximately 500,000 women succumb to these cancers [33]. Health policies and programs often reinforce gender stereotypes and overlook socioeconomic disparities and other diversities among women. Globally, women are increasingly affected by HIV/AIDS. Each year, an estimated 20 million unsafe abortions occur worldwide, resulting in 70,000 deaths among women. Additionally, approximately 585,000 women die annually due to pregnancy and childbirth, equating to more than 1600 deaths every day [12, 36].

According to a WHO report, one in three women under the age of 50 experiences sexual violence perpetrated by an acquaintance or a stranger. Whether physical or sexual, violence has profound implications for a woman's physical and mental health. Addressing these issues requires focused attention in certain areas: providing comprehensive sex education to children and educating both men and women on preventing sexual violence [11]. Consequently, it is essential to sensitize administrators and healthcare professionals to the problem of violence against women.

A 2021 study in *The Lancet* revealed that women account for 71% of global healthcare utilization; however, many women hesitate to seek care at government hospitals due to a lack of awareness and effective government policies. Most women fear being stigmatized for seeking family planning services at government facilities [19]. Nongovernmental organizations (NGOs), self-help groups (SHGs), and Civil Society initiatives collaborate with communities to raise awareness and enhance government support mechanisms [34].

11.3 FUNCTIONING BACKGROUND OF NGOS, NONPROFITS, AND COMMUNITY ORGANIZATIONS

NGOs, SHGs, and Civil Society organizations (Table 11.1) are collective support networks striving to promote social and economic empowerment across diverse populations. In every society and social structure, inherent flaws can result in limited opportunities for certain [27, 28].

TABLE 11.1 Difference Between NGOs, SGHs, and Civil Society

NGOs	SHGs	Civil Society
An NGO is a nonprofit, voluntary group of citizens organized at a local, national, or global level.	The work done by an SHG is generally small in magnitude and is normally limited to the group members.	Civil society is an area of associations, professions, interest groups, classes, families, etc.
NGOs are integral to civil society, often playing a significant and sometimes primary role in driving socioeconomic progress by fostering community engagement in politics and shaping or impacting policy formulation.	Because SHGs operate on the principle of mutual assistance, their efforts are focused on supporting and aiding their group members exclusively.	Civil society is a more inclusive concept that encompasses all organizations and associations existing beyond the scope of the state and the market.
NGO is a relatively new concept.	SHGs are comparatively less organized than their NGO counterparts	Civil society is a comparatively old concept.
The activities undertaken by an NGO are executed on a significant scale, with welfare initiatives extending to the state or national level, thereby garnering greater recognition for their work.	SHGs are predominantly established by women with the dual objectives of promoting women's empowerment and fostering socioeconomic development.	Civil society comprises a network of organizations and groups that operate independently of the state and family, actively contributing to various social, economic, and cultural endeavors positively and dynamically.

This chapter discusses the role of NGOs, SHGs, civil societies, and government agencies to alleviate the disease of gender inequality among women for better health.

11.2 NGOS AND WOMEN'S HEALTH

11.2.1 LEADING NGOS WORKING FOR WOMEN'S HEALTH

There are numerous NGOs around the world that focus on improving women's health [35]. Here are some well-known international NGOs that actively work in the field of women's health:

- Engender health works to enhance the health and well-being of people in underserved communities worldwide, concentrating on family planning, maternal health, and HIV/AIDS prevention.
- Global Fund for Women supports women's rights organizations globally, including those dedicated to health-related issues, by providing grants to empower women and enhance their health and well-being.
- Guttmacher Institute advances sexual and reproductive health and rights through research, policy analysis, and public education, providing evidence-based information to support informed decision-making.
- International Planned Parenthood Federation is a worldwide organization focused on guaranteeing universal access to sexual and reproductive health education, information, and services.
- International Women's Health Coalition advocates for sexual and reproductive health and rights, as well as gender equality, on a global scale. They work to empower women and girls to exercise their rights.
- Planned Parenthood Federation of America is a prominent organization that offers reproductive health services, including family planning, sexual health education, and advocacy for women's health rights.
- UN Women: Although not an NGO, the UN Entity for Gender Equality and the Empowerment of Women (UN Women) plays a significant role in promoting women's health and gender equality worldwide.
- Women Deliver is a global advocacy organization focused on gender equality and the health and well-being of girls and women. They strive to promote women's rights and access to health services.

- Women's Health Foundation focuses on pelvic health issues, particularly pelvic floor disorders, to enhance women's quality of life.
- Women's Refugee Commission is dedicated to improving the well-being and defending the rights of women, children, and youth affected by displacement due to conflict and crises, particularly focusing on the distinct health challenges that displaced women encounter.

These organizations operate at both local and global levels, addressing various aspects of women's health, from reproductive health and family planning to maternal health, gender-based violence, and overall gender equality. Keep in mind that the landscape of NGOs working in women's health is dynamic, and new organizations may emerge over time.

11.2.2 EVIDENCE-GENERATING STUDIES

We conducted a narrative review of research examining the participation of NGOs and their approaches to improving women's health. Our examination indicates that NGOs have been instrumental in addressing gaps in healthcare provision. Despite taking on roles resembling healthcare providers and sharing similar goals with the government, their effectiveness is impeded by governmental inefficiencies and resource constraints (Table 11.2). Our analysis of significant discoveries is discussed within the framework of the dimensions of women's health empowerment.

Achieving better health improvement in women necessitates substantial health system reforms, a task that governments cannot accomplish in isolation. Recognizing and leveraging the strengths and abilities of NGOs, and pooling capital with them, emerges as a potential avenue for realizing health facility enhancement for women. Despite the pivotal role that NGOs play in delivering health services, there remains a relative lack of understanding regarding how to effectively engage these organizations to achieve women's health objectives. Collaborating with NGOs can be instrumental in advancing health facilities for women alongside government efforts and other entities. A comprehensive comprehension of the role played by NGOs and their contribution to health facilities for women is particularly crucial in the homegrown context. Governments should formulate systematic and fundamental strategies for involving

TABLE 11.2 Reviewed Studies Regarding NGOs and Their Approaches to Improving Women's Health

Ref.	Country, Date, and Type	Study Design	Data Collection Method	Intervention(s)
Yagub et al. [37]	Sudan, 2015/ LI	Mix method	Documentation, observation, recordings, and informal interviews	Delivering healthcare services to marginalized populations, particularly focusing on women and children
Albis et al. [2]	Bangladesh, 2019/LMI	Survey	Survey form	Delivering essential healthcare services to economically disadvantaged urban communities
Maio et al. [7]	Italy, 2014/ HI	Descriptive study	Regular program information	Delivering both inpatient and outpatient healthcare services to women experiencing homelessness
Khan et al. [16]	Bangladesh, 2017/ LMI	Survey	Self-reported	Delivering healthcare services focused on maternal, infant, and child health, including preventive and primary care
Khodayari-Zarnaq et al. [15]	Iran, 2019/ UMI	Qualitative study	Semistructured, in-depth qualitative interviews	Setting up and outfitting hospitals, supplying medication and treatment to underserved populations, offering financial assistance to orphans, providing microloans to economically disadvantaged individuals, conducting awareness campaigns, and offering training to vulnerable groups
Sanadgol et al. [28]	Nigeria, 2021/ LMI	Quasiexperimental	A partially structured questionnaire or detailed interview	Enhancing the capacity of 12 NGOs in supporting and advocating for policies related to reproductive health issues
Perry et al. [23]	28 countries	Qualitative study	Analysis of project evaluations, presentations at international health conferences, and articles published in peer-reviewed journals	Delivering healthcare services focused on maternal, neonatal, and child health

TABLE 11.2 *(Continued)*

Ref.	Country, Date, and Type	Study Design	Data Collection Method	Intervention(s)
Chanani et al. [5]	India, 2019/ LMI	Cross-sectional	Android smartphones and the CommCare mobile application	Offering prevention and treatment services, including growth monitoring, referrals to public health facilities, and counseling provided at home
Soe et al. [32]	Myanmar in 2017 was characterized as fragile.	Snapshot descriptive	Regular data	Delivering tuberculosis care within communities to populations that are difficult to access

NGOs in the pursuit of public health goals, facilitating progress toward health facilities for women. With the establishment and development of health services, coupled with a global emphasis on health facilities for women, the presence of NGOs can enhance financial support and elevate the quality of services in underserved and marginalized areas.

11.3 SHGS AND WOMEN'S HEALTH

11.3.1 LEADING SGHS WORKING FOR WOMEN'S HEALTH

SHGs are community-based organizations that bring individuals together for mutual support and empowerment. While they may not always focus exclusively on health, many SHG groups address various aspects of women's well-being, including physical and mental health [26]. Here are some well-known SHGs that function to support women's health:

- Black Women's Health Imperative focuses on the health and well-being of Black women, addressing issues such as reproductive health, chronic diseases, and mental health.
- EmpowHER is an online community and resource center dedicated to women's health, providing information on various topics such as reproductive health, mental health, and overall wellness.
- Global Fund for Widows assists widows worldwide through economic empowerment programs, with a primary emphasis on financial stability. They may also address broader health and social issues impacting widows as part of their initiatives.
- Saheli Women's Group is a community-based organization in India that facilitates SHGs for women. Their main emphasis is on promoting economic empowerment, and these groups also frequently engage with health and social issues.
- SHEROES is an online platform and community offering support and resources tailored for women, covering diverse topics such as health, careers, and relationships.
- The Red Hat Society is a social organization for women over 50 that encourages women to come together for friendship and support, promoting a positive outlook on aging.
- Wellness and Well-being is an online community that provides a platform for women to connect and support each other in various aspects of life, including mental and physical health.

- Widows for Peace Through Democracy works to empower widows globally, addressing their social, economic, and health needs.
- Women's Health Concern is a charity based in the UK that provides information and support on various health issues affecting women. They operate a helpline and online community for women seeking advice and guidance.
- Women's Health Initiative is a major research program in the United States focusing on strategies to prevent heart disease, breast cancer, colorectal cancer, and osteoporotic fractures in postmenopausal women.

These groups provide platforms for women to share experiences, offer support, and access information related to health and well-being. It is essential to note that the effectiveness of SHGs can vary, and individuals may find different groups more suitable based on their specific needs and preferences.

11.3.2 EVIDENCE-GENERATING STUDIES

The studies in Table 11.3 cover various countries and years, focusing on diverse interventions aimed at improving health outcomes through community and group-based approaches.

We analyzed various research papers to assess the role and contribution of SHGs in improving women's health. After analysis, we conclude that SHGs can play a significant role in Women's Health by raising awareness and knowledge about health-related issues, by increasing community participation [24]. However, the road is yet to be paved, and a long journey awaits as most SHGs still focus on economic stability, and health-related topics take a back seat. However, areas with more SHGs overall had better health-related indices, making it evident that SHGs can make an important contribution to women's and children's health if supported well in the long term.

11.4 CIVIL SOCIETIES AND FEMALE HEALTH

11.4.1 LEADING CIVIL SOCIETIES WORKING FOR WOMEN'S HEALTH

Civil societies around the world play a crucial role in advocating for women's rights, including their health and well-being [6]. These

TABLE 11.3 Reviewed Studies Regarding SGHs and Their Approaches to Improving Women's Health

Ref.	Country, Date, and Type	Study Design	Data Collection Method	Intervention(s)
Adedamola et al. [1]	Nigeria, 2017	Survey	In-depth interview	Promoting One Health Practice in Pastoralist Communities
Ruducha et al. [24]	India, 2019	Survey	Pretest and Posttest social network surveys	Enhancing connections and collaboration between SHGs and government healthcare providers
Saggurti et al. [25]	India, 2018	Quasi-experimental	Cluster sampling, structured health messaging	Structured participatory communication on MNCH improves positive health practices better
Hazra et al. [10]	India, 2022	Systematic Review	Review of Intervention Studies	Significance of reporting of implementation intensity of group-based interventions
Saha [26]	India, 2020	Descriptive Study	Data from National Rural Livelihood Mission dataset, National Family Health Survey-4 (2015–16)	Increasing membership in women's groups for better health outcomes
Mehta et al. [20]	California, USA, 2020	Systemic Review	Analysis of annual surveys	Increasing SHG membership improved reproductive, maternal, newborn, and child health and sanitation behavior in women
Hazra et al. [9]	India, 2020	Quasi-experimental	Cross-sectional surveys, discussion-based interventions, and community outreach activities	Reducing inequalities in maternal and newborn health through behavior change communication interventions

organizations work toward policy changes, raise awareness, and provide support services. Here are some well-known civil societies that actively function to promote women's health:

- Association for Women's Rights in Development is an international feminist organization that advocates for women's rights and gender equality. They work on a range of issues, including sexual and reproductive health and rights.
- Center for Reproductive Rights is a worldwide organization committed to promoting reproductive rights as essential human rights. They strive to guarantee women's access to safe and lawful reproductive healthcare services.
- Center for Women's Global Leadership is a leader in global women's rights advocacy. While their focus is broad, they address issues such as gender-based violence and reproductive rights, which are integral to women's health.
- National Women's Health Network is a U.S.-based organization that focuses on women's health advocacy. They work to ensure that women have access to accurate and unbiased information on healthcare and that their health needs are prioritized.
- Women Deliver is recognized as a global advocacy organization that unites diverse voices to champion gender equality and promote the health and well-being of girls and women.
- Women's Environment & Development Organization works at the intersection of gender, environment, and sustainable development. While not exclusively focused on health, they address issues that impact women's overall well-being, including access to healthcare in the context of environmental and development challenges.
- Women's Global Network for Reproductive Rights is an international network that advocates for sexual and reproductive rights. They work to empower women and communities to claim their rights to health, information, and bodily autonomy.
- Women's Health Action is an organization based in New Zealand that focuses on enhancing the health and well-being of women. They offer information, resources, and advocacy on various women's health matters.

- Women's Health and Equal Rights Initiative is a Nigerian-based organization that focuses on promoting women's health and advocating for gender equality. They work on issues such as maternal health, family planning, and women's rights.
- Women's Health Victoria: Based in Australia, it is a state-wide organization that focuses on women's health promotion, policy advocacy, and research. They address a wide range of health issues affecting women.

These civil societies actively contribute to the advancement of women's health through advocacy, research, and community engagement. Their work is instrumental in shaping policies and promoting positive changes that benefit women globally.

11.4.2 EVIDENCE-GENERATING STUDIES

Over the past 40 years, substantial progress has been made in maternal, neonatal, and child health (MNCH), although this improvement has not been uniformed and varies among countries and within them. Additionally, there have been noticeable shifts globally in disease patterns and population demographics. Currently, more than 70% of global deaths are attributed to noncommunicable diseases like hypertension, cancer, diabetes, and chronic respiratory conditions [30]. Civil society plays a vital role in facilitating the health system's outreach to hard-to-reach populations, particularly women, to enhance coverage and access to services (Table 11.4).

We focused on established literature, field data, reports, and published research spanning several years. Our findings highlight the essential role of civil society in enabling the health system to reach marginalized populations, thereby improving overall coverage. Moreover, civil society organizations contribute to the training and development of frontline public health staff through various formal and informal methods [18]. They can propose strategies to reshape the attitudes and motivations of these workers. Leveraging their deep community connections, civil society organizations serve as critical intermediaries and information conduits. Ultimately, they guide individuals to appropriate healthcare facilities, reducing out-of-pocket expenses for healthcare.

TABLE 11.4 Reviewed Studies Regarding Civil Societies and Their Approaches to Improving Women's Health

Ref.	Country, Date, and Type	Study Design	Data Collection Method	Intervention(s)
Jayaraman et al. [13]	India, 2023	Mixed method	Review and Survey	Enhancing primary healthcare systems through the lens of civil society
Samuel et al. [29]	Peru, 2016	Qualitative	Semistructured interviews	Civil society's role in ensuring the state's accountability for providing quality healthcare
Govindasamy et al. [8]	Australia, 2011	Group intervention	Survey	To provide support for Sudanese refugee women
Smith et al [31]	South Africa	Commentary	Illustrative examples	Catalytic role of civil society organizations in achieving Sustainable Development Goal 3
Borzaga et al. [4]	Italy	Qualitative	Survey	The role of third sector organizations in providing healthcare services
Kankya et al. [14]	Uganda	Case study	Cross-sectional survey	The role of civil society organizations in the delivery of healthcare services
Mankell et al. [18]	Sweden, 2021	Qualitative	Semistructured interviews	Aspects of healthcare CSO and collective patient participation in improving quality
Mangone et al. [17]	Italy, 2014	Case study		Critical analysis of the responsibility of Italian civil societies in healthcare
Ndinda et al. [22]	South Africa, 2013	Technical research report	Survey	Civil Society Activism for greater access to healthcare

11.5 SUMMARY

The empowerment of women's health through the collaborative efforts of NGOs, SHGs, and civil societies is imperative for addressing the multifaceted challenges faced by women globally. Despite being half of the world's residents, women often encounter gender disparities that hinder their access to essential healthcare services and information. This necessitates a comprehensive approach to address women's unique health needs across various biological stages and socioeconomic contexts. Evidence from research studies underscores the significant impact of these organizations in improving women's health outcomes. NGOs, SHGs, and civil societies facilitate the delivery of health services, bridge gaps in healthcare access, and advocate for strategy changes to address the root causes of gender disparities in health. In conclusion, collaborative efforts between governments, NGOs, SHGs, and civil societies are essential for advancing women's health and achieving gender equality. By recognizing and leveraging the strengths of these organizations, policymakers can work in the direction of creating comprehensive and equitable healthcare systems that prioritize the health and well-being of all women.

KEYWORDS

- **civil societies**
- **community empowerment**
- **gender inequality**
- **healthcare access**
- **nongovernmental organizations**
- **reproductive health**
- **self-help groups**

REFERENCES

1. Adedamola, F. B. (2017). The impact of self-help groups on pastoral women's empowerment and agency: A study in Nigeria. *Pastoralism*, *7*, 1–12.

2. Albis, M. L. F., Bhadra, S. K., & Chin, B. (2019). Impact evaluation of contracting primary health care services in urban Bangladesh. *BMC Health Services Research, 19*, 1–12.
3. Bauer, I. L. (2021). Healthy, safe and responsible: The modern female traveler. *Tropical Diseases, Travel Medicine and Vaccines*, *7*(1), 14–18.
4. Borzaga, C. (2004). From suffocation to re-emergence: The evolution of the Italian third sector. In: *The Third Sector in Europe* (pp. 45–63). Trento. https://www.researchgate.net/publication/290250989_From_suffocation_to_re-emergence_The_evolution_of_the_italian_third_sector
5. Chanani, S., Waingankar, A., Shah More, N., Pantvaidya, S., Fernandez, A., & Jayaraman, A. (2019). Effectiveness of NGO-government partnership to prevent and treat child wasting in urban India. *Maternal & Child Nutrition*, *15*, e12706.
6. Chilwane, D., Ndinda, C., & Mokomane, Z. (2013). Civil society activism in accessing healthcare in South Africa. In: *Pretoria: Human Science Research Council Technical Report* (p. 94). Codesria and HSRC: Pretoria - SA.
7. De Maio, G., Vanden Bergh, R., Garelli, S., Maccagno, B., Raddi, F., Stefanizzi, A., & Zachariah, R. (2014). Reaching out to the forgotten: Providing access to medical care for the homeless in Italy. *International Health*, *6*(2), 93–98.
8. Hashimoto-Govindasamy, L. S., & Rose, V. (2011). An ethnographic process evaluation of a community support program with Sudanese refugee women in Western Sydney. *Health Promotion Journal of Australia*, *22*(2), 107–112.
9. Hazra, A., Atmavilas, Y., Hay, K., Saggurti, N., Verma, R. K., Ahmad, J., & Irani, L. (2020). Effects of health behavior change intervention through women's self-help groups on maternal and newborn health practices and related inequalities in rural India: A quasi-experimental study. *E Clinical Medicine*, *2020,* 18–22.
10. Hazra, A., Das, A., Ahmad, J., Singh, S., Chaudhuri, I., Purty, A., & Desai, S. (2022). Matching intent with intensity: Implementation research on the intensity of health and nutrition programs with women's self-help groups in India. *Global Health: Science and Practice*, *10*(2), e2100383.
11. Huecker, M. R., King, K. C., & Jordan, G. A. (2023). *Lockdowns during the COVID-19 Pandemic and Domestic Violence Among Virginians*. Doctoral dissertation, Walden University.
12. International Institute for Population Sciences (IIPS) and ICF. (2021). *National FAMILY HEALTH SURVEY (NFHS-5), 2019–21, India (Volume II)*. IIPS: Mumbai. https://main.mohfw.gov.in/sites/default/files/NFHS-5_Phase-II_0.pdf
13. Jayaraman, A., & Fernandez, A. (2023). Role of civil society in health care: Mechanisms for realizing universal health coverage in vulnerable communities of India. *Frontiers in Public Health*, *11*, e1091533.
14. Kankya, C., Akandinda, A., & Rwabukwali, C. (2013). The role of civil society organisations (CSOs) in healthcare delivery system: A case study of child immunization in Kabarole District, Uganda. *Health***,** *5*, 1277–1288. doi: 10.4236/health.2013.58174
15. Khodayari-Zarnaq, R., Kakemam, E., Arab-Zozani, M., Rasouli, J., & Sokhanvar, M. (2020). Participation of Iranian non-governmental organizations in health policy making; Barriers and strategies for development. *International Journal of Health Governance*, *25*(1), 46–56.

16. Khan, J. A., Ahmed, S., MacLennan, M., Sarker, A. R., Sultana, M., & Rahman, H. (2017). Benefit incidence analysis of healthcare in Bangladesh—Equity matters for universal health coverage. *Health Policy and Planning*, *32*(3), 359–365.
17. Mangone, E., & Pace, E. M. (2014). Civil society in the Italian reformed healthcare system: A role or responsibility? *IRPPS Working Papers*, *2014,* 1–20.
18. Mankell, A. (2021). *Collective Patient Participation: Patient Voice and Civil Society Organizations in Healthcare* (Doctoral dissertation, Ersta Sköndal Bräcke högskola).
19. Mousa, M., Boyle, J., Skouteris, H., Mullins, A. K., Currie, G., Riach, K., & Teede, H. J. (2021). Advancing women in healthcare leadership: Systematic review and meta-synthesis of multi-sector evidence on organizational-interventions. *E Clinical Medicine*, *39*, 101084.
20. Mehta, K. M., Irani, L., Chaudhuri, I., Mahapatra, T., Schooley, J., Srikantiah, S., & Ananya Study Group. (2020). Health impact of self-help groups scaled-up statewide in Bihar, India. *Journal of Global Health*, *10*(2), 021006.
21. Mukherjee, S., Mahapatra, B., & Saggurti, N. (2021). Why women do not use contraceptives: Exploring the role of male out-migration. *PloS One*, *16*(3), e0249177.
22. Ndinda, C., Ndhlovu, T. P., Juma, P., Asiki, G., & Kyobutungi, C. (2018). The evolution of non-communicable diseases policies in post-apartheid South Africa. *BMC Public Health*, *18*, 1–12.
23. Perry, H., Morrow, M., Davis, T., Borger, S., Weiss, J., DeCoster, M., & Ernst, P. (2015). Care groups II: A summary of the child survival outcomes achieved using volunteer community health workers in resource-constrained settings. *Global Health: Science and Practice*, *3*(3), 370–381.
24. Ruducha, J., Hariharan, D., Potter, J., Ahmad, D., Kumar, S., Mohanan, P. S., & Long, K. N. (2019). Measuring coordination between women's self-help groups and local health systems in rural India: A social network analysis. *BMJ Open*, *9*(8), e028943.
25. Saggurti, N., Atmavilas, Y., Porwal, A., Schooley, J., Das, R., Kande, N., & Hay, K. (2018). Effect of health intervention integration within women's self-help groups on collectivization and healthy practices around reproductive, maternal, neonatal and child health in rural India. *PLoS One*, *13*(8), e0202562.
26. Saha, S. (2021). Does membership in women's group advance health and empowerment? Evidence from India? *Journal of Family Medicine and Primary Care*, *10*(5), 1829–1834.
27. Sanadgol, A., Doshmangir, L., Majdzadeh, R., & Gordeev, V. S. (2022). Strategies to strengthen non-governmental organizations' participation in the Iranian health system. *Frontiers in Public Health*, *10*, e929614.
28. Sanadgol, A., Doshmangir, L., Majdzadeh, R., & Gordeev, V. S. (2021). Engagement of non-governmental organizations in moving towards universal health coverage: Scoping review. *Globalization and Health*, *17*, 1–19.
29. Samuel, J. (2016). The role of civil society in strengthening intercultural maternal health care in local health facilities, Puno, Peru. *Global Health Action*, *9*(1), e33355.
30. Smith, J., Buse, K., & Gordon, C. (2016). Civil society: The catalyst for ensuring health in the age of sustainable development. *Globalization and Health*, *12*, 1–6.
31. Smith, S. R. (2010). Hybridization and nonprofit organizations: The governance challenge. *Policy and Society*, *29*(3), 219–229.

32. Soe, K. T., Saw, S., van Griensven, J., Zhou, S., Win, L., Chinnakali, P., & Aung, S. T. (2017). International non-governmental organizations' provision of community-based tuberculosis care for hard-to-reach populations in Myanmar, 2013–2014. *Infectious Diseases of Poverty*, *6*, 1–7.
33. United Nations (Department of Economic & Social Affairs). (2020). The World's Women 2020: Trends and Statistics (online). https://www.un.org/en/desa/world%E2%80%99s-women-2020
34. United Nations. (2023). World population day (online). https://www.un.org/en/observances/world-population-day
35. World Bank. (2022). Violence against women and girls – What the data tell us (online). https://genderdata.worldbank.org/data-stories/overview-of-gender-based-violence/
36. World Health Organization. (2021). Abortion (online). https://www.who.int/news-room/fact-sheets/detail/abortion
37. Yagub, A. I., & Mtshali, K. (2015). The role of non-governmental organisations in providing curative health services in North Darfur state, Sudan. *African Health Sciences*, *15*(3), 1049–1055. doi: 10.4314/ahs.v15i3.48

PART III

TECHNOLOGICAL AND INNOVATIVE SOLUTIONS

CHAPTER 12

Digital and Preventive Ecosystems for Female Health

DIDHITI AGARWAL, SAGAR BARAGE, and RAJSHRI SINGH*

*Corresponding author

ABSTRACT

In recent years, the healthcare industry has made tremendous leaps and bounds forward. The expansive realm of digital health involves a diverse array of technologies designed to enhance, facilitate, or bolster the operational aspects of health systems from female health perspectives. This includes mobile health applications, health data analytics, telemedicine, and electronic health records. As healthcare organizations adopt and implement new digital health tools, access to better life quality of the females is expected. The ascent of telehealth and broader acceptance of digital health tools within patients as well as healthcare providers are reshaping female health, enhancing access to crucial life-saving preventive health services. A particularly thrilling facet of the digital health revolution lies in its potential to empower females to attain improved health outcomes.

12.1 INTRODUCTION

The concept of digital health encompasses utilizing technology appropriately to enhance the health and wellness of individuals, while also improving patient care through analysis of clinical information [19]. The utilization of technologies in digital health is on the rise for monitoring, managing, and bolstering well-being. Embracing digital health holds the

Holistic Approaches for Women's Sustainable Health, Volume 2: Advancements, Socioeconomic Impacts, and Innovative Strategies. Junaid Ahmad Malik, Anamika Chauhan, and Megh R. Goyal (Eds)

DOI: 10.1201/9781779641656-15

potential to expand health information accessibility, elevation in the standard of care, minimize errors, and encourage in healthy behaviors [36]. Today, with increasing technology, there are various new digital health tools developed and available for women. "Digital Health" denotes the increasing intersection of digital tools with healthcare provision. The World Health Organization (WHO) defines this term comprehensively, encompassing eHealth alongside emerging disciplines such as advanced computational workflows, big data sciences, artificial intelligence (AI), and genomics [66].

The Ministry of Health and Family Welfare (MoHFW) initiated numerous "e-Gov" ventures, collectively known as "e-Health India," aiming on integrating information and communication technology (ICT) into healthcare. In 2015, within this framework MoHFW proposed a regulatory body that is the National eHealth Authority (NeHA) for promoting standards in health management. NeHA aimed to develop and strengthen an eHealth scenario in India and to promote equitable health facilities [31]. This platform improves centralized access to electronic health records (EHRs). Introduced in 2016, EHR standards aim to establish a consistent model nationwide, facilitating seamless interstate coordination. Additionally, the government has launched "MyHealthRecord," a Personal Health Record Locker, further advancing individual healthcare management [2]. National Health Policy (NHP) was introduced by the MoHFW in 2017 with the objective of achieving widespread implementation of digital healthcare initiatives. The NHP recommended establishing a "Federated National Health Information Architecture" by 2025 to connect health providers, along with a National Health Information Network [45, 56].

In 2018, initial efforts were made by NeHA to execute centralized digital health data for Ayushman Bharat–Pradhan Mantri Jan Arogya Yojana. The Government of India introduced the National Digital Health Mission (NDHM) in 2020 for realization of "Digital India." This pan-country initiative aims to establish a digital framework to improve the productivity, efficacy, and openness of healthcare. Key features include assigning every citizen a unique Health ID and creating a comprehensive Health Facility Registry [22].

Additionally, the NITI Aayog projected the "National Digital Health Blueprint" in 2020 to lay the groundwork for a comprehensive digital health ecosystem, integrating with the NDHM. This blueprint aims to standardize e-Health practices and promote nationwide reach for digitalization [31].

The Indian government plans to implement a standard electronic medical record/EHR system across the nation. With NDHM being implemented nationwide, EHR cards could provide more efficient and quicker surveillance. The nation's comparatively younger population and increasing rate of improvement in digital literacy make it possible for a wider range of digital tools, such as wearables, gadgets, and apps, to be developed and made more widely available to users. These tools can be used for monitoring, screening, adhering to medical guidelines, and tracking risk factors. The "National Family Health Survey 2019–21 (NFHS-5)" data indicate that noncommunicable diseases and lifestyle changes will inevitably become more common due to the changing epidemiology and increased life expectancy in India. Patients' opinions about the treatments they received from both public and affiliated private health facilities are being gathered by the MoHFW, Government of India's MeraAspataal (My Hospital) initiative that functions via a number of communication channels, such as a web portal, a mobile application, outbound dialing, and short message service [53].

The areas that affect women the most are reproductive health and child care. The Reproductive and Child Health (RCH) portal tracks the health of expectant mothers and newborns and is specifically designed for women going through the reproductive lifetime. The nation's vaccine supply chain systems are intended to be supported by the unique technical solution known as the Electronic Vaccine Intelligence Network. The ability to monitor vaccination stock levels and storage temperatures in real time across many locations around the nation is made possible by a combination of trained human resources and an IT infrastructure [20, 21].

12.2 ELEMENTS IN DIGITAL PLATFORM TO IMPROVE AND DEMOCRATIZE HEALTHCARE

People are highly conscious of the digital divide and its unequal effects on many facets of life. Digital accessibility and proficiency are more than just additional "social determinants of health" (SDOH); they actually influence each SDOH and are vital to their functioning or dysfunctioning. Due to the complexity of this gap, addressing it requires joint efforts from governmental entities, private enterprises, social framework, such as healthcare sector, community associations, and citizens [14]. The capacity to locate, comprehend, evaluate, and use resources and information to make decisions about one's health is referred to as health literacy, and it is correlated with health outcomes [47]. Healthcare organizations and governments now prioritize "digital health literacy" (DHL) as a means of successfully involving consumers in their health and well-being, given the growing usage of digital technology in healthcare. DHL has the capacity to identify, comprehend, evaluate, and use health information, especially from digital sources. It includes all abilities necessary for a human to properly interface and engage with digital technology [29, 33]. Particularly, those who are more tech-savvy are better able to manage their health through digital platforms, applications, gadgets, and telemedicine, which are linked with enhanced healthy behaviors and actions [61]. The people with lesser DHL often overlap with those who are already impacted by SDOH and correspond with worse health outcomes [16, 26]. As a result, those who are most impacted by health disparities also typically have lower DHLs, making them more vulnerable to negative consequences from their incapacity to use digital technology. Comprehending these variables is crucial in mitigating the alarming patterns of DHL inequality and will facilitate the creation of focused solutions.

12.2.1 TELEMEDICINE AS A DIGITAL DETERMINANT

Since the start of the COVID-19 epidemic, telemedicine has gained prominence in the medical field to offer conventional clinical assessment and surveillance, which includes virtual consultations, remote patient tracking, and portable healthcare solutions [53]. While telemedicine is frequently effective in meeting the healthcare demands of the normal person, it is frequently not designed with patients with disabilities in mind. These patients are an especially vulnerable group, with significant social, economic, and environmental challenges. Moreover, the majority of telemedicine systems are not made to accommodate users with visual, hearing, or cognitive disabilities. Rather, the user interfaces (UIs) are frequently difficult to use and necessitate reading the fine print contents with great attention [3]. It is imperative to address UI challenges, which include screen reader compatibility, sign language integration, captioning, enlargement options, color and contrast adjustments, alongside developing innovative bio-peripheral devices for physical assessment [57].

12.2.2 AI AS A DIGITAL DETERMINANT

A variety of data-driven technologies are used in the healthcare industry to support patient and individual care in the operation, innovation, and enhancement of health services. AI, a data-driven technology, is still in its early stages in healthcare. Image analysis using AI has been applied in radiology, histology, and dermatology [46, 67]. It serves as the foundation for several clinical decision support technologies that are now in use in the delivery of healthcare, including wearable technology, patient monitors, and symptom checks. AI is also being used for logistical assistance, for example, in automated programs that manage back-office duties, including staff scheduling, clinic visit result prediction, and clinic slot optimization to cut down on patient wait times [15]. AI has great potential for use in healthcare applications, but the majority of research has been directed toward assisting society's more affluent segments. A broad grasp of how these technologies operate and their place in the larger healthcare landscape, as well as enough internet connection and DHL, are necessary for using AI-based technology [38].

12.2.3 DATA ASYMMETRY AS A DIGITAL DETERMINANT

Health data poverty refers to the situation where individuals, groups, or communities cannot fully gain from a breakthrough or innovation because of inadequate representative data sets [28]. Health data encompasses any information pertaining to a patient's physical or mental well-being, spanning biochemical, clinical, radiological, pathological, and molecular. An increasing volume of this data is being stored electronically to facilitate its utilization in forthcoming consultations. Large-scale implementations of this lead to the accumulation of health data sets that serve as the foundation for developing new technologies.

There are many different types of digital health technology, such as mobile applications, telemedicine, AI tools, symptom assessment applications, precision medicine techniques, and robotics. As is the case with many health technologies today, digital inclusion needs to be considered from the very beginning of technology creation and not as an afterthought. To gain deeper insights into the demographic, socioeconomic, and political traits of their consumers and tailor the technology consequently, developers may conduct market research [14].

Governments must prioritize the needs of those with the least power and tackle digital health with an equality and rights-centered approach. One way to do this is to make sure people are prepared for "Digital Health." The term "Digital Health Readiness" describes the varying degree to which people and nations are able to use data and digital technologies to enhance the health and well-being of themselves or their population [35]. By considering the needs and perspectives of minority communities, governments can partner with healthcare professionals and businesses to ensure the ethical and equitable development of digital health technology [44].

Approval of digital technologies is the responsibility of specific national agencies, such as the National Medical Products Administration in China, Food and Drug Administration in the USA, the Central Drugs Standard Control Organization in India, and the Medicines and Healthcare products Regulatory Agency in the United Kingdom. These groups have more potential to oversee health technology. Equality and inclusivity in health technology must be given equal priority in future regulatory agendas, thus, to enable a seamless transition and the exchange of newer technology, data, and ideas, as well as to give development support for digital health in lower- and middle-income countries. Over 120 member states have implemented digital health regulations, as outlined in the WHO global strategy [14]. Proponents of healthcare democratization through digital health technologies reaffirm optimistic expectations regarding their positive impacts [21]. The centralization and empowerment of patients within the healthcare system are intricately linked to the revolutionary role of digital health. This transformation, driven by data-driven technology along with the adoption of mobile health technologies as a catalyst for "institutional recasting" in healthcare, is shifting from clinician-facilitated care to consumer-centric, personalized, and participatory care [4]. The conversation surrounding Digital health democratization celebrates these trends.

12.3 DIGITAL INNOVATIONS TO IMPROVE FEMALE HEALTHCARE

Behavior change interventions leveraging technology have historical origins. The 1940s and 1950s era witnessed the use of mechanical counters to offer real-time, person-specific feedback on behaviors. The instance of such pioneering technology is the pedometer, introduced in 1949 for obesity treatment and subsequently utilized for quantifying physical actions' involvement in behavioral studies in the 1960s. Pedometers provide instant, personalized surveillance of physical activity, serving as a crucial tool for behavior modification. Their affordability and user-friendliness allow for widespread adoption. Public health initiatives incorporating pedometers have proven effective in boosting physical activity levels and are cost-efficient compared to alternative interventions [6].

Advanced iterations in activity sensors emerged, incorporating wrist and ankle-mounted counters, as well as ultrasonic sound measurement, establishing the foundation for present-day wearable fitness bands and smart watches [62].

The devices acquire timing and velocity data for movements at a reduced price in comparison to research-grade accelerometers, which are widely regarded as the standard [17]. Although wearable technology facilitates self-monitoring of physical activity, improving behavior change skills is often essential for effectively promoting and maintaining higher activity levels in adults. These skills could be imparted through traditional in-person interaction interventions or incorporated into web or smartphone applications. Incorporating wearable technology with Just-In-Time or Just-In-Time Adaptive Interventions allows devices to provide intervention content tailored to users' current physical activity behavior, including issuing reminders to walk after extended periods of inactivity [50, 51].

Premium-priced wearable devices primarily attract young and affluent early adopters, but many users quickly lose interest within a short span, leading to notable attrition rates. This trend has led to various initiatives that repurposes unused wearables for underserved communities [24]. The incorporation of social media features into wearable platforms may enhance their effectiveness, but further research is needed to understand the optimal approach. Overall, there is a need for additional research to explore how wearable technology can effectively influence physical activity and additional health benefits. Emerging wearables sectors encompass monitors for diabetes and ultraviolet radiation [24, 27].

Bangladesh and India provide specific examples of how culture affects healthcare platforms tailored for women's health in the digital realm. In these countries, initiatives to enhance maternal health and well-being have resulted in the creation of wearable technology known as the COEL bangle (developed by Grameen Intel), an abbreviation for "Carbon Monoxide

Exposure Limiter." The LED sensor notifies the mother of unsafe carbon monoxide levels in the room and enables her to relocate outdoors until the air quality improves. The bracelet, with its understated appearance, conceals a built-in speaker that delivers a sequence of prerecorded information in native languages to educate women about pregnancy-related topics such as nutrition and diet, prenatal environmental hazards nearby, and antenatal appointment reminders. As a result, in order for the COEL bangle to work, it does not require pairing with a smartphone or internet access [4, 7].

Another breakthrough in maternal health, designed and implemented with cultural considerations, is MomConnect [9, 30, 43]. The countrywide Department of Health in South Africa has implemented a system that uses mobile phones to provide text-based assistance for maternal health on a countrywide scale and has received recognition as a triumph in areas of female health, cultural adjustments, and digital health.

A recent study advocates for the adoption of eHealth in British Columbia's healthcare system. It found that ICOnnecta't, a digital platform, facilitated timely monitoring and intervention for breast cancer patients, potentially preventing the exacerbation of physical and psychological symptoms and reducing healthcare costs [42]. While some patients responded resiliently to their diagnosis, others did not, indicating the need for refined risk assessment to tailor treatments more effectively [5].

A digital health program focused on gender transformation is defined as "Addresses the causes of gender-based health inequities through approaches that challenge and redress harmful and unequal gender norms, roles, and power relations that privilege men over women," in accordance with the definition provided by the WHO. Maternal healthcare outcomes are being improved by gender transformational techniques in digital health programs. The results of the implications study point to the necessity for mHealth research to specifically recognize the methods in which power relations, norms, and values affect maternal health and to deal with these aspects all the way through a mHealth program [65].

The number of research papers proving the usefulness of AI tools or techniques in clinical care has significantly increased in the past several years. Large volumes of clinical data can be quickly synthesized and interpreted by AI algorithms at speeds far faster than those of humans. Furthermore, there may be room to improve how we screen for and prevent diseases, given the development and broad use of several digital technologies.

These resources include smartphone apps for wellness education, patient communication portals, and a range of wearable technology that monitor behavior, physical activity, and biometrics [1]. Even though AI may have a place in the screening process for cardiovascular disease, further study is required to see whether digital technologies live up to the hype and actually enhance patient outcomes and eliminate inequities [37]. International associations have started to develop online tools that can assist physicians in navigating the increasingly complex ecosystem of digital technologies, even if the breadth of these technologies might be intimidating.

The transformative influence of AI in various domains pertinent to fertility and articulate a prospective framework for its integration within assisted reproductive technology [39]. This envisioned integration aims to enhance outcomes, diminish expenses, and foster beneficial advancements in clinical care within the fertility sector.

12.4 TECHNOLOGY ADOPTION, INTEGRATION, AND INTERDISCIPLINARY PARTNERS ACROSS IT LANDSCAPE

Digital health integrates ICT with healthcare, offering tools and services that have the potential to enhance disease management for patients suffering from chronic conditions [31]. The digital transformation of healthcare comprises two main elements: employing technology to provide healthcare services and digitizing medical data. Technology utilization may involve telemedicine, facilitating patients to access medical care remotely without the need for physical interaction with a healthcare provider or facility [64]. Additionally, this transformation may encompass robot-assisted surgery and has prompted an increased emphasis on leveraging AI across multiple facets of healthcare service provision [55]. Digitalization involves the development of EHRs, enabling healthcare providers to access comprehensive patient medical records irrespective of the data's source or collection time. This capability significantly improves the efficiency of medical services [49].

AI mechanisms equipped with data mining and pattern recognition abilities offer a promising approach to explore "Symbolic models of diseases," enabling analysis of their correlation with patient symptoms. This approach facilitates disease management, monitoring, medical protocol development, and drug innovation, with AI tools streamlining tasks conventionally handled by humans, resulting in enhanced efficiency and cost-effectiveness. They hold the potential to revolutionize modern healthcare, as exemplified by various applications such as virtual assistants supporting individuals with Alzheimer's disease or preliminary skin cancer diagnoses [46].

Therefore, prospective technology assessment calls for pertinent methodological and thematic knowledge or abilities that frequently extend beyond the boundaries of well-established scientific specialties. By streamlining data gathering and processing, development in web devices and machine learning apps can offer insightful analyses and forecasts on individual health. However, the flow of information regarding a patient's health status presents a number of technological, legal, and financial issues that require a multidisciplinary approach to be resolved [23, 33]. In numerous countries, including the United States, governments encourage with incentives for the efficient use of e-health technology. In order to create a more thorough knowledge of the digital health transition, there is an urgent need for extensive stakeholder discussion on the management implications of digitalization. In the end, the development of technological information systems, telemedicine, and digital security will all contribute to making sure that the transition to digital health is accepted by all parties. Several suggestions are suggested for every participant in the digital entrepreneurial ecosystem and offer a comprehensive perspective by integrating the results of open future technology, social business, and innovation [58].

This involves promoting the exchange of information and technology through open innovation from the scientific community to all stakeholders working toward achieving the sustainable development goals (SDGs), encompassing more than just businesses, and considering the necessity for financing. There is a need to promote entrepreneurial education and encouragement for social intrapreneurship and/or social enterprise in the potentially influential organizations addressing the SDGs. It suggests seizing the opportunity presented by diversity, particularly in the areas of female entrepreneurship [58]. It is important to have the integration of entrepreneurial ecosystems within the framework of economic as well as regulatory policies for effective adoption and utilization of developing technologies [13].

12.5 DIGITAL HEALTH DATA PROTECTION

The government and other relevant parties must thoroughly assess the current legal and policy frameworks before focusing resources on extensive initiatives to digitize healthcare. This will guarantee a "rights-based" outline covering a premium on user control over data, access to high-quality healthcare, and acknowledgment of informed consent and rights to privacy [31].

Personal health information has to be properly regulated to safeguard patient privacy and safety while promoting innovation. Every person's data record must be precise, current, and organized so that it may be evaluated, changed, and removed upon request. Training should be provided to those who utilize health data, and adequate data privacy controls—like user identification and permission during login—are vital for guaranteeing informed consent, safeguarding privacy, and fostering proficiency in data collection and its processing. Patient record usage should be governed by organized, culturally appropriate processes that provide informed consent. Data should also, if feasible, be aggregated or anonymized. The guidelines pertaining to the use of personal health data by third parties' medical software should address openness, data confidentiality, and cybersecurity. Additionally, the guidelines must include a clear data sharing agreement that protects patient rights [54, 66].

It would be preferable to solve the digital gap and various infrastructure-related concerns in the country primarily, not only from the standpoint of policy but also with regard to its implementation and operation [12].

It is imperative that a thorough legislative layout that adequately handles the concerns of data security, confidentiality, and inclusivity come before any major move toward the digitalization of healthcare. It also has to build the infrastructure required for such a jump to see its advantages materialize on the ground using an intersectional rights-based methodology [31].

Another crucial step is to make it possible for leadership, employees, and trainees from historically underrepresented communities in technology and the health sciences to be hired [10]. The greatest standards of behavior should be expected of organizations that gather health data and researchers who utilize it, including respect for the individuals from whom the data originate and good stewardship of this priceless shared resource. Health information rules ought to take into account the growing number of diverse entities that gather, process, use, transfer, and sell data—sometimes without the contributor's knowledge—as stated by several sources. A learning health system depends on the contributions of both patients and doctors and aims to create "evidence that is both applied and developed as a natural product of the care process" [48].

The COVID-19 epidemic has brought attention to the role that digital health can play. The potential of digital health is recognized in various ways, incorporating the use of digital tools like contact tracing applications to track outbreaks and online consultations to assist in keeping patients and medical staff safe while continuing care. It is crucial to have more leadership in this field and to share information in order to guarantee that people receive quality care and that health systems profit from new technologies [11].

12.6 ADDRESSING ETHICAL ISSUES IN DIGITAL DATA SHARING

The quantity of attention given to the digital ecosystem has increased noticeably for female health, especially with the incorporation of AI and mobile applications for diverse functions, including dietary planning and breast cancer screening. But this development also raises a number of moral and societal issues that warranted to be properly taken into consideration. There are the following ethical issues in the digital ecosystem:

- **Privacy and secrecy:** The use of accelerometers to monitor motion creates significant privacy issues. This technique carries the risk of unintentionally disclosing a person's GPS location, endangering their safety and privacy.
- **Browser history and online behavior:** There is a serious privacy concern when browser history is analyzed to track user behavior online. There are ethical considerations around data use and protection when sensitive information about a person's preferences, interests, and possibly even health is revealed by this data.
- **Call logs and communications:** Privacy issues may also arise from tracking call logs and communications. In-depth conversation logs can make sensitive conversations about health, relationships, and other topics vulnerable to security breaches.
- **Camera usage and geotagging:** Using camera tracking and geotagging capabilities may unintentionally reveal private images or videos of the user. In addition to violating privacy, this also raises questions regarding how such private content may be misused. [60].

Though it presents encouraging improvements in healthcare accessibility and monitoring, the digital ecosystem for female health must negotiate a challenging terrain of moral and societal issues.

12.7 CHALLENGES IN EXPANSION OF DIGITAL ECOSYSTEM

The discipline of digital health aims to enhance patient care through the use of technological tools such as AI, EHRs, mobile health, and telemedicine, while also focusing on its effectiveness and practical implementation. Technologies in digital health have the power to completely change how healthcare is provided, through their ability to improve disease management, facilitate remote monitoring, and provide more personalized treatment. AI, wearable technology, EHRs, telemedicine, and mobile health apps are some of these technologies. A personalized medicine model can be evolved with the use of digital health by collecting information from the vital signs, way of life, and medical background of patients. However, before these technologies are widely used, it is crucial to thoroughly assess their efficacy and safety [18, 63].

There are several barriers that prevent advancements in e-health. These include, among many other challenges, the lack of standards based on evidence, privacy issues, challenges with data governance, and moral conundrums [11, 41]. The sensitivity of health data is a major issue that might result in privacy issues when it is digitized [60]. The permission problem presents additional ethical problems because a large number of users could not completely comprehend the terms of use before agreeing to them [41]. Moreover, there is insufficient data to determine how digital health tactics affect patient outcomes, optimizing expenditure, and system performance. Users' socioeconomic status and earnings may also have an impact on the effective implementation of telehealth platforms [11]. Due to lower levels of health literacy, some groups—who belong to minority groups, are old, are in low-income regions, or are rural residents—may find it challenging to comprehend and use digital health solutions [34].

12.8 FUTURE PROSPECTS IN THE APPLICATION OF DIGITAL FRAMEWORK IN FEMALE HEALTH CARE SCENARIOS

It is imperative to guarantee that telehealth is integrated into national healthcare systems on a long-term basis as opposed to being limited to emergency scenarios [18, 34]. This would make using telemedicine during epidemics more widely possible. The investments in 5G technology and communication framework construction can assist the adoption of telehealth in low-income countries [31]. Connected sensors, smartphones, wearables, and diagnostic algorithms are being used by businesses to collect health information, provide criticism, and advocate proactive treatment approaches. Incorporating digital health into daily routines may encounter various challenges, such as privacy and data security risks, along with potential discordance with patient preferences and values [32, 59]. Addressing these challenges requires the establishment of robust systems with stringent data security and privacy measures. Early involvement of patients and technology developers is imperative to tackle patient concerns during the development of new digital innovations. Furthermore, engaging medical practitioners and adapting healthcare systems to integrate digital health solutions are imperative.

By examining the ways in the engagement of patients and public in digital health innovation—if at all—as well as the main facilitators and hurdles that impede meaningful participation in development, application, and assessment of its innovations, studies fill a recognized vacuum in the body of research [41]. Over the past 10 years, publication numbers have been increasingly rising with patient participation across diverse digital health platforms innovation kinds along with issues, such as cancer, dementia, and mental health [8].

The eminence, occurrence, and extent of patient and public involvement (PPI) are impacted by a number of enablers and barriers, for instance, worries about data security and privacy, financial and time constraints, an unequal power distribution, and traditional, frequently hierarchical working methods that frequently view patient perspectives and recommendations. A large number of study conclusions align with previous studies, stressing the value of collaboration, regular, inclusive communication, and enough funding for PPI initiatives [8].

Concurrently, a growing corpus of bioethics literature highlights the necessity for health technologies and therapies that meet specific requirements for efficacy, safety, and beneficence. This body of work has a strong emphasis on fair, egalitarian, socially responsible, and responsible innovation, proving that health technologies are legitimate breakthroughs with clinically proven potential to improve health, which is largely dependent on this criteria-centric approach [40]. Studies that focus on health innovation standards are considered to be extremely relevant to discussions about democratization because, when evaluating digital health innovations for the purpose of democratizing healthcare, the standard of medical care and technology they allow must be carefully considered. Consequently, if digital health is to achieve its objective of democratizing healthcare, it must not only ensure that each individual user has a reasonable chance of achieving positive and fair health results, but also extend this guarantee to a range of the target group's user demographics, as well as those at the social and global levels when the technology is employed abroad.

Health technologies must be based on information pertinent to the many bodies and health needs of the entire target community, as well as in evidence-based clinical investigations, according to scholars dedicated to health equality and justice [25]. Realizing the promise of technology to empower and democratize requires that the recommendations and health data produced by e-health be accurate, clinically rigorous, and intersectionally effective. Furthermore, in order for digital health to be liberating, it must support material oppression, structural inequality, or regional and global health inequities [52].

12.9 SUMMARY

Digital health leverages technology to revolutionize healthcare by integrating ICTs to enhance wellness and clinical management. In India, the Ministry of Health has pioneered "e-Health India" to integrate ICT into healthcare systems managed by the NeHA. Central to this digital health revolution is DHL, which is crucial for empowering individuals, particularly women, to access and utilize health information from digital platforms effectively. Telemedicine, accelerated during the COVID-19 pandemic, emerged as a pivotal tool but faces accessibility challenges, especially for disabled populations. Improving UIs is pivotal in broadening access to these services.

AI plays a transformative role in healthcare, from image analysis to clinical decision support, yet access remains uneven across socioeconomic divides. Achieving digital health readiness demands inclusive AI development and regulation to ensure equitable distribution of benefits. Innovations in digital health are reshaping female healthcare across regions like India, where wearable technologies and mobile platforms provide educational and support services. The integration of AI in clinical care enhances diagnostics and treatment, yet gender disparities persist, necessitating more inclusive research and implementation strategies. Data protection is critical, and legal frameworks must govern personal health data, emphasizing anonymity, secure handling, and equity. The digital health landscape, particularly for women's health, offers innovations yet raises ethical and societal concerns. Privacy issues from tracking technologies necessitate robust governance, while societal pressures and literacy gaps pose challenges. Overcoming barriers requires enhancing telehealth integration, bolstering infrastructure in underserved regions, and prioritizing privacy and security.

KEYWORDS

- **digital health**
- **preventative healthcare**
- **digital tools**
- **health data analytics**

REFERENCES

1. Adedinsewo, D. A., Pollak, A. W., Phillips, S. D., Smith, T. L., Svatikova, A., Hayes, S. N., & Carter, R. E. (2022). Cardiovascular disease screening in women: Leveraging artificial intelligence and digital tools. *Circulation Research*, *130*(4), 673–690.
2. Aggarwal, L., & Roy, M. (2023). A strategic roadmap to the successful implementation of digital health records. In: *Isabele de Souza Carvalho, Uniting Knowledge Integrated Scientific Research For Global Development, Seven Editora.*
3. Aggarwal, N. K., Pieh, M. C., Dixon, L., Guarnaccia, P., Alegria, M., & Lewis-Fernandez, R. (2016). Clinician descriptions of communication strategies to improve treatment engagement by racial/ethnic minorities in mental health services: A systematic review. *Patient Education and Counseling*, *99*(2), 198–209.
4. Anto-Ocrah, M., Asiedu, M., Rao, S., DeSplinter, L., & Hollenbach, S. (2023). If you build it, they will come or not. Considerations for women's health in the post-pandemic era of digital innovation. *Frontiers in Public Health*, *11*, 1228212.
5. Arigo, D. (2015). Promoting physical activity among women using wearable technology and online social connectivity: A feasibility study. *Health Psychology and Behavioral Medicine*, *3*(1), 391–409.
6. Arigo, D., Jake-Schoffman, D. E., Wolin, K., Beckjord, E., Hekler, E. B., & Pagoto, S. L. (2019). The history and future of digital health in the field of behavioral medicine. *Journal of Behavioral Medicine*, *42*, 67–83.

7. Ashraf, M., Hasin, M. M., Salahuddin, A. B. E., Ahmed, S., Ro, S. C., Ray, P, & Uzir, U. H. (2018). The potential scope of m-health initiative into Grameen renewable energy in Bangladesh. *The International Technology Management Review, 7*, 144–50.
8. Baines, R., Bradwell, H., Edwards, K., Stevens, S., Prime, S., Tredinnick-Rowe, J., & Chatterjee, A. (2022). Meaningful patient and public involvement in digital health innovation, implementation and evaluation: A systematic review. *Health Expectations*, *25*(4), 1232–1245.
9. Barron, P., Peter, J., LeFevre, A. E., Sebidi, J., Bekker, M., Allen, R., & Pillay, Y. (2018). Mobile health messaging service and helpdesk for South African mothers (MomConnect): History, successes and challenges. *BMJ Global Health*, *3*(2), e000559.
10. Bonham, V. L., & Green, E. D. (2021). The genomics workforce must become more diverse: A strategic imperative. *The American Journal of Human Genetics*, *108*(1), 3–7.
11. Bouabida, K., Lebouché, B., & Pomey, M. P. (2022). Telehealth and COVID-19 pandemic: An overview of the telehealth use, advantages, challenges, and opportunities during COVID-19 pandemic. *Healthcare (Basel)*, *10*(11), 2293.
12. Brall, C., Schröder-Bäck, P., & Maeckelberghe, E. (2019). Ethical aspects of digital health from a justice point of view. *European Journal of Public Health*, *29*(3), 18–22.
13. Chesbrough, H. (2019). Open innovation best practices, 1st edn, In: Chesbrough, H. (Ed.). *Open Innovation Results: Going Beyond the Hype and Getting Down to Business* (pp.133–151). Oxford University Press.
14. Chidambaram, S., Jain, B., Jain, U., Mwavu, R., Baru, R., Thomas, B., & Darzi, A. (2024). An introduction to digital determinants of health. *PLOS Digital Health*, *3*(1), e0000346.
15. Department of Health and Social Care. (2019). NHSX: New joint organisation for digital, data and technology. https://www.gov.uk/government/news/nhsx-new-joint-organisation-for-digital-data-and-technology; (accessed on 10 June 2024).
16. Estacio, E. V., Whittle, R., & Protheroe, J. (2019). The digital divide: Examining socio-demographic factors associated with health literacy, access and use of internet to seek health information. *Journal of Health Psychology*, *24*(12), 1668–1675.
17. Evenson, K. R., Goto, M. M., & Furberg, R. D. (2015). Systematic review of the validity and reliability of consumer-wearable activity trackers. *International Journal of Behavioral Nutrition and Physical Activity*, *12*, 1–22.
18. Fagherazzi, G., Goetzinger, C., Rashid, M. A., Aguayo, G. A., & Huiart, L. (2020). Digital health strategies to fight COVID-19 worldwide: Challenges, recommendations, and a call for papers. *Journal of Medical Internet Research*, *22*(6), e19284.
19. Fatehi, F., Samadbeik, M. & Kazemi, A. (2020). What is Digital Health? Review of Definitions. *Studies in Health Technology and Informatics, 23*(275), 67–71.
20. Gopichandran, V., Ganeshkumar, P., Dash, S., & Ramasamy, A. (2020). Ethical challenges of digital health technologies: *Aadhaar*, India. *Bulletin of the World Health Organization*, *98*(4), 277–281.
21. Gurnani, V., Dhalaria, P., Chatterjee, S., Singh, P., Agrahari, K., Kashyap, S., & Haldar, P. (2022). Return on investment of the electronic vaccine intelligence network in India. *Human Vaccines & Immunotherapeutics*, *18*(1), 2009289.

22. Gurumurthy, A., Chami, N., & Thomas, S. (2016). Unpacking digital India: A feminist commentary on policy agendas in the digital moment. *Journal of Information Policy*, *6*, 371–402.
23. Habli, I., Lawton, T., & Porter, Z. (2020). Artificial intelligence in health care: Accountability and safety. *Bulletin of the World Health Organization*, *98*(4), 251.
24. Heintzman, N. D. (2016). A digital ecosystem of diabetes data and technology: Services, systems, and tools enabled by wearables, sensors, and apps. *Journal of Diabetes Science and Technology*, *10*(1), 35–41.
25. Hendl, T., & Shukla, A. (2024). Can digital health democratize health care. *Bioethics*, *38*(6), 491–502.
26. Honeyman, M., Maguire, D., Evans, H., & Davies, A. (2020). *Digital Technology and Health Inequalities: A Scoping Review (2020)*. Public Health Wales NHS Trust: Cardiff.
27. Hussain, M. S., Cripwell, L., Berkovsky, S., & Freyne, J, (2016). Promoting UV exposure awareness with persuasive, wearable technologies. *Studies in Health Technology and Informatics, 227*, 48–54.
28. Ibrahim, H., Liu, X., Zariffa, N., Morris, A. D., & Denniston, A. K. (2021). Health data poverty: An assailable barrier to equitable digital health care. *The Lancet Digital Health*, *3*(4), e260–e265.
29. Islam, M. M. (2019). Social determinants of health and related inequalities: Confusion and implications. *Frontiers in Public Health*, *7*, 11.
30. Jahan, R. (2020). Impact of MomConnect program in South Africa: A narrative review. *On-Line Journal of Nursing Informatics*, *24*(2), 211.
31. Jain, D. (2023). Regulation of digital healthcare in India: Ethical and legal challenges. *Healthcare*, *11*(6), 911.
32. Jain, D., Rastogi, A., Kartik, K., Diwan, A., & Saha, O. (2022). Medical abortion through telehealth in India: A critical perspective. *Sexual and Reproductive Health Matters*, *29*(2), 2107090.
33. Joshi, I., & Morley, J. (Eds.), (2019). Artificial intelligence: How to get it right. In: *Putting Policy into Practice for Safe Data-driven Innovation in Health and Care*. NHSX: London, United Kingdom.
34. Kaihlanen, A. M., Virtanen, L., Buchert, U., Safarov, N., Valkonen, P., Hietapakka, L., & Heponiemi, T. (2022). Towards digital health equity-a qualitative study of the challenges experienced by vulnerable groups in using digital health services in the COVID-19 era. *BMC Health Services Research*, *22*(1), 188.
35. Kickbusch, I., Piselli, D., Agrawal, A., Balicer, R., Banner, O., Adelhardt, M., & Wong, B. L. H. (2021). The Lancet and Financial Times Commission on governing health futures 2030: Growing up in a digital world. *The Lancet, 398*(10312), 1727–1776.
36. Kreps, G. L., & Neuhauser, L. (2010). New directions in eHealth communication: Opportunities and challenges. *Patient Education and Counseling*, *78*(3), 329–336.
37. Krittanawong, C., Rogers, A. J., Johnson, K. W., Wang, Z., Turakhia, M. P., Halperin, J. L., & Narayan, S. M. (2021). Integration of novel monitoring devices with machine learning technology for scalable cardiovascular management. *Nature Reviews Cardiology*, *18*(2), 75–91.

38. Laz, T. H., & Berenson, A. B. (2013). Racial and ethnic disparities in internet use for seeking health information among young women. *Journal of Health Communication*, *18*(2), 250–260.
39. Letterie, G. (2021). Three ways of knowing: The integration of clinical expertise, evidence-based medicine, and artificial intelligence in assisted reproductive technologies. *Journal of Assisted Reproduction and Genetics*, *38*(7), 1617–1625.
40. Lipworth, W., & Axler, R. (2016). Towards a bioethics of innovation. *Journal of Medical Ethics*, *42*(7), 445–449.
41. Manteghinejad, A., & Javanmard, S. H. (2021). Challenges and opportunities of digital health in a post-COVID19 world. *Journal of Research in Medical Sciences*, *26*(1), 11.
42. Medina, J. C., Flix-Valle, A., Rodríguez-Ortega, A., Hernández-Ribas, R., Lleras de Frutos, M., & Ochoa-Arnedo, C. (2022). ICOnnecta't: Development and initial results of a stepped psychosocial eHealth ecosystem to facilitate risk assessment and prevention of early emotional distress in breast cancer survivors' journey. *Cancers*, *14*(4), 974.
43. MomConnect. Department of health republic of South Africa. Available online: https://www.health.gov.za/momconnect/; (accessed on 27 February 2024).
44. Murphy, K., Di Ruggiero, E., Upshur, R., Willison, D. J., Malhotra, N., Cai, J. C., & Gibson, J. (2021). Artificial intelligence for good health: A scoping review of the ethics literature. *BMC Medical Ethics*, *22*, 1–17.
45. National Health Authority National Digital Health Mission. Available online: https://abdm.gov.in:8081/uploads/ndhb_1_56ec695bc8.pdf; (accessed on 26 February 2022).
46. Niazi, M. K. K., Parwani, A. V., & Gurcan, M. N. (2019). Digital pathology and artificial intelligence. *The Lancet Oncology*, *20*(5), e253–e261.
47. Norman, C. D., & Skinner, H. A. (2006). eHealth literacy: Essential skills for consumer health in a networked world. *Journal of Medical Internet Research*, *8*(2), e506.
48. Olsen, L. M., Nabel, E. G., McGinnis, J. M., & McClellan, M. B. (2008). *Evidence-based Medicine and the Changing Nature of Health Care: 2007 IOM Annual Meeting Summary*. National Academies Press.
49. Pai, M. M., Ganiga, R., Pai, R. M., & Sinha, R. K. (2021). Standard electronic health record (EHR) framework for Indian healthcare system. *Health Services and Outcomes Research Methodology*, *21*(3), 339–362.
50. Patel, M. S., Asch, D. A., & Volpp, K. G. (2015). Wearable devices as facilitators, not drivers, of health behavior change. *JAMA*, *313*(5), 459–460.
51. Peake, J. M., Kerr, G., & Sullivan, J. P. (2018). A critical review of consumer wearables, mobile applications, and equipment for providing biofeedback, monitoring stress, and sleep in physically active populations. *Frontiers in Physiology*, *9*, 743.
52. Powers, M. & Faden, R. R. (2006). *Social Justice: The Moral Foundations of Public Health and Health Policy*. Oxford University Press: USA.
53. Ramachandran, A., & Sarbadhikari, S. N. (2021, March). Digital health for the post-COVID-19 pandemic in India: Emerging technologies for healthcare. In: *2021 8th International Conference on Computing for Sustainable Global Development* (pp. 244–249). *(INDIACom)*

54. Ranganathan, S. (2020). Towards a holistic digital health ecosystem in India. *Observer Research Foundation, 2.*
55. Reddy, S. (2018). Use of artificial intelligence in healthcare delivery. In: Heston, T. (Ed.), *eHealth—Making Health Care Smarter*. InTech.
56. Sarbadhikari, S. N. (2019). Digital health in India–As envisaged by the national health policy (2017). *BLDE University Journal of Health Sciences*, *4*(1), 1–6.
57. Scott Kruse, C., Karem, P., Shifflett, K., Vegi, L., Ravi, K., & Brooks, M. (2018). Evaluating barriers to adopting telemedicine worldwide: A systematic review. *Journal of Telemedicine and Telecare*, *24*(1), 4–12.
58. Shamsrizi, M., Pakura, A., Wiechers, J., Pakura, S. & Dauster, D. V. (2020). Digital Entrepreneurship for the "Decade of Action": How entrepreneurs can impact our race towards the sustainable development goals. *Digital Entrepreneurship*. *25*, 303–27.
59. Sharma, A., Harrington, R. A., McClellan, M. B., Turakhia, M. P., Eapen, Z. J., Steinhubl, S., Mault, J. R., Majmudar, M. D., Roessig, L., Chandross, K. J., Green, E. M., Patel, B., Hamer, A., Olgin, J., Rumsfeld, J. S., Roe, M. T., & Peterson, E. D. (2018). Using digital health technology to better generate evidence and deliver evidence-based care. *Journal of the American College of Cardiology*, *71*(23), 2680–2690.
60. Shaw, J. A., & Donia, J. (2021). The sociotechnical ethics of digital health: A critique and extension of approaches from bioethics. *Frontiers in Digital Health*, *3*, 725088.
61. Sieck, C. J., Sheon, A., Ancker, J. S., Castek, J., Callahan, B., & Siefer, A. (2021). Digital inclusion as a social determinant of health. *NPJ Digital Medicine*, *4*(1), 52.
62. Silfee, V. J., Haughton, C. F., Jake-Schoffman, D. E., Lopez-Cepero, A., May, C. N., Sreedhara, M., & Lemon, S. C. (2018). Objective measurement of physical activity outcomes in lifestyle interventions among adults: A systematic review. *Preventive Medicine Reports*, *11*, 74–80.
63. Stoumpos, A. I., Kitsios, F., & Talias, M. A. (2023). Digital transformation in healthcare: Technology acceptance and its applications. *International Journal of Environmental Research and Public Health, 15*, 20(4), 3407.
64. Trocin, C., Mikalef, P., Papamitsiou, Z., & Conboy, K. (2023). Responsible AI for digital health: A synthesis and a research agenda. *Information Systems Frontiers*, *25*(6), 2139–2157.
65. Udenigwe, O., Omonaiye, O., & Yaya, S. (2023). Gender transformative approaches in mHealth for maternal healthcare in sub-Saharan Africa: A systematic review. *Frontiers in Digital Health*, *5*, 1263488.
66. *WHO guideline Recommendations on Digital Interventions for Health System Strengthening*. (2019). World Health Organization. Recommendations on digital interventions for health system strengthening (who.int); (accessed on 10 June 2024)
67. Young, A. T., Xiong, M., Pfau, J., Keiser, M. J., & Wei, M. L. (2020). Artificial intelligence in dermatology: A primer. *Journal of Investigative Dermatology*, *140*(8), 1504–1512.

CHAPTER 13

Role of Internet of Things in Female Healthcare

ANAMIKA CHAUHAN* and MEGH R. GOYAL

*Corresponding author

ABSTRACT

Improved disease management, preventive care, and individualized treatment—especially for women—are the ways that the Internet of Things (IoT) is transforming healthcare. To improve female health outcomes, this chapter explores (1) how important IoT technologies are with emphasis on preventative care, chronic illness management, and reproductive health; (2) how IoT devices have significantly advanced diagnostic precision, continuous health monitoring, and tailored treatment strategies by analyzing the available literature and several case studies; (3) how IoT empowers women to have better health. Additionally, it tackles the important issues that come with IoT use in healthcare, such as security problems, privacy concerns about data, and the possibility of inequities in access. Developing IoT solutions are morally sound and available to all women, regardless of financial background. By providing an in-depth analysis of how IoT applications can specifically address women's needs, this chapter hopes to stimulate additional research and development in this rapidly evolving field, advancing technology-driven healthcare solutions that are fair and considerate of the particularities of women's health.

Holistic Approaches for Women's Sustainable Health, Volume 2: Advancements, Socioeconomic Impacts, and Innovative Strategies. Junaid Ahmad Malik, Anamika Chauhan, and Megh R. Goyal (Eds)

DOI: 10.1201/9781779641656-16

13.1 INTRODUCTION

The Internet of Things (IoT) represents a revolutionary leap in the landscape of female healthcare technology, encompassing a network of interconnected devices to collect, transmit, and analyze data for enhancing healthcare delivery [1]. IoT in healthcare is referred to as the Internet of Medical Things, which includes devices, such as wearable fitness trackers, remote monitoring sensors, and smart medical appliances, to provide critical data points for patient-care management [2]. The application of IoT technologies in healthcare settings promises several transformative benefits. It enables real-time monitoring of patients' physiological parameters, such as heart rate, blood pressure, and glucose levels, thereby facilitating proactive management of chronic conditions and reducing the necessity for in-person visits [4]. Moreover, IoT devices can significantly improve the accuracy and efficiency of healthcare services by automating routine tasks, like patient data entry and medication management, thus allowing healthcare professionals to focus more on patient care rather than administrative duties [3]. The integration of IoT in healthcare is particularly impactful in managing the unique healthcare challenges faced by women. It offers tools for personalized healthcare that can monitor and manage health conditions that predominantly affect women, such as gestational diabetes, breast cancer, and osteoporosis [3, 5]. Furthermore, IoT technologies can enhance access to healthcare services for women, especially in rural or underserved regions, by connecting them with healthcare providers remotely. As IoT continues to evolve, it is poised to become an integral part of healthcare systems globally, driven by the need for more efficient healthcare solutions and the rising demand for personalized care [9].

This chapter explores the diverse applications of IoT in the specific context of female healthcare, highlighting both the advancements it facilitates and the challenges it must overcome. Also, the primary objective of this chapter is to comprehensively explore the impact and potential of the IoT in enhancing healthcare, specifically for women. This chapter aims to systematically evaluate how IoT technologies are currently being utilized to address unique health challenges faced by women, including reproductive health, chronic disease management, mental health, and preventive care. The scope of the chapter extends to examining various IoT devices and systems, such as wearable sensors, remote monitoring devices, and personalized health applications that contribute to improved diagnostic accuracy, effective disease management, and enhanced patient engagement and education. Furthermore, the chapter analyzes both the benefits and the inherent challenges associated with IoT in healthcare, such as issues of privacy, data security, and the potential disparities in technology access among different demographic groups. This chapter seeks to provide a balanced perspective on the transformative capabilities of IoT technologies in fostering better health outcomes for women.

13.2 IMPORTANCE OF IOT IN ADDRESSING UNIQUE NEEDS FOR FEMALE HEALTHCARE

Healthcare Need	IoT Application	Benefits
Breast cancer screening [15]	Smart bras equipped with sensors that detect temperature changes and tissue density variations	Allows for early detection of breast cancer signs, increasing treatment success rates
Chronic disease management [6]	IoT-enabled devices for continuous monitoring of blood pressure, glucose levels, etc.	Provides real-time data to manage chronic conditions like diabetes and hypertension more effectively
Mental health tracking [10]	Apps and wearables that monitor mood, stress levels, and sleep patterns	Supports mental health by identifying patterns and triggers and facilitating timely interventions
Osteoporosis management [27]	Sensors that monitor movement and predict risk of falls, integrating with alert systems for caregivers	Prevents fractures by alerting users and caregivers of high-risk activities, crucial for osteoporosis management
Pregnancy monitoring [23]	Wearables track vital signs and fetal heart rate, sending data directly to healthcare providers	Enhances prenatal care and early detection of potential complications
Reproductive health [12, 14]	IoT devices monitor menstrual cycles and predict fertility windows	Improves family planning and identifies reproductive health issues earlier

13.3 IOT TECHNOLOGIES IN FEMALE HEALTHCARE

The integration of IoT technologies into female healthcare encompasses a broad spectrum of devices and systems designed to monitor, manage, and improve health outcomes for women. Wearable devices such as smartwatches and fitness trackers monitor vital signs like heart rate and sleep patterns, which are crucial for assessing overall health and detecting potential health issues early. Smart bras and patches specifically designed for women can monitor signs related to breast health, such as temperature fluctuations and tissue density, which are instrumental in early breast cancer detection [10]. Additionally, IoT-enabled applications in reproductive health include devices like fertility trackers that use sensors to monitor physiological parameters relevant to menstrual cycles and ovulation periods, aiding in both conception and general reproductive health monitoring [21]. During pregnancy, specialized wearable devices can track fetal movements and heart rate, as well as maternal health parameters, providing critical data to healthcare providers remotely [23]. For chronic conditions, such as osteoporosis and autoimmune diseases, IoT devices can offer continuous monitoring of relevant health indicators. For instance, devices to monitor bone density and inflammatory markers can alert patients and doctors to changes that may require intervention, thus managing the condition more effectively [17].

The use of IoT in mental healthcare, such as mood trackers and stress management applications, also plays a significant role. These tools help in identifying patterns in behavior and triggers for stress or depression, enabling timely therapeutic interventions [7].

13.4 EXAMPLES OF IOT APPLICATIONS IN REPRODUCTIVE HEALTH, PRENATAL AND POSTNATAL CARE

- **Postnatal care:** Postnatal IoT applications focus on both maternal and infant health. Smart breast pumps connected to apps help mothers track milk volume and pumping sessions and provide tips for improving breast milk production [19]. For infants, IoT-enabled baby monitors detect breathing patterns, sleep quality, and even predict sickness before visible symptoms appear, ensuring immediate medical attention if needed [25].

- **Prenatal care:** In prenatal care, wearable IoT devices play a critical role. Smart belly bands and patches monitor fetal heart rates and maternal health metrics, such as blood pressure and weight, transmitting data directly to healthcare providers. This continuous monitoring helps in the early detection of potential issues like preeclampsia or gestational diabetes, enabling timely interventions [26]. Another innovative application is the use of ultrasound patches that pregnant women can use at home to get real-time images of the fetus, shared instantly with their doctors [24].

- **Reproductive health:** IoT technologies significantly enhance the management and understanding of reproductive health. Smart fertility devices, such as connected thermometers and hormone monitoring kits, leverage IoT to track ovulation cycles, and predict fertility windows accurately. These devices sync data to a smartphone app, providing users with real-time insights into their reproductive health [29]. Additionally, IoT vaginal rings deliver localized medication while monitoring uterine health, offering a promising avenue for treating conditions like endometriosis [23].

13.5 BENEFITS OF IOT IN FEMALE HEALTH

- **Improved diagnostic accuracy through real-time data collection**: One of the primary benefits of IoT in women's health is the enhancement of diagnostic accuracy facilitated by real-time data collection. IoT devices equipped with sensors can continuously monitor various physiological parameters, such as heart rate, blood pressure, glucose levels, and more, which are essential for diagnosing and managing health conditions specific to women [22]. For example, smart wearables and implants can track hormonal changes throughout the menstrual cycle, providing valuable data that can help diagnose disorders like polycystic ovary syndrome (PCOS) and endometriosis more accurately [28]. Real-time data collection via IoT devices also plays a crucial role in prenatal care. Wearable devices can monitor fetal heart rates and maternal blood pressure continuously, allowing for the early detection of conditions like preeclampsia, which, if left untreated, can lead to serious health issues for both mother and child [20]. This instantaneous flow of data ensures that healthcare providers can make informed decisions quickly, potentially saving lives and preventing complications. Furthermore, IoT technologies contribute to the accuracy of chronic disease management in women, such as diabetes and cardiovascular diseases, by providing continuous, real-time monitoring. This capability allows for adjustments in treatment plans on an as-needed basis, rather than relying solely on periodic doctor visits [8].

- **Empowerment through increased health literacy and self-management tools**: The IoT has significantly empowered women by increasing health literacy and providing robust self-management tools. These technologies offer users unprecedented access to their health information, fostering a deeper understanding of personal health needs and enabling informed decision-making [20]. For instance, IoT applications like health-tracking apps and wearable devices provide feedback on a wide range of health metrics such as physical activity, nutritional intake, sleep quality, and more. This data empowers women to make lifestyle adjustments proactively, rather than reacting to health issues as they occur [28]. Moreover, IoT devices specialized for women's health issues, such as smart breast pumps and menstrual cycle trackers, not only provide critical health data but also offer guidance and educational content. These tools help women understand their bodies better and manage specific conditions like breastfeeding challenges or menstrual irregularities effectively [19]. By integrating these devices with mobile apps, women can receive personalized health tips and reminders, further enhancing their capability to manage their health independently. IoT technology also plays a critical role in chronic disease management. Devices that monitor blood pressure, glucose levels, and other critical health indicators can automatically adjust medication dosages or notify healthcare providers if intervention is needed. This not only improves treatment outcomes but also gives patients, particularly women managing multiple family health needs, a sense of control and reassurance [18].
- **Enhanced preventive care with personalized health monitoring**: The IoT has revolutionized preventive care in women's health through personalized health monitoring. By continuously collecting and analyzing data specific to an individual's health metrics, IoT devices enable early detection and intervention, which are critical for preventing serious health issues [11]. For example, wearable devices that monitor cardiovascular functions can detect

irregular heartbeats or changes in blood pressure, alerting users and healthcare providers to potential risks before they escalate into more severe conditions [13]. In the realm of reproductive health, IoT technologies like smart menstrual cups and fertility trackers provide insights into menstrual health and reproductive patterns, helping in the early identification of irregularities such as abnormal cycle lengths or ovulation patterns. This data not only aids in preventive care but also enhances the management of fertility issues and menstrual-related disorders like endometriosis [16]. For pregnant women, IoT devices such as smart belly bands track vital statistics, including weight, blood pressure, and fetal heart rate. This monitoring allows for personalized care plans, early warnings about potential prenatal complications, and adjustments to lifestyle or medication based on real-time data, thus enhancing the overall prenatal care experience [12]. Moreover, IoT applications extend to postnatal care, where devices like smart scales and sleep monitors can help new mothers manage their health and recovery more effectively. These devices can track sleep patterns, weight changes, and other health metrics, providing personalized data that assists in adjusting postpartum care plans [26].

13.6 CASE STUDIES

- **Case study 1—IoT in managing chronic diseases among women:** This case study explores the implementation of IoT technologies in managing type 2 diabetes, a chronic disease that disproportionately affects women, especially in middle and older age groups. The focus is on a pilot program launched in an urban community health center aimed at enhancing patient self-management and improving health outcomes. The program equipped 100 women with IoT-enabled glucose monitors that continuously tracked their blood sugar levels. These devices were connected to a smartphone app that provided real-time feedback and personalized dietary and exercise recommendations based on the data collected. Additionally, the app allowed for remote consultations with endocrinologists who could adjust medication dosages and treatment plans based on the collected data. Over the course of one year, participants showed significant improvement in their glycemic control, evidenced by a 20% decrease in average Hemoglobin A1c levels. Furthermore, the real-time monitoring enabled early identification of hyperglycemic episodes, reducing emergency room visits by 30%. Participants also reported increased satisfaction with their healthcare management, noting particularly the convenience and reassurance provided by the continuous monitoring and support [6, 17].

The success of this program highlights the potential of IoT technologies to transform chronic disease management in women by fostering greater patient engagement and enhancing the precision of care. The real-time data collection and analysis facilitate a more responsive and personalized approach to healthcare, which is crucial for conditions like diabetes.

- **Case study 2—IoT Innovations in Reproductive Health Monitoring:** This case study examines the implementation of an IoT-based system designed to monitor and manage reproductive health issues among women in a suburban community. The project focuses on the use of smart devices that integrate with mobile health applications to provide continuous monitoring and data-driven insights into reproductive health. The program involved 150 women who used smart menstrual cups connected to a mobile application that tracked menstrual cycle data, including flow volume, cycle length, and associated symptoms such as pain and mood changes. This information was analyzed by the app to predict and identify issues like irregular cycles or symptoms indicative of conditions such as PCOS or endometriosis. After six months of participation, the data collected led to a 40% increase in the diagnosis accuracy of menstrual-related conditions compared to traditional methods. The program also improved participants' understanding of their reproductive health, leading to better-informed discussions with healthcare providers. Additionally, 75% of participants reported feeling more in control of their reproductive health and more satisfied with the management of their conditions [10, 30].

This case study highlights the transformative potential of IoT in reproductive health monitoring. By providing continuous, personalized data directly to users and healthcare providers, IoT devices can significantly enhance the diagnosis and management of reproductive health conditions, leading to better health outcomes and increased patient empowerment.

- **Discussion on the outcomes and lessons learned from each case study:** In the first case study, implementing IoT-enabled glucose monitors led to improved management of type 2 diabetes among women, with outcomes showing enhanced glycemic control, reduced emergency room visits, and increased patient satisfaction due to real-time health monitoring and feedback. Lessons learned highlighted the importance of real-time data in improving compliance and the effectiveness of personalized care, though challenges in technology adoption among older participants underscored the need for user-friendly designs and better training. The second case study focused on IoT innovations in reproductive health monitoring using smart menstrual cups, which improved diagnostic accuracy for conditions like PCOS and endometriosis, and increased patient engagement and empowerment. This study demonstrated the potential of IoT to provide precise, personalized health insights, while also revealing a greater acceptance of health monitoring technologies among younger demographics. Both studies underscore the transformative potential of IoT in enhancing women's healthcare by offering personalized, data-driven insights and interventions, but they also stress the importance of addressing technological and educational barriers to maximize benefits.

13.7 CHALLENGES AND ETHICAL CONSIDERATIONS

- **Privacy and data security concerns specific to IoT in healthcare:** One of the foremost challenges in the adoption of IoT technologies in healthcare is ensuring privacy and data security. As IoT devices collect, transmit, and store an immense volume of personal health information, they become prime targets for data breaches and cyberattacks, which can lead to unauthorized access to sensitive data. The implications of such breaches are particularly severe in healthcare, where the exposure of personal health information can result in privacy violations, discrimination, and even personal harm.

Privacy concerns stem from the potential for continuous surveillance and data collection by IoT devices without explicit patient consent or awareness. For instance, wearable health monitors and connected medical devices can collect data far beyond what is necessary for medical treatment, including location tracking and lifestyle habits, which could potentially be used for purposes other than healthcare, such as marketing or insurance assessments. Data security is another critical issue, as many IoT devices lack robust security features, making them vulnerable to hacking and unauthorized access. This vulnerability is exacerbated by the decentralized nature of IoT networks, where data often traverses multiple networks and devices, each with potentially different security protocols and standards.

To address these challenges, strict regulatory compliance with health data protection standards such as Health Insurance Portability and Accountability Act in the United States, General Data Protection Regulation in Europe, or similar regulations in other jurisdictions is essential. Moreover, the development and implementation of advanced security technologies, such as end-to-end encryption, secure authentication methods, and regular security updates, are critical to safeguarding patient data. Additionally, healthcare providers and IoT device manufacturers must work together to improve the transparency of data collection practices and enhance patient trust by clearly communicating how patient data is used, stored, and protected. These privacy and security issues not only pose technical challenges but also ethical ones, demanding a balance between leveraging technological advances in healthcare and protecting individual privacy rights. The integration of IoT in healthcare, therefore, requires careful consideration of both ethical imperatives and practical implementations to ensure that the benefits of these technologies are realized without compromising patient trust or safety.

- **Issues of accessibility and the digital divide:** The integration of IoT technologies in healthcare highlights critical issues of accessibility and the digital divide, which pose significant challenges for equitable healthcare delivery. Economic barriers, technological literacy, and geographic limitations often prevent vulnerable populations from accessing these innovations, potentially exacerbating existing health disparities. For instance, the high costs of IoT devices and the infrastructure required for their operation can exclude low-income families, while individuals in rural areas may struggle with insufficient internet connectivity which is crucial for the functionality of these devices. Moreover, older adults and less educated individuals might find the technology intimidating or difficult to use, further widening the gap. To bridge these divides, it is essential to implement supportive policies that subsidize costs for underprivileged groups, invest in infrastructure improvements, enhance digital literacy through targeted educational programs, and ensure that IoT healthcare technologies are designed with universal accessibility in mind. Such measures are vital not only for advancing healthcare technology but also for ensuring that its benefits are distributed fairly across all segments of society.

- **Ethical implications of continuous health monitoring:** The ethical implications of continuous health monitoring through IoT technologies in healthcare are multifaceted and provoke considerable debate. On one hand, continuous monitoring offers substantial benefits, such as the ability to track patient health metrics in real-time, which can lead to earlier detection of potential health issues, more timely interventions, and overall better patient outcomes. However, these advantages also come with ethical concerns, primarily related to privacy and autonomy. Continuous health monitoring can be perceived as invasive, as it often involves the constant collection of personal health data that might be shared with various stakeholders, including healthcare providers, insurance companies, and technology providers, sometimes without the full consent or awareness of the individuals being monitored. This raises significant questions about the ownership of health data and the potential for misuse or unauthorized access. Moreover, there is the concern of dependency, where patients might become overly reliant on technology for health management, potentially diminishing personal agency and decision-making capabilities. To navigate these ethical challenges, it is crucial to implement robust data protection measures, ensure transparent communication about how data is used, and maintain a balance that respects patient privacy while harnessing the benefits of technology for enhanced healthcare outcomes.

13.8 FUTURE DIRECTIONS

- **Potential technological advancements in IoT for enhancing women's health:** The future of IoT in enhancing women's health holds immense potential, characterized by rapid technological advancements that promise to further personalize and improve healthcare delivery. Innovations on the horizon include the development of more advanced wearable devices that can track a broader range of physiological parameters with greater accuracy, such as hormonal levels across different phases of the menstrual cycle or during pregnancy, potentially offering earlier diagnostics and more tailored treatment plans. Additionally, the integration of artificial intelligence (AI) with IoT devices is expected to significantly enhance the capability of these technologies to analyze vast amounts of data in real-time, enabling predictive analytics that can forecast health issues before they manifest clinically. This could be particularly transformative for conditions like ovarian cancer or gestational diabetes, where early detection is crucial. Moreover, advancements in nanotechnology could lead to the creation of even smaller, more comfortable, and less invasive devices that could continuously monitor health metrics without impacting daily activities or privacy. Blockchain technology is also anticipated to play a crucial role in enhancing data security and privacy, providing a decentralized and tamper-proof platform for managing health data, thus addressing some of the primary concerns around the use of IoT in healthcare. Collectively, these technological advancements aim to create a more connected, responsive, and efficient healthcare system that is better equipped to meet the unique needs of women at various stages of their health journey.
- **Integration of AI with IoT for predictive analytics in female health issues:** The integration of AI with the IoT in healthcare,

particularly for female health issues, represents a significant advancement in predictive analytics. This synergy allows for the aggregation and analysis of large volumes of real-time data collected from IoT devices such as wearable health monitors, smart implants, and other medical devices. AI algorithms are particularly adept at recognizing patterns and anomalies in data, which can be crucial for early detection of conditions that disproportionately affect women, like breast cancer, ovarian cancer, and osteoporosis. For instance, AI can analyze data from a smart bra that monitors tissue temperature and stiffness to predict early signs of breast cancer with greater accuracy and speed than traditional methods.

Moreover, AI-driven predictive analytics can enhance the management of chronic conditions such as diabetes and cardiovascular diseases by forecasting potential health risks based on continuous monitoring of vital signs and lifestyle data. This proactive approach facilitates timely medical interventions, potentially preventing the escalation of conditions and improving overall health outcomes. In reproductive health, AI integrated with IoT devices can predict fertility windows and potential complications during pregnancy with higher precision, offering personalized healthcare recommendations to the user. As this technology continues to evolve, it is poised to transform women's healthcare by enabling more personalized, efficient, and preemptive healthcare solutions. However, the implementation of these technologies must be handled with care to ensure privacy, consent, and data security, addressing the ethical concerns associated with extensive data collection and analysis. The goal is to empower women with better insights into their health and wellness, paving the way for a more informed and proactive approach to healthcare.

- **Policy recommendations for ensuring safe and equitable use of IoT in healthcare**: To ensure the safe and equitable use of IoT in healthcare, policy recommendations should focus on several key areas: *privacy and security*, *accessibility*, and *ethical use of technology*. First, stringent data protection laws must be enacted and enforced to safeguard patient privacy and ensure that data collected by IoT devices is used responsibly and securely. This includes mandatory encryption of health data, regular security audits, and strict penalties for data breaches. Second, policies should address the digital divide by promoting equitable access to IoT technologies. This could involve subsidizing IoT healthcare devices for low-income populations, investing in internet infrastructure in underserved areas, and ensuring that IoT devices are designed to be user-friendly for all demographic groups, including those with limited technological literacy. Furthermore, policy frameworks should encourage the development of open standards for IoT in healthcare to foster interoperability among devices from different manufacturers, facilitating a cohesive ecosystem that benefits all users. Ethical guidelines should also be established to govern the development and implementation of IoT technologies, ensuring that they enhance rather than undermine patient autonomy and do not lead to discrimination or unequal treatment. Finally, ongoing collaboration between governments, healthcare providers, technology developers, and patient advocacy groups is crucial to continuously monitor the impact of IoT on healthcare and adjust policies as necessary to address emerging challenges and opportunities. This collaborative approach ensures that the benefits of IoT in healthcare are maximized, while minimizing potential risks, leading to a healthcare system that is both innovative and inclusive.

13.9 SUMMARY

The impact of IoT on female healthcare is profound and multifaceted, reflecting a significant shift toward more personalized, precise, and proactive healthcare solutions. IoT technologies have enhanced the ability to monitor and manage health in real-time, leading to improved diagnostic accuracy and more effective disease prevention and management, specifically tailored to the unique needs of women. Devices such as wearable health monitors, smart reproductive health trackers, and connected prenatal care tools have empowered women to take an active role in their healthcare, fostering greater health literacy and enabling self-management of health conditions. The continuous data collection capabilities of IoT devices provide healthcare providers with detailed insights into their patients' health status, allowing for earlier intervention in diseases that disproportionately affect women, such as breast cancer and osteoporosis. This has the potential to improve outcomes and reduce healthcare costs by catching problems before they develop into more serious conditions. However, the deployment of IoT in female healthcare also presents challenges and ethical considerations, particularly concerning privacy and data security, the accessibility of technology, and the risk of exacerbating health disparities due to the digital divide. Addressing these issues requires robust policy frameworks, ethical guidelines, and ongoing collaboration among stakeholders to ensure that the benefits of IoT technologies are realized equitably and responsibly. In conclusion, while IoT technologies hold transformative potential for enhancing female healthcare, their implementation must be handled with careful consideration of the associated challenges. With the right approaches, IoT can significantly contribute to a more responsive, efficient, and patient-centered healthcare system, ultimately improving health outcomes for women globally.

Reflection on the importance of continuing innovation in this area: The ongoing innovation in the realm of IoT for female healthcare is not just a technological imperative but a societal necessity. As healthcare demands become more complex and nuanced, particularly in addressing the specific needs of women, continuous innovation ensures that healthcare solutions evolve accordingly. This is crucial for several reasons:

- First, women's health issues often require nuanced approaches due to the physiological and hormonal differences that influence disease presentation and progression. IoT technologies have the potential to cater to these specific needs by providing personalized data and healthcare solutions, from reproductive health to chronic disease management. Innovation in this area can lead to more accurate diagnostics and tailored treatment plans that address the root causes of health issues rather than just the symptoms. Second, the dynamic nature of technology and healthcare regulations demands perpetual innovation. As new challenges and vulnerabilities emerge, particularly in cybersecurity and data privacy, continuous technological advancement is essential to safeguard patient data and ensure compliance with changing regulations. This also includes adapting to new medical knowledge and practices, ensuring that IoT applications in healthcare remain relevant and effective.

- Second, innovation is critical for bridging existing gaps in healthcare access and quality, especially in underserved or low-resource settings. Advancements in IoT can democratize healthcare by making it more accessible and affordable, breaking down barriers related to geography, socioeconomic status, and educational disparities. Lastly, the reflection on the importance of innovation in IoT for female healthcare underscores a broader commitment to gender equity in healthcare provision. It recognizes that enhancing women's healthcare contributes significantly to overall societal health and well-being, supporting better outcomes not only for women but for families and communities at large. Hence, the imperative for ongoing innovation in IoT for female healthcare is clear. It is not merely about maintaining pace with technology but about ensuring that advancements are meaningful and equitable, truly enhancing the health and quality of life for women around the world. This requires a concerted effort from technologists, healthcare providers, policymakers, and communities to foster an environment where sustained innovation leads to tangible improvements in healthcare.

Call to action for researchers, practitioners, and policymakers: The rapid evolution of the IoT in healthcare demands coordinated action from researchers, practitioners, and policymakers to harness its full potential while addressing associated risks, particularly in female healthcare. Researchers should continue to innovate and validate IoT technologies through rigorous, interdisciplinary studies that enhance device efficacy and patient safety. Practitioners are encouraged to integrate these technologies into clinical practice responsibly, educating patients about their benefits and risks, and providing critical feedback to developers. Policymakers must develop robust regulatory frameworks that ensure device safety, data privacy, and equitable access to these technologies, preventing any exacerbation of existing health disparities. Collectively, these efforts should focus on ethical considerations, including patient consent and autonomy, to foster a healthcare environment where IoT tools not only advance medical care but also uphold the dignity and rights of every patient. Engaging in these concerted efforts will ensure that IoT's impact on healthcare is both transformative and benevolent, aligning technological advancements with the highest standards of care and ethical responsibility.

KEYWORDS

- **data security**
- **health monitoring**
- **Internet of Things**
- **personalized healthcare**
- **women's health**

REFERENCES

1. Abdulmalek, S., Nasir, A., Jabbar, W. A., Almuhaya, M. A. M., Bairagi, A. K., Khan, M. A., & Kee, S. H. (2022). IoT-based healthcare-monitoring system towards improving quality of life: A review. *Healthcare (Basel, Switzerland), 10*(10), 1993. doi:10.3390/healthcare10101993
2. Ahmed, L. J., Madhumitha, R., Oviya, K., & Sharmila, M. (2022, March). A survey of IoT based pregnancy woman health monitoring system. In: *8th IEEE International Conference on Advanced Computing and Communication Systems (ICACCS), 1,* 2089–2094. doi:10.1109/ICACCS54159.2022.9785324
3. Amine, R., & Oumnad, A. (2018). Challenges and opportunities of Internet of Things in healthcare. *International Journal of Electrical and Computer Engineering (IJECE), 8*, 2753–2761. doi:10.11591/ijece.v8i5.pp2753-2761
4. Chataut, R., Phoummalayvane, A., & Akl, R. (2023). Unleashing the power of IoT: A comprehensive review of IoT applications and prospects in healthcare, agriculture, smart homes, smart cities, and Industry 4.0. *Sensors (Basel, Switzerland), 23*(16), 7194. doi:10.3390/s23167194
5. Cochrane, S., Smith, C. A., Possamai-Inesedy, A., & Bensoussan, A. (2014). Acupuncture and women's health: An overview of the role of acupuncture and its clinical management in women's reproductive health. *International Journal of Women's Health, 6*, 313–325. doi:10.2147/IJWH.S38969
6. Dadkhah, M., Mehraeen, M., Rahimnia, F., & Kimiafar, K. (2021). Use of Internet of Things for chronic disease management: An overview. *Journal of Medical Signals & Sensors, 11*, 138–157. doi:10.4103/jmss.JMSS_13_20
7. Ejiyi, C., Qin, Z., Ejiyi, M., Nneji, G., Monday, H., Agu, F., Ejiyi, T., & Diokpo, C. (2023). The Internet of Medical things in healthcare management: A review. *Journal of Digital Health, 2*, 30–62. doi:10.55976/jdh.22023116330-62
8. Farooq, M. S., Riaz, S., Tehseen, R., Farooq, U., & Saleem, K. (2023). Role of Internet of Things in diabetes healthcare: Network infrastructure, taxonomy, challenges, and security model. *Digital Health, 9*, 20552076231179056. doi:10.1177/20552076231179056

9. Farooq, S., Masooma, A., Omer, U., Tehseen, R., Gilani, S., & Atal, Z. (2023). The role of IoT in woman's safety: A systematic literature review. *IEEE Access, 11*, 69807–69825; doi:10.1109/ACCESS.2023.3252903
10. Friedlander, A. (2023). Menstrual tracking, fitness tracking and body work: Digital tracking tools and their use in optimising health, beauty, wellness and the aesthetic self. *Youth, 3*(2), 689–701. doi:10.3390/youth3020045
11. Gruebner, O., van Haasteren, A., Hug, A., Elayan, S., Sykora, M., Albanese, E., Stettner, G. M., Waldboth, V., Messmer-Khosla, S., Enzmann, C., Baumann, D., von Wyl, V., Fadda, M., Wolf, M., & von Rhein, M. (2023). Mental health challenges and digital platform opportunities in patients and families affected by paediatric neuromuscular diseases - experiences from Switzerland. *Digital Health, 9*, 20552076231213700. doi:10.1177/20552076231213700
12. Hossain, M. M., Kashem, M. A., Islam, M. M., Sahidullah, M., Mumu, S. H., Uddin, J., Aray, D. G., de la Torre Diez, I., Ashraf, I., & Samad, M. A. (2023). Internet of Things in pregnancy care coordination and management: A systematic review. *Sensors (Basel, Switzerland), 23*(23), 9367. doi:10.3390/s23239367
13. Huhn, S., Axt, M., Gunga, H. C., Maggioni, M. A., Munga, S., Obor, D., Sié, A., Boudo, V., Bunker, A., Sauerborn, R., Bärnighausen, T., & Barteit, S. (2022). The impact of wearable technologies in health research: Scoping review. *JMIR mHealth and uHealth, 10*(1), e34384. doi:10.2196/34384
14. Khademioore, S., Ebrahimi, E., Khosravi, A., & Movahedi, S. (2023). The effect of an mHealth application based on continuous support and education on fear of childbirth, self-efficacy, and birth mode in primiparous women: A randomized controlled trial. *PLoS ONE, 18*(11), e0293815. doi:10.1371/journal.pone.0293815
15. Khooshebast Baghsangani, M., & Gush, M. (2022). Breast cancer detection using machine learning and IoT: A review. In: *Conference on Recent Research in Science and Technology.* https://sid.ir/paper/950015/en
16. Kumar, M., Kumar, A., Verma, S., Bhattacharya, P., Ghimire, D., Kim, S.-h., & Hosen, A. S. M. S. (2023). Healthcare Internet of Things (H-IoT): Current trends, prospects, applications, challenges, and security issues. *Electronics, 12*(9), 2050. doi:10.3390/electronics12092050
17. Li, X., Lu, Y., Fu, X., & Qi, Y. (2021). Building the Internet of Things platform for smart maternal healthcare services with wearable devices and cloud computing. *Future Generation Computer Systems, 118*, 282–296.
18. Mathur, P., Mishra, S., Awasthi, R., Khanna, A., Maheshwari, K., Papay, F., Naylor, A., Abdallah, N., Weight, C., Bhattacharyya, A., Khare, A., Singh, G., Reddy, S., Cha, J., Anand, A., Nguyen, H., Tandon, A., Mamillapalli, C., Pozdeyev, N., & Cywinski, J. (2022). Artificial intelligence in healthcare: 2021 year in review. doi:10.13140/RG.2.2.25350.24645/1
19. Meier, P., Patel, A., Hoban, R., & Engstrom, J. (2016). Which breast pump for which mother: An evidenced-based approach to individualizing breast pump technology. *Journal of Perinatology: Official Journal of the California Perinatal Association, 36*, 493–499. doi:10.1038/jp.2016.14
20. Nikbakht-Nasrabadi, A., Sabzevari, S., & Negahban-Bonabi, T. (2015). Women empowerment through health information seeking: A qualitative study. *International Journal of Community Based Nursing and Midwifery, 3*(2), 105–115.

21. Pandey, S. K., Hart, J. J., & Tiwary, S. (2003). Women's health and the internet: Understanding emerging trends and implications. *Social Science & Medicine, 56*(1), 179–191. doi:10.1016/s0277-9536(02)00019-9
22. Prieto-Avalos, G., Cruz-Ramos, N. A., Alor-Hernández, G., Sánchez-Cervantes, J. L., Rodríguez-Mazahua, L., & Guarneros-Nolasco, L. R. (2022). Wearable devices for physical monitoring of heart: A review. *Biosensors, 12*(5), 292. doi:10.3390/bios12050292
23. Priyanka, B., Kalaivanan, V. M., Pavish, R. A., & Kanageshwaran, M. (2021). IoT-based pregnancy women health monitoring system for prenatal care. In: *2021 International Conference on Advances in Computing, Communication and Security,* (pp. 1264–1269). doi:10.1109/ICACCS51430.2021.9441677
24. Sarhaddi, F., Azimi, I., Labbaf, S., Niela-Vilén, H., Dutt, N., Axelin, A., Liljeberg, P., & Rahmani, A. M. (2021). Long-term IoT-based maternal monitoring: System design and evaluation. *Sensors (Basel, Switzerland), 21*(7), 2281. doi:10.3390/s21072281
25. Sator, P., Mamat, R., Syed Abdul Rahim, S. S., Geok-Chan, K., Saimon, R., Kaur, S., & Sawatan, W. (2022). The health and wellness benefits of traditional postnatal practice (TPC) on postnatal mothers: A systematic review. *Malaysian Journal of Medical Sciences, 18*, 286–294. doi:10.47836/mjmhs18.6.37
26. Shmerling, A., Hoss, M., Malam, N., Staton, E. W., & Lyon, C. (2022). Prenatal care via telehealth. *Primary Care, 49*(4), 609–619. doi:10.1016/j.pop.2022.05.002
27. Sözen, T., Özışık, L., & Başaran, N. Ç. (2017). An overview and management of osteoporosis. *European Journal of Rheumatology, 4*(1), 46–56. doi:10.5152/eurjrheum.2016.048
28. Srinivasan, M., Mathew, G., Mathew, N., Kumar, M., Goyal, N., & Kamath, M. (2024). Technologies that empower women for better access to healthcare in India – A scoping review. *Global Public Health, 19*, 2318240. doi:10.1080/17441692.2024.2318240
29. Thilakarathne, N., Kagita, M. K., & Gadekallu, T. (2020). The role of the Internet of Things in health care: A systematic and comprehensive study. *International Journal of Engineering and Management Research, 10*, 145–159. doi:10.31033/ijemr.10.4.22
30. Verdejo Espinosa, Á., Lopez Ruiz, J., Mata Mata, F., & Estevez, M. E. (2021). Application of IoT in healthcare: Keys to implementation of the Sustainable Development Goals. *Sensors, 21*(7), 2330. doi:10.3390/s21072330

CHAPTER 14

Machine Learning Model to Detect Ovarian Cancer Cells Through Image Processing

MOHAMMAD AWDE, MOHAMMAD ALI MTAIREK, AYA KAWSSAN, ALI JAWAD, JAD MAJED, and HAIDAR KANSO*

*Corresponding author

ABSTRACT

Globally, ovarian cancer is a complicated illness that impacts a large number of people. This chapter thoroughly investigates the challenges posed by detecting ovarian cancer using image processing and machine learning (ML) models, underlying causes and contributing factors, diagnosis methods, and, in particular, the role of artificial intelligence (AI) models in cancer cell detection, primarily ML tools. This overview begins with ovarian cancer terminology, its prevalence and incidence across different age groups, its influence on women's lives, common symptoms and manifestations, and their staging and gradings. Meanwhile, the authors have extensively highlighted ovarian cancer diagnosis and the value of early detection in life improvement, using numerous types of methods for diagnosis as physical examination, blood tests, pelvic ultrasound, computerized tomography scan, positron emission tomography scan, and colonoscopy. Furthermore, the image processing models used in the diagnosis of ovarian cancer have been briefly described, including their aims, challenges, and accuracy. In addition, ML models were also defined and listed, putting to the reader their progress in the detection field. Finally, the purpose of this research is to give significant insights into ovarian cancer

Holistic Approaches for Women's Sustainable Health, Volume 2: Advancements, Socioeconomic Impacts, and Innovative Strategies. Junaid Ahmad Malik, Anamika Chauhan, and Megh R. Goyal (Eds)

DOI: 10.1201/9781779641656-17

diagnosis utilizing AI, namely, ML algorithms. By addressing the many facets of this illness, the authors intend to increase the trust in ML models in ovarian cancer detection, ensuring early diagnosis and improving life quality women with ovarian cancer.

14.1 INTRODUCTION

Many tools, such as AI and machine learning (ML), have recently made their way into the realm of medicine for medical diagnosis. These models are frequently employed in the detection of malignant cells, such as ovarian cancer (OC) [53, 124]. AI tools, by definition, are computational tools that can mimic human behavior in order to produce similar outcomes, but ML models are a subtype of AI that is distinguished by the ability to learn automatically from past data in order to build its own classifications [26]. According to Shrestha et al. [93], AI techniques are extremely useful in the early differentiation between benign and malignant cells. Yet, OC, with an annual mortality rate of 151,900, is thought to be the most fatal malignancy, according to a study published in Global Cancer Statistics, the year 2012 [105]. Because the symptoms produced by OC are not very distinct and are frequently neglected or assigned to other illnesses, identification will occur at the latest stages of disease development. Furthermore, there is currently no effective screening method for this type of cancer, making early detection more difficult [23, 38]. This makes OC diagnosing a great challenge for usual diagnosing methods and new ones, AI and ML.

The purpose of this review is to elucidate the significance of these novel models and how they help in the process of OC identification. Using the knowledge gained from the past, we look ahead to the technological and infrastructure advancements that will enable OC diagnosis techniques, particularly AI and ML, to achieve the earliest detection and ensure a rise in the standards of life for women with OC.

14.2 OVARIAN CANCER: UNDERSTANDING THE CHALLENGE

Ovarian cancer is an important health issue that affects numerous women globally, and understanding the different aspects of this disease is essential.

The term ovarian cancer describes the aberrant cell proliferation in female reproductive organs, particularly the ovaries. It can develop from a variety of cells, resulting in three major types: *epithelial* (the most common), *germ cell*, and *sex-cord-stromal*, with the latter two comprising only approximately 5% of all ovarian malignancies. *Epithelial* OC has four primary histologic subtypes: serous (classified into two types: high-grade serous carcinomas and low-grade severe carcinomas), *endometrioid*, *mucinous*, and *clear cell* [97].

This cancer can occur at any age, but it is more common in older women. Women under forty are less likely to develop OC, and germ cell tumors account for the majority of malignancies in this age group. Over 90% of tumors in women older than forty are *epithelial*, and the risk increases with age, reaching a peak in the late 1970s [110].

Early detection of OC depends on being aware of its symptoms and signs. With a median diagnostic age of 63 years, OC impacts most women later in life [72]. This is due to the fact that symptoms of OC might be initially missed or attributed to other disease processes because they are general and nonspecific. Generally, women present with a dominant pelvic mass, ascites, and marked abdominal distension. Other signs and symptoms include stomach bloating, abdominal and/or pelvic pain, tachycardia, and decreased breath sounds [78].

Such malignancy can have a significant impact on a woman's quality of life. For example, some patients may reevaluate their attitudes toward relationships, work, and day-to-day life following an OC diagnosis [68].

Ovarian cancer is staged and graded to evaluate the degree of the disease and help guide treatment decisions. The International Federation of Gynecology and Obstetrics (FIGO) staging approach is used in the pathological examination and tumor staging of OC. This method is based on surgical assessment of the malignancy at initial diagnosis, including excision of lymph nodes, tissue sample, and abdominal fluid. A consistent method for classifying the degree of illness based on clinical, radiographic, and surgical findings is provided by the FIGO staging classification for cancer of the ovary, fallopian tube, and peritoneum. The staging method has four primary stages, identified as I–IV. Each stage is further classified into smaller groups according to the unique features of the tumor and its dissemination. With subgroups dependent on the degree of tumor involvement, stage I denotes cancer that has only spread to the ovary or fallopian tube. Stage II refers to dissemination to adjacent pelvic tissues, while stage III refers to dissemination to the abdominal lining and lymph nodes. Stage IV denotes metastases that are far from the abdomen. The FIGO staging classification plays a critical role in prognostication, treatment planning, and enabling healthcare practitioners to communicate about the degree of the disease [12].

14.3 CAUSES AND CONTRIBUTING FACTORS

Understanding the causes of OC aids in the prediction of the group at the greatest risk of development, allowing us to strive to eliminate modifiable factors and perform appropriate screening for these people [110]. Ovarian cancer (OC) has been linked to a higher number of ovulatory cycles in older women, where cellular divisions related to the development of OC are much higher; these women are particularly those with an early *menarche* (first occurrence of *menstruation*) and a late *menopause* [33]. Actually, 80% of women diagnosed with OC are over 50 years old, indicating a higher frequency in postmenopausal women [88]. The risk is also associated to ethnic groups, with white and Caucasian women having the largest connection (12 per 100,000), followed by Hispanic (10.3 per 100,000), Asian (9.2 per 100,000), and finally African–American (0.4 per 100,000) [9, 33]. Ashkenazi Jewish European ancestry carries genes associated with breast and OC (over a 2% frequency), such as *BRCA1* and *BRCA2*, and this community is genetically examined due to the high prevalence of ethnic-related OC, even in those with no personal history [21, 99]. *BRCA1* and *BRCA2* tumor suppressor genes, which are located on *chromosomes 17 and 13*, respectively, are susceptible to more than 140 autosomal dominant mutations that boost the risk of *breast and* OC by 5–15% [36, 73, 99]. Regardless of regional or racial background, family history appears to be a substantial risk factor for OC [88]. There is a high lifetime risk of acquiring hereditary *ovarian malignancies* (approximately 40–50%) in families where two or more incidences of OC have been discovered at an early stage in first-degree relatives, compared to the risk in the general population, which is 2% [88]. Some hereditary disorders, such as *Lynch syndrome*, which includes an inherited germline mutation in *DNA* mismatch repair system genes called *MLH1*, *MSH2*, *PMS2*, and *MSH6*, are capable of increasing the risk of a wide range of cancers, including OC, with patients carrying these mutations having a mean presentation age of OC of 48 years compared to the normal population's median age of 68 years [68]. According to data collected from 21 studies on 1.3 million women and 5584 OCs from the Ovarian Cancer Cohort Consortium, oral contraceptive use has been associated with a significant reduction in almost all types of OC except mucinous OC [112]. Women who use oral contraception often for five years or more have about half the risk of OC as those who have never used contraception [82]. However, because oral contraceptives are rarely used in the general population, their chemopreventive effects cannot aid in the prevention of OC [80]. Infertility and nulliparity (having no children), on the other hand, seem to enhance the risk since they are associated with greater ovarian activity [27].

In addition to oral contraceptives, breastfeeding and pregnancy also limit *ovulatory cycles*, which reduces the risk of OC [41, 47]. While full-term births are valuable toward minimizing OC, a series of 15 case-control studies suggests that even partial pregnancies (less than 6 months) can reduce OC [45]. Pregnancy is associated with a 21%, 42%, 49%, and 51% reduction in OC risk for one, two, three, and four pregnancies, respectively, when compared to nulligravid women (women with no pregnancies) [45]. Pregnancy's preventive effect against OC has been explained by a number of concepts; "the incessant ovulation hypothesis" clarifies how many ovulation cycles are inhibited throughout the course of pregnancy [27], "the gonadotropin hypothesis" emphasizes the blocked effects of pituitary gonadotropins during pregnancy [63], and "the cell clearance hypothesis" demonstrates the removal of accumulated premalignant cells during pregnancy [4]. Many studies have been conducted to investigate the effect of breastfeeding in the prevention of OC, with some claiming that it plays a crucial part [9]. According to a study [62], every five months of breastfeeding reduces the incidence of OC by around 8%, indicating an important inverse relationship between them. Another study found that breastfeeding reduced the odds of *invasive tumors* by 14% and high-grade *serous tumors* by 16% [9].

Obesity (or high BMI [55]) has been reported as a probable risk factor for the development of postmenopausal OC in a number of studies; a meta-analysis revealed an increased risk of 13% in women with a 5-kg weight gain and no or low usage of postmenopausal hormone replacement therapy [68]. Cigarette smoking is a double-edged sword, given that it considerably reduces the risk of *clear-cell carcinoma*, while raising the possibility of *mucinous carcinoma* [112]. Other factors that could contribute to OC include talc powder [71] (often used in ceramics, paints, and roofing materials), flavonoids and black tea [17], *NSAIDs* [103], and persistent depression, according to Nurse's Health Study [44].

14.4 CANCER DIAGNOSING

Diagnostic tests allow the detection of diseases in patients having risk factors or symptoms for a certain disease [74]. On the other hand, screening tests, also referred to as medical surveillance, assess the possibility of having a certain disease in a population which is perceived as asymptomatic. Usually, a comparison is made between diagnostic tests and a "gold standard," which refers to a diagnostic test that is comparable with the true measure of the pathologic, biochemical, or physiologic, biochemical, or pathological state the test is assessing [74].

A test's validity allows us to distinguish between people who have a disease and those who do not [98], and it is estimated objectively by two measures: specificity and sensitivity [94]. A test is considered accurate if both sensitivity and specificity are high [98], allowing their use for screening decisions [106]. High sensitivity classifies patients as having the condition, with confidence, if their test result is negative. However, high specificity allows regarding patients, with confidence, as having the condition if their test result is positive [106]. The cut-off value is the value, which determines the limit between positive and negative test results. It is directly proportional to false negatives but inversely proportional to false positives [98]. Furthermore, misdiagnosis is possible in case the clinician lacks sufficient education to analyze the test results [69].

Positive predictive value (PPV) of a test is the probability of having the condition in question when the screening test result is positive, whereas negative predictive value (NPV) is the probability of the absence of the condition in question when the screening test result is negative [106]. Sensitivity and specificity do not permit the estimation of the probability of having the disease in patients [5]. Thus, it is more practical to use PPV and NPV [106]. Moreover, PPV and NPV vary with the disease prevalence among populations. A rise in prevalence causes the PPV to rise while the NPV falls. Consequently, physicians cannot utilize published PPV and NPV numbers with their patients [5].

14.4.1 ROLE OF EARLY DIAGNOSIS

The five-year survival rate for OC in the early stages (I, II) is approximately 90%, but that of the late stages (III, IV) ranges from 20% to 40%

[122]. Tumor classification is necessary since different types of tumors possess distinguished characteristics, prognoses, and treatment regimens. Consequently, early diagnosis of OC is essential for follow-up treatment and prognosis [59]. Late diagnosis may lead to unrespectable disease [43]. Thus, early recognition of neoplastic tissue allows for excellent surgical attempts [32].

14.4.2 DIAGNOSING METHODS

When diagnosing epithelial OC, 80% of the cases are in the late stages, during which the cancer has metastasized [22]. Diagnostic biomarkers allow for a diagnosis that is more accurate, and they may be stage- and subtype-specific [18]. An ideal biomarker is one that is exclusively secreted by cancerous tissues but not normal tissues. It can also be tumor-specific antigen that can be detected in body fluids [18]. Considering the disease's low prevalence, it is an objective to reach a PPV value of at least 10% for early-stage detection strategies, which must have a high specificity (99.6%) and a high sensitivity (>75%) [10]. This high specificity cannot be currently obtained using existing screening methods and is less likely to be obtained by selecting a singular testing strategy [18].

14.4.2.1 PSYCHOLOGICAL EXAMINATION

Clinical investigations are a source of uncertainty and threat to women and provoke anxiety [39]. After being diagnosed with OC, a woman may experience a range of emotions, such as despair, helplessness, and shock. Psychological anguish affects around one-third of individuals with newly diagnosed or recurring cancer [58].

14.4.2.2 BLOOD TESTS

Cancer antigen *125 (CA-125)* or carcinoma antigen *125*, also known as *Mucin 16 (MUC16)*, is a glycosylated transmembrane mucin protein [18, 64]. The FDA-approved *CA-125* test has been used to diagnose and screen for various stages of OC [22]. On the surface of mesothelial cells and surfaces of mullerian-origin, *CA-125* is expressed and gets released from there by proteolytic cleavage to enter the bloodstream [85]. High levels of *CA-125* may be observed only in 50% of OCs during the early stages [22]. The reference [8] value for *CA-125* is 0–35 units/mL in the serum under normal conditions in most laboratories.

However, a major disadvantage of *CA-125* test is that it lacks enough sensitivity to detect for early-stage epithelial OC. This is because the five-year survival rate rises as the OC is treated earlier [81]. Furthermore, the sensitivity and specificity of *CA-125* levels can be limited since menopause can affect normal *CA-125 serum* levels [82], and some diseases, such as uterine fibroids, gastrointestinal cancer, liver cirrhosis, and endometriosis can show higher concentrations [18, 31, 49, 81, 96]. In addition, it has been noted that pregnancy and pelvic masses such as cysts may elevate *CA-125* levels. Moreover, it is possible not to observe an increase in those levels in 20% of OCs in the late stages [31, 36, 49, 81].

Another biomarker used in diagnosis of OC is human epididymis protein 4, or *HE4 protein*, isolated from the epididymis originally, but is also expressed in the respiratory and reproductive routes. Five to six months before the detection of *CA-125* levels, *HE4* levels may already be present [16]. Besides, *HE4* has shown, respectively, a pooled sensitivity and specificity of 80% and 91.6%, in comparison with 66% and 87.1% for *CA-125* [117]. It has been demonstrated that *HE4* with *CA-125* is a more reliable advanced screening marker method than *CA-125* alone [16, 25, 29]. Nonetheless, *HE4* levels vary between nonsmokers (20%) and smokers (30%) [14], and oral contraceptive users were found to have lower *HE4* levels [28].

14.4.2.3 PELVIC ULTRASOUND

Gynecologists can conduct a vaginal or abdominal ultrasound, which is a common method to discern benign cysts from malignant ones. Vaginal and abdominal ultrasound images have distinct features [43]. Moreover, benign and malignant masses show a variation in textures [2]. The diagnostic accuracy depends on radiologist's clinical experience as well as their interpretation of the images [2]. In clinical practice, tumors are not present in the majority of ultrasound images [43].

According to the International Ovarian Tumor Analysis group, the Simple Rules to evaluate tumors and predict their status are split between benign tumors (B features) and malignant tumors (M features). Regarding the former, B1 indicates a unilocular cyst, B2 signifies a solid component having a diameter less than 7 mm, B3 suggests the presence of acoustic shadows, B4 shows a smooth multilocular tumor having a maximum diameter of 10 mm, and B5 proposes no detectable color Doppler signal. Regarding the latter, M1 shows an irregular solid tumor, M2 indicates ascites, M3 suggests papillary structures, M4 demonstrates an irregular multilocular mass with a diameter greater than 10 mm M4, and M5 proposes a strong color Doppler signal [43].

In addition, some general features to interpret the images are employed by radiologists, such as dark areas having low-intensity pixel values indicating fluid cysts, extensive areas of higher intensities indicating solid mass, and high-intensity lines inside dark areas showing the perimeters multilocular cysts, and so on [107]. Additionally, nonadditive speckle noise from ultrasonic scans can alter the textural features of the image and degrade its quality [34, 35, 95].

14.4.2.4 CT SCAN

Computerized tomography, referred to as CT scan, produces cross-sectional images of the anatomic structures using special X-ray equipment, creating a three-dimensional volume of images of the internal structures of the body [19, 48, 89]. CT scan is a standard imaging tool in OC diagnosis, decision-making for treatment and surgery, and follow-up of cancer survivors, including both primary OC and metastatic disease, which originated from multiple primary tumors [46, 54].

CT is conducted to assess for occult intraabdominal malignancy or ascites. Moreover, advanced OC on CT typically presents as cysts with thick walls, septations, and papillary projections that are more clearly seen after contrast administration [46]. Additionally, the CT provides extremely precise information on the amount of ovarian tumors and abdominal dissemination, including peritoneal carcinomatosis [90].

The peritoneal carcinomatosis index (PCI) is an established, structured score that quantifies and assesses the carcinomatosis in CT (CT-PCI) and/or at surgery (surgical-PCI [S-PCI]). Reduced OC survival and a higher clinical stage were linked to increased CT-PCI [90]. However, PCI estimation from a preoperative CT scan (CT-PCI) is not a component of standard guidelines for OC diagnostics [7].

However, CT has some limitations that affect the diagnosis and clinical decision-making. It cannot directly explain tumor heterogeneity, which is considered a crucial characteristic of malignant tumors [75]. CT features of masses can be used to localize and detect the condition of interest, but the analysis of images by radiologists may lead to interobserver variability and can be time-consuming [65]. Although CT represents an optimal tool to diagnose advanced disease, its potential to detect tiny lesions is limited. Therefore, the possibility of micrometastatic disease in ovaries and the limited sensitivity of CT in detecting small lesions could serve as an explanation for its modest performance in the detection of secondary tumors of the ovary (STOs) [54].

14.4.2.5 PET SCAN

Using positron emission tomography (PET), medical conditions can be examined visually inside the patient's body noninvasively. In PET imaging, a radiotracer, which is a radioactive substance, is injected into a patient. The chemical releases a radioactive signal that can be tracked using special scanners from inside the patient's body to create a three-dimensional image of the tracer's location. A radioisotope and a portion that targets the illness are a radiotracer's two primary parts. Since a radioisotope cannot naturally travel to the location of the disease, it needs to be joined to a chemical substance that targets something unique about the disease. A commonly used radioisotope is fluorine-18, which comprises the "signaling part" of many PET radiotracers. [F]FDG, known as fluorodeoxyglucose, is used to diagnose cancer, and it resembles a sugar molecule that has been radiolabeled with F. Because they require more energy and proliferate and replicate more quickly than normal cells, cancer cells use more [F]FDG [77].

The combination of contrast-enhanced CT and fluorine-18 fluorodeoxyglucose positron emission tomography (PET) allows for assessing recurrence of ovarian carcinoma with a higher accuracy than contrast-enhanced CT alone, both in asymptomatic and symptomatic individuals, and stratification of malignancy stages [1, 30, 37, 46, 76]. In comparison with other traditional imaging methods like MRI and CT, PET/CT has a greater sensitivity and specificity [56, 76], both of which can reach up to 91% and 100%, respectively [30, 46, 76]. However, this method is not recommended if used for the initial identification of epithelial OC but is more useful postoperatively [30, 46, 76]. Recurrence of ovarian tumor is common, with 75–80% of all individuals and 90–95% of those with advanced disease (FIGO stage III/IV) relapsing within two years following primary treatment [6].

It has been demonstrated that the CA-125 threshold values of 17 UI/mL are the best balance between sensitivity and specificity in identifying either positive or negative PET/CT results, allowing linkages across various diagnostic techniques [24].

Additionally, PET/CT results have been noted in 40–60% of patients to change the treatment course for recurrent ovarian carcinoma, and the available evidence supports FDG PET/CT usage in individuals having a negative CT or MRI, with increasing CA-125 levels. In theory, extra-abdominal disease may be ruled out by PET/CT scan [76].

A drawback observed in F-FDG PET/CT imaging is when hypermetabolic ovarian uptake, seen in premenopausal women during the late follicular-early luteal cyst, has been mistakenly identified as metastases to the pelvic sidewall nodes or ovaries. On the contrary, hypermetabolic ovarian uptake in a postmenopausal woman can be suspected of malignancy since it is abnormal. Ovarian tracer uptake ought to be linked with the women's menstrual status and phase [46]. Another disadvantage is that misdiagnosis is possible when F-FDG is uptaken by physiologically normal structures, such as thyroid, myocardium, and skeletal muscle. Although PET/CT permits to precisely localize the site of F-FDG uptake, improving the differentiation between normal and abnormal uptake, physiologic F-FDG uptake can be challenging, especially in the pelvis and abdomen due to the excretion of F-FDG through the urinary system and the presence of many structures showing different F-FDG uptake, such as the bowel [51].

14.4.2.6 COLONOSCOPY

A colonoscopy is an invasive procedure that includes visual inspection of the colon's internal canal and is used for a number of diagnostic purposes [50]. According to the National Comprehensive Cancer Network guideline, recently diagnosed individuals of a pelvic mass suspected of OC ought to be regarded as candidates for gastroscopy/colonoscopy. This strategy is due to two reasons. First, about 3.2–7.0% of *ovarian tumors* can result from metastasis from the stomach or colon, and for these patients, therapeutic decisions should not be made by gynecologists but rather by surgical oncologists. Second, OC may disseminate in the abdominal cavity, and preoperative evaluation is deemed necessary [57].

Clinicians may consider, when diagnosing individuals with pelvic masses, hypothesizing the presence of STOs derived from colorectal origin [54]. It is noted that the presence of a giant ovarian tumor encompasses patients with primary ovarian carcinoma, those with metastatic tumor, and others with pathologically benign tumor that mimics malignancy. Metastatic ovarian tumors, or STOs, have been identified to account for around 20–30% of all malignant tumors of the ovary [54]. About 65% of ovarian metastases are a result of colorectal cancer (CRC), and this percentage has been increasing recently over the years [66]. Moreover, whereas STOs have a high prevalence relative to other cancers, as many as 45% of ovarian metastases emerging from CRC are primarily recognized as primary OC. Moreover, it has been documented that the most prevalent tumors that mimic primary ovarian tumors are STOs from a CRC, with 32–36% of STOs identified as primary OC. Compared to postmenopausal patients, premenopausal women having CRC have a higher risk of developing ovarian metastases [54].

It has been documented in clinical practice that the results of gastrointestinal endoscopy have led to the alteration of few patients' diagnoses and treatment regimens. Moreover, the present guidelines do not clearly recommend using gastroscopy/endoscopy in case OC is suspected [57]. However, as colon cancer is far more common than OC, a routine colonoscopy ought to be deemed essential in each instance with massive ovarian tumor prior to therapy [65].

14.5 IMAGE PROCESSING OVARIAN CANCER IDENTIFICATION

In the constantly evolving field of oncology, the development of sophisticated tools and software for image processing marks a pivotal stride toward more effective cancer diagnostics and treatment. These distinctive improvements, powered by cutting-edge computational intelligence, are made to handle the complexity of tumor morphology and response to treatment. In the attempt to identify OC, the principal objective of these image-processing tools is to assist healthcare professionals in spotting the tumor at its early stages in the ovary. For therapy to be effective and for the outcomes of patients to get better, early identification is essential. By automating the analysis of medical images, these tools aim to provide a rapid and reliable assessment, aiding medical professionals in making informed decisions about patient care.

Convolutional neural networks (CNNs) are a type of deep learning (DL) algorithm that have demonstrated exceptional performance in recent years on issues like image interpretation and computer vision. In order to create feature maps of images and extract the best features for network model training in image classification, a CNN is utilized. There have been several proposed CNN designs, and they differ in how they extract features. DenseNet reduces the vanishing-gradient issue and enhances feature propagation, ResNet employs a residual learning framework, and GoogLeNet employs an inception network design [43].

The accurate identification of images containing tumor cells and the differentiation from those without tumor can be achieved through the application of CNNs. This technique is capable for discernment of specific regions, such as serous ovarian carcinoma areas, from unaffected regions within the ovaries. The histopathology grade signifies the degree of differentiation in serous ovarian adenocarcinoma tissue, and it correlates with the prognosis of individuals with OC. The utility of quantitative histopathology analysis on determining tumor grade can be examined by employing CNNs to classify image patterns of patients with different histopathology grades. Yu et al.'s CNN approach was able to predict how well patients with serous OC will respond to platinum-based treatment, as it successfully differentiated between the histopathology images of patients with shorter platinum-free interval (PFI) from those with longer PFI [116].

In the last 30 years, a number of computer-aided diagnostics (CADs) have been created, utilizing ultrasound, blood test results [87], and mass spectrometry data [83, 100, 101], to accurately predict the risk of OC. These methods often include the selection of predetermined characteristics that quantify the differences in gray-scale intensity in the images, which are then utilized to create classifiers that can automatically identify the presence of illness [3]. They also have the potential to be cost-effective since they can help radiologists evaluate pictures and extract characteristics from medical images that are invisible to the human eye [13, 104, 123].

However, in comparison to other medical disciplines, these techniques are still fairly new in the field of gynecologic oncology [54]. Wang et al. recently presented a project in the area of gynecological cancers, wherein a CAD method had been created to classify ovarian cells as being malignant, benign, borderline, and typical. The technique combined an automated ML tree-based pipeline optimization tool with the visualization of secondary harmonics development and the *k*-nearest neighbors' predictor [108].

Deep learning and other recent developments in omics and computational technologies have promoted research in integrated multiomics analysis for cancer and precision medicine [42]. Ovarian cancer has been the subject of a few integrated multiomics analysis including di-omics [119, 120] and tri-omics [11, 119]-based studies. Due to the increasing availability of large-scale multiomics cancer data, ML approaches, especially DL approaches [20, 60, 121] are becoming very useful and effective in integrated multiomics analysis of cancer data.

Multiphoton microscopy (MPM) is one of several optical techniques that have shown efficacy in the detection of aberrant ovarian tissue [109, 111]. The basis of MPM is the simultaneous interaction of multiple photons with tissue molecules, which enables the creation of signals at a greater energy than that of the illuminating light. Second-harmonic generation (SHG) is a particular type of MPM in which nonlinear scattering of noncentrosymmetric structures forms contrast [15]. MPM produces contrast that illustrates how OC affects changes in collagen structure (SHG) and endogenous cellular fluorescence (two-photon excited fluorescence) [52, 70, 113].

As demonstrated, ML and AI tools promise enhanced accuracy in early detection, accurate characterization, and personalized treatment planning. However, their predictive value is limited due to various factors. Although ovarian tumor categorization using the currently available imaging prediction models is highly effective, user experience and subjective evaluation have a significant impact on the models. Consequently, a more thorough analysis of the various imaging modalities' separate tactics to identify. For instance, it has been found that grade annotations exhibit interrater variability when using CNNs [67, 79]. Therefore, more objective prediction models are needed. Modern deep CNNs possess millions of parameters, making them very difficult to interpret.

Despite the vast and varied advancements that CAD has made since the dawn of computers, there are still several issues that CAD systems must deal with [102]. Numerous algorithmic limits, including input data installation, pretreatment, interpretation, and system assessments, are present in CAD programs [40]. Nevertheless, in earlier studies in the area of CAD-based ovarian tumor classification, it was found that the classification accuracy could be further improved. Thus, using a variety of texture features based on basic data, including the gray level cooccurrence matrix and run length matrix, another CAD technique called GyneScan was proposed in this investigation. GyneScan is capable of effectively capturing the subtle variations in the gray-level intensity differences in the ultrasound images of benign as well as malignant tumors in the ovaries [3].

With regard to multiomics, high-dimensional omics data typically have an imbalance between the quantity of accessible samples with clinical labeling and the number of molecular attributes, thus complicating DL-based integrated multiomics analysis, particularly in individual cancer cases [42].

Concerning MPM, it is still categorized as an emerging technology because of its limited use and difficulty in adapting due to the expense and complexity of the pulsed lasers needed for it, despite its obvious appeal to biomedical scientists, particularly since MPM is present in commercially available instruments [115]. Additionally, the capacity to efficiently label thick samples, such as tissues, limits the depth of penetration and image quality of MPM in 3D tissue imaging, in spite of its benefits. It gets more challenging to introduce fluorescent markers into deeper tissues [61].

14.6 ML MODELS

ML encompasses a range of tools, methodologies, and approaches utilized across diverse sectors, including the medical field. Its application extends to addressing diagnostic challenges in various medical realms such as medical imaging, cancer detection, and wearable sensor technologies. ML is instrumental in scrutinizing crucial clinical parameters, involving tasks like extracting medical data and forecasting diseases and their progression stages. Consequently, it contributes to the planning and support of patient well-being. Additionally, ML facilitates effective healthcare monitoring through its role in data analysis, issuing intelligent alerts when necessary. On a broader scale, ML, rooted in the AI movement of the 1950s, is a field within computer science dedicated to enabling computers to learn autonomously, emphasizing practical objectives like prediction and optimization [84, 92].

In the realm of healthcare, AI denotes the utilization of software, specifically "machine-learning algorithms," to emulate human "cognition" for the analysis, representation, and comprehension of intricate health and medical data. The primary goal of AI applications in healthcare is to scrutinize correlations between patient outcomes and clinical procedures, distinguishing itself from traditional methods by its capacity to gather, process, interpret, and deliver definitive outputs based solely on input data. This is achieved through AI's adoption of DL techniques and ML methodologies, enabling these systems to discern behavioral patterns and autonomously formulate reasoning. Presently, AI-driven information finds application in diagnostic processes, pharmaceutical development, personalized medicine, patient monitoring, and the formulation of treatment protocols [105, 118].

OC stands as a prevalent gynecological malignancy on a global scale, affecting over 10,000 individuals annually [88]. When considering other gynecological malignancies, this one has a significantly worse prognosis and a higher death rate. Despite notable advancements in OC treatment modalities, including debulking surgery, chemotherapy, immunotherapy, and targeted therapy, the five-year survival rate hovers around a mere 30% [86].

Precise anticipation and identification of cellular tumors play a pivotal role in ensuring accurate prognosis and treatment, thereby enhancing overall survivability. The advantages of employing DL in this context encompass the ability to process vast datasets and generate highly accurate predictions, consequently minimizing erroneous diagnoses. Furthermore, it facilitates the early identification of ovarian carcinoma, contributing to increased treatment efficacy. Another noteworthy aspect is its capacity to enable personalized treatment plans by predicting the varied impacts of treatments on individual women, thus fostering tailored and efficient care. Ultimately, the integration of DL holds the potential to enhance patient outcomes and reduce mortality rates through its contributions to early detection and personalized treatment strategies. The use of ML algorithms for the early detection and diagnosis of OC has been the focus of recent research [124].

ML empowers computers to acquire knowledge from historical data without the need for creating algorithms that encompass an infinite array of potential feature combinations. Distinct from conventional methods reliant on manual labeling, DL techniques undertake a unique approach. DL methods acquire insights into the features of incoming images seamlessly, bypassing the necessity for feature extraction or engineering. CNNs serve as a means to grasp the intrinsic representation of images, employing interconnected layers and weight sharing in a partial manner [91].

ML brings together and scrutinizes high-throughput molecular experiments to formulate novel biomarkers for comprehending diseases. Through the amalgamation of data in ML analysis, biologically significant biomarker candidates can be uncovered, notwithstanding alterations occurring at various omics levels. Using AI research, it is anticipated that OC precision medicine will develop. These gains are also facilitated by the use of DL to picture evaluation and the comparative analysis of DL and ML methods [124].

Utilizing ML techniques, AI algorithms play a pivotal role in the early detection and diagnosis of OC by analyzing extensive patient data, including medical imaging, pathology reports, and genetic information. These algorithms excel in identifying subtle patterns indicative of the disease at an early stage, enabling timely intervention. Studies demonstrate the high accuracy of AI models in predicting the pathological diagnosis of *ovarian tumors*. Furthermore, the application of AI extends to the enhancement of image-based diagnosis, as meta-analyses highlight the significant benefits of AI algorithms in interpreting medical images more accurately. Trained on extensive datasets, these algorithms contribute to improved diagnostic precision, thereby accelerating the diagnostic process and enhancing overall diagnostic outcomes in the context of OC [114, 124].

14.7 SUMMARY

The chapter looks at how AI and ML can be used to improve the diagnosis of OC, which is notorious for being detected late. AI and ML models have the potential to distinguish between benign and malignant cells early on, addressing the need for better screening. The severity of OC is highlighted by a lack of efficient screening methods. Causes and risk factors, including age, ethnicity, genetic variations, and lifestyle, are investigated, with a focus on protective and increased components. It is emphasized how crucial it is to understand these factors in order to identify high-risk populations and provide targeted screening. Excellent survival rates need early identification of OC. While diagnostic tests like HE4 and CA-125 aim for accuracy, CA-125 is not sensitive enough in the early stages of the disease. Imaging techniques such as pelvic ultrasound, CT, and PET scans aid in diagnosis, and colonoscopy is advised for cancers suspected of having colorectal origin. The chapter also discusses advances in image processing, including CNNs and CADs, which seek to automate medical picture analysis for early OC identification. Despite the limitations, the study is optimistic about the ability of AI and ML to improve accuracy in early diagnosis, characterization, and tailored treatment planning. This integration is a significant step forward in improving patient outcomes in OC care, showing a more effective and sophisticated diagnostic environment.

KEYWORDS

- **artificial intelligence**
- **cancer screening**
- **computer-aided diagnostics**
- **convolutional neural networks**
- **machine learning**
- **ovarian cancer**
- **photo processing**

REFERENCES

1. Abdelhafez, Y., Tawakol, A., Osama, A., Hamada, E., & El-Refaei, S. (2016). Role of 18F-FDG PET/CT in the detection of ovarian cancer recurrence in the setting of normal tumor markers. *The Egyptian Journal of Radiology and Nuclear Medicine, 47*(4), 1787–1794.
2. Acharya, U. R., Sree, S. V., & Krishnan, M. M. R. (2012). Ovarian tumor characterization using 3D ultrasound. *Technology in Cancer Research & Treatment, 11*(6), 543–552.

3. Acharya, U. R., Sree, S. V., Kulshreshtha, S., et al. (2014). GyneScan: An improved online paradigm for screening of ovarian cancer via tissue characterization. *Technology in Cancer Research & Treatment, 13*(6), 529–539.
4. Adami, H. O., Hsieh, C. C., Lambe, M., et al. (1994). Parity, age at first childbirth, and risk of ovarian cancer. *Lancet, 344*(8932), 1250–1254.
5. Akobeng, A. K. (2007). Understanding diagnostic tests 1: Sensitivity, specificity and predictive values. *Acta Paediatrica, 96*(3), 338–341.
6. Antunovic, L., Cimitan, M., Borsatti, E., et al. (2012). Revisiting the clinical value of 18F-FDG PET/CT in detection of recurrent epithelial ovarian carcinomas. *Clinical Nuclear Medicine, 37*(8), e184–e188.
7. Asp, M., Malander, S., Wallengren, N. O., et al. (2022). The role of computed tomography in the assessment of tumour extent and the risk of residual disease after upfront surgery in advanced ovarian cancer (AOC). *Archives of Obstetrics and Gynecology, 306*(4), 1235–1243.
8. Atallah, G. A., Abd. Aziz, N. H., Teik, C. K., Shafiee, M. N., & Kampan, N. C. (2021). New predictive biomarkers for ovarian cancer. *Diagnostics, 11*(3), 465.
9. Babic, A., Sasamoto, N., Rosner, B. A., et al. (2020). Association between breastfeeding and ovarian cancer risk. *JAMA Oncology, 6*(6), e200421.
10. Bast, R. C., Hennessy, B., & Mills, G. B. (2009). The biology of ovarian cancer: New opportunities for translation. *Nature Reviews Cancer, 9*(6), 415–428.
11. Bell, D., et al. (2011). Integrated genomic analyses of ovarian carcinoma. *Nature, 474*, 609–615.
12. Berek, J. S., Renz, M., Kehoe, S., Kumar, L., & Friedlander, M. (2021). Cancer of the ovary, fallopian tube, and peritoneum: 2021 update. *International Journal of Gynaecology and Obstetrics, 155*(Suppl 1), 61–85.
13. Biagiotti, R., Desii, C., Vanzi, E., & Gacci, G. (1999). Predicting ovarian malignancy: Application of artificial neural networks to transvaginal and color Doppler flow US. *Radiology, 210*(2), 399–403.
14. Bolstad, N., Øijordsbakken, M., Nustad, K., & Bjerner, J. (2012). Human epididymis protein 4 reference limits and natural variation in a Nordic reference population. *Tumor Biology, 33*(1), 141–148.
15. Campagnola, P. J., & Loew, L. M. (2003). Second-harmonic imaging microscopy for visualizing biomolecular arrays in cells, tissues and organisms. *Nature Biotechnology, 21*(11), 1356–1360.
16. Capriglione, S., Luvero, D., Plotti, F., et al. (2017). Ovarian cancer recurrence and early detection: May HE4 play a key role in this open challenge? A systematic review of literature. *Medical Oncology, 34*(9), 164.
17. Cassidy, A., Huang, T., Rice, M. S., Rimm, E. B., & Tworoger, S. S. (2014). Intake of dietary flavonoids and risk of epithelial ovarian cancer. *American Journal of Clinical Nutrition, 100*(5), 1344–1351.
18. Chakraborty, S., Shenoy, P. S., Mehrotra, M., et al. (2023). Through the looking glass: Updated insights on ovarian cancer diagnostics. *Diagnostics, 13*(4), 713.
19. Chau, S., & Hayre, C. M. (2022). Computed tomography in medical imaging. In: Hayre, C. M. (Ed.), *Computed Tomography* (pp. 3–5). CRC Press.

20. Chaudhary, K., Poirion, O. B., Lu, L., & Garmire, L. X. (2018). Deep learning-based multi-omics integration robustly predicts survival in liver cancer. *Clinical Cancer Research, 24*(6), 1248–1259.
21. Daly, M. B., Pilarski, R., Yurgelun, M. B., et al. (2020). NCCN Guidelines insights: Genetic/familial high-risk assessment: Breast, ovarian, and pancreatic, version 1.2020. *Journal of the National Comprehensive Cancer Network, 18*(4), 380–391.
22. Davis, M. (2018). A comprehensive review of the diagnostic and treatment methods for ovarian cancer. *European Journal of Engineering Research and Science, 3*(2), 13.
23. Della Pepa, C., Tonini, G., Santini, D., et al. (2015). Low grade serous ovarian carcinoma: From the molecular characterization to the best therapeutic strategy. *Cancer Treatment Reviews, 41*(2), 136–143.
24. Dondi, F., Albano, D., Bertagna, F., & Giubbini, R. (2022). [18F] FDG PET/CT and CA-125 in the evaluation of ovarian cancer relapse or persistence: Is there any correlation? *Nuclear Medicine Review, 25*(2), 78–84.
25. Drapkin, R., von Horsten, H. H., Lin, Y., et al. (2005). Human Epididymis Protein 4 (HE4) is a secreted glycoprotein that is overexpressed by serous and endometrioid ovarian carcinomas. *Cancer Research, 65*(6), 2162–2169.
26. Erickson, B. J., Korfiatis, P., Akkus, Z., & Kline, T. L. (2017). Machine learning for medical imaging. *Radiographics, 37*(2), 505–515.
27. Fathalla, M. F. (1971). Incessant ovulation—A factor in ovarian neoplasia? *The Lancet, 2*(7716), 163.
28. Ferraro, S., Schiumarini, D., & Panteghini, M. (2015). Human epididymis protein 4: Factors of variation. *Clinical Chimica Acta, 438*, 171–177.
29. Fortner, R. T., Schock, H., Le Cornet, C., et al. (2018). Ovarian cancer early detection by circulating CA 125 in the context of anti-CA 125 autoantibody levels: Results from the EPIC cohort. *International Journal of Cancer, 142*(7), 1355–1360.
30. Foti, P. V., Attinà, G., Spadola, S., et al. (2016). MR imaging of ovarian masses: Classification and differential diagnosis. *Insights into Imaging, 7*(1), 21–41.
31. Fruscio, R., de Haan, J., Van Calsteren, K., Verheecke, M., Mhallem, M., & Amant, F. (2017). Ovarian cancer in pregnancy. *Best Practice & Research Clinical Obstetrics & Gynaecology, 41*, 108–117.
32. Gajjela, C. C., Brun, M., Mankar, R., et al. (2023). Leveraging mid-infrared spectroscopic imaging and deep learning for tissue subtype classification in ovarian cancer. *Analyst, 148*(12), 2699–2708.
33. Gaona-Luviano, P., Medina-Gaona, L. A., & Magaña-Pérez, K. (2020). Epidemiology of ovarian cancer. *Chinese Clinical Oncology, 9*(4), 47.
34. Garg, A., & Khandelwal, V. (2018). Combination of spatial domain filters for speckle noise reduction in ultrasound medical images. *Advances in Electrical and Electronic Engineering, 15*(5), 857–865.
35. Garg, A., & Khandelwal, V. (2016). Speckle noise reduction in medical ultrasound images using coefficient of dispersion. In: *2016 International Conference on Signal Processing and Communication (ICSC)* (pp. 208–212). IEEE.
36. Gayther, S. A., & Pharoah, P. D. (2010). The inherited genetics of ovarian and endometrial cancer. *Current Opinion in Genetics & Development, 20*(3), 231–238.

37. Ghosh, J., Thulkar, S., Kumar, R., Malhotra, A., Kumar, A., & Kumar, L. (2013). Role of FDG PET-CT in asymptomatic epithelial ovarian cancer with rising serum CA-125: A pilot study. *National Medical Journal of India, 26*(6), 327–331.
38. Goff, B. A., Mandel, L., Muntz, H. G., & Melancon, C. H. (2000). Ovarian carcinoma diagnosis. *Cancer, 89*(10), 2068–2075.
39. Gonçalves, V., Jayson, G., & Tarrier, N. (2010). A longitudinal investigation of psychological disorders in patients prior and subsequent to a diagnosis of ovarian cancer. *Journal of Clinical Psychology in Medical Settings, 17*(2), 167–173.
40. Guo, Z., Xie, J., Wan, Y., et al. (2022). A review of the current state of the computer-aided diagnosis (CAD) systems for breast cancer diagnosis. *Open Life Sciences, 17*(1), 1600–1611.
41. Hennessy, B. T., Coleman, R. L., & Markman, M. (2009). Ovarian cancer. *The Lancet, 374*(9698), 1371–1382.
42. Hira, M. T., Razzaque, M. A., Angione, C., Scrivens, J., Sawan, S., & Sarker, M. (2021). Integrated multi-omics analysis of ovarian cancer using variational autoencoders. *Scientific Reports, 11*(1), 6265.
43. Hsu, S. T., Su, Y. J., Hung, C. H., Chen, M. J., Lu, C. H., & Kuo, C. E. (2022). Automatic ovarian tumors recognition system based on ensemble convolutional neural network with ultrasound imaging. *BMC Medical Informatics and Decision Making, 22*(1), 298.
44. Huang, T., Poole, E. M., Okereke, O. I., et al. (2015). Depression and risk of epithelial ovarian cancer: Results from two large prospective cohort studies. *Gynecologic Oncology, 139*(3), 481–486.
45. Husby, A., Wohlfahrt, J., & Melbye, M. (2022). Pregnancy duration and ovarian cancer risk: A 50-year nationwide cohort study. *International Journal of Cancer, 151*(10), 1717–1725.
46. Iyer, V. R., & Lee, S. I. (2010). MRI, CT, and PET/CT for ovarian cancer detection and adnexal lesion characterization. *American Journal of Roentgenology, 194*(2), 311–321.
47. Jensen, A., Sharif, H., Frederiksen, K., & Kjaer, S. K. (2009). Use of fertility drugs and risk of ovarian cancer: Danish Population Based Cohort Study. *BMJ, 338*, b249.
48. Kamble, P. D., & Attar, V. (2022). Predicting parameter values of CT scanner using machine learning techniques. In: *2022 4th International Conference on Advances in Computing, Communication Control and Networking (ICAC3N)*, (pp. 438–442). IEEE.
49. Katchman, B. A., Chowell, D., Wallstrom, G., et al. (2017). Autoantibody biomarkers for the detection of serous ovarian cancer. *Gynecologic Oncology, 146*(1), 129–136.
50. Kelly, L. (2022). Colonoscopy: An evidence-based approach. *Nursing Standard, 37*(4), 77–82.
51. Kim, S. K., Kang, K. W., Roh, J. W., Sim, J. S., Lee, E. S., & Park, S. Y. (2005). Incidental ovarian 18F-FDG accumulation on PET: Correlation with the menstrual cycle. *European Journal of Nuclear Medicine and Molecular Imaging, 32*(7), 757–763.
52. Kirkpatrick, N. D., Brewer, M. A., & Utzinger, U. (2007). Endogenous optical biomarkers of ovarian cancer evaluated with multiphoton microscopy. *Cancer Epidemiology, Biomarkers & Prevention, 16*(10), 2048–2057.

53. Koh, D. M., Papanikolaou, N., Bick, U., et al. (2022). Artificial intelligence and machine learning in cancer imaging. *Communications Medicine, 2,* 133.
54. Kubeček, O., Laco, J., Špaček, J., et al. (2021). Clinicopathological characteristics and prognostic factors in ovarian metastases from right- and left-sided colorectal cancer. *Current Oncology, 28*(4), 2914–2927.
55. La Vecchia, C. (2017). Ovarian cancer: Epidemiology and risk factors. *European Journal of Cancer Prevention, 26*(1), 55–62.
56. Limei, Z., Yong, C., Yan, X., Shuai, T., Jiangyan, X., & Zhiqing, L. (2013). Accuracy of positron emission tomography/computed tomography in the diagnosis and restaging for recurrent ovarian cancer: A meta-analysis. *International Journal of Gynecological Cancer, 23*(4), 598–607.
57. Liu, G., Yan, J., Long, S., et al. (2021). Is routine gastroscopy/colonoscopy reasonable in patients with suspected ovarian cancer: A retrospective study. *Frontiers in Oncology, 11*, 608999.
58. Liu, J., & Holland, J. C. (2003). Psychological aspects of ovarian cancer and BRCA testing. In: *Diagnosis and Management of Ovarian Disorders*, (pp. 545–553). Elsevier.
59. Liu, P., Liang, X., Liao, S., & Lu, Z. (2022). Pattern classification for ovarian tumors by integration of radiomics and deep learning features. *Current Medical Imaging Reviews, 18*(14), 1486–1502.
60. Liu, Q., & Hu, P. (2019). Association analysis of deep genomic features extracted by denoising autoencoders in breast cancer. *Cancers (Basel), 11*(4), 494.
61. Liu, E., Vega, S. L., Treiser, M. D., Sung, H. J., & Moghe, P. V. (2011). *Fluorescence Imaging of Cell–biomaterial Interactions*. Elsevier eBooks.
62. Luan, N. N., Wu, Q. J., Gong, T. T., Vogtmann, E., Wang, Y. L., & Lin, B. (2013). Breastfeeding and ovarian cancer risk: A meta-analysis of epidemiologic studies. *American Journal of Clinical Nutrition, 98*(4), 1020–1031.
63. Lukanova, A., & Kaaks, R. (2005). Endogenous hormones and ovarian cancer: Epidemiology and current hypotheses. *Cancer Epidemiology, Biomarkers & Prevention, 14*(1), 98–107.
64. Luo, L. Y., Katsaros, D., Scorilas, A., et al. (2001). Prognostic value of human kallikrein 10 expression in epithelial ovarian carcinoma. *Clinical Cancer Research, 7*(8), 2372–2379.
65. Lusk, J. F., Miranda, C., Howell, M., Chrest, M., Eshima, J., & Smith, B. S. (2019). Photoacoustic flow system for the detection of ovarian circulating tumor cells utilizing copper sulfide nanoparticles. *ACS Biomaterials Science & Engineering, 5*(3), 1553–1560.
66. Maeda, Y., Minagawa, N., Shoji, H., Kobayashi, T., & Yamamoto, K. (2022). Giant ovarian tumor with colorectal cancer: Suggestion concerning the need for colonoscopy screening in cases with large ovarian tumor—a report of three cases. *BMC Surgery, 22*(1), 111.
67. Matsuno, R. K., Sherman, M. E., Visvanathan, K., Goodman, M. T., Hernandez, B. Y., Lynch, C. F., Ioffe, O. B., Horio, D., Platz, C., Altekruse, S. F., et al. (2013). Agreement for tumor grade of ovarian carcinoma: Analysis of archival tissues from the Surveillance, Epidemiology, and End Results residual tissue repository. *Cancer Causes & Control, 24*(4), 749–757.

68. Matulonis, U. A., Sood, A. K., Fallowfield, L., Howitt, B. E., Sehouli, J., & Karlan, B. Y. (2016). Ovarian cancer. *Nature Reviews Disease Primers, 2,* 16061.
69. Merrill, R. (2010). *Introduction to Epidemiology*, 5th ed., Jones & Bartlett Learning.
70. Nadiarnykh, O., LaComb, R. B., Brewer, M. A., & Campagnola, P. J. (2010). Alterations of the extracellular matrix in ovarian cancer studied by Second Harmonic Generation imaging microscopy. *BMC Cancer, 10,* 94.
71. Narod, S. A. (2016). Talc and ovarian cancer. *Gynecologic Oncology, 141*(3), 410–412.
72. National Cancer Institute. (2016). *SEER Stat Fact Sheets: Ovarian Cancer*. SEER. Retrieved from http://seer.cancer.gov/statfacts/html/ovary.html
73. Negri, E., Pelucchi, C., Franceschi, S., et al. (2003). Family history of cancer and risk of ovarian cancer. *European Journal of Cancer, 39*(4), 505–510.
74. Nolan-Kenney, R. C., Wang, Y., & Liu, M. (2020). Diagnostic test basics: A primer for neuro-ophthalmologists. *Journal of Neuro-Ophthalmology, 40*(4), 445–449.
75. Nougaret, S., McCague, C., Tibermacine, H., Vargas, H. A., Rizzo, S., & Sala, E. (2021). Radiomics and radiogenomics in ovarian cancer: A literature review. *Abdominal Radiology (New York), 46*(6), 2308–2322.
76. Nunes, R. L., Teixeira, F. R., Diniz, T. P., et al. (2023). The value of PET/CT for cytoreductive surgery selection in recurrent ovarian carcinoma. *Journal of Gynecologic Oncology, 34*(3), e31.
77. O'Malley, M. G., & Inkster, J. A. H. (2022). Looking inside the human body using radioactive atoms. *Frontiers for Young Minds, 10*, 689970.
78. Orr, B., & Edwards, R. P. (2018). Diagnosis and treatment of ovarian cancer. *Hematology/Oncology Clinics of North America, 32*(6), 943–964.
79. Papp, E., et al. (2018). Integrated genomic, epigenomic, and expression analyses of ovarian cancer cell lines. *Cell Reports, 25*, 2617–2633.
80. Parazzini, F., Chatenoud, L., Chiantera, V., Benzi, G., Surace, M., & La Vecchia, C. (2000). Population attributable risk for ovarian cancer. *European Journal of Cancer, 36*(4), 520–524.
81. Park, Y., Lee, J. H., Hong, D. J., Lee, E. Y., & Kim, H. S. (2011). Diagnostic performances of HE4 and CA125 for the detection of ovarian cancer from patients with various gynecologic and non-gynecologic diseases. *Clinical Biochemistry, 44*(10–11), 884–888.
82. Pasalich, M., Su, D., Binns, C. W., & Lee, A. H. (2013). Reproductive factors for ovarian cancer in southern Chinese women. *Journal of Gynecologic Oncology, 24*(2), 135–140.
83. Petricoin, E. F., Ardekani, A. M., Hitt, B. A., Levine, P. J., Fusaro, V. A., Steinberg, S. M., Mills, G. B., Simone, C., Fishman, D. A., Kohn, E. C., & Liotta, L. A. (2002). Use of proteomic patterns in serum to identify ovarian cancer. *The Lancet, 359,* 572–577.
84. Bi, Q., Goodman, K. E., Kaminsky, J., & Lessler, J. (2019). What is machine learning? A primer for the epidemiologist. *American Journal of Epidemiology, 188*(12), 2222–2239.
85. Razmi, N., & Hasanzadeh, M. (2018). Current advancement on diagnosis of ovarian cancer using biosensing of CA 125 biomarker: Analytical approaches. *Trends in Analytical Chemistry, 108,* 1–12.

86. Reid, B. M., Permuth, J. B., & Sellers, T. A. (2017). Epidemiology of ovarian cancer: A review. *Cancer Biology & Medicine, 14*, 9–32.
87. Renz, C., Rajapakse, J. C., Razvi, K., & Liang, S. K. C. (2002). In neural information processing, 2002. ICONIP '02. In: *Proceedings of the 9th International Conference on* (pp. 809–813, vol. 802).
88. Rooth, C. (2013). Ovarian cancer: Risk factors, treatment and management. British *Journal of Nursing, 22*(17), S23–S30.
89. Saad, M. S., & Moore, S. (2022). Computed tomography scan. In: *A Medication Guide to Internal Medicine Tests and Procedures* (pp. 78–84). Elsevier.
90. Sartor, H., Bjurberg, M., Asp, M., et al. (2023). Imaging ovarian cancer – From baseline characteristics to high-risk image factors. *Journal of Ovarian Research, 16*(1), 78.
91. Sarvamangala, D. R., & Kulkarni, R. V. (2022). Convolutional neural networks in medical image understanding: A survey. *Evolutionary Intelligence, 15*(1), 1–22.
92. Shehab, M., Abualigah, L., Shambour, Q., Abu-Hashem, M. A., Shambour, M. K. Y., Alsalibi, A. I., & Gandomi, A. H. (2022). Machine learning in medical applications: A review of state-of-the-art methods. *Computers in Biology and Medicine, 145*, 105458.
93. Shrestha, P., Poudyal, B., Yadollahi, S., et al. (2022). A systematic review on the use of artificial intelligence in gynecologic imaging—Background, state of the art, and future directions. *Gynecologic Oncology, 166*(3), 596–605.
94. Singh, A. S., & Masuku, M. B. (2012). Understanding and applications of test characteristics and basic inferential statistics in hypothesis testing. *European Journal of Applied Sciences, 4*(2), 90–97.
95. Singh, K., Ranade, S. K., & Singh, C. (2017). A hybrid algorithm for speckle noise reduction of ultrasound images. *Computer Methods and Programs in Biomedicine, 148,* 55–69.
96. Skates, S. J., Mai, P., Horick, N. K., et al. (2011). Large prospective study of ovarian cancer screening in high-risk women: CA125 cut-point defined by menopausal status. *Cancer Prevention Research, 4*(9), 1401–1408.
97. Stewart, C., Ralyea, C., & Lockwood, S. (2019). Ovarian cancer: An integrated review. *Seminars in Oncology Nursing, 35*(2), 151–156.
98. Stojanovic, M., Andjelkovic-Apostolovic, M., Stojanovic, D., et al. (2014). Understanding sensitivity, specificity and predictive values. *Vojnosanitetski Pregled, 71*(11), 1062–1065.
99. Struewing, J. P., Hartge, P., Wacholder, S., et al. (1997). The risk of cancer associated with specific mutations of BRCA1 and BRCA2 among Ashkenazi Jews. *New England Journal of Medicine, 336*(20), 1401–1408.
100. Tan, T. Z., Quek, C., Ng, G. S., & Razvi, K. (2008). Ovarian cancer diagnosis with complementary learning fuzzy neural network. *Artificial Intelligence in Medicine, 43*, 207–222.
101. Tang, K. L., Li, T. H., Xiong, W. W., & Chen, K. (2010). Ovarian cancer classification based on dimensionality reduction for SELDI-TOF data. *BMC Bioinformatics, 11,* 109.
102. Tate, J. E., Burton, A. H., Boschi-Pinto, C., & Parashar, U. D.; World Health Organization–Coordinated Global Rotavirus Surveillance Network. (2016). Global,

regional, and national estimates of rotavirus mortality in children <5 years of age, 2000–2013. *Clinical Infectious Diseases, 62*(2), S96–S105.

103. Terry, K. L., Karageorgi, S., Shvetsov, Y. B., et al. (2013). Genital powder use and risk of ovarian cancer: A pooled analysis of 8,525 cases and 9,859 controls. *Cancer Prevention Research, 6*(8), 811–821.
104. Timmerman, D., Verrelst, H., Bourne, T. H., De Moor, B., Collins, W. P., Vergote, I., & Vandewalle, J. (1999). Artificial neural network models for the preoperative discrimination between malignant and benign adnexal masses. *Ultrasound in Obstetrics and Gynecology*, *13*(1), 17–25.
105. Torre, L. A., Bray, F., Siegel, R. L., Ferlay, J., Lortet-Tieulent, J., & Jemal, A. (2015). Global cancer statistics, 2012. *CA: A Cancer Journal for Clinicians*, *65*(2), 87–108.
106. Trevethan, R. (2017). Sensitivity, specificity, and predictive values: Foundations, pliabilities, and pitfalls in research and practice. *Frontiers in Public Health*, *5*, 307.
107. Van Calster, B., Van Hoorde, K., Froyman, W., Kaijser, J., Wynants, L., Landolfo, C., & Timmerman, D. (2015). Practical guidance for applying the ADNEX model from the IOTA group to discriminate between different subtypes of adnexal tumors. *Facts, Views & Vision in ObGyn*, *7*(1), 32.
108. Wang, G., Sun, Y., Jiang, S., et al. (2021). Machine learning-based rapid diagnosis of human borderline ovarian cancer on second-harmonic generation images. *Biomedical Optics Express, 12*(9), 5658–5669.
109. Watson, J. M., et al. (2013). Two-photon excited fluorescence imaging of endogenous contrast in a mouse model of ovarian cancer. *Lasers in Surgery and Medicine, 45,* 155–166.
110. Webb, P. M., & Jordan, S. J. (2017). Epidemiology of epithelial ovarian cancer. *Best Practice & Research Clinical Obstetrics & Gynaecology, 41*, 3–14.
111. Welge, W. A., DeMarco, A. T., Watson, J. M., Rice, P. S., Barton, J. K., & Kupinski, M. A. (2014). Diagnostic potential of multimodal imaging of ovarian tissue using optical coherence tomography and second-harmonic generation microscopy. *Journal of Medical Imaging, 1*(2), 025501.
112. Wentzensen, N., Poole, E. M., Trabert, B., et al. (2016). Ovarian cancer risk factors by histologic subtype: An analysis from the Ovarian Cancer Cohort Consortium. *Journal of Clinical Oncology, 34*(24), 2888–2898.
113. Williams, R. M., Flesken-Nikitin, A., Ellenson, L. H., et al. (2010). Strategies for high-resolution imaging of epithelial ovarian cancer by laparoscopic nonlinear microscopy. *Translational Oncology, 3*(3), 181–194.
114. Xu, H. L., Gong, T. T., Liu, F. H., Chen, H. Y., Xiao, Q., Hou, Y., Huang, Y., Sun, H. Z., Shi, Y., Gao, S., Lou, Y., Chang, Q., Zhao, Y. H., Gao, Q. L., & Wu, Q. J. (2022). Artificial intelligence performance in image-based ovarian cancer identification: A systematic review and meta-analysis. *EClinicalMedicine, 53,* 101662.
115. Yamada, M., Lin, L. L., & Prow, T. W. (2014). Multiphoton microscopy applications in biology. Chapter 13; In: Cornea, A., & Michael Conn, P. (Eds.), *Fluorescence Microscopy*, (pp. 185–197), Academic Press: USA. https://doi.org/10.1016/B978-0-12-409513-7.00013-0
116. Yu, K. H., Hu, V., Wang, F., et al. (2020). Deciphering serous ovarian carcinoma histopathology and platinum response by convolutional neural networks. *BMC Medicine, 18*(1), 236.

117. Yu, S., Yang, H. J., Xie, S. Q., & Bao, Y. X. (2012). Diagnostic value of HE4 for ovarian cancer: A meta-analysis. *Clinical Chemistry and Laboratory Medicine, 50*(8), 1439–1446.
118. Zhang, B., Shi, H., & Wang, H. (2023). Machine learning and AI in cancer prognosis, prediction, and treatment selection: A critical approach. *Journal of Multidisciplinary Healthcare, 16,* 1779–1791.
119. Zhang, H., et al. (2016). Integrated proteogenomic characterization of human high-grade serous ovarian cancer. *Cell, 166,* 755–765.
120. Zhang, Z., et al. (2016). Molecular subtyping of serous ovarian cancer based on multi-omics data. *Scientific Reports, 6,* 26001.
121. Zhang, X., Zhang, J., Sun, K., Yang, X., Dai, C., & Guo, Y. (2019, November). Integrated multi-omics analysis using variational autoencoders: Application to pan-cancer classification. In: *2019 IEEE International Conference on Bioinformatics and Biomedicine (BIBM)* (pp. 765–769). IEEE.
122. Zhou, R., Liu, Y., Wang, Y., Huo, X., Zhu, J., & Zhang, T. (2020). Clinicopathological characteristics and prognosis analysis of ovarian metastases in colorectal cancer: A single-center experience. *International Journal of Clinical Oncology, 25*(10), 1822–1829.
123. Zimmer, Y., Tepper, R., & Akselrod, S. (1999). Computerized quantification of structures within ovarian cysts using ultrasound images. *Ultrasound in Medicine & Biology, 25*(2), 189–200.
124. Ziyambe, B., Yahya, A., Mushiri, T., et al. (2023). A deep learning framework for the prediction and diagnosis of ovarian cancer in pre- and post-menopausal women. *Diagnostics (Basel), 13*(10), 1703.

CHAPTER 15

Role of IoT, AI, Chatbot, and ChatGPT in the Diagnosis and Treatment of Female Health Conditions

PANKAJ SHARMA,* SALONI JAIN, ADITI BHARDWAJ, SANDEEP SHARMA, and VINAY JAIN

*Corresponding author

ABSTRACT

Through a dynamic fusion of Internet of Things, artificial intelligence (AI), Chatbots, and Chat Generative Pretrained Transformer (ChatGPT), it was observed that there is notable potential for these innovations to revolutionize diagnosis and treatment methods for various female health conditions. In the past several months, researchers and medical professionals have begun to consider the potential uses of AI-related big language models in health care. In this chapter, the thorough analysis focused on providing a summary of Chatbots and ChatGPT as well as their applications in health care. Initially, a broad overview of Chatbots, their development, design, and potential applications in medicine are covered. Second, ChatGPT's applications in medicine are highlighted, along with their design and instructional techniques, medical diagnosis and therapy, ethical concerns in research, and a comparison of ChatGPT with other natural language processing models. The review also covered ChatGPT's possibilities and limits. These massive model languages along with ChatGPT have vast potential for the healthcare industry in the decades to come. Yet, further study in this technology is required.

Holistic Approaches for Women's Sustainable Health, Volume 2: Advancements, Socioeconomic Impacts, and Innovative Strategies. Junaid Ahmad Malik, Anamika Chauhan, and Megh R. Goyal (Eds)

DOI: 10.1201/9781779641656-18

15.1 INTRODUCTION

In recent times, there have been significant advancements in artificial intelligence (AI) in many forms, including Chatbots. A linguistic model for discussion is called Chat Generative Pretrained Transformer (ChatGPT). On November 30, 2022, open AI published an early version of this Chatbot [7]. After which, ChatGPT has drawn many users from a variety of disciplines due to its ability to offer thorough and human-like replies to nearly any query. It is said that ChatGPT is used for several medical purposes, including medical writing, monitoring, recordkeeping, and teaching. According to published reports, ChatGPT can successfully complete the most difficult US medical test, indicating that it may have important uses in health care [32].

According to Kashefi and Mukerji [29], ChatGPT can write numerical algorithm code for programming. According to Perkel [52], an AI-based large language model (LLM) can troubleshoot and annotate codes. It is capable of translating software across different programming languages.

It is necessary to give precise description of Chatbot and ChatGPT, though a Chatbot is an automatic software program designed to mimic human–user discussions. These Chatbots understand user requests and can provide informal, intelligent responses by utilizing machine learning (ML) and natural language processing (NLP) techniques. An AI-derived Chatbot called ChatGPT processes input using deep learning (DL) techniques. OpenAI Inc. (San Francisco, CA, USA) used NLP to generate text-based answers for customer inputs. Built on the GPT construction, this Chatbot can perform a wide range of language-based activities. The GPT is also known as an LLM. But in terms of health care, the query was: Would ChatGPT alter medical treatment? The issue was addressed, and it was affirmed by an article in *Nature Medicine* that this LLM will improve medical treatment, the standard of life, and the provision of health care. It has a great deal of opportunity to support clinical requirements. It was concluded that language assessment of models will revolutionize the medical domain [14]. Khan et al. [30] shared their perspectives on the clinical leadership and medical schooling functions of AI-powered chatbots. Like a smartphone mental wellness app, Graber-Stiehl [17] indicated that this technology can be utilized as a counselor.

Yang [82] also mentioned about the application of this technology for medical education. Researchers are investigating the tool's potential applications in a variety of domains, including programming for computers, classroom instruction, health care, and heritage preservation. The tool is now widely used. However, out of all the new Chatbot innovations driven by DL-based models of language, ChatGPT has emerged as the leader. A computer software has been created for chatting with humans as the user in a Chatbot format. It can recognize queries and offer automated answers. More specialized areas of AI, such as DL and NLP, are used in modern Chatbot technology. It can communicate verbally and in writing using graphical languages to interface with individuals [1, 21]. Chatbot techniques are defined as AI-driven illustrations of a human–computer interface. Virtual aids, interacting representatives, cleverbots, and intelligent conversational beings are some well-known names for Chatbots.

15.2 TECHNOLOGICAL ADVANCEMENTS IN FEMALE HEALTH CARE

Processing and analyzing vast volumes of or big data, clinical data, from sources such as imaging tests, results of laboratory tests, and medical records, is one of ML's main advantages. This method helps to find correlations and danger indicators that human specialists would overlook. Studies indicate that AI may be able to diagnose illness just as well as or perhaps more effectively than people [42]. Early illness detection and identification, that is especially crucial for female health, can be facilitated by technologies. A sophisticated type of ML, for instance, that uses neural networks or deep learning has shown encouraging results in the detection of breast cancer.

Through the analysis of mammograms and the identification of questionable regions for additional investigation, scientists have discovered how this kind of imaging can assist radiologists with the faster and more precise detection of breast cancer [33]. Until these technologies become more extensively used, further clinical studies are required, even if this may result in quicker intervention and improved results. Crucially, technology is required to be able to identify more complicated breast tumors and provide reliable findings on women of diverse ages, races, and body shapes.

Personalized medicine is yet another way AI may help women's health. Customized insights and suggestions may be obtained by analyzing vast amounts of data related to women's health requirements, which vary greatly depending on aspects such as weight, age, reproductive circumstance, and medical background. AI facilitates this process. The quickly growing femtech or female technological sector is likely where this use is most visible. For instance, the telemedicine startup Nurx employs AI algorithms in its "competent question" function to identify each woman's optimal birth control method. Upon completing the digital form to obtain a prescription for contraception, the platform employs AI algorithms to examine the user's medical background, lifestyle choices, and inclinations, subsequently furnishing tailored suggestions for birth control alternatives [22]. As an additional illustration, the wearable technology created by the fertility monitoring business Ava Science monitors physiological data, including body temperature and heart rate variation, using a mixture of devices and ML algorithms [15]. After analyzing the data, AI algorithms offer individualized information regarding a woman's reproduction, ovulation, and duration of cycle.

15.3 OVERVIEW OF CONVERGENCE BETWEEN INTERNET OF THINGS (IOT), AI, CHATBOTS, AND FEMALE HEALTH

Prenatal care has benefited greatly from AI in the past few years, since it has made easier to diagnose diseases, plan treatments, and keep track of patient's health. This has improved the health of both the mother and the fetus. By using large datasets, AI models can recognize people who are more likely to have negative consequences, which helps healthcare practitioners to make precise and prompt judgments. Recent research has highlighted the promise of AI in utilizing a variety of biological markers and AI models to foresee issues, such as preterm delivery, preeclampsia, and gestational diabetes, during pregnancy [73]. Furthermore, while acceptability rates are impacted by education and knowledge with AI technology, a significant population of pregnant women are receptive to incorporate AI into maternal health care. This change indicates that AI may play a significant role in improving maternity health care [15] and various other advantages in healthcare industry (Figure 15.1).

Also, the area has seen a tremendous transformation with the addition of robots, which has greatly enhanced imaging for medicine, fertility treatments, and surgical precision. The advent of virtual reality (VR) technologies that provide models of laparoscopic and robotic procedures has completely changed the way healthcare providers receive their education. This development has the potential to refine abilities to previously unheard-of levels of precision and efficacy. Future advancements in medical technology might be far more extensive and easily available with telemedicine and VR. Imagine a world in which wearable technology tracks health indicators for pregnancies at elevated risk and robots aid in birthing, allowing for prompt intervention. ChatGPT along with other AI Chatbots with advanced modeling of languages are kind of augmented companions that are eager to accompany and guide new mothers throughout the process [18].

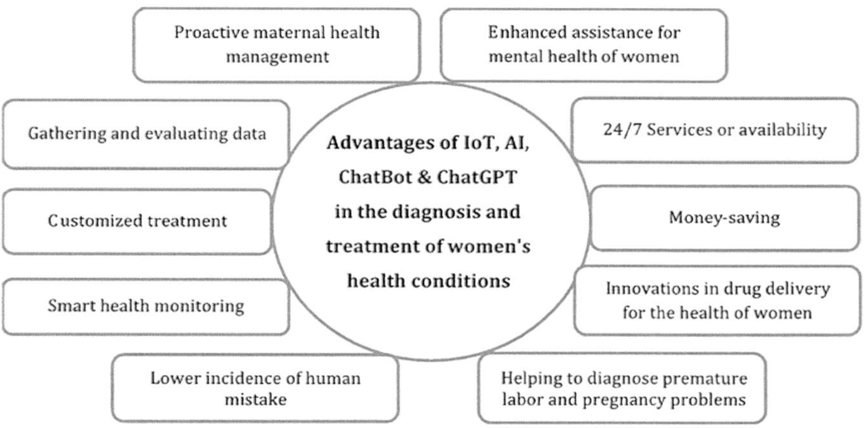

FIGURE 15.1 Advantages of IoT, AI, Chatbot and ChatGPT in the diagnosis and treatment of female health conditions.

Thanks to modern standards and algorithms, the IoT is emerging as a major worldwide communication channel. Numerous objects, particularly electrical equipment and household appliances with wireless sensors, are connected to the internet through it [67]. Considering the next big technical revolution, the IoT has become increasingly common during the past 10 years, making things inherently linked. One example of an IoT application is an intelligent health tracking system [66].

IoT refers to the practice of using networks and objects to link computers to the internet. Health-monitoring devices can make use of these interrelated components. Afterward, the data is transmitted to distant locations using machine-to-machine communication, utilizing mobile phones, desktops, and handheld electronics [67]. It is an easy way to monitor and optimize treatment for any health concern that is also adaptable, energy-efficient, much smarter, and accessible. Adaptable interfaces, mental health tracking, and helper gadgets are examples of modern technology that make life easier for humans [64].

15.4 METHODOLGY

A thorough review of the literature was done to find pertinent research on ChatGPT and Chatbots in the healthcare industry. Utilizing Scopus, PubMed, and Google Scholar, articles published during the last 3 years were selected. The most popular search phrases were “ChatGPT,” “Chatbot,” “artificial intelligence,” “healthcare Chatbot,” “medical Chatbot,” and “machine learning.” The query plan was modified to consider the needs and features of every database. Publications on ChatGPT and Chatbots in health care or medical were selected based on certain criteria. Consideration was given to publications that covered the advantages, restrictions, difficulties, and potential applications of Chatbot technologies in medicine, diagnostic assistance, and communication with patients. The use of Chatbots and ChatGPT for healthcare programs, as well as their effectiveness and results, was examined in the chosen publications. A summary of recent studies in this field was created by extracting and summarizing pertinent material. A lot of helpful knowledge on the deployment and efficacy of Chatbots and ChatGPT in medicine was observed.

Under two major topics, this chapter covered the general environment for Chatbots and ChatGPT. Authors first glanced over a general review of Chatbots and then determined ChatGPT’s application in medicine. The authors of this chapter provided an introduction, history, architecture, technologies employed, and applications of Chatbots in medicine in the initial part to help readers understand the basic concepts of Chatbots. The subsequent half of the discussion focused on ChatGPT’s applications in medicine, including medical diagnosis and therapy, architecture and training methodologies, research ethics related to ChatGPT in medicine, and the contrast of ChatGPT with other NLP models utilized in the field. Authors also observed any prospects and constraints.

15.5 APPLICATIONS OF IOT FOR DIAGNOSIS OF FEMALE HEALTH CONDITIONS

An interconnected network of computers having unique IDs and the capacity to send data across a network without requiring human-to-computer or human-to-human contact is called the IoT. The idea of a "smart home," which consists of several gadgets maintaining an integrated ecosystem and is managed by related devices such as smartphones, is arguably the most well-known instance of the IoT.

15.5.1 WEARABLE DEVICES FOR CONTINUOUS MONITORING

Completing the current generation of digital health care is wearable and nearable technology. Wearables include smart contact lenses, wristbands, and smart bras (Figure 15.2).

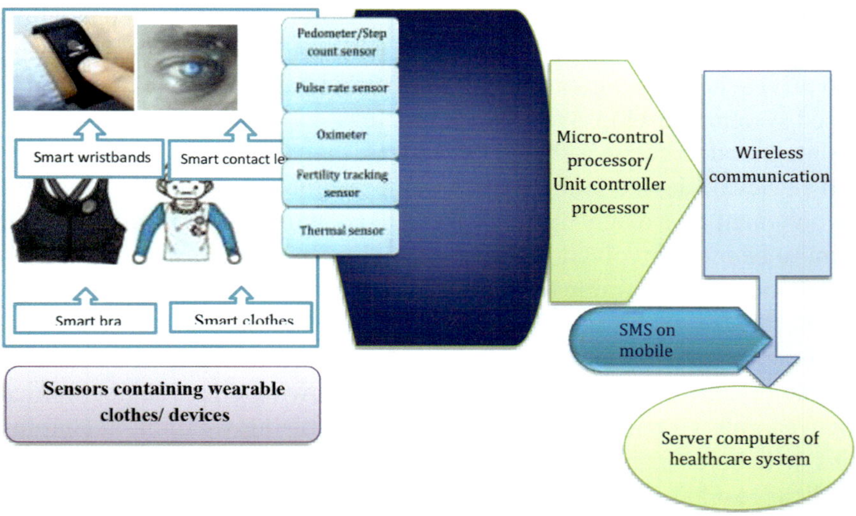

FIGURE 15.2 Wearable devices for continuous monitoring.

The term "wearables" refers to miniature wireless devices having sensors that may transfer data. These will get past the complex and ineffective institution-based treatment and, where necessary, replace the present rigid delivery methods with independent tailored medication. The biosensors (implantable or invisible biological sensors) will interface with supplier networks and handheld devices. When costly, intrusive therapy is required, they will promote prompt communication between healthcare provider and patient and action. Such devices include chips that enable ongoing tracking of vital signs, bionic eyes that enable vision for the blind, cardioverter-defibrillators that cure abrupt cardiac arrest, and smart medications that wirelessly transfer medical information to the healthcare practitioner [31].

15.5.1.1 TRACKING VITAL SIGNS

Wearable technology promotes "relevant" conversations with close companions and caregivers while reviving consumer awareness of oneself. Now, wearable technology is becoming increasingly medically oriented for integrating information with medical facilities for tracking chronic diseases. Wearable technology measures several elements of a patient's health in a contemporary fashion; thus, it provides deeper, useful information outside bodily diagnostics. More smartphone connection with workplace applications, portals for patients, digital medical records, and private health information will be possible as smartphones and cloud-based systems develop. Wearable technology and better, safer clouds will be integrated to create a shared framework that allows for data archiving and retrieval, device and system interoperability, and increased patient involvement and diagnostics accuracy [31]. Women who are in midlife want to be more involved in health-related matters. According to studies, people perceive wearable technology to be efficient, economic, cozy, and handy [85].

Senior citizens who are getting older, caregivers, and women with ongoing medical conditions are among the growing client demographics for wearable technology. Clinical techniques using wearable technologies will be used in novel companies that involve patients. Improved medical results, prompt intervention, and mutual responsibility are the goals [85].

Ava transforms the way women view reproductive health and is the perfect companion for women. This serves as a wearable fertility monitoring gadget that has received the Food and Drug Administration (FDA) approval. The Ava bracelet tracks five physiological markers while it is worn in slumber by utilizing ML techniques. It considers nine physiological factors to accurately and simply forecast when a woman will ovulate and when her next viable window will occur. Ava has demonstrated an 89% accuracy rate in identifying 5.3 fertile days on average every cycle. First results have been released in a peer-reviewed publication *Scientific Reports* after a year-long investigation at the University Hospital of Zurich. Ava has a CE certification and has been registered with the FDA [13].

15.5.1.2 COLLECTING BIOMETRIC DATA

Human features such as the fingerprints and face are used by systems that recognize biometric data to identify or authenticate identity. As sensing technology progresses, it becomes increasingly commonplace and solves the disadvantage of authentication using passwords [83]. While password-based authorization is less secure when using biometric systems, biometric data saved as pattern data in centralized databases or electronic devices is susceptible to hacking since, unlike passwords, no one's biometric characteristics can be altered or duplicated. Security lapses and privacy violations are likely to happen if biometric template information gets hacked, and the damage is irreversible. Sensitive information or records kept in IoT devices may be seriously jeopardized if a competitor uses biometric templates that have been obtained to gain entry to the devices. Thus, there are two reasons why biometrics template data protection is important. Initially, user identification needs to be secured, so that the initial biometric data cannot be obtained. Second, only authorized individuals should have possession of private or sensitive information saved on IoT devices [84].

15.6 AI-ASSISTED DIAGNOSIS FOR FEMALE HEALTH ISSUES

These days, there is a lot to explore in the application of AI in health care, particularly when it comes to the diagnosis or prediction evaluation of medical information. More clinical health data has been produced and will be produced annually as information technology for healthcare advances. The biggest information category is made up of information on medical personnel mental health, information from clinical trials, and diagnostic information in tandem. These days, AI may generate algorithms for clinical studies for diagnosis and therapy [27].

15.6.1 ML ALGORITHMS FOR EARLY DETECTION OF DISEASES

A method for monitoring, detecting, and analyzing data was described by Otoom et al. [45]. This suggested technology was able to monitor and detect coronary artery disease. Using the naive Bayes method, Vembandasamy et al. [77] conducted research for diagnosing cardiac disease (Figure 15.3). In naive Bayes, the Bayes hypothesis is applied. naive Bayes has strong independent assumptions as a result. One of the top diabetes study centers in Chennai provided the used dataset. Five hundred individuals make up the dataset. By utilizing decision chains and naive Bayes, Iyer et al. [24] conducted research to predict the onset of diabetes. When there is inadequate insulin synthesis or inappropriate insulin utilization, diseases develop. Vijayarani and Dhayanand [78] used support vector machines and naive Bayes categorization methods to predict liver illness.

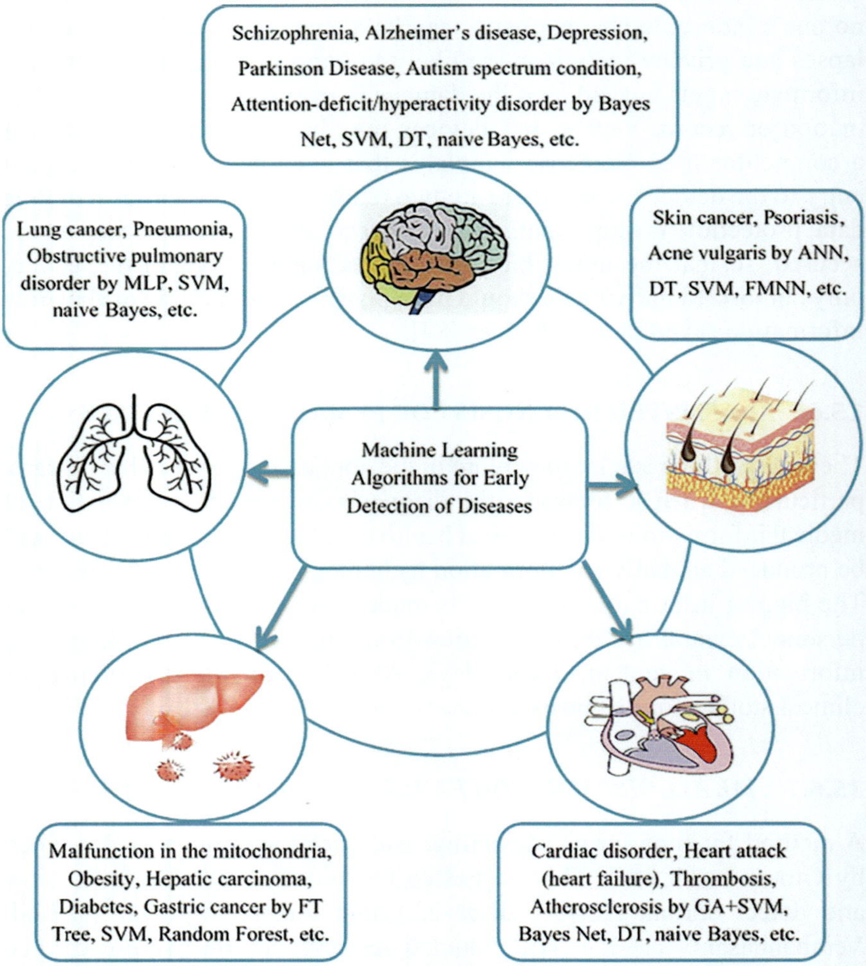

FIGURE 15.3 Early disease detection using various ML methods.

In addition to providing evaluation and therapy, healthcare organizations are attempting to use ChatGPT to support medical facilities, identify possible research subjects, and notify healthcare professionals, including nurses, physicians, and medical school students, regarding new advancements in their respective fields [11, 26, 55]. Scientists have employed it in several fields of medicine. Among the applicable fields are healthcare imaging, clinical administration, education in medicine, hepatocellular carcinoma and cirrhosis, clinical reports, clinical toxicology, and research on diabetes.

15.6.1.1 BREAST CANCER SCREENING USING AI

Based on the pathophysiology of breast cancer, there are several variables that might contribute to an individual's risk of developing breast cancer, including gender, inheritance, environmental factors, genetics, and employment. The best approach to treating the illness is to use early screening techniques [3, 5].

AI integration improves the efficacy rate of therapy when used in screening processes such as biopsy slides inspection. Among the essential AI components needed for breast cancer diagnosis are ML and DL. A popular method in AI systems is radiomics. It takes what is known as feature—quantitative aspects—from a picture [76]. AI is being used in the realm of breast cancer therapy to enable early diagnosis through the utilization of data from biopsy specimens and radiomics.

The most common technique for monitoring breast cancer is mammography [40, 79]. It produces a high-resolution picture that may be stored and utilized in the future without regard to age or type of body. Technologies for full-field digital mammograms have two different kinds: (1) inputs (raw pictures) and (2) outputs (postprocessing). AI uses image analysis to identify mammary masses, density of the breasts, mass division, and likelihood of cancer. One of the most crucial stages in computer-aided diagnosis is identifying mammary masses, which are frequently found in patients with breast cancer [49].

15.6.1.2 CERVICAL CANCER SCREENING THROUGH AUTOMATED SYSTEMS

As a major cause of cancer-related mortality for women, cervical cancer continues to pose a substantial danger to their emotional and physical well-being. With early detection and diagnosis, this malignancy is easily prevented. While technological developments have made it possible to diagnose cervical cancer much earlier, there are still several variables that make a precise diagnosis challenging. Uses for AI in healthcare diagnostics have grown in popularity recently, and they are very applicable to the detection and diagnosis of cervical cancer. They have the advantage of requiring less time, requiring less skilled and competent employees, and not being biased due to subjective variables. To increase the effectiveness of early detection, we specifically wanted to talk about how AI may be applied to cancer of the cervical cavity detection and screening [23].

15.7 CHATBOTS AS VIRTUAL ASSISTANTS IN PROVIDING SUPPORT TO FEMALES

By providing patients with round-the-clock medical guidance and support, virtual assistants may be utilized in the medical field to enhance patient care. Chatbots are computer programs that mimic human conversation and are intended to assist users in managing their health and corresponding with healthcare professionals. Other domains where Chatbots could prove useful include processes, tracking, medical care, and health advocacy. Medical facilities are becoming easier to access, more useful, and more efficient thanks to Chatbots [8].

15.7.1 PERSONALIZED INFORMATION DELIVERY THROUGH CONVERSATIONAL INTERFACES

Car et al. [74] carried out a scoping review. Through the aim of finding the terms "conversational agents," "conversational AI," "Chatbots," and related equivalents, Excerpta Medica Database; Ovid, Medical Literature Analysis and Retrieval System Online; Ovid, Scopus, PubMed, and Cochrane Central were searched for pertinent research for their systematic research exploration. In April 2019, they also conducted a search of obscure literature utilizing resources such as ResearchGate and the WorldCat directory maintained by the Online Computer Library Center. The authors of this chapter looked through pertinent articles' lists of references to find further articles. Two reviewers worked simultaneously on the evaluation and information extraction processes. Using the concepts of theme evaluation, a narrative examination of the provided material was conducted [74].

Most of the research that they have read on conversational machines related to health care is qualitative in nature, focusing on tracking, therapy, and assistance for medical facilities. It mostly covers text-based, AI-powered, and mobile app-delivered conversational bots. Strong evaluations of the acceptance, safety, and efficacy of various medical conversational agent forms are desperately needed [74].

15.7.2 MENTAL WELL-BEING SUPPORT VIA INTERACTIVE CHATBOTS

AI Chatbots are conversational software applications with cognitive ability that can process information, make decisions, and perform tasks on their own or in conjunction with individuals. They use ML; NLP; and big data to increase their capacity, boost output, and help, direction, and conversations [6].

There are instances in which AI Chatbots can offer more perceptive answers than people can. They might nevertheless be devoid of a personalized and sympathetic touch. It is suggested that human–artificial intelligence (HAI) might assist in overcoming these constraints by allowing people and AI to complement one another's skills to work together toward a shared objective for effective, secure, long-lasting, and pleasurable work and lifestyles. The Center for the Development of Humane Technology's efforts to include human principles into HAI, including compassion, empathy, and accountability, are in line with the AI idea [9].

A major issue that impacts millions of individuals globally is mental health. For instance, around 20% of adult Australians suffer from a mental disease. If cumulative experiences with mental illness are considered, this number rises to 44%, spending the economy billions of dollars [81] due to deteriorated health and shorter life expectancies. Unfortunately, several obstacles, including stigma, expense, and limited availability of mental health offerings, prevent many individuals from getting the assistance they require. Young adults who make use of technology for mental health evaluation, assistance, avoidance, and therapy are the target audience for digital mental health services [25]. For instance, Chatbots powered by AI are used to provide psychological assistance, while AI and ML models are utilized to detect mental disease. Nevertheless, the moral and legal ramifications of these instruments are unclear.

15.8 ROLE OF CHATGPT IN FEMALE HEALTH CARE

The most well-known AI Chatbot today is called ChatGPT, and it was created by California-based OpenAI, a study and implementation business for AI [44]. This cutting-edge AI approach, which is based on transformer neural networks, can produce writing that appears human-like by using its understanding of contextual clues in conversations. ChatGPT, which went live on November 30, 2022, has amassed over 100 million users in a short period of time [70].

15.8.1 UTILIZING NLP MODELS TO IMPROVE COMMUNICATION

ChatGPT is a game-changer in the field of health care, as the amount of medical expertise is expanding exponentially [72]. It transforms how experts obtain the most recent findings from studies by making it easier to retrieve accurate and current information [37]. Because ChatGPT makes complicated medical language easier to understand and facilitates efficient interaction with patients, its impact goes outside the field of medicine and into specialist medical domains such as pathology, radiology, and genomics [41].

In oncology, ChatGPT is very revolutionary. Numerous difficulties arise in the detection, therapy, and scientific study of cancer. The field of cancer has seen significant developments recently because of advances in AI and natural language processing, with ChatGPT leading the way [75]. A potential chance to improve healthcare decision-making, patient education, and research in medicine exists when ChatGPT is integrated into cancer [71].

15.9 ETHICAL CONSIDERATIONS AND PRIVACY CONCERNS

The rapid growth of healthcare Chatbots as conversational tools for patient usage during the global epidemic has accelerated the creation and application of suitable moral frameworks for this novel technology by healthcare ethical thinkers. Healthcare Chatbots have so far raised several ethical and legal issues that require attention and resolution [35]. They involve safety for patients, information security, data utilization, confidentiality and integrating, Chatbot information format, and mutual trust and openness between all parties. Because it depends on patient input and frequent updates from the Chatbot, creating appropriate ethical standards would take effort. Negotiations between different parties are also very important. Consider responsibility for information about patients as a case study. The development of ChatGPT as a Chatbot for health care is happening so quickly that the current state of such guidelines for ethical installation is not keeping up. The need to integrate this kind of technological disruption in the healthcare sector in such a brief period will put increasing demands on medical personnel.

15.9.1 ENSURING DATA SECURITY AND CONFIDENTIALITY DURING REMOTE CARE

ChatGPT has the potential to change investigations, clinical procedures, and medical training. When used to medicine, it raises potential ethical problems that need to be solved. In order to improve its language-generating capabilities, ChatGPT requires a large amount of data. However, this data frequently contains private information that needs to be protected in order to maintain privacy, including medical records [46, 59]. The model may not be capable to manage sensitive medical data appropriately; thus, there are additional security and safety issues to consider. While practitioners may quit utilizing their clinical judgment in favor of the model's recommendations, there is a greater demand for technologies [10, 51, 58]. The absence of human connection in health care, the requirement for informed permission, and the possibility that the model would replace actual physicians and cause layoffs are some ethical issues. AI will never be able to completely substitute human doctors in real life, though, as they lack human comprehension, empathy, and a feeling of responsibility. Possible prejudices in health care and medicine raise further ethical concerns. If the initial data is skewed toward a specific demographic category, ChatGPT's performance may suffer. Additionally, there are legal and moral issues associated with the use of ChatGPT along with other AI techniques in medical literature. These include the possibility of copyright violations, difficulties in medicolegal situations, and the need for transparency in text written by AI [36, 60]. Because they have such heavy obligations, it follows that the potential replaceability for human doctors is restricted.

An AI doctor cannot take the place of a human physician. To tackle these issues, it is essential to comprehend the possible risks, limitations, and implications of using these advances in the medical field. Several suggestions and best practices might help to allay the present moral dilemmas. Among them is making sure that proper precautions are taken to ensure confidentiality for patients while using ChatGPT; one such precaution is to safeguard user privacy by using text ambiguation systems. To prevent biases in ChatGPT's language creation, the next step is to make sure that the data for training it uses is accurate to the population and varied. It is also crucial to guarantee that appropriate legal safeguards are in place to protect the confidentiality of patients while utilizing ChatGPT in the medical field.

15.10 CASE STUDIES: SUCCESSFUL IMPLEMENTATIONS

The main uses of IoT in health care are via apps and services. Notifications and monitoring of medications are two of the primary IoT applications. On the other hand, services have many different use cases [53, 65]. In the field of IoT and health care, there are many review articles accessible. A significant contribution giving a thorough, systematic review that covers IoT patterns, uses, and methodologies for the healthcare industry was done by the researchers of Kashani et al. [28]. Through a thorough evaluation process that kindly contributed to the body of literature in this field, Selvaraj and Sundaravaradhan [56] tried to highlight the potential and difficulties that exist in IoT-based healthcare systems. In their evaluation of smart health, tracking, and observation management, Panchatcharam and Vivekanandan [47] also examined IoT designs and security analysis for data transmission in IoT devices in the healthcare sector [57].

15.10.1 REAL-LIFE EXAMPLES HIGHLIGHTING BENEFITS AND OUTCOMES

We discovered an app that tracks fetal development, an essential component of prenatal care. This app monitors heart rate, movements of the fetus, temperature, and labor pain. Accelerometers, force sensors, microcontrollers, Global System for Mobile Communication, sweat sensors, heart rate sensors, and temperature gauges are only a few of the sensors and IoT technologies that are used by the gadget [20, 63, 68]. This application's thorough monitoring has numerous advantages, one of which is that routine fetal surveillance is now more convenient and effective. Nevertheless, it is crucial to recognize that possible challenges to external reliability, including fictitious labor pain or differences in ambient circumstances, such as excessive sweating, may have an impact on the system's precision in real-world settings [16]. It is imperative that further research and improvement can be focused on these issues to guarantee the system's dependability in a variety of scenarios [61, 62].

Sarhaddi et al. [54] described an IoT-based system that provides extensive maternal health surveillance over the course of pregnancy and after delivery. Numerous gathering devices in the framework monitor the state of motherhood, particularly those which measure anxiety, insomnia, and activity levels. After discussing how to integrate the technology that was given with the healthcare system that is currently in place, respondents will get a self-reported questionnaire that was created using an app that is cross-platform to gather their background information. The purpose of the survey is to collect data on their standard of existence, perceived anxiety level, past miscarriages or premature births, and documented ailments. The lack of contrast between standard treatment and health results is the main reason for the investigation's low generalization.

A device named "NEO" was presented by Singh et al. [69], and it comprises of three components: (1) a data getting component, (2) a data transmission component, and (3) a display interface component. By incorporating multiple sensors and devices attached to newborns in the neonatal intensive care unit, the gadget could collect crucial data instantaneously. They failed to consider the risk of privacy, in addition to the substantial integration prices and infrastructure difficulties.

A newborn incubator apparatus was developed by El-Aziz and Taloba [12] to give neonates the same ideal conditions as they would in the womb: optimal humidity, ideal temperature, optimal light, and the right amount of oxygen. An Arduino UNO microprocessor and several IoT sensors that can measure temperature and humidity make up this setup. One of the constraints of the investigation is that the investigator was supposed to make a comparison in terms of cost integrating and effectiveness.

IoT-based drug recognition and prescription tracking system were suggested by Jara et al. [38]. In the system they had, radio frequency identification and near-field communication were the primary components. But as a matter of urgency for everyone involved, scientists should discuss confidentiality and ethical problems. The devices also need a thorough examination into repeatable scalability, even if they are appropriate for initial planning and simulation.

Eswari and Priya [39] both focused on medication identification processes and provided the ability to identify abnormalities in health from indicators of health. According to their opinion, two of the most significant problems in the healthcare industry pertaining to patient protection are drug adherence and adverse drug reactions (ADRs). Nevertheless, the study found no empirical support for the viability and efficacy of the suggested approach in raising adherence to medication and lowering ADR.

A system for IoT-based smart health tracking and fog-assisted surveillance was presented by Beri et al. [4], and it can obtain and process a pregnant woman's temperature, electrocardiogram, blood pressure, and pulse oximeter data. To examine their method, they employed fog computing-related real-time series data and rule-based algorithms. Given the continued sensitivity of the material, security and moral issues are significant and were anticipated by the people who wrote it.

15.11 RESTRICTIONS AND PROSPECTS FOR THE FUTURE

According to Yeung et al. [2], ChatGPT has demonstrated proficiency in the theoretical portion of the US medical licensure test; however, it still requires further training or comprehensive medical schooling. However, the use of ChatGPT along with other AI tools for medical literature presents ethical and legal issues, such as the requirement for openness regarding AI-generated content and possible infringements on intellectual property. Considerable promise exists for ChatGPT to enhance patient-centered treatment in radiography along with other medical specialties; however, further research is necessary to ascertain any potential drawbacks. Reports have surfaced of potentially harmful consequences and misleading remarks. Thus, while using ChatGPT and other foundational designs, especially in the medical field, it is imperative to take their drawbacks into account [80]. Numan et al. [43] demonstrated how incorporating external frameworks into social VR can provide novel opportunities for collaboration using ChatGPT as an embodiment conversational agent within the system.

It shows how versatile ChatGPT is as an instrument for enhancing consumer experiences in a range of contexts. ChatGPT will be very helpful for mental health in the years to come. In a research project, Koko, a psychological software beginning, provided those who participated with a therapy conversation environment in which they may discuss their mental health problems via ChatGPT [19, 48]. Additionally, Chatbots can provide health-related services and data, including aiding smokers in quitting.

According to Li et al. [34], ChatGPT has the potential to provide personalized and precise medical information, which might result in reduced mistakes and problems, enhanced outcomes for patients, more patient engagement, as well as more economic delivery of health care. Yet, further study is needed to evaluate ChatGPT's effectiveness in medicine since the reports under examination must be of higher caliber. Notwithstanding this, there is a lot of promise for ChatGPT's application in the medical field. Its performance, dissemination methods, and theoretical foundations should all be fully documented in future study [50].

15.12 SUMMARY

In conclusion, the use of ChatGPT and other Chatbots in the medical field has demonstrated potential to enhance medical instruction and patient care. Medical professionals have discovered that ChatGPT is useful for several tasks, including patient tracking, evaluation, and study. It can also be a useful tool for increasing knowledge about health, especially among youth and teenagers. The need for Chatbot-based products that assess complaints with AI has increased significantly. These applications leverage natural interactions to suggest potential illnesses and assist users in self-triaging using AI. It is also crucial to take ethical issues into account, such as the veracity and quality of the data offered, the possibility of prejudice, the requirement for transparency and responsibility, and other elements. While ChatGPT and other Chatbots can increase the efficiency of medical care, they are not a complete replacement for physicians.

More studies and developments are needed in the potential study areas of ChatGPT and Chatbots in medicine. Subsequent investigations ought to focus on developing and optimizing ever-more complex and advanced Chatbots that can handle a wide range of medical questions and issues. Given the patient's specific information and health history, these bots must provide tailored advice. It is highly recommended that a comprehensive investigation and examination should be carried out to fully examine and assess the possibilities of Chatbots in enhancing patient involvement and elevating their standard of life. Furthermore, fostering cooperation between tech firms, government agencies, and healthcare providers may aid in the creation of foreseeable and next-generation Chatbots having characteristics that are responsible. Here, the best course of action should be decided in collaboration with governmental organizations, computer programmers, ethicists, researchers, medical experts, patients, assistance suppliers, and other governing bodies with their supporters and inspectors. It could be a very difficult process. To enhance patients' happiness with life, the project will contribute to the development of next-generation, DL-based Chatbots that are more legal, accountable, and free of mistakes.

ACKNOWLEDGMENTS

The authors acknowledge Shri Ram College of Pharmacy, Banmore, Morena, Madhya Pradesh, India for encouraging us and providing necessary facilities.

KEYWORDS

- **artificial intelligence**
- **cancer**
- **Chatbot**
- **ChatGPT**
- **IoT**
- **pregnancy**
- **woman's health**

REFERENCES

1. Adamopoulou, E., & Moussiades, L. (2020). Chatbots: History, technology, and applications. *Machine Learning with Applications*, *2*, e100006. doi: 10.1016/j.mlwa.2020.100006
2. Au Yeung, J., Kraljevic, Z., Luintel, A., Balston, A., Idowu, E., Dobson, R. J., & Teo, J. T. (2023). AI chatbots not yet ready for clinical use. *Frontiers in Digital Health*, *5*, 60–65. doi: 10.3389/fdgth.2023.1161098
3. Baxi, V., Edwards, R., Montalto, M., & Saha, S. (2022). Digital pathology and artificial intelligence in translational medicine and clinical practice. *Modern Pathology*, *35*(1), 23–32.
4. Beri, R., Dubey, M. K., Gehlot, A., Singh, R., Abd-Elnaby, M., & Singh, A. (2022). A novel fog-computing-assisted architecture of E-healthcare system for pregnant women. *The Journal of Supercomputing*, *2022*, 1–25.
5. Bray, F., Ferlay, J., Soerjomataram, I., Siegel, R. L., Torre, L. A., & Jemal, A. (2018). Global cancer statistics: GLOBOCAN estimates of incidence and mortality worldwide for 36 cancers in 185 countries. *CA: A Cancer Journal for Clinicians*, *68*(6), 394–424.
6. Caldarini, G., Jaf, S., & McGarry, K. (2022). A literature survey of recent advances in chatbots. *Information*, *13*(1), 41–46.
7. ChatGPT. (2023). ChatGPT: Optimizing language models for dialogue. https://openai.com/blog/chatgpt/; (accessed on 28 January 2024).
8. Chow, J. C., Sanders, L., & Li, K. (2023). Impact of ChatGPT on medical chatbots as a disruptive technology. *Frontiers in Artificial Intelligence*, *6*, e1166014. doi: 10.3389/frai.2023.1166014
9. Clement, S., Schauman, O., Graham, T., Maggioni, F., Evans-Lacko, S., Bezborodovs, N., & Thornicroft, G. (2015). What is the impact of mental health-related stigma on help-seeking? A systematic review of quantitative and qualitative studies. *Psychological Medicine*, *45*(1), 11–27.
10. Corsello, A., & Santangelo, A. (2023). May artificial intelligence influence future pediatric research? The case of ChatGPT. *Children*, *10*(4), 757–761. doi: 10.3390/children10040757
11. Dave, T., Athaluri, S. A., & Singh, S. (2023). ChatGPT in medicine: An overview of its applications, advantages, limitations, future, and ethical considerations. *Frontiers in Artificial Intelligence*, *6*, e1169595. doi: 10.3389/frai.2023.1169595
12. El-Aziz, R. M. A., & Taloba, A. I. (2021). Real time monitoring and control of neonatal incubator using IOT. *arXiv preprint arXiv:2112.02071*.
13. Empowering women's health with AI. https://www.biopharmatrend.com/post/701-notable-companies-empowering-womenshealthwithai/#:~:text=Ava%20has%20 been%20 shown %20to,registered%20device%20and% 20CE%2Dcertified; (accessed on 29 January 2024).
14. Gates, B. (2023). Will ChatGPT transform healthcare? *Nature Medicine*, *29*, 505–506. doi: 10.1038/s41591-023-02289-5
15. Goodale, B. M., Shilaih, M., Falco, L., Dammeier, F., Hamvas, G., & Leeners, B. (2019). Wearable sensors reveal menses-driven changes in physiology and enable

prediction of the fertile window: Observational study. *Journal of Medical Internet Research*, *21*(4), e13404. doi: 10.2196/13404

16. Gopalakrishnan, D., Warale, P., & Bhaumik, R. (2021). Design of a maternal healthcare monitoring device for pregnant women. In: *Design for Tomorrow, Volume 3: Proceedings of ICoRD 2021*, (Volume 3, pp. 495–509). Springer: Singapore.
17. Graber-Stiehl, I. (2023). Is the world ready for ChatGPT therapists? *Nature*, *617*(7959), 22–24. doi: 10.1038/d41586-023-01473-4
18. Grewal, H., Dhillon, G., Monga, V., Sharma, P., Buddhavarapu, V. S., Sidhu, G., & Kashyap, R. (2023). Radiology gets chatty: The ChatGPT saga unfolds. *Cureus*, *15*(6), e40135.
19. Grodniewicz, J. P., & Hohol, M. (2023). Therapeutic conversational artificial intelligence and the acquisition of self-understanding. *The American Journal of Bioethics*, *23*(5), 59–61. doi: 10.1080/15265161.2023.2191021
20. Haliima, N., Rushingabigwi, G., & Nzanywayingoma, F. (2022, March). Design of an IoT based monitoring system for expectant rural women in developing countries. In: *International Conference on Computer Science and Software Engineering (CSASE)*, (pp. 41–47). IEEE.
21. Haque, M. R., & Rubya, S. (2023). An overview of Chatbot-based mobile mental health apps: Insights from app description and user reviews. *JMIR mHealth and uHealth*, *11*(1), e44838. doi: 10.2196/44838
22. Hawkins, L. (2021, April 20). Nurx: Breaking down barriers to women's healthcare. https://healthcare-digital.com/ digital-healthcare/nurx-breaking-down-barriers-womenshealthcare; (accessed on 28 January 2024).
23. Hou, X., Shen, G., Zhou, L., Li, Y., Wang, T., & Ma, X. (2022). Artificial intelligence in cervical cancer screening and diagnosis. *Frontiers in Oncology*, *12*, e851367. doi: 10.3389/fonc.2022.851367.
24. Iyer, A., Jeyalatha, S., & Sumbaly, R. (2015). Diagnosis of diabetes using classification mining techniques. *arXiv preprint arXiv:1502.03774*. doi: 10.5121/ijdkp.2015.5101
25. Iyortsuun, N. K., Kim, S. H., Jhon, M., Yang, H. J., & Pant, S. (2023, January). A review of machine learning and deep learning approaches on mental health diagnosis. *Healthcare*, *11*(3), 285–290.
26. Jeblick, K., Schachtner, B., Dexl, J., Mittermeier, A., Stüber, A. T., Topalis, J., & Ingrisch, M. (2023). ChatGPT makes medicine easy to swallow: An exploratory case study on simplified radiology reports. *European Radiology*, *2023*, 1–9. doi: 10.1007/s00330-023-10213-1
27. Jiang, F., Jiang, Y., Zhi, H., Dong, Y., Li, H., Ma, S., & Wang, Y. (2017). Artificial intelligence in healthcare: Past, present and future. *Stroke and Vascular Neurology*, *2*(4), 230–243. doi: 10.1136/svn-2017-000101. PMID: 29507784.
28. Kashani, M. H., Madanipour, M., Nikravan, M., Asghari, P., & Mahdipour, E. (2021). A systematic review of IoT in healthcare: Applications, techniques, and trends. *Journal of Network and Computer Applications*, *192*, e103164.
29. Kashefi, A., & Mukerji, T. (2023). ChatGPT for programming numerical methods. *Journal of Machine Learning for Modeling and Computing*, *4*(2), online. doi: 10.1615/JMachLearnModelComput.2023048492

30. Khan, R. A., Jawaid, M., Khan, A. R., & Sajjad, M. (2023). ChatGPT-Reshaping medical education and clinical management. *Pakistan Journal of Medical Sciences*, *39*(2), 605–610. doi: 10.12669/pjms.39.2.7653
31. Krohn, R., Metcalf, D., & Salber, P. (2017). *Connected Health: Improving Care, Safety, and Efficiency with Wearables and IoT Solution*. CRC Press: Boca Raton.
32. Kung, T. H., Cheatham, M., Medenilla, A., Sillos, C., De Leon, L., Elepaño, C., & Tseng, V. (2023). Performance of ChatGPT on USMLE: Potential for AI-assisted medical education using large language models. *PLOS Digit Health, 2*(2), e0000198. doi: 10.1371/journal.pdig.0000198. PMID: 36812645..
33. Leibig, C., Brehmer, M., Bunk, S., Byng, D., Pinker, K., & Umutlu, L. (2022). Combining the strengths of radiologists and AI for breast cancer screening: A retrospective analysis. *The Lancet Digital Health*, *4*(7), e507–e519.
34. Li, W., Zhang, Y., & Chen, F. (2023). ChatGPT in colorectal surgery: Promising tool or a passing fad? *Annals of Biomedical Engineering*, *51*(9), 1892–1897.
35. Liebrenz, M., Schleifer, R., Buadze, A., Bhugra, D., & Smith, A. (2023). Generating scholarly content with ChatGPT: Ethical challenges for medical publishing. *The Lancet Digital Health*, *5*(3), e105–e106.
36. Liu, J., Wang, C., & Liu, S. (2023). Utility of ChatGPT in clinical practice. *Journal of Medical Internet Research*, *25*, e48568. doi: 10.2196/48568
37. Lubowitz, J. H. (2023). ChatGPT, an artificial intelligence chatbot, is impacting medical literature. *Arthroscopy*, *39*(5), 1121–1122.
38. Lyu, P., Peng, M., Lyu, Y., Chen, Y., & Yang, J. (2013, October). A multi-communication-fusion based mobile monitoring system for maternal and fetal information. In: *IEEE 15th International Conference on e-Health Networking, Applications and Services* (*Healthcom,* pp. 559–563). IEEEexplore. Lisbon, Portugal, doi: 10.1109/HealthCom.2013.6720739.
39. Macones, G. A., Hankins, G. D., Spong, C. Y., Hauth, J., & Moore, T. (2008). The 2008 National Institute of Child Health and Human Development workshop report on electronic fetal monitoring: Update on definitions, interpretation, and research guidelines. *Journal of Obstetric, Gynecologic, & Neonatal Nursing*, *37*(5), 510–515.
40. McDonald, E. S., Oustimov, A., Weinstein, S. P., Synnestvedt, M. B., Schnall, M., & Conant, E. F. (2016). Effectiveness of digital breast tomosynthesis compared with digital mammography: Outcomes analysis from 3 years of breast cancer screening. *JAMA Oncology*, *2*(6), 737–743.
41. Mese, I., Taslicay, C. A., & Sivrioglu, A. K. (2023). Improving radiology workflow using ChatGPT and artificial intelligence. *Clinical Imaging*, *2023*, e109993.
42. Mirbabaie, M., Stieglitz, S., & Frick, N. R. (2021). Artificial intelligence in disease diagnostics: A critical review and classification on the current state of research guiding future direction. *Health and Technology*, *11*(4), 693–731.
43. Numan, N., Giunchi, D., Congdon, B., & Steed, A. (2023, March). Ubiq-genie: Leveraging external frameworks for enhanced social VR experiences. In: *2023 IEEE Conference on Virtual Reality and 3D User Interfaces Abstracts and Workshops (VRW)*, (pp. 497–501). IEEE.
44. OpenAI, online. https://openai.com/about; (accessed on June 2023).

45. Otoom, A. F., Abdallah, E. E., Kilani, Y., Kefaye, A., & Ashour, M. (2015). Effective diagnosis and monitoring of heart disease. *International Journal of Software Engineering and Its Applications*, *9*(1), 143–156.
46. Ovalle, A., Beikzadeh, M., Teimouri, P., Chang, K. W., & Sarrafzadeh, M. (2023). ChatGPT for us: Preserving data privacy in ChatGPT via dialogue text ambiguation to expand mental health care delivery. arXiv preprint arXiv:2306.05552.
47. Panchatcharam, P., & Vivekanandan, S. (2019). Internet of things (IOT) in healthcare–smart health and surveillance, architectures, security analysis and data transfer: A review. *International Journal of Software Innovation (IJSI)*, *7*(2), 21–40.
48. Pankaj, S., Ashish, D., Dheerendra, R., Yogendra, R., Ramakant, J. K. S., & Kuldeep, S. (2015). Formulate and evaluate oro-dispersible tablets of Primaquine. *Indo American Journal of Pharmaceutical Research*, *5*(5), 1625–1632.
49. Parvathavarthini, S., & Shanthi, S. (2019). Breast cancer detection using crow search optimization based Intuitionistic fuzzy clustering with neighborhood attraction. *Asian Pacific Journal of Cancer Prevention (APJCP)*, *20*(1), 157–162.
50. Payton, E., Khubchandani, J., Thompson, A., & Price, J. H. (2017). Parents' expectations of high schools in firearm violence prevention. *Journal of Community Health*, *42*, 1118–1126.
51. Pennestrì, F., & Banfi, G. (2022). Artificial intelligence in laboratory medicine: Fundamental ethical issues and normative key-points. *Clinical Chemistry and Laboratory Medicine (CCLM)*, *60*(12), 1867–1874.
52. Perkel, J. M. (2023). Six tips for better coding with ChatGPT. *Nature*, *618*(7964), 422–423.
53. Rayan, R. A., Tsagkaris, C., & Zafar, I. (2021). *IoT-Integrated Robotics in the Health Sector. Biomedical and Robotics Healthcare Series.* CRC Press: Oxon.
54. Sarhaddi, F., Azimi, I., Labbaf, S., Niela-Vilén, H., Dutt, N., Axelin, A., & Rahmani, A. M. (2021). Long-term IoT-based maternal monitoring: System design and evaluation. *Sensors*, *21*(7), e2281.
55. Sedaghat, S. (2023). Early applications of ChatGPT in medical practice, education and research. *Clinical Medicine*, *23*(3), 278–279.
56. Selvaraj, S., & Sundaravaradhan, S. (2020). Challenges and opportunities in IoT healthcare systems: A systematic review. *SN Applied Sciences*, *2*(1), 139–142.
57. Sharma, P. (2021). Modification of human behavior due to coronavirus outbreak: A brief study on current scenario. *Asian Journal of Pharmaceutics (AJP)*, *15*(3), online
58. Sharma, P. (2022). Applications of statistical tools for optimization and development of smart drug delivery system. *Smart Drug Delivery.* London: Intech Open, 2022, 183 (online).
59. Sharma, P. (2023). Nanostructured biomaterials in drug delivery: Current trends and upcoming possibilities. In: *Engineered Biomaterials: Synthesis and Applications* (pp. 261–280). Springer Nature: Singapore.
60. Sharma, P., & Jain, V. (2023). An overview of current advances and pharmaceutical uses of 3D and 4D printing. *Exploration of Medicine, 24*, 560–575.
61. Sharma, P., & Tailang, M. (2017). Opportunities and challenges to develop transdermal patch with nanocarrier. *WJPR*, *6*(15), 392–400.

62. Sharma, P., & Tailang, M. (2020). Design, optimization and evaluation of buccal drug delivery system of propranolol for hypertension treatment. *International Journal of Pharmaceutical Sciences and Research*, *11*(1), 301–311.
63. Sharma, P., Jain, V., & Jain, S. (2021). Fabrication, optimization and evaluation of chronotropic drug delivery system of captopril. *International Journal of Pharmaceutical Sciences and Research*, *12*, 2203–2210.
64. Sharma, P., Jain, V., & Tailang, M. (2022). Swarm intelligence and machine learning algorithms for cancer diagnosis. *Swarm Intelligence and Machine Learning: Applications in Healthcare*, *2022*, 34–40.
65. Sharma, P., Jain, V., & Tailang, M. (2022). *Selection and Role of Polymers for Deigning of a Drug Carrier (online)*. IntechOpen. doi: 10.5772/intechopen.103125
66. Sharma, P., Jain, V., & Tailang, M. (2023). How artificial intelligence is transforming medicine: The future of pharmaceutical research. In: *Industry 4.0 and Healthcare: Impact of Artificial Intelligence* (pp. 133–150). Springer Nature: Singapore.
67. Sharma, P., Jain, V., Jain, A., & Tailang, M. (2022). Role of swarm intelligence for health monitoring and related actions. *Internet of Things and Fog Computing-Enabled Solutions for Real-Life Challenges*, *6*, 95–99.
68. Shermi, S. C. S. S. D., Soundarya, S., & Manickavasagam, M. R. (2020). Smart maternal real time monitoring using IoT-technique. *International Research Journal of Engineering and Technology*, *7*(3), online.
69. Singh, H., Kaur, R., Gangadharan, A., Pandey, A. K., Manur, A., Sun, Y., & Kumar, P. (2018). Neo-bedside monitoring device for integrated neonatal intensive care unit (iNICU). *IEEE Access*, *7*, 7803–7813.
70. Singh, O. P. (2023). Artificial intelligence in the era of ChatGPT: Opportunities and challenges in mental health care. *Indian Journal of Psychiatry*, *65*(3), 297–301.
71. Thapa, S., & Adhikari, S. (2023). ChatGPT, bard, and large language models for biomedical research: Opportunities and pitfalls. *Annals of Biomedical Engineering*, *51*(12), 2647–2651.
72. Thirunavukarasu, A. J., Ting, D. S. J., Elangovan, K., Gutierrez, L., Tan, T. F., & Ting, D. S. W. (2023). Large language models in medicine. *Nature Medicine*, *29*(8), 1930–1940.
73. Togunwa, T. O., & Babatunde, A. O. (2023). Deep hybrid model for maternal health risk classification in pregnancy: Synergy of ANN and random forest. *Frontiers in Artificial Intelligence*, *6*, 16–21.
74. Tudor-Car, L., Dhinagaran, D. A., Kyaw, B. M., Kowatsch, T., Joty, S., Theng, Y. L., & Atun, R. (2020). Conversational agents in health care: Scoping review and conceptual analysis. *Journal of Medical Internet Research*, *22*(8), e17158.
75. Uprety, D., Zhu, D., & West, H. (2023). ChatGPT: A promising generative AI tool and its implications for cancer care. *Cancer*, *129*(15), 2284–2289. doi: 10.1002/cncr.34827. PMID: 37183438.
76. Van Timmeren, J. E., Cester, D., Tanadini-Lang, S., Alkadhi, H., & Baessler, B. (2020). Radiomics in medical imaging—"how-to" guide and critical reflection. *Insights into Imaging*, *11*(1), 1–16.
77. Vembandasamy, K., Sasipriya, R., & Deepa, E. (2015). Heart diseases detection using naive Bayes algorithm. *International Journal of Innovative Science, Engineering & Technology*, *2*(9), 441–444.

78. Vijayarani, S., & Dhayanand, S. (2015). Liver disease prediction using SVM and Naïve Bayes algorithms. *International Journal of Science, Engineering and Technology Research (IJSETR)*, *4*(4), 816–820.
79. Welch, H. G., Prorok, P. C., O'Malley, A. J., & Kramer, B. S. (2016). Breast-cancer tumor size, overdiagnosis, and mammography screening effectiveness. *New England Journal of Medicine*, *375*(15), 1438–1447.
80. Wen, J., & Wang, W. (2023). The future of ChatGPT in academic research and publishing: A commentary for clinical and translational medicine. *Clinical and Translational Medicine*, *13*(3), e1207.
81. Wies, B., Landers, C., & Ienca, M. (2021). Digital mental health for young people: A scoping review of ethical promises and challenges. *Frontiers in Digital Health*, *3*, 697072.
82. Yang, H. (2023). How I use ChatGPT responsibly in my teaching. *Nature*, *317*.
83. Yang, W., Hu, J., & Wang, S. (2013, December). A Delaunay triangle group based fuzzy vault with cancellability. In: *2013 6th International Congress on Image and Signal Processing (CISP)*, (3, pp. 1676–1681). IEEE.
84. Yang, W., Wang, S., Sahri, N. M., Karie, N. M., Ahmed, M., & Valli, C. (2021). Biometrics for internet-of-things security: A review. *Sensors*, *21*(18), 6163.
85. Yoldemir, T. (2020). Internet of things and women's health. *Climacteric*, *23*(5), 423–425.

CHAPTER 16

Text Mining and Natural Language Processing for Reproductive Health

ANANYA VERMA, RAJSHRI SINGH, and SAGAR BARAGE*

*Corresponding author

ABSTRACT

Reproductive health is currently undergoing a significant transformation in the context of the contemporary digital era, owing to the advent of artificial intelligence, machine learning, and data science. Given the vast amount of unstructured data that is already accessible, text mining and natural language processing methodologies present a significant opportunity to extract meaningful insights, increase healthcare outcomes, and deepen our comprehension of several elements related to reproductive health. This chapter provides a comprehensive introduction to text mining, encompassing its concept, procedural aspects, and practical implementations in real-world reproductive health scenarios, along with the ethical considerations and potential developments and prospects in the field, which encompass the emergence of increasingly sophisticated artificial intelligence-powered models and tools in reproductive healthcare.

16.1 INTRODUCTION

Text Mining was defined as "the non-trivial extraction of hidden, previously unknown, and potentially useful information from (large

Holistic Approaches for Women's Sustainable Health, Volume 2: Advancements, Socioeconomic Impacts, and Innovative Strategies. Junaid Ahmad Malik, Anamika Chauhan, and Megh R. Goyal (Eds)

DOI: 10.1201/9781779641656-19

amount of) textual data" by Daniel Waegel in his thesis describing the first version of long-short term memory (LSTM) (TextMOLE) system for textual data mining [32]. It is an essential component of natural language processing (NLP) which is a subfield of artificial intelligence (AI) that aims to understand human language and extract useful information from available data to assist in patient care and clinical research through the identification of patterns and trends in sexual and reproductive health issues by facilitating the extraction, processing, and derivation of structured data from unstructured data found in electronic medical records (EMRs), medical literature, and patient notes. In the context of reproductive medicine, NLP can be applied to analyze EMRs, extract relevant information for clinical decision-making, and support research studies by processing and summarizing medical literature. By leveraging NLP techniques, healthcare providers can improve the efficiency of information retrieval, enhance clinical decision support systems, and ultimately contribute to better patient care and outcomes in reproductive health [2].

16.2 MODES OF TEXT CLASSIFICATION

For efficient categorization of data, several text classification techniques encompassing deep learning models such as neural networks, decision trees, K-nearest neighbors, support vector machines (SVMs), and Bayesian classification. Decision trees facilitate data interpretation by constructing tree-like structures with nodes representing features and branches representing decision rules, while SVMs delineate decision boundaries between classes by maximizing the margin, thus accommodating both linear and nonlinear separation through kernels. Co-occurring terms are identified to predict classes in association-based classification, whereas in centroid-based classification, centroids are clustered by assigning labels on the basis of the proximity of data points. Moreover, K-nearest neighbor classification involves the assignment of labels via measurement of similarities among the k-nearest neighbors in a feature space as per majority classes, and Bayesian classification uses Bayesian theory to predict a class value for a given set of features. Each method offers distinct advantages and is selected based on the nature of the data and the specific classification task at hand.

16.3 METHODS

16.3.1 TERM BASED

"Term" refers to any expression having a significant meaning and may denote a specific concept. Documents are assessed on the basis of a term in this method, offering efficient computing performance and benefits from well-established weighting theories [25]. However, one cannot solely rely on term-based methods due to issues like polysemy (a word can have multiple meanings), synonymy (multiple terms may refer to a singular concept), and the extraction of terms whose meaning is uncertain, often obscuring information desired by the user.

16.3.2 PHRASE BASED

As the name suggests, phrase-based methods involve the analysis of phrases or groups of words at a single stretch, rather than individual terms, as in the case of term-based methods. This method makes the access and interpretation of information much more contextual [21]. Nevertheless, he phrase-based method has its own set of limitations, including increased phrase redundancy, poor statistical attributes, low frequency of occurrence of specific phrases, and escalated amounts of noisy phrases.

16.3.3 CONCEPT BASED

Concept-based method is not only capable of distinguishing between redundant and significant terms that encompass a sentence but also statistically analyzes words and phrases, thus eliminating noise and redundancy, subsequently overcoming the hurdles of the phrase-based method. Concept-based models run on three key steps—sentences' semantic structure evaluation, semantic structure description via construction of a conceptual ontological graph, and extraction of featured concepts using a vector space model [9].

16.3.4 PATTERN TAXONOMY

The pattern taxonomy approach is employed to analyze documents, organizing them into a taxonomy using "is-a" relationships. Techniques like rule mining and frequent item set mining refine patterns, providing superior performance compared to concept-based and term-based methods. In text mining, challenges arise with applying discovered patterns due to issues like misinterpretations and low-frequency patterns. A proposed pattern-based methodology addresses these challenges by deploying and evolving patterns. Experimental results highlight the enhanced performance of the pattern-based model in text analysis compared to alternative data mining and concept-based approaches [36].

16.4 APPROACHES

16.4.1 TEXT PROCESSING

Text processing refers to the handling and examination of text data to perform functions, including breaking up text into single words or tokens (tokenization), reducing words to their basic or root form (stemming), and combining variations of a specific word (lemmatization).

16.4.2 NAMED ENTITY RECOGNITION (NER)

The identification and classification of specific entities (like patient names, age, location, medical anomalies) in clinical reports for the extraction of relationships or any other information necessary for retrieval or organization of data with respect to the patient's reproductive health concern is known as NER. It assists in the mining of biomedical abbreviations and synonyms, rearrangement of literature searches, and establishment of links between concepts, thereby leading to the enhancement of data quality and facilitating the creation of structured knowledge bases.

16.4.3 SUMMARIZATION

Condensation of large volumes of content into concise and short summaries; this approach in data mining is used to extract key information from extensive research articles or medical reports.

16.4.4 CATEGORIZATION/CLASSIFICATION

As the name suggests, it refers to the sorting of textual data into predefined classes or labels; in the field of reproductive healthcare, it can be employed in triaging of patient inquiries, classification of medical literature, and identification of disease-related research publications.

16.4.5 VISUALIZATION

The representation of data in visual form through the use of maps, graphs, word clouds, and charts to provide an effective and quick summary of not just keywords but also patterns and trends observed in papers, including clinical notes, journals, records, etc.

16.4.6 RELATION EXTRACTION (RE)

A method within information extraction that aims at establishing meaningful relations between keywords, concepts, or phenomena, followed by their classification and labelling. RE forms an important component of methodologies aiming at disease diagnosis or novel clinical discoveries.

16.4.7 CLUSTERING

Grouping of similar keywords, terms, or concepts, which helps in combining documents relevant to a particular health concern, is known as clustering. There are various machine learning (ML) models, such as k-means clustering, hierarchical clustering, and density-based clustering that can be used for clustering.

16.4.8 TOPIC TRACKING

It is the process of examining conversations or exchanges between two or more parties for the purpose of understanding and identifying topics, patterns, and trends. Topic tracking may be used in the compilation of research documents regarding a specific ailment or the development of clinical databases.

16.4.9 QUESTION ANSWERING

Often one of the key features of chatbots, question answering systems to assimilate information given by the user and provide appropriate responses to the same in human-like language or in natural conversational style, thus facilitating smooth retrieval of information from large volumes of data.

16.4.10 SENTIMENT ANALYSIS

Sentiment analysis refers to the determination of emotions expressed in text; it may be used for the analysis of patient feedback for counselling purposes, public sentiments via social media posts, and patient experiences for the development of new strategies when dealing with sensitive topics pertaining to reproductive healthcare (Figure 16.1).

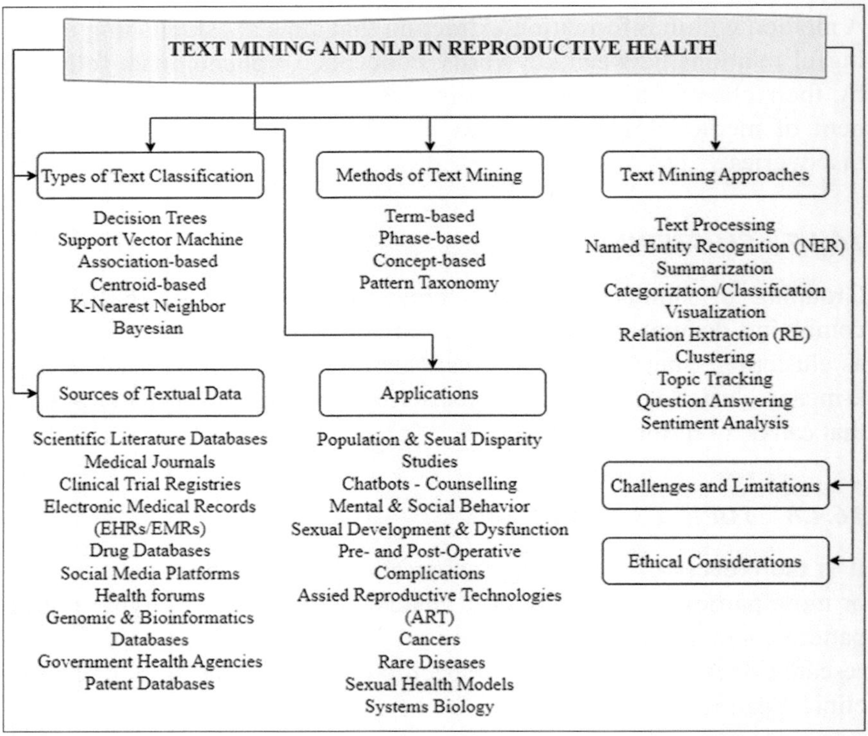

FIGURE 16.1 Basic concepts in text mining and NLP in reproductive health.

16.5 ROLE OF TEXT MINING AND NLP IN AI, ML, AND BIG DATA

Big data analytics offers a cost-effective approach to acquiring and analyzing data by employing computational techniques like text mining, which can be used to extract and expound upon valuable medical concepts from unstructured information sources like free-text documents in electronic health records (EHRs) and streamline processes to achieve efficiency and low-labor intensity. NLP techniques are utilized by AI models to contain information that can be used for pretraining, subsequently contributing to clinical decision support, predictive modeling, and individualized treatment strategies in reproductive medicine. Ultimately, this leads to enhanced treatment results and improved patient care. Furthermore, within ML models, it facilitates tasks such as information retrieval, sentiment analysis, and document classification, which aid in decision-making and driving intelligent insights. In a nutshell, AI in reproductive medicine holds the potential to revolutionize clinical practice, improve patient outcomes, and contribute to the advancement of reproductive and sexual healthcare [20].

16.6 DATA SOURCES FOR RESEARCH AND CLINICAL STUDIES

In addition to its applications, text mining and knowledge extraction leverage various sources of biomedical data to advance research, decision-making, and knowledge discovery; these include scientific literature databases such as Google Scholar and PubMed, medical journals like The Lancet and Journal of the American Medical Association, and clinical trial registries like ClinicalTrials.gov to stay abreast with completed and clinical trials all over the world. Moreover, patient data, history, and clinical notes contained in EMRs, along with drug databases, such as DrugBank, facilitate recognition patterns and establishment of comprehensive effective treatment strategies. Nowadays, social media platforms and health forums are too considered as sources since they not only report outcomes and experiences but also help uncover population trends, while genomic and bioinformatics databases like GenBank, UniProt, and National Center for Biotechnology Information contain genomic data and associations with diseases, informing research on the genetic basis of diseases and therapeutic targets. Government health agencies (National Institutes of Health and Centers for Disease Control and Prevention (CDC) in the USA, Central Bureau of Health Intelligence in India) and patent databases (Patent database of India, United States Patent and Trademark Office) also offer valuable datasets and reports related to public health, epidemiology, and intellectual property in healthcare.

16.7 APPLICATIONS OF TEXT ANALYTICS IN REPRODUCTIVE HEALTHCARE

16.7.1 POPULATION AND SEXUAL DISPARITY STUDIES

The analysis of clinical notes from the MIMIC III dataset in the EMR of atherosclerotic cardiovascular disease patients was done with the application of NLP within the clinical bidirectional encoder representations from transformers (Clinical BERT) deep learning model by Witting et al. [35]. The NLP training's gold standard was developed by manual annotation of clinical notes chosen randomly to distinguish between prescription and nonprescription of statins, and the study of reasons behind the latter; this step was followed by splitting of the dataset into test and training sets. The model created was validated via 10-fold cross-validation, and the hyperparameters were fine-tuned. After the comparison of metrics, including precision recall, F1 score, and area under the curve (AUC) for the assessment of the model performance, the highest performing model was implemented in the determination of primary and secondary outcomes within the clinical notes.

Xie et al. used NLP to identify the status of homelessness and housing instability among seriously ill patients by processing clinical records accompanying medical encounters within the period of 6 months prior and after the diagnosis. Chart review iterations and conclusions drawn from them were utilized for algorithm refinement to ensure uniformity within population data, subsequently converting medical records to structured data for determining patients who were homeless or at risk of homelessness [38].

16.7.2 CHATBOTS AND THEIR ROLE IN COUNSELLING

Ever since conversation-stimulating internet-based computer programs have seen the light, efforts have been taken to tailor-stitch chatbots' personality traits in accordance with users or their preferences to facilitate engaging conversations that promote empathy, provide anonymous nonjudgmental emotional support (especially when tackling sensitive subjects such as infertility or life-threatening diagnosis), respond at a human-like pace, and iterate according to user-fed responses [30].

User experiences with chatbots have suggested the possible advancements in women's health by providing round-the-clock improved and immediate access to information, enhancing the understanding of concept within women's health, maintaining strong relations with regular users, building self-concept among women conscious about their issues, integrating, sharing, and extracting information to and from various networks and people, and addressing sexual and reproductive health (SRH)-related stigmas [18].

Chatbots not only find application in the field of women's health and related disorders but also in male sexual well-being. The AI-powered ChatGPT chatbot has proven to be capable of responding to practitioners' queries on common urological matters, including but not limited to infertility in males, decreased testosterone levels, and Peyronie's disease, thereby acting as an instantaneous, accessible, and reliable source of information to not just urologists but also suspecting patients or general information seekers [27].

Text mining and NLP techniques involving the use of computational tools and algorithms to extract and analyze linguistic features such as the frequency of specific words (e.g., positive and negative affect words, sexual words, emotion words), syntactic patterns, and semantic content were utilized to study the language used by women with or without childhood sexual abuse history in writing essays in the research by Pulverman et al. [22]. Essays were written by participants on neutral as well as sexually ambiguous or sexual self-schema-related topics. They were able to quantitatively assess the language used in the essays and identify differences in linguistic patterns between women with and without histories of CSA. This approach allowed for a more objective and systematic analysis of the women's expressive writing, providing insights into the cognitive processes and emotional experiences related to sexuality in the context of childhood sexual abuse, which could be later used for counselling purposes.

In a study by Chervenak et al., VADER (Valence Aware Dictionary and sEntiment Reasoner), which operates as a rule-based model, was utilized for the sentiment analysis of responses given by ChatGPT for fertility-related questions [5]. VADER assigned polarity and intensity scores to words or phrases based on a predefined sentiment lexicon, hence allowing analysis of clinical narratives, patient feedback, or online discussions regarding all sorts of reproductive health concerns. Similarly, Textblob, a Python library for text processing, which has been used to assess the function of ChaGPT as a counselling tool by conducting sentiment analysis, was also utilized [10]. Within the same study by Chervenak et al., ChatPGT was used over three domains—Response to CDS FAQs on infertility, Cardiff Fertility Knowledge Scale, and the Fertility and Infertility Treatment Knowledge Score (FIT-KS), with an objective of establishing its use as a fertility counseling tool. Although the answers generated by ChatGPT were comparable to CDC in terms of facts described, length, and subjectivity, it outperformed it by providing more facts for approximately half of the queries at an error rate of 6.12% and 0.68% assertions having their references cited. Not only did the chatbot attain higher scores than published population data in FKS and FIT-KS surveys, but it also managed to replicate facts missing from the American Society for Reproductive Medicine committee opinion on “Optimizing Natural Fertility” with perfect accuracy. Although ChatGPT shows tremendous potential in fertility-related interactions, concerns remain regarding data corruption, result manipulation, and suboptimal model performance.

The ANA Chatbot played a pivotal role in the “Chup! Jom Sembang Seks” (loosely translated to “Let’s Talk about Sex!”) campaign in Malaysia, which was developed by the Federation of Reproductive Health Associations, UNICEF, and R.AGE to address common misconceptions and educate youth and young adults regarding various aspects of SRH [17]. Liew et al. explored the effect of certain AI attributes (perceived intelligence and anthropomorphism) on intention, trust, and engagement of users and their subsequent behavioral and attitude change toward the ANA chatbot, thereby providing insights and reporting knowledge gaps to the concerned authorities.

Wang et al. developed a safe, nonjudgmental platform for the discussion on sensitive SRH-related topics, including contraception, family planning, and safe sex in the form of the SnehAI chatbot, which not only offers reliable information in the form of open, honest, and engaging conversations but also gives personalized responses pertaining to the users’ queries [33]. The chatbot shares necessary information on local services (helplines for counseling or reporting sexual assault) that they can access, thus allowing individuals to take independent and informed decisions on their SRH-related issues. Similarly, the AdolescentBot, as discussed in the paper by Rahman et al., serves as a vital resource for adolescents in Bangladesh by focusing on reproductive health support and information sharing [23].

16.7.3 MENTAL AND SOCIAL BEHAVIOR TOWARD SRH

The study by Valdez et al. utilized the unsupervised NLP Latent Dirichlet Allocation topic models to examine content and common themes of Spanish tweets associated with abortion-themed identity labels within Spanish tweets like "proelección," "derecho a decider," "proaborto," "provida," "antiaborto," and "derecho a vivir," which mean pro-choice, right to choose, pro-abortion, pro-life, antiabortion, and right to life, respectively [31]. It was revealed that direct translation of keywords such as pro-choice and pro-life may not be adequate to conduct surveys in either English or Spanish, since the Spanish labels were not as forthright as their English counterparts, thus leading to confusion, further harming quality of data. The study inferred that labelling, survey generation, and data generation should be done keeping in mind the nation of origin of participants such that when tackling issues concerning multicultural and multilingual individuals, the tasks at hand can be clearly and concisely explained to those involved.

16.7.4 SEXUAL DEVELOPMENT AND DYSFUNCTION

The Mayo clinical Text Analysis and Knowledge Extraction System (cTAKES) may be employed in various applications in women's health, including conditions like polycystic ovary syndrome (PCOS) through which valuable information from clinical narratives related to disorders, such as symptoms, diagnostic criteria, treatment options, and patient outcomes, could be extracted. It could involve developing specific modules or customizing existing components to recognize relevant entities and relationships within the clinical text [4]. This can aid in automating the extraction of PCOS-related information from EMRs, research studies, and other healthcare documents. Overall, 32 terms were used to build an algorithm for the identification of PCOS cases by processing clinical text notes using cTAKES; an AUC of 0.87, positive predictive value of 91%, and cutoff value as 0.392 for PCOS were attained, resulting in the classification of 6295 candidates in the given set as those suffering from PCOS [4].

Google Trends data offers valuable insights into public health behaviors related to sexual and reproductive health by analyzing query patterns over time, thus complementing standard data collection methods for researchers by widening scope of knowledge discovery, helps guide practitioners in clinical-decision making, and policymakers in weighing women's health issues [13]. It allows authorities to determine common interests, developing interests and problems faced, and concerns of the population and predict trends in health behaviors, such as forecasting unplanned pregnancies or abortions during specific periods like the COVID-19 pandemic. Evidence-based decision-making not only aids in the implementation of measures but also in the development of educational programs and SRH kits for the public good.

16.7.5 PRE- AND POSTOPERATIVE COMPLICATIONS

Text mining techniques also find applications in the detection of post- and preoperative complications. Between the years 2009 and 2020, at the Kaiser Permanente Southern California (KPSC), Xie et al. implemented an algorithm that was established and corroborated using data extracted from EHRs for the classification of preterm labor evaluation visits for the exploration of preterm labors such as physiological descriptions, medications prescribed, ultrasound, abdominal pain, uterine contractions, fetal fibronectin tests [37]. The data generated was further compared with the studies on retrospective studies on live births and pregnancies during that time period at KPSC hospitals. It was discovered that the algorithm created was highly specific and sensitive in determining preterm labor evaluation visits and their methods of evaluation, thereby succeeding in achieving accurate results.

16.7.6 ASSISTED REPRODUCTIVE TECHNOLOGIES

Extracting key concepts and trends from textual data on reproductive medicine through text mining enables researchers and practitioners to not only gain knowledge in the form of medical guidelines, clinical studies, research papers, and scientific literature and keep up with latest advancements in the field of artificial reproductive technologies but also gain clarity through patient data (medical records and notes) analysis to cater to their specific needs for patient, their management, personalized treatment strategies, and medication choices. Moreover, text mining, when combined with image analysis, assists in the evaluation of reproductive cells (oocytes, embryos, and sperms) offering in-depth perceptions into morphology, genetic characteristics, and viability and assisting in candidate selection for fertilization and implantation. Treatment outcomes, patient consultations, and fertility histories can be studied by text mining algorithms for the prediction of artificial reproductive technologies, subsequently predicting pregnancies. Thus, NLP-powered artificial reproductive technologies facilities have the potential to enhance reproductive medicine [34].

16.7.7 INFERTILITY

Language models might transform research in gynecology and infertility by providing quick access to pertinent data, formulating diagnostic hypotheses, integrating information sources, improving decision-making, and discovering new perceptions. In a letter to the editor, Wang et al. elucidated on the potential and differences between advanced learning language models ChatGPT 3.5 and ChatGPT 4 in not just text generation but also contextual understanding of reproductive health issues, customization, and synthesis of gynecological data [26]. ChatGPT 3.5 demonstrated enhanced natural language creation in comparison to its predecessor, while ChatGPT 4 continued to enhance this capability. ChatGPT 4 improved upon its predecessor by not only improving long-term memory but also offering more comprehensive user-driven fine-tuning and domain adaption. ChatGPT 3.5 demonstrated skill in combining complex gynecological research data, whereas ChatGPT 4 stood out in creating coherent summaries of study findings. Hence, it can be established that with time active efforts are being made to augment user interface and experiences of women with respect to infertility and other gynecological issues.

16.7.8 CANCER OF SPECIFIC TISSUES

By investigating information from EMRs, text mining provides valuable support to clinical decision-making in cancer care, including identification of cancer risk factors, cancer, recognition of patterns in treatment outcomes, and optimization of patient management [28]. In a study by Labrosse et al., text mining technologies were used to perform text-based and phrase-based methods to pinpoint pregnancy cases post breast cancer diagnosis within large volumes of EMR. Data curated was further investigated, thereby establishing a smooth workflow and efficient method for cancer-related clinical decision making [12]. NLP techniques have also been used in thyroid cancer analysis [15].

16.7.9 RARE DISEASES

Timely diagnosis is crucial for enhancing patient outcomes, averting permanent damage, and enabling efficient disease care for patients with rare disorders. As per the study by Liévin et al., the FindZebra search engine improves search capabilities by leveraging NLP techniques to assist practitioners to attain precise diagnoses; it does so by initially collecting a large variety of data on the detection of uncommon illnesses with elaborate phenotypes through clinical reports available on PubMed, followed by usage of Apache Solr for the creation of search indices for every condition incorporating numerous criteria (age, gender, clinical traits) through textual dissemination, thereby enhancing the specificity of the search results obtained, which are further retrospectively validated by health specialists using real-world outcomes survey data on patients with illnesses like Gaucher and Fabry to ensure their clinical significance and practicality [16]. Thus, FindZebra has the potential to help medical professionals examine the search results to determine their clinical significance for certain patient groups, helping identify strengths and limits in aiding clinicians in detecting uncommon illnesses.

16.7.10 SEXUAL HEALTH MODELS

Sexual health models are structured frameworks that encompass treatment, policy advocacy, education, prevention, diagnosis, and support services with the aim of fostering sexual wellness. In order to prevent unintended pregnancies and venereal disorder, educational awareness programs are conducted to emphasize safe sex practices and vaccinations, whereas diagnosis and treatment services equip individuals with healthcare access to address sexually transmitted infections, infertility, and sexual dysfunction. Psychosocial support systems encompassing counseling for relationship difficulties and sexual trauma, and advocacy for policy initiatives that promote gender equality, LGBTQ+ inclusion, reproductive health rights, and access to sexual health services also form a part of sexual health models [7]. Various models such as the biopsychosocial model, the WHO sexual health model, and the PLISSIT model provide distinct viewpoints on sexual health by focusing on biological processes, individual rights, counseling treatments, and socioecological impacts. A number of models developed emphasize on the use of NLP to augment access to imperative reproductive health services such as the Recognition Model, as proposed by Couldrick et al., which aims to cater to disabled individuals and their treatment as sexual beings with distinct desires and needs like any other individual [6]. The authors emphasized on the promotion of an environment that is conducive to addressing the needs of the disabled requires practitioners to acknowledge the sexual identity of service users and give priority to their sexual requirements when developing service plans, which involves team-work, validation, normalization, and affirmation.

16.7.11 INTEGRATION OF SYSTEMS BIOLOGY WITH EMR

Due to enhanced clinical genomic understanding and analytical techniques like next-generation sequencing, there has been an advancement in genetic research. Moreover, the increase in access and the decrease in genotyping costs have led to the involvement of larger demographic groups and widened the scope of research projects. The comprehension of diseases and conception of treatments facilitated by the evolution of computational methodologies required in genomic data analysis has resulted in the discovery of genetic links and tailored medical strategies. The adoption of NLP techniques in extracting structured data from unstructured text present in genomic and pharmacogenomic research contained in EMRs enables the identification of pertinent phenotypic traits and the establishment of high-validity collections of cases and controls for specific conditions in precision medicine and personalized healthcare initiatives.

16.7.12 OTHER TOOLS

16.7.12.1 BIDIRECTIONAL ENCODER REPRESENTATIONS FROM TRANSFORMERS (BERT)

BERT is a deep learning language model that is pretrained on clinical records from various datasets and provides an upper hand during biomedical text mining through its improved performance, area-specific comprehension and answering capabilities, and quicker analysis of bulky reproductive health data. It has been implemented in the detection of infertility as well as PCOS. There are multiple versions of BERT that have been employed in the study of patterns and further in clinical decision-making; these include MedBERT, BioBERT, and ClinicalBERT [3, 11, 24].

16.7.12.2 FERTILOME® MULTIGENE PANEL TEST

By analyzing about 4758 studies to identify genetic regions linked to female reproductive conditions, Strom et al. developed this genetic test to aid reproductive endocrinologists in the evaluation of infertile couples through the identification of genetic factors linked to perpetual female reproductive disorders. The Fertilome® Multigene Panel Test examines genetic variations in 32 genes involved in immune response regulation, hormone regulation, and DNA replication, which are strongly associated with conditions like endometriosis, PCOS, and recurrent pregnancy loss [29].

16.7.12.3 DRUGEX

The DrugEx system proposed in the study by Alfattni et al. involves the employment of two text mining methods—NER for the identification of drugs, their strength, their dosage, frequency, form, route, and reason for administration, and rule-based RE for determining the relationship of the of the entities identified via NER to the concerned ailment, which was further assessed against a content-aware LSTM model using the 2018 n2c2 shared task data. It utilizes advanced deep learning techniques such as bidirectional LSTM with conditional random fields and many types of embeddings (word, character, and semantic feature) to analyze the impact of different embeddings on performance [1]. The suggested comprehensive system successfully obtained positive results and showed the possibility of using deep learning techniques to extract drug details from unstructured text input.

16.7.12.4 BREAST AND OVARIAN ANALYSIS OF DISEASE INCIDENCE AND CARRIER ESTIMATION ALGORITHM

This prediction model estimates one's risk of developing breast cancer by collecting and integrating data on a large number of genetic factors–common genetic variants selected according to their SNP-based polygenic risk scores and rare pathogenic variants (ATM, BRCA1, BRCA2, CHEK2, and PALB2) and nongenetic risk factors such mammographic density, hormonal factors, lifestyle factors, and reproductive history. The risk subsequently calculated forms the basis of categorizing individuals and allowing the determination of their need for screening, prevention, consultation, or risk management [14] (Figure 16.2).

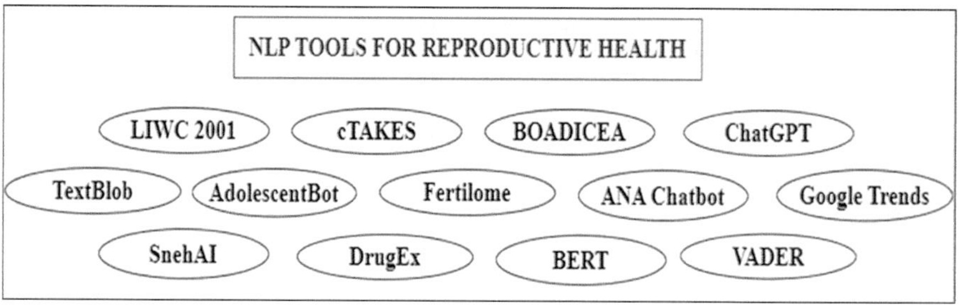

FIGURE 16.2 Some text mining tools and their applications.

16.8 CHALLENGES, LIMITATIONS, AND ETHICAL CONSIDERATIONS

There are several key data management challenges that need to be addressed when delving into women's health research. Historical data bias due to greater male attention and limited female representation in biomedical research in the past has impeded comprehensive study and created research gaps in feminine health anomalies and their effective treatment, especially in minority populations. Hence, it is necessary to take into account factors (race, age, gender identity, medical history, or ethnicity) that may affect calculations and biochemical levels during analysis and the changes they may result in during data interpretation. Besides equitable data access, it is also necessary to ensure promotion, support, and smooth functioning of studies dealing with women's health; since it has been found that in comparison to their male counterparts, female researchers struggle with resource allocation and attaining funding for their projects, subsequently leading to disparity, inconsistency, and incoherence in women-centric projects [19]. To guarantee uniform and precise results for treatment or further research on a specific reproductive health concern, one could use a standardized coding system that would facilitate the integration of information from various medical databases, consider sensitive details, as well as tend to ethical considerations. Besides protecting patient privacy and data security, the use of cutting-edge ML techniques for data mining could overcome the challenges faced when performing statistical methods, thus maintaining accuracy, consistency, and integrity, especially when various data sources, and impending processing of data have to be considered [8].

16.9 SUMMARY

The digital age is reshaping reproductive health by leveraging data science, ML, and AI. Text mining and NLP methodologies play a pivotal role, offering opportunities for valuable insights, improved healthcare outcomes, and a deeper understanding of reproductive health. This transformation spans various domains, including counseling, population studies, analysis of sexual disparities, mental and social behaviors, sexual development, assessment of complications, ART, and infertility examination. The utilization of models and tools such as TextBlob, Clinical BERT, GPT, and VADER is explored, alongside considerations of ethical implications and potential advancements in AI-driven reproductive healthcare.

KEYWORDS

- **text mining**
- **natural language processing**
- **chatbot**
- **reproductive health**

REFERENCES

1. Alfattni, G., Belousov, M., Peek, N., & Nenadic, G. (2021). Extracting drug names and associated attributes from discharge summaries: Text mining study. *JMIR Medical Informatics, 9*(5), e24678.
2. Bansod, A. R., Jha, R. K., More, A., & Fadnavis, R. A. (2022). Artificial intelligence in reproductive medicine. *Journal of Datta Meghe Institute of Medical Sciences University*, *17*(2), 499–503.
3. Borole, Y. D., Agrawal, A. V., Tesfayohanis, M., Thakkar, D., Abonazel, M. R., & Awwad, F. A. (2022). [Retracted] BERT-based clinical name entity reorganization model for health diagnosis. *Disease Markers*, *2022*(1), 2297063.
4. Castro, V., Shen, Y., Yu, S., Finan, S., Pau, C. T., Gainer, V., Keefe, C. C., Savova, G., Murphy, S. N., Cai, T., & Welt, C. K. (2015). Identification of subjects with polycystic ovary syndrome using electronic health records. *Reproductive Biology and Endocrinology*, *13*, 1–8.

5. Chervenak, J., Lieman, H., Blanco-Breindel, M., & Jindal, S. (2023). The promise and peril of using a large language model to obtain clinical information: ChatGPT performs strongly as a fertility counseling tool with limitations. *Fertility and Sterility*, *120*(3), 575–583.
6. Couldrick, L., Sadlo, G., & Cross, V. (2010). Proposing a new sexual health model of practice for disability teams: The Recognition Model. *International Journal of Therapy and Rehabilitation*, *17*(6), 290–299.
7. Curchoe, C. L., Malmsten, J., Bormann, C., Shafiee, H., Farias, A. F. S., Mendizabal, G., & Rosenwaks, Z. (2020). Predictive modeling in reproductive medicine: Where will the future of artificial intelligence research take us. *Fertility and Sterility*, *114*(5), 934–940.
8. Dong, T., Zhu, M., Li, R., & Wang, X. (2022). Challenges of utilizing medical big data in reproductive health research. *Frontiers in Reproductive Health*, *4*, 800760.
9. Gaikwad, S. V., Chaugule, A., & Patil, P. (2014). Text mining methods and techniques. *International Journal of Computer Applications*, *85*(17), 42–45.
10. Hazarika, D., Konwar, G., Deb, S., & Bora, D. J. (2020). Sentiment analysis on twitter by using TextBlob for natural language processing. *ICRMAT*, *24*, 63–67.
11. Kawazoe, Y., Shibata, D., Shinohara, E., Aramaki, E., & Ohe, K. (2021). A clinical specific BERT developed using a huge Japanese clinical text corpus. *PLoS One*, *16*(11), e0259763.
12. Labrosse, J., Lam, T., Sebbag, C., Benque, M., Abdennebi, I., Merckelbagh, H., Osdoit, M., Priour, M., Guerin, J., Balezeau, T., Grandal, B., Coussy, F., Bobrie, A., Ferrer, L., Laas, E., Feron, J.-G., Reyal, F., & Hamy, A.-S. (2019). Text mining in electronic medical records enables quick and efficient identification of pregnancy cases occurring after breast cancer. *JCO Clinical Cancer Informatics*, *3*, 1–12. doi: 10.1200/CCI.19
13. Larki, M., Manouchehri, E., & Latifnejad Roudsari, R. (2022). Using google trends in infodemiological studies in sexual and reproductive health research. *Journal of Midwifery and Reproductive Health*, *10*(4), 3529–3533.
14. Lee, A., Mavaddat, N., Wilcox, A. N., Cunningham, A. P., Carver, T., Hartley, S., Babb de Villiers, C., Izquierdo, A., Simard, J., Schmidt, M. K., Walter, F. M., Chatterjee, N., Garcia-Closas, M., Tischkowitz, M., Pharoah, P., Easton, D. F., & Antoniou, A. C. (2019). BOADICEA: A comprehensive breast cancer risk prediction model incorporating genetic and nongenetic risk factors. *Genetics in Medicine*, *21*(8), 1708–1718.
15. Lian, R., Hsiao, V., Hwang, J., Ou, Y., Robbins, S. E., Connor, N. P., Macdonald, C. L., Sippel, R. S., Sethares, W. A., & Schneider, D. F. (2023). Predicting health-related quality of life change using natural language processing in thyroid cancer. *Intelligence-based Medicine*, *7*, 100097.
16. Liévin, V., Hansen, J. M., Lund, A., Elstein, D., Matthiesen, M. E., Elomaa, K., Zarakowska, K., Himmelhan, I., Botha, J., Borgeskov, H., & Winther, O. (2023). FindZebra online search delving into rare disease case reports using natural language processing. *PLoS Digital Health*, *2*(6), e0000269.
17. Liew, T. W., Tan, S. M., Yoo, N. E., Gan, C. L., & Lee, Y. Y. (2023). Let's talk about Sex!: AI and relational factors in the adoption of a chatbot conveying sexual and reproductive health information. *Computers in Human Behavior Reports*, *11*, 100323.

18. Mills, R., Mangone, E. R., Lesh, N., Mohan, D., & Baraitser, P. (2023). Chatbots to improve sexual and reproductive health: Realist synthesis. *Journal of Medical Internet Research*, *25*, e46761.
19. Mirin, A. A. (2021). Gender disparity in the funding of diseases by the US National Institutes of Health. *Journal of Women's Health*, *30*(7), 956–963.
20. Murdoch, T. B., & Detsky, A. S. (2013). The inevitable application of big data to health care. *JAMA*, *309*(13), 1351–1352.
21. Bhattarai, P. (2022). Introduction to text mining with R. RPubs by R studio. https://rpubs.com/vipero7/introduction-to-text-mining-with-r
22. Pulverman, C. S., Kilimnik, C. D., & Meston, C. M. (2018). The impact of childhood sexual abuse on women's sexual health: A comprehensive review. *Sexual Medicine Reviews*, *6*(2), 188–200.
23. Rahman, R., Rahman, M. R., Tripto, N. I., Ali, M. E., Apon, S. H., & Shahriyar, R. (2021, May). AdolescentBot: Understanding opportunities for chatbots in combating adolescent sexual and reproductive health problems in Bangladesh. In: *Proceedings of the 2021 CHI Conference on Human Factors in Computing Systems* (pp. 1–15).
24. Rasmy, L., Xiang, Y., Xie, Z., Tao, C., & Zhi, D. (2021). Med-BERT: Pretrained contextualized embeddings on large-scale structured electronic health records for disease prediction. *NPJ Digital Medicine*, *4*(1), 86.
25. Reddy, S., Rotker, K. L., Honig, S. C., & Harnisch, B. (2023). High capability of ChatGPT to answer common patient questions encountered by reproductive urologist. *Fertility and Sterility*, *120*(4), e254.
26. Salton, G., & Buckley, C. (1988). Term-weighting approaches in automatic text retrieval. *Information Processing & Management*, *24*(5), 513–523.
27. Sengupta, P., Dutta, S., Chakravarthi, S., Jegasothy, R., Jeganathan, R., & Pichumani, A. (2023). Comparative efficacy of ChatGPT 3.5, ChatGPT 4, and other large language models in gynecology and infertility research. *Gynecology and Obstetrics Clinical Medicine*, *3*(4), 203–206.
28. Spasić, I., Livsey, J., Keane, J. A., & Nenadić, G. (2014). Text mining of cancer-related information: Review of current status and future directions. *International Journal of Medical Informatics*, *83*(9), 605–623.
29. Strom, C. B., Northrop, L. E., & Beim, P. Y. (2019). Introducing the Fertilome® multigene panel test: A genetic test for female reproductive health and fertility. *Reproductive BioMedicine Online*, *38*, e7.
30. Technology, I. D. P. M., & Cycle, S. (2018). Women's experience of a sexual and reproductive health chatbot Women's experience of a sexual and reproductive health chatbot Women's experience of a sexual and reproductive health chatbot.
31. Valdez, D., Jozkowski, K. N., Montenegro, M. S., Crawford, B. L., & Jackson, F. (2022). Identifying accurate pro-choice and pro-life identity labels in Spanish: Social media insights and implications for comparative survey research. *Perspectives on Sexual and Reproductive Health*, *54*(4), 166–176.
32. Waegel, D. (2006). *The Development of Text-Mining Tools and Algorithms*. Ursinus College.
33. Wang, H., Gupta, S., Singhal, A., Muttreja, P., Singh, S., Sharma, P., & Piterova, A. (2022). An artificial intelligence chatbot for young people's sexual and reproductive

health in India (SnehAI): Instrumental case study. *Journal of Medical Internet Research*, *24*(1), e29969.
34. Wang, R., Pan, W., Jin, L., Li, Y., Geng, Y., Gao, C., Chen, G., Wang, H., Ma, D., & Liao, S. (2019). Artificial intelligence in reproductive medicine. *Reproduction*, *158*(4), R139–R154.
35. Witting, C., Azizi, Z., Gomez, S. E., Zammit, A., Sarraju, A., Ngo, S., Hernandez-Boussard, T. & Rodriguez, F. (2023). Natural language processing to identify reasons for sex disparity in statin prescriptions. *American Journal of Preventive Cardiology*, *14*, 100496.
36. Wu, S. T., Li, Y., Xu, Y., Pham, B., & Chen, P. (2004). Automatic pattern-taxonomy extraction for web mining. In: *IEEE/WIC/ACM International Conference on Web Intelligence (WI'04)*, (pp. 242–248). IEEE.
37. Xie, F., Khadka, N., Fassett, M. J., Chiu, V. Y., Avila, C. C., Shi, J., & Getahun, D. (2022). Identification of preterm labor evaluation visits and extraction of cervical length measures from electronic health records within a large integrated health care system: Algorithm development and validation. *JMIR Medical Informatics*, *10*(9), e37896.
38. Xie, F., Wang, S., Viveros, L., Rich, A., Nguyen, H. Q., Padilla, A., & Nau, C. L. (2023). Using natural language processing to identify the status of homelessness and housing instability among serious illness patients from clinical notes in an integrated healthcare system. *JAMIA Open*, *6*(3), ooad082.

PART IV

HOLISTIC AND TRADITIONAL APPROACHES TO FEMALE HEALTH

CHAPTER 17

Role of Religious Beliefs, Yoga, and Meditation in Empowering Female Health: Polycystic Ovarian Syndrome (PCOS)

MOUMITA DAS,[1] RITIKA RASAILY,[1] and AYAN CHATTERJEE[2*]

*Corresponding author

ABSTRACT

The women's health is of particular concern as the female reproductive system is a complex and fragile system. It is important to adapt a healthy lifestyle and protect it from long-term and life-threatening health issues. This review chapter focuses on polycystic ovarian syndrome (PCOS), which is an emerging endocrinopathy associated with multifaceted metabolic syndrome. It is caused by the formation of multiple sacs of fluid, which leads to an enlarged ovary. PCOS is characterized by hyper-androgenism and an imbalance hormonal level. It is both psychogenic and lifestyle disorder and is strongly associated with obesity, stress, and diabetes. This review focuses on the management of PCOS through yoga and meditation to lower the testosterone level and manages the stress and anxiety level, thereby balancing the hormones. The review also includes the dietary pattern in PCOS, which can manage blood sugar level to help combat the insulin resistance. It explores the physiological relationship between food and PCOS. The aim of this review is to provide valuable information for the management of PCOS through

Holistic Approaches for Women's Sustainable Health, Volume 2: Advancements, Socioeconomic Impacts, and Innovative Strategies. Junaid Ahmad Malik, Anamika Chauhan, and Megh R. Goyal (Eds)

DOI: 10.1201/9781779641656-21

simple lifestyle modification and its physiological changes and benefits to the body thereby prioritizing the reproductive health. By addressing the different aspects of PCOS and providing the scientific evidence on the relationship between yoga, meditation, dietary pattern, and the PCOS, the authors hope to contribute to the health and well-being of the female reproductive system.

17.1 INTRODUCTION

The biological makeup of a woman is molded by her unique surroundings as well as her societal, cultural, and physical factors. Health inequity is still prevalent, and women's health continues to be underfunded, undervalued, and under-researched, thus creating serious obstacles and deepening social and economic inequalities as well as gender differences. Despite recent advancements in medical science, there are considerable breaches in our knowledge of and ability to treat illnesses that affect women differently than they do men, including menstruation and maternal health issues. These differences may lead to serious health issues and avoidable treatment inequalities.

One such health issue with increasing incidence is infertility in couples at reproductive age. However, society holds the female responsible for this. Out of many, one of the reasons for female infertility is the increasing evidence of poly cystic ovarian syndrome (PCOS).

This chapter focuses on the physical (yoga and meditation) and nutritional approaches to ameliorate PCOS, one of the common gynecological problems in our society.

Prevalence of female infertility in the World and India: Infertility is of major concern in both males and females which is mainly failure to achieve pregnancy after an unprotected intercourse for over a year; however, it has a greater impact on female health. According to World Health Organization (WHO), one in six people are affected by infertility, which accounts for around 17.5% of the total population. The fertility rate of India also shows a significant decline over the past years from 2022 to 2024, ranging from 0.92% to 0.79% [64–66]. Figure 17.1 represents the fertility rate across the globe, which shows a decline in the fertility rate over time [63].

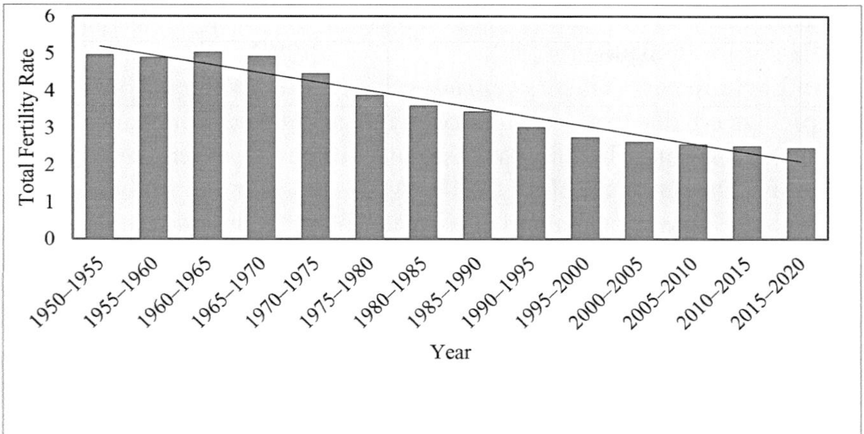

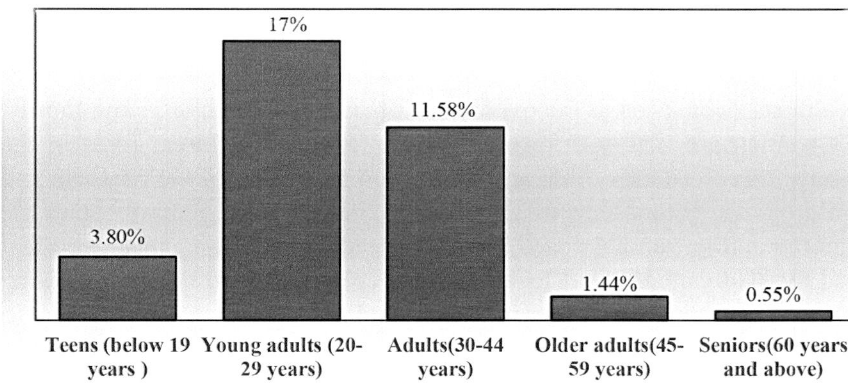

FIGURE 17.1 Graphical representation of total fertility rate across the globe (1950–2020), top; and global prevalence of PCOS in 2022 among different age groups, bottom.

Infertility issue is of concern among women, which is caused by tubal disorder, endocrine system disorder, uterine disorder, and ovarian disorder (such as PCOS), which is associated with poor lifestyle and unhealthy eating patterns. PCOS is a common cause of anovulation and infertility that may lead to obesity, cardiovascular diseases, diabetes, hypercholesterolemia, and eventually involve multiple organs. The core treatment for PCOS is lifestyle adjustment, which has been scientifically proven for managing hormones and treating infertility. Women with PCOS are at risk of abortion, spontaneous miscarriage, anovulation, the quality of oocytes decreases, insulin resistance, and prolonged hyperplasia, which may be a risk factor for implantation [56].

Importance of women's reproductive health: Women's health is of utmost concern due to several disadvantages and gender dominance rooted in our sociocultural beliefs. Women and girls at their reproductive age are in increased susceptibility to HIV/AIDS and prone to iron deficiency due to blood loss every month and greater blood supply demands during pregnancy. Certain socioeconomic factors such as inequality among men and women, sexual, physical and emotional violence, illiteracy rate among girls, and devoid of employment prevent women from getting the quality health services, which makes them more vulnerable and ignorant about the consequences of the diseases and the importance of their health [67].

Women's reproductive and sexual health issues are related to menstruation, fertility, contraception, pregnancy, cervical screening, sexually transmissible illnesses, chronic reproductive problems like PCOS, endometriosis, menopause, unplanned pregnancies, and abortions [7]. Women's health is the epitome of the family. Ensuring her with quality health services leads to the overall well-being of the children and family. As women are tied with responsibilities and play different roles in the family, therefore they often are focused on the health of their spouse and children, neglecting their own. Under such conditions, many diseases are ignored and left undiagnosed, therefore leading to breast cancer, cervical and ovarian cancer, heart diseases, gynecological conditions, pregnancy issues, autoimmune diseases, and hormonal imbalances, which can lead to anxiety and depression [55].

An overview of PCOS among women at reproductive age: PCOS is one of the most common disorders faced by females at their reproductive age; it affects around 6–12% of the total population at present. It is an endocrine disorder and is marked by hormonal imbalance. The endocrine, pituitary, hypothalamic, ovarian, adrenaline, and peripheral adipose tissues are among the glands that contribute to the imbalance associated with PCOS. It is associated with irregular menstruation and anovulation. People with PCOS are frequently associated with hyperinsulinemia, insulin resistance, and are prone to type 2 diabetes and impaired glucose tolerance. PCOS is characterized by an elevated level of testosterone, Dehydroepiandrosterone (DHEA-S), androstenedione, prolactin, higher or lower level of estrogen hormone, and higher luteinizing hormone (LH) to follicle-stimulating hormone (FSH) ratio. In PCOS, more than 10 follicles are seen as compared to the normal ovary. The cysts present in the ovary are not harmful but can be a risk factor for future diseases and lead to anovulation and complications in pregnancy along with the hormonal imbalance [39, 58, 59, 65].

Although the precise origin of PCOS is still unknown, internal factors such as insulin resistance, obesity, hyperandrogenism, environmental factors, genetics, and epigenetics may be to blame. Managing PCOS is critical since it can exacerbate conditions including metabolic syndrome, heart disease, type 2 diabetes, depression, and anxiety. The most crucial step in managing PCOS is reduction in the weight and lifestyle modification and dietary pattern which balances the hormone and regulates the menstrual cycle [22–38].

The prevalence of PCOS among women: According to the WHO article, PCOS affects 8–13% of reproductive aged women, out of which 70% is left undiagnosed [52, 65, 66]. There is a worldwide prevalence of 6–26%, and India accounts for 3.7–22.5% [45, 65]. As per the large survey conducted in India in 2020, young adults between the age group of 20–29 years are mostly affected by PCOS [65, 66]. However, there has been limited study on the prevalence of PCOS by region or ethnicity, but the recent study of 2022 shows that PCOS was common among the southern United States, followed by North Central, West, and the Northeast [34–36].

17.1.1 AN OVERVIEW OF THE STRUCTURE OF THIS REVIEW CHAPTER

The aim of this review is to provide scientific information, and the consequences of PCOS and its management through simple lifestyle modifications and healthy dietary patterns. This review connects yoga, meditation, nutrition, and PCOS. The review further discusses the role of yoga and certain yoga postures and their benefits in PCOS and its physiological and psychological changes in response to it and the positive impact and its association with PCOS. The review also covers the role of meditation and its impact on hormonal balance, thereby controlling anxiety and depression, which is commonly seen in women with PCOS. Furthermore, this review gives an insight into the importance of dietary patterns and their relationship with PCOS. Ultimately, the review provides a holistic approach in the management of PCOS and thereby promotes health and well-being.

17.2 ROLE OF YOGA IN PCOS

PCOS is merely an endocrine disorder, whose actual cause is not known, but many researchers have reported the cause of PCOS to be hormonal imbalance, stress, depression, unhealthy eating patterns, or sedentary lifestyle, and untreated PCOS can lead to cardiovascular disease, diabetes, infertility, and even cancer. Various alternative medications are available in the treatment of PCOS, which may have a faster recovery rate but are temporary and may lead to some side effects due to the chemical treatment and the dosage requirements. Moreover, using natural treatments has zero side effects and lifelong prevention of the disease.

Yoga can naturally heal the symptoms and help in the management of stress and hormonal balance, which is thought to be the main cause of PCOS. It has a superior beneficial effect than the drugs, and it purifies the body from the inside out both mentally and physically [40, 45]. Some effective yoga postures (Figure 17.2) for the management of PCOS are listed below:

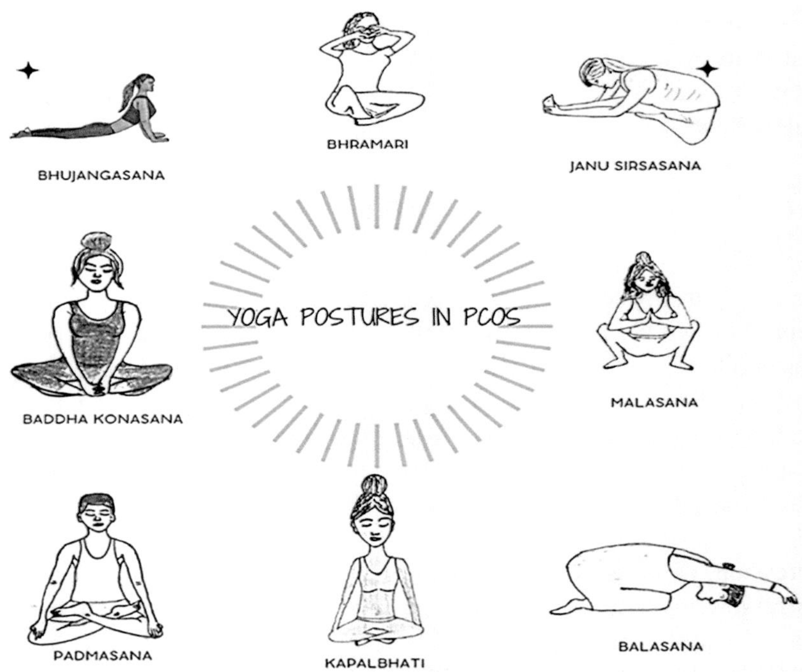
BHUJANGASANA
BHRAMARI
JANU SIRSASANA
BADDHA KONASANA
YOGA POSTURES IN PCOS
MALASANA
PADMASANA
KAPALBHATI
BALASANA

FIGURE 17.2 A visual guide for the different postures of yoga and its impact on women with PCOS.

- ***Pranayama:*** (1) ***Kapalbhati*** is a wonderful breathing technique that is associated with toning of abdominal muscles and purification of blood. The kapalbhati is practiced with normal air inhalation and forced exhalation from the abdominal musculature. The abdominal musculature is not usually involved in normal breathing; however, in kapalbhati, the involvement of the abdomen during forceful expiration produces a slow yet large tidal volume, thereby managing to cope with a stressful environment, mental and emotional stability, and better supply of oxygen in the brain and heart [60]. The women with PCOS are prone to diabetes, hypertension, atherosclerosis, cardiovascular disease, insulin resistance, and obesity, and pranayama plays a vital role in controlling the diabetes and aids in weight management and stress control, which are commonly seen in women with PCOS [2]. (2) ***Bhramari pranayama*** is best practiced in the early morning, after 5 min of defecation till 20 min. It is practiced by sitting in a comfortable position, followed by deep inhalation through the nose and exhalation with a sound "hmm" which is also referred to as humming like a bee [9]. As we see a major drift in the ratio of FSH to LH in the women with PCOS, therefore the *Bhramari pranayama* inhibits estrogen biosynthesis by preventing the hypothalamus from receiving the negative feedback of estrogen, thereby increasing the FSH level and maintaining the FSH and LH ratio and promoting ovulation and maintaining the menstrual cycle [11].

- ***Malasana*** is the strengthening of the abdominal core and pelvic floor, thereby increasing the blood flow in the pelvic region in women with PCOS [9]. It is practiced by sitting in the squat position with two knees wider apart and bringing the hands together in namaskar position by pressing the knees gently with elbows, making it wider with chest opened up and spine elongated and gently bringing the hips downward [9].

- ***Bhujangasana*** aids in regulating the menstrual cycle by exerting pressure on the stomach and improving ovarian function. It is practiced by lying down on your stomach, facing downward and placing both palms behind the chest and gently lift the head and upper body and face upward and hold the position. This pose is best for PCOS as it increases the blood flow in the pelvic region and enhances flexibility [9].

- ***Badakonasana*** is also known as a butterfly pose, which strengthens and opens the pelvic region and reduces stress. It is practiced by sitting in a comfortable position with both the knees bent and both the soles of the feet touching each other and slowly bringing the feet close to the genitals. Press the thigh downward toward the floor with a deep breath and flap both the legs for a minute and come to a halt [9].
- ***Balasana*** plays a vital role in treating PCOS. To practice the asana, kneel down on both the knees and separate both the knees apart and bring the head toward the floor with the torso between the thighs and the shoulders stretched behind the torso and relax in this position for 30 seconds to 1 minute and revert back to the normal position. This *asana* brings about control of the mind by targeting the central nervous system and regulating the menstrual cycle and bringing relief in the premenstrual syndrome and menstrual cramps, thereby regulating the blood flow throughout the body [9].
- ***Janu Sirsasan*** helps the women with PCOS. It is also known as head to knee forward bend. As PCOS is an endocrine disorder that involves a major hormonal imbalance, therefore this asana is helpful in maintaining the emotional stability, lowers the testosterone level, aids in weight management, and releases the stress and lowers anxiety and depression [9]. This asana is practiced by bending the right leg and bringing the sole of the right feet to the inner left thigh and bringing the upper body toward the left thigh and try to take hold of the feet or ankle with the hands stretched forward and hold the pose for 5–10 breaths [9].

17.2.1 PHYSIOLOGICAL AND PSYCHOLOGICAL CHANGES IN THE BODY: IMPACT OF YOGA

Practicing yoga provides several benefits to our body, both physically and mentally. Yoga helps to relieve depression, which is one of the vital problems faced by the current generation. It holds prime position in alleviating PCOS symptoms. The common problems seen in women with PCOS are stress, anxiety, and depression, which can be controlled by the simple yogic postures. The symptoms associated with PCOS are widely associated with a response to stress. The response of the human body to stress is a significant disruption of the immune function and endocrine systems, which triggers the activation of the sympathetic nervous system, the hypothalamic-pituitary-adrenal (HPA) axis, and other inflammatory responses. Depression affects the metabolism of noradrenaline, serotonin, and dopamine. Gamma-aminobutyric acid (GABA) also plays a vital role in depression. Yoga facilitates reducing the activity of the HPA axis and vagal nerve stimulation and activates the parasympathetic activity by decreasing the sympathetic activity. Yoga also regulates the release of catecholamine and cortisol, thereby decreasing the release of stress hormones and increasing the dopamine level, plasma serotonin, and boost melatonin production and is involved in the positive modification of gene expression, all of which help in reducing stress in the body and promote emotional stability and peace of mind [42, 51].

PCOS can lead to type 2 diabetes mellitus (T2DM), which is caused by insulin resistance where the cells of the organs do not respond to the insulin adequately, and it results in excessive sugar level in the blood or absolute insulin deficiency. T2DM is associated with a modern sedentary lifestyle that results in a major hormonal imbalance in women with PCOS. High level of stress in the body promotes higher sugar level in the blood and metabolic dysfunction. The stress and diabetes work bidirectionally, that is, one can influence the effect of the other [60]. Diabetes causes chronic action of HPA axis, an increase in the release of inflammatory cytokines, and an increase in the action of the sympathoadrenal system all of which are associated in response to the stress. Yoga helps in decreasing the action of HPA axis and also aids in glycemic control, which is mainly impaired in diabetes, vagal stimulation, and acts parasympathetically. It also helps in the reduction of inflammatory cytokines, blood pressure, and cardiac disease. Yoga also shows an improvement in nerve conditions and cognitive functions [50].

Yoga has direct control over the hypothalamus, pituitary, and ovarian axis, which shows a beneficial effect in women with PCOS [32]. Yogic posture regulates blood flow to the uterus and opens the pelvic region, thereby soothing the inflammation and promoting the blood flow [3]. It also helps in controlling sugar cravings and reduces the blood sugar level which is mainly associated with balancing the major hormones involved in the menstrual cycle [32]. The random experimental study was conducted between two groups to study the effect of yoga therapy in women with PCOS, and it showed a decreased LH and FSH ratio among the women who performed yoga therapy than the control group [3].

17.3 ROLE OF MEDITATION

17.3.1 STRESS AND ANXIETY IN MODERN LIFESTYLE: IMPACT OF MEDITATION

Stress is a biological response to external or internal stimulus. The pathophysiological condition changes in the body in response to stress, which can lead to various complications and can be a triggering factor for aggravating many diseases [67, 68]. Today, most of the people adapt a sedentary lifestyle and rely more on ready-to-eat, packaged, and processed foods, which can be a major factor for cardiovascular diseases, diabetes, PCOS, cancer, depression, all of which are strongly associated with lifestyle disorders. People nowadays have started adapting to stress and anxiety as a part of their daily life. Antidepressants have now become a common medication around the globe, but these kinds of medications in the long run can lead to adverse effects and can be life-threatening conditions. Lifestyle modification has a promising approach in the treatment of stress and anxiety [46]. Research suggests that 60–70% of the subjects are prone to chronic diseases due to lifestyle choices, according to the individual and certain environmental factors. Lifestyle medicine is a branch of medicine science aimed at treating and preventing diseases, focusing mainly on chronic disease through evidence-based therapeutic approaches to existence. The American College of Lifestyle Medicine has adapted six factors, such as eating whole food predominately plant-based diet, regular exercise, managing stress, avoiding abusive substances, maintaining social and physical connection, and sleep management and practicing mindfulness. These lifestyle modifications have shown a beneficial effect to treat depression [25–29]. To practice mindfulness and have control over the stress hormones, the best proven treatment is meditation, which have control both the mind and body.

Meditation can be performed through several techniques, such as transcendental meditation (TM), mindfulness meditation, walking meditation, relaxation response, moving meditation, progressive meditation, and by chanting certain guided *mantras*. Meditation brings about relaxation of mind and body by increasing the brain's alpha waves. Meditation also works on the nervous system and regulates the functioning of digestive system and blood pressure, which otherwise is impaired by chronic stress in the body. Stress causes inflammation and disruption of the immune functioning, thereby affecting the digestive system, and regular meditation helps in controlling the genes responsible for inflammation and proper functioning of the immune system [20].

Continuous meditation works on training the mind to be aware of the current situation, and instead of generating a response to the reaction in the body, it focuses on accepting and experiencing the feeling observed in the body and work on reacting differently to a negative thought, thereby decreasing the negative energy, which helps in decreasing the stress in the body [20].

Amygdala and medial prefrontal cortex are two regions of the brain that cause depression. The medial prefrontal cortex generates a response to stress encountered in the body, and cortisol is escalated to a peak by the amygdala region of brain, but the regular practice of meditation prevents the interaction of both regions of brain, thereby managing the stress in the body [20].

17.3.2 IMPACT ON HORMONAL BALANCE

Meditation has a wide impact on the endocrine system. The endocrine system consists of various glands which are responsible for producing hormones that assist in the proper functioning of the body [46]. The improper functioning of the endocrine system leads to an imbalance in the release of hormones, and in response to that, the body produces stress [54].

The hormones released in response to stress are cortisol and adrenaline that are produced in hypothalamus and pituitary glands [44]. Cortisol is an important hormone, which is responsible for the conversion of protein into energy, managing inflammation and storing the glucose as glycogen. The optimal level of cortisol is essential for the body, but higher level of cortisol affects the proper functioning of digestive system and endocrine system; disrupts muscle and bone; impairs metabolic activity, hypertension; increases the blood sugar level; weakens the immune system; and affects psychological function [14–26]. The experimental study reported on the decreased level of cortisol among the participants who practiced TM [14].

Meditation also helps in regulating the sleep cycle by boosting melatonin, which is a hormone that induces sleep and is highly activated during the night, and it is reduced during daytime. Melatonin regulates sleep, prevents depression, and boosts the overall immune functioning of the body. Meditation has control over serotonin, which is also associated with the release of cortisol, and serotonin is a monoamine neurotransmitter that helps synthesize melatonin. It is referred to as happy neuroendocrine, and it regulates sleep; relaxes the mind; works on brain cells enhances mood; decreases depression, anxiety, and stress; and aids in weight management [13, 44].

DHEA is a hormone, which synthesizes steroid hormone estrogen and testosterone, and it decreases with age. One of the experimental studies reported a higher level of DHEA among men and women, who performed meditation [14]. DHEA helps in boosting the immune system, prevents heart diseases, decreases aging, supports bone and muscle, and enhances psychological functions [44].

Meditation also increases GABA (a neurotransmitter) that is responsible for calmness, relaxation, reduces stress, anxiety, depression, and enhances brain function. Lack of GABA is one of the main reasons for addiction to abusive substances. According to the research, the population which performed meditation was detected with a 27% increase in the GABA level after 60 minutes of practice [13–19].

Meditation was effective in increasing the endorphins naturally, which is another neurotransmitter to reduce the feeling of pain and stress and gives the feeling of joy and contentment [44].

17.3.3 SPIRITUALITY AND SCIENCE

Science is the study of the external world through observations, experimentation, and theories and its interaction with the biological system, and it leads to the discoveries of facts and creates wonders [47]. An intriguing implication is that science might offer a source of meaning and overall well-being apart from religious spirituality if it can function as a source of spirituality and religiosity. It is frequently stated that greater psychological well-being is linked to religiosity [17], and religion provides a source of existential support. Meditation connects you to your inner self, giving control over the conscious mind and inspiring individuals to greater and nobler causes. Connecting to self reduces mental stress as the saying goes a healthy mind resides in a healthy body.

17.3.4 TRANSCENDENTAL MEDITATION

TM was founded by Maharishi Mahesh Yogi. TM is performed using silent mantras or sound for almost 15–20 minutes twice a day in a comfortable sitting position [57]. It is a best technique to keep the mind in calm, relaxed state, and be aware of the current situation and attain a state of pure consciousness. The theoretical aspect of TM originated from Vedic philosophy [57]. TM has derived its foundation from Hinduism. TM is explained more effectively in a religious aspect than scientifically [61].

TM has proven beneficial in heart health. One of the experimental studies reported a 48% reduction in the risk of developing stroke or mortality rate among the group who performed TM and 24% drop in the possibility of developing hypertension, cardiovascular-related mortality, stress, and other factors related to lifestyle behavior [54]. The effects of TM on the anxiety level were found to be more efficacious than the usual treatment among the people with anxiety [41]. One of the studies was designed to investigate the blood flow pattern among the group who practiced TM and has proven to increase the blood flow in the attention area and reduced blood flow in the arousal area, thereby activating the attention area with minimal effort; this type of change is only observed in the case of TM as compared with other meditation practitioners [33].

TM works by stimulation of the alpha wave of the brain (prefrontal and temporal area) and helps in enhancing the dopamine and serotonin level, thereby promoting the feeling of pleasure and well-being. It reduces the stress by decreasing the cortisol and noradrenaline level and shifts from sympathetic stimulation to parasympathetic stimulation, thereby reducing the inhibition of the release of the GABA system and maintaining the gastrointestinal system, cardiovascular health, and blood pressure, enhancing psychological health and reducing stress and anxiety [38].

17.3.5 IMPACT OF MEDITATION ON PCOS

Understanding PCOS is a complex metabolism as it involves deeper understanding of hormonal-related mechanism and metabolism that has a wide effect on developing several diseases. The major cause of PCOS is associated with psychological distress; as per the research, PCOS women are more prone to greater level of stress than healthy women. Stress is the major contributor that can disrupt various metabolisms in the body such as insulin resistance, obesity, hirsutism, hyperandrogenism, infertility, acne; all are related to PCOS. Therefore, stress being the important factor is essential to control the stress-inducing hormone and to align the mind in a relaxed and calm state. As per the research, women with PCOS have increased cortisol level, HPA activity, adrenocorticotropic hormone, and heart rate; all of these are stress-inducing hormone [43].

Meditation is one of the naturally healing techniques in women with PCOS. It works by balancing the hormone by decreasing the cortisol level, enhancing the melatonin production [43], boosting the production of antibody, reducing inflammation, and enhancing the overall immune functioning [43].

TM works on the parasympathetic stimulation and reduces the Vanillylmandelic acid excretion, catecholamines, and DHEA sulfate, all of which is responsible for stress and shows an increase in serotonin level and dopamine level; both of which helps in regulating mood, digestion, appetite, enhances sleep, and sexual behavior, and lower level of these hormones is linked with the higher level of stress and anxiety. MRI of the brain shows that meditation increases attentiveness through enhanced blood flow. TM works at the genetic level by increasing the lifespan of lymphocytes through preventing cell death by regulating the antiapoptosis gene. It also reduces the release of interleukin 6 (IL-6), thereby reducing the inflammation associated with PCOS [32].

Women with PCOS are prone to insulin resistance; therefore, TM works by lowering the blood sugar level by reducing stress and induces sleep, thereby controlling the person from overeating at night because snacking at night leads to a spike in the sugar level [28]. A recent study reported that the TM practitioners among teenage girls suffering from PCOS have improved quality of life as compared to the control group that confirms the effectiveness of TM in the women with PCOS.

17.4 ROLE OF NUTRITION

17.4.1 DIETARY PATTERNS IN PCOS

Nutrient intake is an essential factor in women with PCOS, and it is very important to understand the interaction between the intake of nutrients and the PCOS. The modern lifestyle is accompanied with a job in a sitting position for several hours; with lack of movement and body exercise, people adapt sedentary lifestyle; with the increase in work load and mental pressure, around half of the population are stressed in the current generation, which leads to stress eating mainly consuming all the junks and processed food which is easily available in the market; leading such lifestyle is the hub for developing many diseases in future; and one of those widely faced in women in the current scenario is PCOS.

According to the research, women with PCOS shows higher glucose level, fasting glucose, low-grade chronic inflammation, and obesity that can further aggravate the condition. Women with PCOS was found to consume less virgin oil, seafood, PUFA, MUFA, and nuts and more of indulged in an unhealthy lifestyle [4]. It is very essential to formulate a diet in such a way that supports the reproductive health and manages the symptoms associated in PCOS.

An experimental study explored the influence of diet on PCOS. The women who consumed low starch and dairy diet showed reduced fasting insulin, HbA1C, and testosterone levels. The diet with carbohydrate that contains low glycemic index, meat and dairy product, lean protein, healthy fats, fruits, and vegetable showed the release of inflammatory mediators but not enough to combat the inflammatory reactions [21]. Mediterranean diet was effective in PCOS women as it reduces insulin resistance, hyper-androgenemia, and inflammatory markers. Diet loaded with lean meat, low-fat dairy, low starch, vegetable oil, restricted fast food, and low-salt diet has shown improvement in insulin resistance, improved menstruation, reduces testosterone, and increase in sex hormone binding protein. Mediterranean and Dash diet have shown a decrease in follicles; low-sodium diet has shown decreased insulin resistance, glucose regulation, and weight management. High fiber diet, minerals, macronutrients, vitamins, and antioxidant have proven to be beneficial in regulating FSH. Ketonic Mediterranean with high protein and low carbs has shown a decrease in insulin resistance, cholesterol level, and triglyceride level and balances the FSH/LH ratio along with androgen, thereby balancing and maintaining the hormone homeostasis [66].

According to the research, the diet in PCOS should include high in fiber, such as green leafy vegetable, almonds, lentils, berries, which support gastrointestinal health and does not increase the sugar level instantly and prevents the insulin resistance, and addition of anti-inflammatory foods, such as tomatoes, olive oil, nuts, fish, that help reduce the inflammation;

it is essential to add plenty of fruits and vegetables as it is loaded with antioxidant and reduces the oxidative stress. Complex carbohydrate can be added, but refined carbohydrate like pasta, white bread, and noodles should be avoided as it leads to an increase in sugar level and weight gain [18]. Spices like ginger, clove, turmeric, cinnamon should be added as it has anti-inflammatory properties and antibacterial properties and aid in management of sugar level [18].

17.4.2 ROLE OF INTAKE OF DAIRY PRODUCTS ON PCOS

As PCOS is associated with major hormonal imbalance, the intake of dairy product and its role in PCOS is a well-known topic which needs to be discussed. According to a study, the intake of calcium, vitamin D, magnesium, dry fruits, nuts, and seeds was seen less in women with PCOS as such the level of calcium, vitamin D, adiponectin was found to be less and increase in the thyroglobulin level. The study shows an increase in insulin secretion with the increase in calcium and vitamin D [48].

A descriptive cross-sectional study was conducted in 400 women with PCOS and showed a direct relationship between the milk intake and PCOS when the intervening variable was modified, which shows that with one unit intake of milk there is 1% increment in risk factor [48].

The protein metabolism produces insulin secretion same as that of carbohydrates. The milk contains a high amount of branched-chain amino acid which is linked with the increase in insulin resistance and risk for T2DM. However, some components present in the milk such as calcium, magnesium, potassium, carbohydrate with low glycemic index help in regulating glucose homeostasis. The consumption of low-fat dairy product has seen beneficial in homeostatic model assessment for insulin resistance (HOMA-IR), which is an assessment technique that estimates the amount of glucose and insulin present in the body to assess insulin resistance, weight management, and reduction in diabetes mellitus [50]. However, consumption of yogurt has a beneficial effect in reduction of T2DM [24].

According to the study, the consumption of dairy products has seen increase in the insulin resistance by 30% among black women, and 38% increase among white women and also an increase in HOMA-IR values, but the women who had less consumption of milk have shown 13% decrement in the HOMA-IR values. Daily intake of dairy content in larger amount has seen an association with hyperinsulinemia and insulin resistance [24].

Dairy product is also associated with modulating the hormones, which show an increase in the dairy product; LH also increases by 2.9%. The increase in dairy product has a beneficial effect in fertility as with the increase in the lactose the fertility rate increases, and the risk of female fertility reduces by 70%. However, it also has some negative effects as it increases the insulin-like growth factor, which otherwise has a negative effect in ovarian function and antral follicular count. The intake of dairy product has seen beneficial in PCOS women along with some negative effects [24].

17.4.3 THE EFFECT OF RED MEAT, GLUTEN FOOD, FRIED FOOD, AND PROCESSED JUNK FOOD ON PCOS

Read meat is a meat with a higher content of protein myoglobin and contains large amount of iron, zinc, phosphorus, creatine, and B vitamins. According to the research, the beef meat has shown an increase in the androgen hormone, which otherwise present in excess in women with PCOS can lead to impairment in ovarian function [1].

Red meat is associated with an increase in risk of colorectal cancer as it contains heme iron which affects the formation of carcinogenic N-nitroso compound [5]. The study also reported that the consumption of red meat has 16% increased risk in the coronary heart disease and stroke. Another study reported on the consumption of plant protein which shows a decrease in the low-density lipoprotein (LDL) cholesterol and non-high-density lipoprotein (HDL) cholesterol level [6].

Red meat [62] has been seen to increase HOMA which is directly associated with insulin resistance, which develops a risk factor for T2DM. However, some studies also show no significant impact on the risk of T2DM [53]. The consumption of red meat for a prolonged time has shown an increase in heart diseases, but no such changes are observed in inflammation and glycemic control [40]. The consumption of red meat and the risk factor for T2DM needs further research to understand the relationship between them [30]. Red meat is also involved in hormonal effects as it decreases the progesterone level, increases weight, and causes more inflammation in the body; therefore, it is advised to avoid the consumption of red meat in PCOS women [65–67].

Gluten is a wheat protein that mainly consists of gliadin and gluten [8]. Women with PCOS are encountered with chronic inflammation, and according to the study, gluten contributes to inflammation by initiating an immune response [16].

Autoimmune thyroid disease (AITD) is seen in 18–40% of the women with PCOS. A study was conducted to investigate the AITD and PCOS relationship, which shows 26.03% of women with PCOS are diagnosed with AITD and 9.72% among the control group [53]. Gluten-free diet has been beneficial in reducing the thyroid antibody titers and an increase in 25-hydroxy vitamin D level and Structure Parameter Inference Approach–Thyroid's Secretory Capacity for Thyroxine index which is associated with AITD [27].

Women with PCOS considerably contain lower level of progesterone hormone which leads to overstimulation of immune function that leads to an increase in the estrogen hormone, which accounts for the production of various autoantibodies which has seen to be associated with different autoimmune conditions [35]. Therefore, gluten should be taken in a considerable amount in women with PCOS (Figure 17.3).

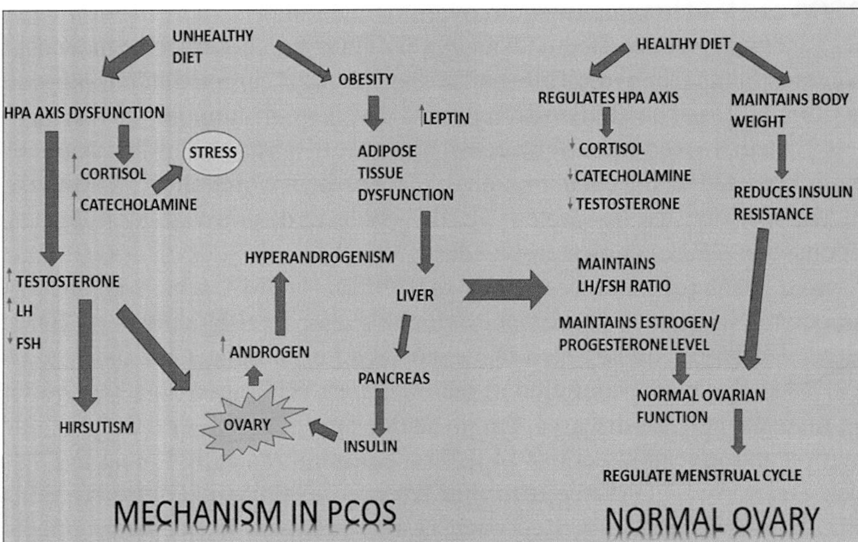

FIGURE 17.3 A flowchart exploring the metabolic shift during dietary management of PCOS.

Junk food is high in calories with an abundance of fats and sugar with little nutritive content [12]. A cross-sectional study was conducted with 200 girls, and with the consumption of junk food, the girls reported menstrual abnormalities. Junk food reduces the metabolism of the body and affects the function of androgen level, thereby affecting the insulin and increasing the sex hormone binding protein, which lowers the androgenic activity, leading to hyperandrogenism in women with PCOS [12].

Processed foods and junk food impact hormonal balance. Loss of control, persistent craving, and overeating in the absence of satiety lead to addiction to junk food. Junk food leads to downregulation of dopamine receptors, which reduces the pleasurable response and can only be fulfilled by the consumption of junk food that gives pleasure with the increase in the dopamine. Stress and emotional dysfunction can also lead to overeating. PCOS is associated with inflammatory response and increases oxidative stress which is further aggravated by the consumption of junk food that increases the reactive oxygen species and lowers antioxidant defense which damages the cell. Oxidative stress is also associated with the increase in ovarian follicle in women with PCOS [12].

Junk food also alters the gut–brain axis, which is the interaction between the gut and the HPA axis and the other associated regulatory pathways. The consumption of the processed and unhealthy food loaded with fats, sugar and high in calories leads to the disruption in the intestinal microbiota that is also associated with obesity, insulin resistance, and metabolic dysfunction, which is the common underlying cause of PCOS [12].

The intake of high level of saturated fats and processed food can lead to increase in the androgen level, thereby reducing the fertility in women with PCOS. The increase in the estrogen level is also seen with the consumption of unhealthy food that affects the reproductive health mainly the menstrual cycle. Consumption of junk food in excess also results in an increase in the cortisol level, which is associated with stress and depression; therefore, women with PCOS are prone to psychological distress. Higher level of cortisol also affects the progesterone level, a hormone which regulates the menstrual cycle and results in irregular menstrual cycle [12].

17.4.4 THE IMPORTANCE OF SEED CYCLING IN PCOS

Seed cycling is use of different types of seeds in each phase of the menstrual cycle. It is one of the natural remedies in balancing the hormone mainly progesterone and estrogen level in women with PCOS. The seeds which are used are dense in zinc and magnesium tryptophan, which are involved in balancing the hormones [10]. Most of the women with PCOS are associated with obesity which is caused by dysfunction of the adipose tissue, which further leads to improper functioning of the metabolism. Women with PCOS and obesity reported lower level of polyunsaturated fatty acid, mainly omega-3 fatty acid, and low level of DHA. Adipose tissue secretes adipokines, which releases leptin/ghrelin and inflammatory cytokines (IL-6). Therefore, due to the improper functioning of leptin/ghrelin in women with PCOS, they are more prone to overeating and eventually leads to weight gain. The seeds which are used in seed cycling are rich in PUFA and increase DHA level and enhance the metabolic activity, which helps in body weight management.

To understand seed cycling, first understanding the two phases of menstrual cycle is important. The period from the start of the menstrual blood till ovulation, that is, from 0 to 14 days is the follicular phase where the egg matures in the ovary. In the follicular phase, the estrogen hormone rises, followed by the luteal phase, which starts from ovulation till the start of the next menstrual cycle, that is, from 15 to 28 days, where the progesterone level peaks. Imbalance in these hormones results in irregular menstruation, PMS, cramps, and the symptoms associated in PCOS [10].

The different types of seeds in use are flax and pumpkin seeds in the follicular phase, followed by the sesame and sunflower seeds in the luteal phase (Figure 17.4). Pumpkin seed is enriched with omega-3 fatty acid and vitamin E (such as alpha tocopherol and gamma tocopherol). Phytoestrogen present in plants has estrogenic properties that help in binding the excess estrogen. The study has reported that due to estrogenic properties of phytoestrogen and tocopherol, it helps to control the cholesterol, lipids metabolism, bone function, decreases the LDL, increases HDL, and maintains triglyceride level [23]. Pumpkin seed is also rich in zinc which improves the functioning of corpus luteum, which is responsible in boosting the progesterone level for menstruation and preparing the uterus for implantation [10].

Flax seed is rich in lignans, alpha linoleic acid, and dietary fiber. It also contains phytoestrogen which helps in estrogen production and lignans present in the flax seed binds to extra estrogen, thereby reducing the excess of estrogen. Flax seed helps in reduction of the free testosterone by increasing the sex hormone binding protein. It is associated with increase

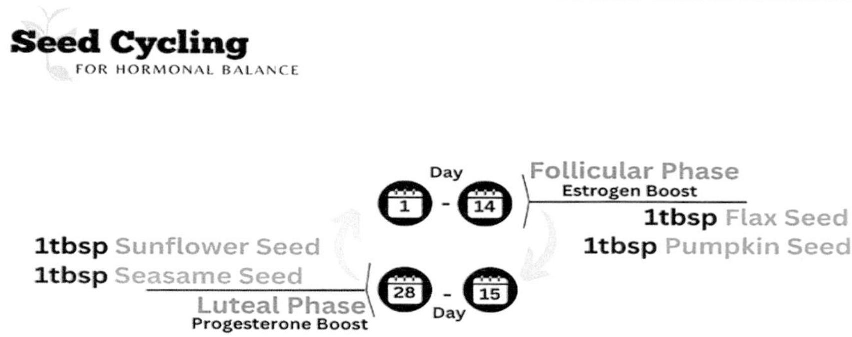

FIGURE 17.4 The potential benefits of specific seeds symmetrical with the menstrual cycle phase that assists in management of PCOS.

in the duration of luteal phase improving the ovulation process and reduces the pain associated in the menstruation. A study was conducted among 41 women who consumed 30 g of flax seed for 12 weeks with certain lifestyle changes that resulted in reduce in the body weight, insulin resistance, C-reactive protein level, leptin, decrease in LDL, and increase in HDL [23]. Flax seed is also rich in omega-3 fatty acid, which enhances the blood flow in the uterus and increases the progesterone for next phase of the cycle [10].

Sesame seed is rich in calcium, magnesium, zinc, and considerable amount of good fats, which aid in controlling the glucose level. It is also a good source of antioxidant, sex hormones, and blood lipids, which has shown beneficial effect in postmenopausal women. It is also associated with blocking excess estrogen level by boosting the progesterone level in the luteal phase.

Sunflower seed contains amino acid such as glutamic acid, aspartic acid, cysteine, arginine, and linoleic acids. Sunflower seed is enriched with protein, fiber, unsaturated fats, vitamin E, folate, copper, zinc, iron, and phytochemicals. It is also rich in vitamin E and selenium, which detoxifies the liver with excess estrogen. Sunflower seed also helps in progesterone production [10, 23]. An experiment was conducted which showed a decrease in the LH in the experimental group than the control group; therefore, seed cycling is seen effective in treating PCOS by hormonal balance [49].

17.5 HOLISTIC APPROACH FOR MANAGEMENT OF PCOS

PCOS can be prevented by simple lifestyle modification, and adapting yoga and meditation in our daily routine can be an icing to a cake. The underlying condition associated with PCOS is stress which is the major factor for aggravating many conditions. Management of stress is a crucial factor in PCOS which can be controlled by simple yogic postures, which is not only beneficial in reducing the stress hormone but also shows ample benefits in the reproductive health. Yoga being the sole bearer in aligning the mind and body helps in lowering the catecholamine and cortisol level and increasing the dopamine and serotonin level, which considerably reduces stress and enhances mood. It also helps in controlling the blood glucose level, inflammation, and enhances sleep quality by the secretion of melatonin. Meditation comes with various techniques in which one of the effective techniques in PCOS discussed above is TM that uses certain mantras and postures effective in inflammation and has a phenomenal effect in the changing the brain waves and acts upon certain brain regions associated with stress.

Apart from yoga and meditation, diet also plays a major role in PCOS. Consumption of processed and junk food has seen an increase in the sugar level, cholesterol, lipids, triglyceride level, and obesity. Obesity being the underlying cause of PCOS further aggravates the condition. Diet with high fiber, low salt, fruits, vegetables, nuts, seeds, and lentils has shown beneficial effects in alleviating the symptoms associated with PCOS. Therefore, a mixture of the three components helps in the biochemical and metabolic functions associated with PCOS.

17.6 SUMMARY

Among women of reproductive age, 6–12% suffer from PCOS, a prevalent endocrine condition. The major symptom associated with PCOS is the hormonal imbalance, which results in an imbalance in the progesterone and estrogen hormone that regulates the menstrual cycle. The FSH and LH show an improper ratio and are also associated with higher level of androgen and testosterone hormone, which results in hyperandrogenism, hirsutism, and acne in women with PCOS. PCOS can be managed with medication; however, it has various side effects on long-term usage, but

PCOS can be treated naturally with simple lifestyle modification with zero side effects. The ancient practice of yoga and meditation has a wide range of benefits in the women with PCOS from balancing the hormones to regulation of psychological health. It has the power to control over the regions of the brain by stimulating the alpha waves and parasympathetic action. Further, it has control over stress-inducing hormones and mood enhancement, thereby reducing depression in women with PCOS. Diet along with the yoga and meditation helps in controlling the hormonal-related issues and aids in weight management. The chapter covers insight into the mechanism of how certain yogic postures; meditation, mainly TM; and diet are involved in managing the hormonal imbalance and associated metabolic diseases, which are the underlying cause of PCOS; further, it explores the effect of gluten, junk food, dairy intake, and importantly seed cycling in each phase of menstrual cycle and the management of PCOS through dietary pattern. The integration of yoga, meditation, and diet has shown a remarkable approach in treating PCOS, and adapting these simple changes can save the lives of a thousand women.

KEYWORDS

- **female infertility**
- **hormonal imbalance**
- **meditation**
- **nutrition**
- **polycystic ovarian syndrome**
- **woman's health**
- **yoga**

REFERENCES

1. Abedal-Majed, M. A., Springman, S. A., Jafar, H. D., Bell, B. E., Kurz, S. G., & Wilson, K. E. (2022). Naturally occurring androgen excess cows are present in dairy and beef herds and have similar characteristics to women with PCOS. *Journal of Animal Science, 100*(6), 1–12.

2. Ansari, R. M. (2016). Kapalabhati Pranayama: An answer to modern day polycystic ovarian syndrome and coexisting metabolic syndrome? *International Journal of Yoga*, *9*(2), 163–167.
3. Balasubramani, S. (2022). Efficacy of yoga therapy on serum creatinine and LH-FSH ratio among adult women suffering with polycystic ovarian syndrome. *International Journal of Humanities, Law and Social Sciences*, *9*(5), 135–142.
4. Barrea, L., Arnone, A., Annunziata, G., Muscogiuri, G., Laudisio, D., & Salzano, C. (2019). Adherence to the Mediterranean diet, dietary patterns and body composition in women with polycystic ovary syndrome (PCOS). *Nutrients*, *11*(10), 1–21.
5. Bastide, N. M., Pierre, F. H. F., & Corpet, D. E. (2011). Heme iron from meat and risk of colorectal cancer: A meta-analysis and a review of the mechanisms involved. *American Association for Cancer Research*, *4*(2), 177–184.
6. Bechthold, A., Boeing, H., & Hoffmann, G. (2019). Food groups and risk of coronary heart disease, stroke and heart failure: A systematic review and dose-response meta-analysis of prospective studies. *Critical Reviews in Food Science and Nutrition*, *59*(7), 1071–1090.
7. Bhasin, S., Shukla, A., & Desai, S. (2020). Services for women's sexual and reproductive health in India: An analysis of treatment-seeking for symptoms of reproductive tract infections in a nationally representative survey. *BMC Women's Health*, *20*, 156–162.
8. Biesiekierski, J. R. (2017). What is gluten? *Journal of Gastroenterology and Hepatology, 32*(S1), 78–81.
9. Bijendar, S., Badola, J., Laxmi, V., & Ijmtst, E. (2021). The Positive effects of Asanas and Pranayama on PCOS and How to deal with hormonal imbalance? *International Journal of Modern Trends in Science and Technology*, 7(7), 190–195.
10. Bippen, J. (2020). Seed cycling for hormone balance. *Nourished by Nutrition*; https://nourishedbynutrition.com/seed-cycling-for-hormone-balance/; (accessed on 3 February 2024).
11. Birajdar, D. V. A. (2023). Management of PCOS with Bhramari Pranayam: Case study. *International Journal of Scientific Development and Research*, *8*(5), 877–879.
12. Chapman, A. G. (1993). Junk food and healthy food: Meanings of food in adolescent women's culture. *Journal of Nutrition Education*, *25*(3), 108–113.
13. Chen, K. W., & Berger, C. C. (2012). Meditative therapies for reducing anxiety: A systematic review and meta-analysis of randomized controlled trials. *Depression and Anxiety*, *29*(7), 545–562.
14. Daube, W. C., & Jakobsche, C. E. (2015). Biochemical effects of meditation - a literature review. *Scholarly Undergraduate Research Journal at Clark*, *1*(1), 80–85. https://commons.clarku.edu/cgi/viewcontent.cgi?article=1017&context=surj
15. DelMonte, M. M. (1985). Biochemical indices associated with meditation practice—A literature review. *Neuroscience & Biobehavioral Reviews*, *9*(4), 557–561. doi: 10.1016/0149-7634(85)90002-8
16. DePunder, K., & Pruimboom, L. (2013). The dietary intake of wheat and other cereal grains and their role in inflammation. *Nutrients*, *5*(3), 771–787. doi: 10.3390/nu5030771.

17. Diener, E., & Tay, L., & Myers, D. G. (2011). The religion paradox: If religion makes people happy, why are so many dropping out? *Journal of Personality and Social Psychology*, *101*(6), 1278–1290.
18. Douglas, C., & Norris, E. (2006). Difference in dietary intake between women with polycystic ovary syndrome and healthy controls. *Fertility and Sterility, 86*(2), 411–417.
19. Glaser, J. L., Brind, J. L., & Vogelman, J. H. (1992). Elevated serum dehydroepiandrosterone sulfate levels in practitioners of the transcendental meditation (TM) and TM-Sidhi programs. *Journal of Behavioral Medicine*, *15*(4), 327–341.
20. Goyal, M., Singh, S., Sibinga, E. M., Gould, N. F., Rowland-Seymour, A., Sharma, R., Berger, Z., Sleicher, D., Maron, D. D., Shihab, H. M., Ranasinghe, P. D., Linn, S., Saha, S., Bass, E. B., & Haythornthwaite, J. A. (2014). Meditation programs for psychological stress and wellbeing: A systematic review and meta-analysis. *JAMA Internal Medicine*, *174*(3), 357–368. doi: 10.1001/jamainternmed.2013.13018.
21. Farshchi, H., Rane, A., Love, A., & Kennedy, R. L. (2007). Diet and nutrition in polycystic ovary syndrome: Pointers for nutritional management. *Journal of Obstetrics and Gynaecology, 27*(8), 762–773.
22. Hosna, M. S., Ida, A., & Daniela. C. (2022). Polycystic ovary syndrome: A comprehensive review of pathogenesis, management, and drug repurposing. *International Journal of Molecular Science, 23*(2), 583–590.
23. Irfan, T., Seher, K., Rizwan, B., Fatima, S., & Sani, A. (2021). Role of seed cycling in polycystic ovaries syndrome. *Pakistan Biomedical Journal*, *4*(2) 121–130.
24. Janiszewska, J., Ostrowska, J., & Szostak-Węgierek, D. (2020). Milk and dairy products and their impact on carbohydrate metabolism and fertility—A potential role in the diet of women with polycystic ovary syndrome. *Nutrients*, *12*(11), 1–17.
25. Khademi, A., Alleyassin, A., Aghahosseini, M., Tabatabaeefar, L., & Amini, M. (2010). The effect of exercise in PCOS women who exercise regularly. *Asian Journal of Sports Medicine*, *1*(1), 35–40.
26. Krishnakumar, D. (2015). Meditation and yoga can modulate brain mechanisms that affect behavior and anxiety—A modern scientific perspective. *Ancient Science of Life, 2*(1), 13–19.
27. Krysiak, R., Szkróbka, W., & Okopień, B. (2019). The effect of gluten-free diet on thyroid autoimmunity in drug-naïve women with Hashimoto's thyroiditis—A pilot study. *Experimental Clinical Endocrinology Diabetes*, *127*(7), 417–422.
28. Labrador, M. P., & Polk, D. (2006). Effects of a randomized controlled trial of transcendental meditation on components of the metabolic syndrome in subjects with coronary heart disease. *Archives of Internal Medicine*, *166*(11), 1218–1224.
29. Lee, J. S., Jaini, P. A., & Papa, F. (2022). An epigenetic perspective on lifestyle medicine for depression: Implications for primary care practice. *American Journal of Lifestyle Medicine*, *16*(1), 76–88.
30. Lescinsky, H., Afshin, A., Ashbaugh, C., Bisignano, C., Brauer, M., & Ferrara, G. (2022). Health effects associated with consumption of unprocessed red meat: A burden of proof study. *Natural Medicine, 28*(10), 2075–2082.
31. Lucchetti, G. (2021). Spirituality, religiousness, and mental health: A review of the current scientific evidence. *World Journal of Clinical Cases, 9*(26), 7620–7631.

32. Mahajan, A. S. (2014). Role of yoga in hormonal homeostasis. *International Journal of Clinical and Experimental Physiology*, *1*(3), 173–178.
33. Mahone, M. C., Travis, F., Gevirtz, R., & Hubbard, D. (2018). fMRI during transcendental meditation practice. *Brain and Cognition*, *123*(1), 30–33.
34. Michelmore, K. F., Balen, A. H., Dunger, D. B., & Vessey, M. P. (1999). Polycystic ovaries and associated clinical and biochemical features in young women. *Clinical Endocrinology (Oxf)*, *51*(6), 779–786. doi: 10.1046/j.1365-2265.1999.00886.x
35. Mobeen, H., Afzal, N., & Kashif, M. (2016). Polycystic ovary syndrome may be an autoimmune disorder. *Scientifica, 2016*(5), 1–7.
36. Moran, C. (2010). Prevalence of polycystic ovary syndrome and related disorders in Mexican women. *Gynecologic and Obstetric Investigation*, *69*, 274–280.
37. Moro, C., Pasarica, M., Elkind-Hirsch, K., & Redman, L. M. (2009). Aerobic exercise training improves atrial natriuretic peptide and catecholamine-mediated lipolysis in obese women with polycystic ovary syndrome. *The Journal of Clinical Endocrinology and Metabolism*, *94*(7), 2579–2586.
38. Mosini, A. C., Saad, M., Braghetta, C. C., Medeiros, R. D., Peres, M. F. P., & Leão, F. C. (2019). Neurophysiological, cognitive-behavioral and neurochemical effects in practitioners of transcendental meditation—Literature review. *Revista da Associacao Médica Brasielera, 65*(5), 706–713.
39. Muhas, C., Nishad, K. M., Ummunnoora, K. P., Jushna, K., Saheera K. V., & Dilsha, K. P. (2018). Polycystic ovary syndrome (PCOS)—An overview. *International Journal of Current Pharmaceutical Research*, *10*(6), 5–9. doi: 10.22159/ijcpr.2018v10i6.30969
40. Muhas, C., & Naseef, P. P. (2017). A review article—Gestational *diabetes mellitus*. *International Journal of Current Pharmaceutical Research*, *9*(1), 1. doi: 10.22159/ijcpr.2017v9i1.16615
41. Muhas, C., Sruthy, S. A., & Naseef, P. P. (2021). Factors that favor the spread of bacterial resistance. *International Journal of Current Pharmaceutical Research*, *13*(5). doi: 10.22159/ijcpr.2021v13i5.1905
42. O'Connor, L. E., Kim, J. E., Clark, C. M., Zhu, W., & Campbell, W. W. (2020). Effects of total red meat intake on glycemic control and inflammatory biomarkers—A meta-analysis of randomized controlled trials. *Advances in Nutrition*, *12*(1), 115–127.
43. Okoroh, E. M., Hooper, W. C., Atrash, H. K., Yusuf, H. R., & Boulet, S. L. (2012). Prevalence of polycystic ovary syndrome among the privately insured, United States 2003–2008. *American Journal of Obstetrics and Gynecology, 207*(4), 299–305.
44. Orme-Johnson, D. W., & Barnes, V. A. (2014). Effects of the transcendental meditation technique on trait anxiety: A meta-analysis of randomized controlled trials. *Journal of Alternative and Complementary Medicine, 20*(5), 330–341.
45. Padmavathi, R., Kumar, A. P., Dhamodhini, K. S., Venugopal, V., Silambanan, S., & Maheshkumar, K. (2023). Role of yoga in stress management and implications in major depression disorder. *Journal of Ayurveda and Integrative Medicine*, *14(*5), 2–6.
46. Panjrath, Y. (2023). PCOS and meditation: A review paper. *International Journal of Indian Psychology, 16*(11), 2349–3429.
47. Pascoe, C., Thompson, R, D., & Ski, C. F. (2020). Meditation and endocrine health and wellbeing. *ScienceDirect, 31*(7), 469–477.

48. Pavithra, L. (2023). Identification of phytoconstituents for combating polycystic ovarian syndrome through in silico techniques. *Indian Journal of Biophysics and Biochemistry*, *60*(2), 99–107.
49. Piotrowski, M. C., Lunsford, J., & Gaynes, B. N. (2021). Lifestyle psychiatry for depression and anxiety: Beyond diet and exercise. *Lifestyle Medicine*, *2*(1), 1–12.
50. Preston, J. L., Coleman, T. J., & Shin, F. (2023). Spirituality of science: Implications for meaning, well-being, and learning. *Personality and Social Psychology Bulletin, 51*(4), 632–643, article ID 01461672231191356. doi: 10.1177/01461672231191356.
51. Rajaeieh, G., Marasi, M., Shahshahan, Z., Hassanbeigi, F., & Safavi, S. M. (2014). The relationship between intake of dairy products and polycystic ovary syndrome in women who referred to Isfahan University of Medical Science Clinics in 2013. *International Journal of Preventive Medicine, 5*(6), 687–694.
52. Rasheed, N., & Ahmed, A. (2023). Effectiveness of combined seeds (pumpkin, sunflower, sesame, flaxseed): As adjacent therapy to treat polycystic ovary syndrome in females. *Food Science and Nutrition*, *11*(6), 3385–3393.
53. Raveendran, A. V., Deshpandae, A., & Joshi, S. R. (2018). Therapeutic role of yoga in type 2 diabetes. *Endocrinology and Metabolism*, *33*(3), 307–317.
54. Romitti, M., Fabris, V. C., Ziegelmann, P. K., Maia, A. L., & Spritzer, P. M. (2018). Association between PCOS and autoimmune thyroid disease—A systematic review and meta-analysis. *Endocrine Connect*ions, *7*(11), 1158–1167.
55. Sadeghi, H. M., Adeli, I., Calina, D., Docea, A. O., Mousavi, T., & Daniali, M. (2022). Polycystic ovary syndrome: A comprehensive review of pathogenesis, management, and drug repurposing. *International Journal of Molecular Science*, *23(*2), 1–33.
56. Sanders, L. M., Wilcox, M. L., & Maki, K. C. (2023). Red meat consumption and risk factors for type 2 diabetes—A systematic review and meta-analysis of randomized controlled trials. *European Journal of Clinical Nutrition*, *77*(2), 156–160.
57. Schneider, H. R. (2012). Stress reduction in the secondary prevention of cardiovascular disease: Randomized, controlled trial of transcendental meditation and health education in Blacks. *American Heart Association Journals*, *5*(6), 750–758.
58. Scott, R. W. S. (2022). The importance of women's health. *Journal of Clinical Investigation, 12*(3), 75–76.
59. Segal, T. R., & Giudice, L. C. (2019). Before the beginning: Environmental exposures and reproductive and obstetrical outcomes. *Fertility and Sterility*, *112*(4), 613–621.
60. Singh, P., & Singh, A. K. (2024). Transcendental meditation—A path to holistic wellbeing. *The International Journal of Indian Psychology*, *12*(1), 643–653.
61. Singh, V. P., & Khandelwal, B. (2020). Effect of yoga and exercise on glycemic control and psychosocial parameters in type 2 diabetes mellitus: A randomized controlled study. *International Journal of Yoga*, *13*(2), 144–151.
62. Sochol, K. M., Johns, T. S., Buttar, R. S., Randhawa, L., Sanchez, E., & Gal, M. (2019). The effects of dairy intake on insulin resistance: A systematic review and meta-analysis of randomized clinical trials. *Nutrients*, *11*(9), 2–20.
63. Thakur, D., Singh, D. S. S., Tripathi, D. M., & Lufang, D. (2021). Effect of yoga on polycystic ovarian syndrome: A systematic review. *Journal of Bodywork and Movement Therapies*, *1*(27), 281–286.
64. Trama, S., & Cheema, N. (2016). Transcendental meditation: Nature and perspectives. *Indian Journal of Health and Wellbeing*, *7*(9), 928–933.

65. World Health Organisation (WHO). (2023). Polycystic ovary syndrome. Polycystic ovary syndrome (who.int); (accessed on 3 February 2024).
66. World Health Organisation (WHO), Women's health. Women's health (who.int); (accessed on 3 February 2024).
67. Xenou, M., & Gourounti, K. (2021). Dietary patterns and polycystic ovary syndrome—A systematic review. *Maedica (Bucur)*, *16*(3), 516–521. doi: 10.26574/maedica.2020.16.3.516.
68. Yang, J. (2021). *The Human Microbiome Project—Extending the Definition of What Constitutes a Human*. National Human Genome Research Institute, NIH: Washington, DC.

CHAPTER 18

Innovative Time Management Techniques for Female Health

SASMITA DASH* and JAYANTA KUMAR PANDA

*Corresponding author

ABSTRACT

Women often have many responsibilities, such as work, family, and personal well-being, so time management is critical to maintaining optimal health. The chapter explores various strategies, such as prioritization, delegation, and technology integration, to help women efficiently manage their time and prioritize health-related activities. It also examines the impact of stress and lifestyle factors on female health and suggests practical ways to mitigate these effects through effective time management. By implementing these innovative techniques, women's well-being can be enhanced and attain a better professional work and personal life balance. Innovative time-management techniques can empower women to prioritize their health and well-being amidst their busy lives. Women who incorporate these ideas into their everyday routines can achieve a healthy balance and lead more fulfilling lives. This chapter focuses on the specific strategies and techniques tailored to help women effectively manage their time and prioritize their health needs.

18.1 INTRODUCTION

Time management is a critical aspect of modern life, allowing individuals to balance various responsibilities effectively [4]. However, for women, managing time extends beyond professional and personal obligations

Holistic Approaches for Women's Sustainable Health, Volume 2: Advancements, Socioeconomic Impacts, and Innovative Strategies. Junaid Ahmad Malik, Anamika Chauhan, and Megh R. Goyal (Eds)

DOI: 10.1201/9781779641656-22

to include aspects of health and well-being unique to their gender. The intersection of time management and female health presents a complex landscape that requires innovative approaches. Women often face distinct challenges related to health and time management due to societal expectations, biological factors, and lifestyle demands [19]. These challenges are further exacerbated for working women, who are often the primary caregivers and face additional health issues such as stress-related conditions, respiratory problems, and social constraints [2]. Factors such as menstrual health, reproductive health, caregiving responsibilities, and hormonal changes can significantly impact how women manage their time and prioritize their health. Recently, there has been an increasing awareness of the significance of tackling these issues and creating new time-management strategies specifically designed for women's health [29]. The goal of these methods is to give women the ability to manage their health and time effectively, ultimately improving their well-being and quality of life. This book chapter explores the unique time-management challenges faced by women in relation to their health and introduces innovative techniques and strategies to address these challenges. By highlighting the importance of integrating health into the broader framework of time management, this chapter provides practical insights and solutions that can help women achieve a healthier, more balanced lifestyle. Figure 18.1 presents innovative time-management techniques for female health.

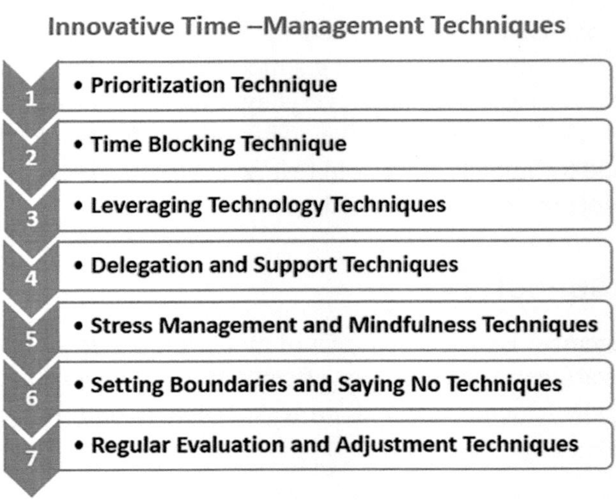

FIGURE 18.1 Innovative time-management techniques.

18.1.1 OVERVIEW OF THE UNIQUE TIME-MANAGEMENT CHALLENGES FACED BY WOMEN

Women face a myriad of unique time-management challenges that stem from societal expectations, gender roles, and often, the disproportionate burden of caregiving and household responsibilities [19]. These challenges can significantly impact their ability to efficiently organize their time and achieve their personal and professional objectives. Women are often expected to juggle multiple roles, including those of caregiver, homemaker, and professional. This can result in feelings of being overwhelmed and exhausted, which can make it difficult to effectively manage time for each role [22]. Women are more likely to be caregivers for children, ageing parents, or other loved ones. Caregiving can take a lot of time, leaving less time for hobbies or career growth [31]. Women find work–life balance is especially difficult and often feel the pressure to perform at a high level in both areas of their lives. This can result in feelings of guilt or shame when they feel they are not meeting expectations in one area or the other [7]. When it comes to time management, women often struggle with unconscious bias and lack of access to career opportunities, which can affect their ability to effectively manage their time while working toward their professional goals [38]. Women are more prone to experiencing "time poverty," where they feel overwhelmed by the amount of work they have to do and the amount of time they do not have to do it. Societal expectations around gender roles can influence how women prioritize their time [11]. For example, women may feel pressured to prioritize caregiving and household responsibilities over their own personal or professional pursuits. Women may also face a lack of support in managing their time effectively, whether in the form of access to affordable childcare, flexible work arrangements, or support from their partners and communities. Women confront unique time-management issues that impair their capacity to attain objectives and gain a proper balance between professional work and personal life [30]. Addressing these difficulties necessitates both societal change, such as a more equitable division of caregiving obligations, and individual time management measures.

18.1.2 IMPORTANCE OF PRIORITIZING HEALTH AMIDST VARIOUS RESPONSIBILITIES

Prioritizing health is crucial, especially when juggling numerous responsibilities. Good health allows us to perform daily tasks efficiently.

Neglecting health can lead to illnesses, reducing our ability to fulfill responsibilities. Depression, anxiety, and fatigue can result from neglecting one's mental health. Making mental health a priority enhances overall well-being, focus, and mood. Healthy individuals are more productive [5].

Prioritizing health can lead to better time management and higher quality work [41]. Prioritizing health sets a positive example for others, especially children, encouraging them to adopt healthy habits. Healthy habits contribute to a longer, more fulfilling life. Prioritizing health ensures longevity to enjoy time with loved ones and pursue goals. Good health enhances quality of life. It enables participation in activities that bring joy and fulfillment. Prioritizing health includes preventive measures. Regular checkups and healthy habits can prevent serious health issues. Overall, prioritizing health ensures individuals can fulfill responsibilities effectively while enjoying a better quality of life. Figure 18.2 shows the importance of prioritizing health.

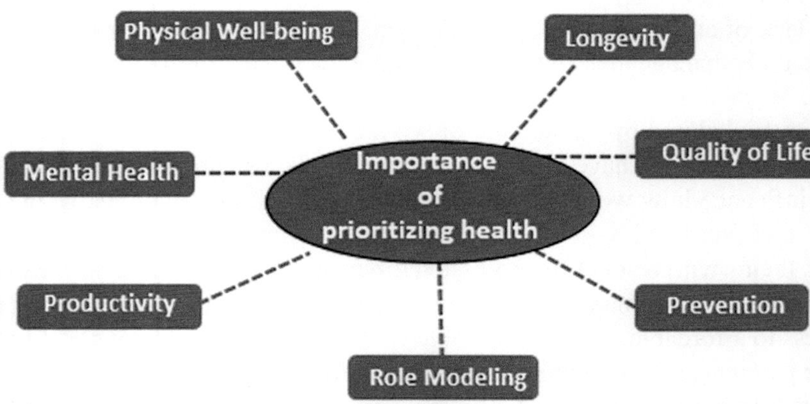

FIGURE 18.2 The importance of prioritizing health.

18.2 PRIORITIZATION TECHNIQUES

Effective time management is essential, especially for women who frequently juggle multiple responsibilities. Time management becomes even more complex when considering the unique health needs and challenges faced by women. The intersection of time management and female health requires innovative approaches to ensure that women can prioritize their well-being amidst various demands. This section focuses on prioritization techniques tailored to meet the unique health requirements of women. By understanding and implementing these techniques, women can better manage their time while ensuring that their health remains a top priority. From identifying key health goals to utilizing time blocking and stress management techniques, this section also provides practical strategies to help women achieve a balanced and healthy lifestyle. By highlighting the importance of integrating health into the broader framework of time management, this aims to empower women to take control of their well-being. Through innovative prioritization techniques, women can enhance their overall health and quality of life. Prioritization Techniques for Innovative Time-Management for Female Health are given below:

1. **Identify key health goals:** Begin by identifying your key health goals, whether they are related to physical fitness, mental well-being, or preventive care. This will help you prioritize activities that directly contribute to these goals.
2. **Use the Eisenhower matrix:** According to their importance and urgency, tasks are divided into four quadrants by the Eisenhower Matrix. Both urgent and important task is given priority.
3. **Implement the "Eat That Frog!" Technique:** Initiating your day by addressing your most difficult or significant task can boost your sense of achievement and motivation to handle subsequent tasks.
4. **Utilize time blocking:** Time blocking is important to efficiently utilize time. This technique requires setting aside dedicated time blocks for various activities or tasks. Time slots in the daily routine are to be allocated for exercise, self-care, mindfulness, and other health-related activities.
5. **Mindfulness practice:** Integrate mindfulness practice into everyday schedule in order to decrease stress levels and enhance concentration. Practices like meditation, controlled breathing, and yoga are effective ways to cope with stress and enhance your overall state of well-being.
6. **Establish smart goals:** Make sure your health objectives are clearly defined, quantifiable, realistic, pertinent, and have a set deadline. This approach will enable you to maintain concentration and monitor your advancements as time goes by.

7. **Create a support system:** Ensure that you are surrounded by a caring and helpful circle of family members, friends, or medical experts who can provide the necessary support and inspiration to help you make your health a top priority.
8. **Regular evaluation:** Regularly assess your time-management techniques and health objectives to guarantee they are in line with your priorities, and make any necessary changes.

18.2.1 IDENTIFYING IMPORTANT HEALTH-RELATED ACTIVITIES

Identifying important health-related activities is a critical step toward achieving optimal well-being. By recognizing and prioritizing these activities, time can be efficiently used and concentrated on actions that hold the utmost importance for their well-being.

This section explores the importance of identifying important health-related activities and provides practical guidance on how to prioritize them. Understanding the significance of physical activity, healthy eating, stress management, and preventive care is essential for maintaining overall well-being [18]. By integrating these practices into their daily routines, individuals can empower themselves to improve their health and elevate their quality of life. By devoting time and energy to engaging in activities that enhance health and well-being, individuals can experience a healthier and more satisfying life. Table 18.1 presents the health-related activities. It is crucial to engage in regular physical exercise in order to maintain good health. Determine the type of physical activity that suits women best, whether it be a gym workout, yoga, dance, or outdoor activities. Make sure to allocate time in a daily or weekly routine for exercise to ensure that you remain active. Nutrition is also important for female health [24]. Identify the diet that needs improvement and make it more nutritious. Planning and preparing meals can assist in making healthier food choices and saving time. Quality sleep is highly needed for overall well-being [32]. Identify factors that may be affecting sleep quality, such as screen time before bed or a busy schedule, and make adjustments to improve sleep hygiene. Chronic stress can have a negative impact on female health.

TABLE 18.1 Health-Related Activities

Health-Related Activity	Description
Exercise	Engaging in physical activity to improve fitness
Healthy eating	Making nutritious food choices for optimal health
Sleep	Getting sufficient rest for physical and mental health
Stress management	Practicing techniques to reduce stress and anxiety
Preventive care	Regular examinations and screenings for timely identification
Mental health	Activities to support mental well-being
Self-care	Practices that promote relaxation and self-compassion

Identify sources of stress in life and practice meditation, yoga, deep breathing exercises, and spending time with nature to help relax and unwind. Regular health examination is essential for detecting health problems early [23]. Identify the recommended preventive care measures based on age, gender, and health history, and schedule appointments accordingly. Mental well-being holds equal importance to physical well-being. Recognize activities that enhance mental health, such as pursuing hobbies, connecting with family, or seeking professional support if needed. Participating in self-care practices is crucial for overall health and wellness. Recognize activities that promote relaxation and rejuvenation, like reading, bathing, practicing mindfulness, and prioritize them in daily schedule.

18.2.2 STRATEGIES FOR PRIORITIZING HEALTH WITHOUT NEGLECTING OTHER RESPONSIBILITIES

In the modern era of rapid advancements, it can be quite demanding to give due importance to one's health, particularly when managing various obligations like professional duties, familial responsibilities, and personal commitments. Nevertheless, disregarding one's health can result in enduring repercussions, affecting both the physical and mental state of well-being. Hence, it is imperative to devise effective approaches that enable individuals to prioritize their health while fulfilling other responsibilities. This section explores effective strategies for prioritizing health while managing other responsibilities. From setting clear priorities and using time-blocking techniques to practicing efficient work habits and incorporating health into daily routines, these strategies are designed to help individuals strike a balance between their health and other obligations [36]. By implementing these strategies, individuals can prioritize their health without feeling overwhelmed by their other responsibilities. Strategies for prioritizing health without neglecting other responsibilities are mentioned below:

1. **Set clear priorities:** Determine your most important health goals and make sure to schedule time for them in your daily routine. This could involve incorporating consistent physical activity, planning nutritious meals, and engaging in stress-relieving practices.
2. **Utilize time blocking:** Schedule designated time slots for various tasks, such as those related to your well-being, to guarantee that you prioritize your health while still managing your other obligations.
3. **Multitask mindfully:** Look for opportunities to combine health-promoting activities with other tasks. For example, listen to educational podcasts while exercising or prepare healthy meals in bulk to save time.
4. **Delegate responsibilities:** Assigning tasks that can be accomplished by others is a prudent approach to create more time for prioritizing your well-being. This may include asking family members for help with household tasks or seeking support from co-workers in the workplace.
5. **Practice efficient work habits:** Improve your efficiency at work to free up time for health-related activities. This may involve prioritizing tasks, minimizing distractions, and setting realistic deadlines.
6. **Establish attainable objectives:** Establish health objectives that are within reach and align with your current lifestyle. This approach will enhance your motivation and prevent any sense of being overwhelmed.
7. **Integrate health into daily schedule:** Seek opportunities to integrate activities that promote good health into your daily routine. For instance, opt for taking the stairs instead of the elevator or engage in stretching exercises while watching television.
8. **Engage in self-care:** Give importance to engaging in self-care activities that aid in your relaxation and rejuvenation. This may involve practicing meditation, indulging in reading, or spending quality time outdoors.

9. **Stay flexible:** Be open to adapting your schedule whenever necessary to accommodate unforeseen circumstances or shifts in priorities. This adaptability will assist you in maintaining a harmonious equilibrium between your well-being and other obligations.
10. **Reach out for assistance:** Do not hesitate to seek assistance from your loved ones, friends, or healthcare professionals. They can offer support, encouragement, and help you stay committed to your health objectives.

18.3 TIME BLOCKING FOR HEALTH

In the current fast-paced environment, finding time can be difficult for activities that promote good health. With work, family, and other responsibilities, neglecting self-care can happen easily. Prioritizing health is crucial for females' overall well-being. One effective method for ensuring that time is made for female health is through time blocking. This is a time management technique where specific periods for various tasks or activities are allocated [17, 33]. Dedicating a period for health-related activities like exercise, meal planning, and self-care, one can ensure that these important tasks are not overlooked amidst a busy schedule. This section covers the concept of time blocking for health and provides practical advice and strategies for incorporating this technique into daily life. Time blocking technique can be particularly effective when it comes to prioritizing activities that promote good health. It allows to allocate focused time for exercise, meal planning, self-care, and other health-promoting activities. Time blocking for female health can be utilized in the following ways:

1. **Identify health priorities:** Start by identifying the main aspects of health that require attention, like physical activity, nutritious eating, and stress relief.
2. **Create time blocks:** Allocate specific blocks of time in daily or weekly schedule for each health priority. For example, one can set aside 30 minutes every morning for exercise and one hour every Sunday for meal planning and preparation.
3. **Be specific:** Clearly define what each time block will involve. For instance, if a female can dedicate time to exercise, specify the

type of exercise she will be doing, whether it's running, yoga, or strength training.

4. **Stick to your schedule:** Once time blocks are created, commit to sticking to them. Treat these blocks of time as non-negotiable appointments and prioritize them accordingly.

By implementing time blocking for female health, one can ensure that she makes time for activities that promote well-being. This technique will help in maintaining a healthy balance in life and prioritize female health amidst a busy schedule, and effectively allocating time for exercise, meal planning, and self-care, leading to a healthier lifestyle. It is crucial to incorporate health-focused time blocks into daily routines in order to maintain a healthy lifestyle and overall well-being. By giving priority to these activities and including them in schedules, one can enhance physical and mental health. By implementing these strategies, we can establish a well-rounded and sustainable routine that allows us to prioritize our health alongside our other responsibilities. Whether we are professionals with demanding careers, parents with busy family lives, or individuals juggling multiple roles, it is possible to find time for health-focused activities with the right approach. Integrating health-focused time blocks into a busy schedule is vital for maintaining a healthy lifestyle.

18.4 LEVERAGING TECHNOLOGY FOR HEALTH MANAGEMENT

In recent times, the rapid progress of technology has brought about significant changes in numerous aspects of our lives, including the way we handle our health. From keeping track of our fitness to utilizing telemedicine, technology has completely transformed how individuals monitor, track, and enhance their health. This section explores the various ways in which technology can be utilized for managing health, providing valuable insights into the tools and strategies that are shaping healthcare. By enhancing the accessibility and convenience of health management, technology has enabled individuals to adopt a proactive approach toward their well-being [14]. Whether it is through wearable devices that monitor fitness levels, mobile applications that track vital signs, or virtual coaching platforms that offer personalized guidance, technology is enabling people to make informed decisions about their health. This section explores the important technologies that are driving advancements in health management, highlighting their benefits and potential impact on improving health outcomes. By embracing these technologies, individuals can better understand their health, make healthier choices, and ultimately lead happier and more fulfilling lives.

In the modern era of technology, the role of technology in effectively managing one's health cannot be overstated. There are various ways in which technology can support and enhance health management, including fitness trackers, telemedicine services, health monitoring apps, and coaching platforms [34]. Here are some important ways in which technology can be utilized for health management:

1. **Tracking fitness:** Fitness trackers and smartwatch wearable devices have the capability to track activity levels and other health metrics. The Wearable devices provide instant data, empowering users to monitor their progress and make informed choices about their health and fitness goals.
2. **Health monitoring apps:** There is a wide range of apps available that assist individuals in monitoring their health metrics. These apps offer valuable insights into health trends and patterns, empowering individuals to make proactive choices about their well-being.
3. **Telemedicine services:** Telemedicine enables people to remotely consult with healthcare providers, eliminating the necessity for in-person appointments. This service is advantageous for people with limited mobility or those who have limited access to healthcare facilities.
4. **Virtual coaching platforms:** Virtual coaching platforms provide personalized guidance and support for various health goals, including fitness, nutrition, and stress management. These platforms offer tailored advice based on individual needs and preferences.
5. **Health information management:** Electronic health record (EHR) systems assist individuals and healthcare providers in efficiently managing health information. EHRs can store medical history, test results, and treatment plans, facilitating better coordination of care.
6. **Medication management apps:** These apps aid individuals in keeping track of their medications, including dosage instructions and refill reminders. This can enhance medication adherence and reduce the risk of medication errors.

7. **Remote monitoring devices:** These allow healthcare professionals to monitor vital signs and other health indicators remotely for individuals with chronic conditions. This allows for timely intervention if necessary.
8. **Health education and awareness:** Technology can be utilized to educate and raise awareness about health issues. Apps, websites, and social media platforms can disseminate information on preventive measures, healthy lifestyle choices, and disease management. By utilizing these tools, individuals can actively participate in their health journey, making informed decisions, monitoring their progress, and staying engaged in their well-being.

Overall, technology has revolutionized health management by providing with apps, devices, and resources to manage their well-being. By leveraging these technological advancements, individuals can lead healthier lives.

18.4.1 HEALTH-TRACKING APPS AND DEVICES

In the modern digital era, health-tracking apps and devices have transformed the process by which individuals monitor and control their health [34]. These innovative tools utilize technology to monitor different health aspects, offering users insightful feedback to assist them in making informed decisions regarding their well-being [25]. A wide array of health-tracking apps and devices, including fitness trackers, blood pressure monitors, and heart rate monitors, are readily available to empower individuals in taking charge of their health. This section presents an overview of some prevalent types of health-tracking apps and devices, emphasizing their unique features, advantages, and how they can contribute to enhancing health outcomes. By comprehending the functionalities of these tools, individuals can make the right decisions about selecting the most suitable options based on their requirements and objectives. As technology progresses, health-tracking apps and devices are anticipated to assume a more significant role in preventive healthcare and personalized medicine [28]. Through the utilization of technology, individuals can effectively monitor their health, ultimately leading to an enhancement in their overall health and well-being. Figure 18.3 presents some common types of health-tracking apps& devices, and Table 18.2 provides a concise overview of each health-tracking app and devices, outlining its primary purpose and functionality.

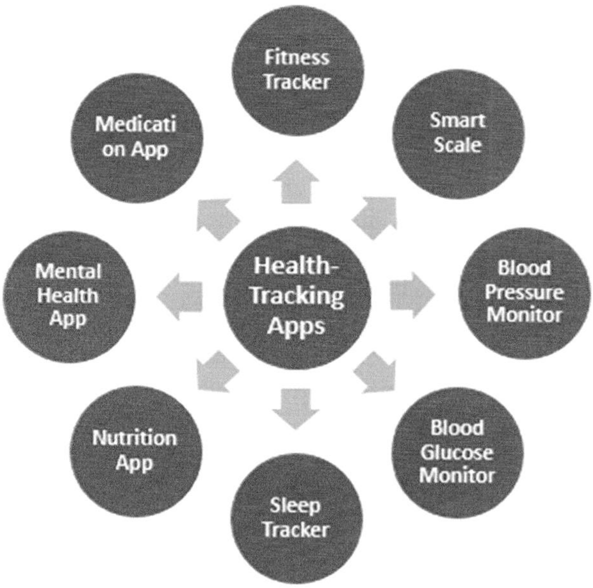

FIGURE 18.3 Some common types of health-tracking apps and devices.

TABLE 18.2 The Overview of Health-Tracking Apps and Devices

Health-Tracking Device/App	Description
Fitness trackers	Wearable digital devices that track physical activity, such as step count, distance covered, and heart rate
Smart scales	Devices that measure weight, body fat, muscle mass, and other metrics related to body composition
Blood pressure monitors	Digital devices that enable to track the blood pressure of people from home
Blood glucose monitors	Devices used by individuals with diabetes to monitor their blood sugar levels
Sleep trackers	Devices that monitor sleep patterns and quality, including total sleep time and sleep stages
Nutrition apps	Smartphone apps that help users track their food intake, calorie consumption, and nutritional content
Mental health apps	Apps offering tools and resources for coping with stress and other mental issues
Medication management apps	Apps that assist users in managing their medications, including the amount and frequency of dose instructions and reminders for refills

Fitness trackers are wearable devices that track physical activity such as step count, distance travelled, burned calories, and heart rate. They often synchronize with smartphone applications to offer users detailed activity data and insights into their fitness levels [15]. Smart scales measure weight, fat, and other metrics related to body composition. They can synchronize data with smartphone applications, enabling users to monitor changes in their body composition over time. Blood pressure monitors enable tracking the blood pressure of people from home. These devices provide accurate readings and assist users in tracking their blood pressure trends over time. Blood glucose monitors are utilized by individuals with diabetes to monitor their blood sugar levels. Continuous glucose monitors offer real-time glucose readings and trends, aiding users in effectively managing their diabetes. Sleep trackers monitor sleep patterns and quality, including total sleep time, sleep stages, and sleep disruptions. They can provide insights into sleep habits and overall sleep health. Nutrition apps help users track their food intake, calorie consumption, and nutritional content. Mental health applications help to effectively handle stress, anxiety, and other mental health conditions. These apps often incorporate features such as meditation, mindfulness exercises, and relaxation techniques to assist users in finding relief. Medication management applications assist users in effectively monitoring their medications. These apps offer features like dosage instructions and refill reminders, which can greatly enhance medication adherence and minimize the likelihood of medication errors. Furthermore, health-tracking apps and devices offer users valuable insights into their overall well-being.

18.4.2 TIPS FOR USING TECHNOLOGY TO STREAMLINE HEALTH-RELATED TASKS

The advancement of technology has revolutionized the manner in which we oversee our well-being, presenting inventive solutions to simplify health-related responsibilities and enhance our general state of wellness. From mobile apps to wearable devices, there are countless ways technology can be leveraged to make health management more efficient and effective [3]. This section discusses tips for using technology to streamline health-related tasks, providing practical advice on how to leverage digital tools to simplify and enhance your health routine. By integrating these tips into everyday routine, overall health and wellness can be enhanced. Fitness objectives can be monitored by handling persistent ailments or simply maintaining a healthy lifestyle. Technology provides a wide range of instruments and materials to assist in attaining the targets [13]. Tips for using technology to streamline health-related tasks include the following:

1. **Set reminders:** Use apps or devices to set reminders for medications, appointments, and health-related tasks to ensure you stay on track.
2. **Use health apps:** Utilize health apps to track your diet, exercise, and overall health.
3. **Telemedicine services:** Consider using telemedicine services for nonemergency medical consultations. This can save you time and eliminate the need for travel to a healthcare facility.
4. **Online prescription refills:** Use online platforms to refill prescriptions. Many pharmacies offer online services that allow you to order refills and have them delivered to your door.
5. **Virtual workouts:** Take advantage of virtual workout classes and fitness apps to stay active from the comfort of your home. This can save you time and eliminate the need for travel to a gym.
6. **Use wearable and health monitoring devices:** Wearable and health monitoring devices help to monitor health metrics.
7. **Digital health records:** Use digital health record systems to access your medical records and share them with healthcare providers.
8. **Automate tasks:** Look for opportunities to automate health-related tasks, such as setting up automatic prescription refills or ordering groceries online for healthier meal options.

18.5 DELEGATION AND SUPPORT SYSTEMS

Delegation and support systems are essential components of effective management and teamwork, serving as pillars that enable individuals and organizations to achieve their goals efficiently and successfully. Delegation involves the transfer of tasks and responsibilities from one individual to another, typically based on their skills, expertise, and availability. Support systems, on the other hand, encompass the resources, guidance, and assistance provided to individuals to help them succeed in their roles. Support systems are crucial for building confidence and competence among team members, empowering them to take on new challenges and excel in their work. Together, delegation and support systems have a vital role in building a strong and capable team. By delegating tasks appropriately and providing the necessary support, managers can create a culture of collaboration and empowerment within their teams. In the workplace, effective delegation and support systems can lead to several benefits. They can enhance productivity by ensuring that tasks are allocated efficiently and completed on time. They can also promote skill development by providing individuals with opportunities to take on new responsibilities and learn from their experiences. Delegation and support systems offer several benefits, including improved efficiency, skill development, enhanced teamwork, reduced stress, and improved job satisfaction.

The importance of delegating tasks to free up time for health, highlighting the numerous benefits of this approach, is discussed in this section. It also provides practical tips and strategies for effective delegation, helping individuals incorporate this practice into their daily lives. By recognizing the value of delegation and implementing strategies to delegate tasks effectively, individuals can create a balanced and sustainable lifestyle that prioritizes health and happiness. Delegating tasks is crucial for freeing up time to prioritize health [13]. When individuals take on too many responsibilities, especially in a professional setting, they often neglect their health due to lack of time. Delegating tasks allows individuals to redistribute workload, ensuring that they have time to focus on their well-being [37]. By effectively assigning tasks to others, individuals can achieve a harmonious equilibrium between their professional and personal lives. This enables them to participate in activities that foster good health, such as physical exercise, maintaining a balanced diet, and engaging in relaxation techniques. Moreover, delegating tasks can serve as a preventive measure against burnout and can enhance mental well-being, as individuals have more opportunities to rest and rejuvenate. In essence, delegating tasks to create time for health is important for maintaining a balance between work and life and ensuring long-term well-being [13]. It empowers individuals to prioritize their health and invest in activities that contribute to their overall happiness and sense of fulfillment.

It is imperative to establish support systems that can effectively manage both health and responsibilities in order to maintain a well-rounded and satisfying life. In today's fast-paced society, Females are often feeling burdened due to heavy loads of work at both professional and family levels, leaving little time or energy to prioritize their own health and well-being. However, with the appropriate support systems in place, it is possible to successfully navigate both aspects of life and attain a sense of equilibrium and contentment. One of the primary advantages of establishing support systems is that they provide individuals with the necessary tools, guidance, and encouragement to overcome the challenges associated with managing both health and responsibilities [16]. For instance, seeking professional support from healthcare providers can assist individuals in developing personalized strategies for managing their health conditions and staying on track with their health objectives. Building support systems can also aid individuals in prioritizing their health and well-being amidst competing demands [39]. By creating a support system that includes accountability partners or wellness coaches, individuals can remain motivated and focused on their health goals. Additionally, support systems can help individuals establish boundaries and decline tasks or commitments that may hinder their health. Establishing support systems for managing both health and responsibilities is vital for maintaining a healthy balance between work and life [9]. By acknowledging the significance of support systems and taking proactive measures to build and sustain them, females can effectively manage their health and responsibilities, leading to a more fulfilling life.

18.6 STRESS MANAGEMENT AND MINDFULNESS

The demands of work, family, and various obligations frequently result in sensations of being overwhelmed, anxious, and exhausted. Nevertheless, the techniques of stress management and mindfulness offer individuals the means to better handle stress and enhance their general state of being. Through acquiring effective stress management skills and nurturing mindfulness, individuals can elevate their quality of life, boost their emotional well-being, and attain a greater sense of tranquility and equilibrium [6].

1. **Stress management:** Stress management requires the identification of stressors and the implementation of strategies to minimize or deal with them efficiently. This can involve methods like time management, relaxation techniques, and problem-solving abilities. By mastering stress management, individuals can avoid the adverse impacts on their physical and mental well-being, boost productivity, and elevate their overall quality of life [14].

2. **Mindfulness:** Practicing mindfulness entails focusing on the current moment with openness, curiosity, and acceptance. By fully immersing oneself in the present moment and observing thoughts, feelings, and sensations without judgment, females can reduce stress, increase self-awareness, and cultivate a deeper sense of peace and well-being through techniques like meditation, deep breathing, and body scans [35].
3. **Interconnection:** Stress management and mindfulness are closely interconnected, as mindfulness techniques can be powerful tools for managing stress. Through the practice of mindfulness, women can enhance their understanding of what causes them stress and acquire the ability to address these stressors with a sense of tranquility and focus. Mindfulness can also help individuals develop resilience to stress by cultivating a mindset of acceptance and nonreactivity [40].
4. **Benefits:** There are numerous advantages to integrating mindfulness into stress management techniques. Studies have demonstrated that interventions based on mindfulness can effectively decrease stress, anxiety, and depression, enhance the quality of sleep, boost cognitive function, and promote overall well-being. Through regular mindfulness practice, individuals can cultivate better emotional regulation, enhance their coping abilities, and experience a heightened sense of inner peace and equilibrium.

18.6.1 TECHNIQUES FOR REDUCING STRESS

Mindfulness meditation is a highly effective technique for alleviating stress and enhancing mental wellness [35]. Through consistent practice of mindfulness meditation, women can develop the ability to monitor their emotions and thoughts without being consumed by them, resulting in a heightened state of tranquility and mental clarity. Deep breathing exercises are a proven technique to effectively alleviate stress [20]. By engaging in deep breathing exercises, women can feel relaxed, counteracting the negative effects of mental stress and fostering a sense of tranquility and relaxation. By taking slow, deliberate breaths and focusing on the sensation of breathing, individuals can effectively decrease their mental stress and anxiety levels and improve their mental health. In addition to deep breathing exercises, physical activity also has an important role in managing stress and promoting mental health [21]. The activities, including walking, exercising, or practicing yoga, are particularly beneficial in reducing stress and enhancing mental well-being.

Furthermore, maintaining a balanced and nutritious diet is essential for promoting mental well-being. A diet that includes ample amounts of vegetables, fruits, lean proteins, and whole grains is required for brain health and decreases the mental health issues [10]. It is also important to limit the consumption of excessive caffeine, sugar, and processed foods, as they can contribute to stress and hinder mental well-being. In addition to these techniques, reaching out for social support from friends, family, and community members can aid in alleviating stress and enhancing mental health [39]. Social support fosters a feeling of belonging and connection, ultimately diminishing feelings of isolation and enhancing mental well-being. By integrating these practices into your daily life, you can effectively manage stress, improve mental well-being, and enhance overall quality of life. Figure 18.4 illustrates different technique for reducing stress.

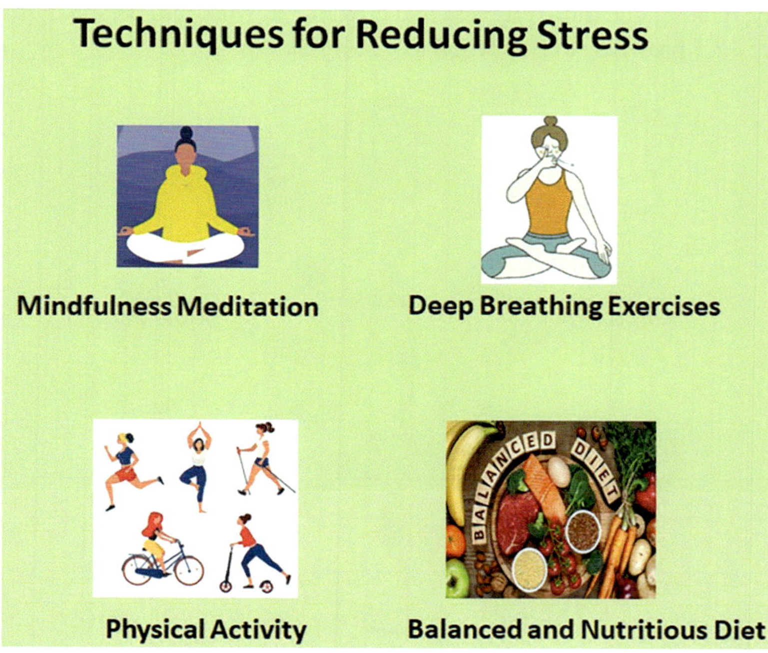

FIGURE 18.4 Techniques for reducing stress.

18.6.2 INTEGRATING MINDFULNESS PRACTICES INTO DAILY LIFE FOR BETTER TIME MANAGEMENT

The responsibilities of work, family, and other obligations may lead to feelings of being inundated and anxious. Yet, through incorporating mindfulness techniques into everyday routines, the ability to manage time effectively is enhanced and alleviates stress and tension. Practicing mindfulness entails being completely attentive and involved in the present moment, free from any form of judgment. It requires observing the thoughts, emotions, and environment with a sense of receptiveness and interest. By cultivating mindfulness, the ability to concentrate on the current activity is enhanced, improving decision-making skills, and optimizing time management [6]. Incorporating mindfulness techniques into daily routine can significantly enhance both general well-being and time management capabilities [12]. Mindfulness entails being completely engaged in the present moment, conscious of thoughts, emotions, and environment, without any form of criticism. Through the development of mindfulness, it enhances concentration and decision-making skills and better organizes time. Mindfulness helps in approaching tasks with greater focus and clarity, making one more efficient and effective in work and personal life [6]. Figure 18.5 presents several benefits of mindfulness.

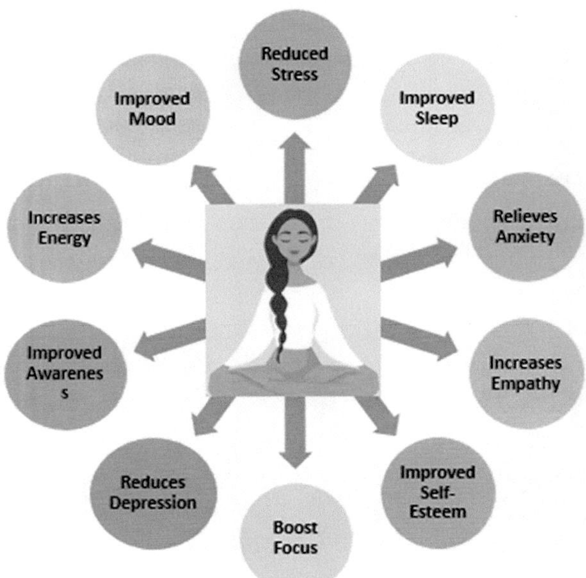

FIGURE 18.5 Benefits of mindfulness.

18.7 SETTING BOUNDARIES AND SAYING NO

Setting boundaries and learning to say no are crucial skills for work–life balance and female well-being [8]. Boundaries are the limits we set to protect our physical, emotional, and mental health, while saying no is a way of respecting those boundaries and prioritizing our own needs. However, many people struggle with setting boundaries and saying no, often feeling guilty or afraid of disappointing others. This section discusses the importance of setting boundaries and saying no, highlighting the benefits of these practices and providing practical tips for incorporating them into daily life. From recognizing one's limits to communicating the boundaries effectively, there are many strategies you can use to establish healthy boundaries and assert your needs. By learning to set boundaries and say no, we can protect our time, energy, and emotions [26]. These are crucial for maintaining wellness in work and life and protecting well-being. Boundaries are like invisible lines that define what acceptable and unacceptable behavior from others is. They help in establishing limits and protecting time, energy, and emotions. Saying no is a way of enforcing those boundaries and prioritizing needs and values [8]. Setting boundaries and saying no may feel uncomfortable at first, but they are essential for maintaining well-being and preventing burnout. By prioritizing needs and values, a healthier and more balanced life can be created. The following points describe how to effectively set boundaries and say no:

1. **Identify limits:** Determine what is important and where you need to set boundaries. This could include time, energy, emotions, or physical space.
2. **Recognize needs:** Understand needs and prioritize self-care.
3. **Saying no practice:** The practice of saying No essential skill for maintaining balance and well-being.
4. **Set priorities:** Determine priorities and align commitments with them. This helps to make decisions about whether to say yes or no.
5. **Be prepared for reactions:** Not everyone will respect boundaries, and some people may react negatively. Stay firm and remember that well-being is important.
6. **Evaluate and adjust:** Regularly evaluate boundaries and adjust them as needed. Boundaries may change depending on circumstances and needs.

Setting boundaries is a vital aspect of health and well-being. Boundaries help us establish limits on what is acceptable and unacceptable in various areas of our lives, including work, relationships, and personal time. Figure 18.6 illustrates the key strategies for setting boundaries in life. By setting boundaries, we protect our physical, emotional, and mental health and ensure that our needs are met. From establishing physical boundaries to protecting emotional well-being, there are many ways to set boundaries that support health and well-being. By setting boundaries in these areas of life, health and well-being will be protected, prevent burnout, and make a balanced work–life and healthy well-being [26]. Few strategies for setting boundaries in various areas of life are given below:

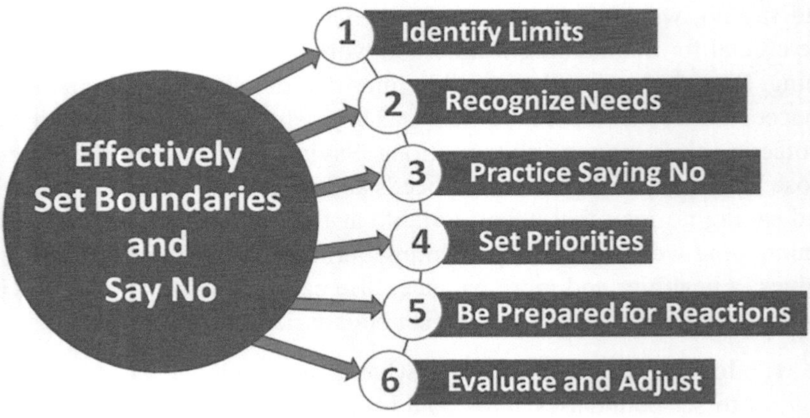

FIGURE 18.6 Effectively set boundaries and say no.

Physical boundaries: Set boundaries around your physical space and time, ensuring you have time for rest and relaxation, and creating a comfortable and safe environment for yourself.

Emotional boundaries: Protect your emotional well-being by setting boundaries. This might involve saying no to requests that require you to provide excessive emotional support or setting limits on how much you share about your own emotions with others.

Social boundaries: Establish boundaries in your social interactions to ensure that your relationships are healthy and respectful.

Work boundaries: Establishing clear boundaries in your professional life is crucial for a harmonious balance between work and life. This may entail defining the number of hours you dedicate to work, establishing specific times when you are accessible for work-related inquiries, and determining the tasks you are willing to undertake.

Digital boundaries: It is important to set boundaries regarding your technology usage in order to safeguard your mental well-being. This may involve establishing restrictions on the amount of time spent on social media or email, as well as determining specific times when you are available via phone or computer.

Self-care boundaries: It is important to establish boundaries around self-care activities, including time for physical exercise, meditation, pursuing hobbies, or immersing oneself in nature.

Assertive communication: Practice assertive communication to clearly express your boundaries to others. Be firm and respectful when stating your limits, and be willing to enforce them if they are not respected.

Self-reflection: Regularly reflect on your boundaries and assess whether they are serving you well. Adjust them as needed to ensure they continue to support your health and well-being.

Saying no to commitments can be challenging, especially when we fear disappointing or letting down others. This often leads to feelings of guilt, which can be difficult to overcome. However, learning to overcome this guilt is essential for maintaining healthy boundaries and prioritizing our own well-being. This section explores strategies for overcoming guilt associated with saying no to certain commitments. It highlights the importance of setting boundaries and prioritizing self-care, and provides practical tips for managing guilt and asserting your needs. By learning to navigate these feelings of guilt, you can establish boundaries that support your well-being and lead to healthier, more fulfilling relationships. Overcoming guilt associated with saying no to certain commitments can be challenging, but it is an important skill to learn for maintaining your well-being.

18.8 REGULAR EVALUATION AND ADJUSTMENT

Regular evaluation and adjustment are important components for maintaining well-being and achieving goals, allowing one to stay on track and make necessary changes for progress [27]. Whether in personal or professional lives, the ability to assess progress, identify areas for improvement, and adapt strategies accordingly can lead to greater success and satisfaction. This section explores the importance of regular evaluation and adjustment in achieving a balanced and fulfilling life.

Efficient time management is essential for reaching objectives, handling duties, and sustaining a harmonious work–life equilibrium. Yet, merely applying time-management techniques is insufficient; it is equally vital to consistently evaluate and modify these techniques to guarantee their efficacy. These openings highlight the significance of routinely assessing time-management techniques and their productivity, goal attainment, and general well-being. Regularly assessing time-management strategies is essential for optimizing the use of time, achieving goals, and maintaining a balanced and fulfilling life [1]. It is essential to consistently evaluate time-management strategies for a variety of important reasons.

Identifying effectiveness: Regular assessment helps in determining which time-management strategies are working well and which are not. This allows us to focus on the methods that are most effective.

Adapting to changes: Life is dynamic, and circumstances change. Regular assessment helps you adapt your time-management strategies to new situations, such as changes in workload, personal responsibilities, or goals.

Improving efficiency: By evaluating your time-management strategies, you can identify inefficiencies and areas where you can improve. This can lead to better use of your time and increased productivity.

Setting realistic goals: Regular assessment helps in designing realistic goals based on current circumstances and priorities. This prevents you from overcommitting and feeling overwhelmed.

Maintaining balance: Evaluating your time-management techniques can assist you in guaranteeing that you are maintaining a harmonious equilibrium between your professional commitments, personal life, and self-care.

Staying motivated: Regular assessment allows tracking the progress and celebrating successes, which helps in staying motivated.

In the ever-evolving landscape of work and life, the ability to adjust strategies based on changing priorities and circumstances is a crucial skill. Whether it's a shift in professional responsibilities, a change in personal circumstances, or unexpected events, being able to adapt and realign your strategies is essential for maintaining productivity and achieving your goals. This introduction explores effective strategies for adjusting your approach in response to changing priorities and circumstances, ensuring that you remain focused and effective in the face of change.

18.9 CONCLUSION

Effective time management is crucial for maintaining optimal health, particularly for women who often encounter unique challenges in juggling multiple responsibilities. Women frequently prioritize the needs of others above their own, but it is vital to remember that self-care is fundamental for overall well-being. This encompasses allocating time for regular exercise, sufficient sleep, nutritious eating, and relaxation. Allocating dedicated time for self-care activities can contribute to improving physical and mental health. Women often assume numerous roles and responsibilities, both at home and in the workplace. It is important to establish realistic goals that consider these responsibilities, as well as any health requirements or limitations. Establishing attainable goals can help prevent burnout and alleviate feelings of being overwhelmed. Women are often expected to shoulder an unequal share of household and caregiving responsibilities. Delegating tasks to family members, friends, or hired assistance can help create more time for self-care and other important activities. Clearly communicating your needs and boundaries is crucial to ensure that others comprehend and respect them. Technology is now a valuable tool for effective time management. The benefit of using technology, such as apps or digital calendars, is to improve organization and productivity. By utilizing these tools, females can create to-do lists, set reminders for important deadlines or appointments, and track their progress toward achieving their goals. This can help individuals stay focused, manage their time more effectively, and ultimately, increase their chances of success. Technology can also facilitate staying connected with your support network and accessing resources that can assist in managing time more efficiently. Mindfulness practices, such as meditation or yoga, help in decreasing stress, enhancing focus, and improving overall females' mental health. Devoting time to practicing mindfulness helps women remain grounded and present, even during busy or stressful periods. Establishing boundaries to safeguard your time and energy is important. This may involve declining less priorities or values commitments, or setting limits on the amount of time you allocate to certain activities. Establishing clear boundaries is essential in avoiding burnout and prioritizing what truly matters to you. Cultivating a robust support system consisting of friends, family, and healthcare providers can assist in better time management. This network can offer motivation, guidance, and hands-on assistance during challenging times. Remember, it is important to seek help, when necessary, without hesitation.

Implementing these strategies enables women to effectively manage their time and give priority to their health, resulting in a more balanced and satisfying life. It is common to feel overwhelmed by the numerous responsibilities and demands of daily life, often neglecting one's own health and well-being. However, it is crucial to remember that prioritizing women's health is not only beneficial for them but also for those who rely on them. Women deserve to prioritize their health and well-being, just like anyone else. Despite the countless tasks and responsibilities women handle each day, taking care of herself should not be considered a luxury but rather a necessity. Women's health is an investment for her future, ensuring that women can continue to care for others and lead a fulfilling life. By giving priority to her health, women set a positive example for those around her, including her family and friends. Demonstrating the importance of self-care can inspire them to do the same, creating a ripple effect of well-being. A healthy lifestyle not only benefits her physically but also mentally and emotionally. It provides the energy and strength to confront life's challenges head-on, making one stronger and more resilient. Remember, self-care is not selfish; it is an important part of maintaining physical and mental health. Females do not have to make drastic changes to prioritize their health. Small, consistent actions such as consuming nutritious meals, staying active, and getting sufficient rest can make a significant difference in how you feel. These small steps are acts of self-love that can have a profound impact on her health and happiness.

KEYWORDS

- **female health**
- **technique**
- **time-management**
- **work–life balance**
- **happiness**

REFERENCES

1. Akhmarov, A. V., Potapov, P., & Kaimova, F. A. (2023). Effective time management: Methods and techniques. *Ekonomika I Upravlenie: Problemy, Resheniya*, *10/5*(139), 151–157.
2. Ali, S. (2016). Quality of human resources in organized and unorganized sectors with special reference to health issue management of working women. *Al-Barkaat Journal of Finance & Management*, *8*(1), 82–91.
3. Altamimi, R., & Skinner, G. (2018, March). Evaluating contemporary physical activity self-monitoring technology performance. In: *2018 12th International Symposium on Medical Information and Communication Technology (ISMICT)*, (pp. 1–8). IEEE.
4. Alvarez Sainz, M., Ferrero, A. M., & Ugidos, A. (2019). Time management: Skills to learn and put into practice. *Education+ Training*, *61*(5), 635–648.
5. Burton, W. N., Schultz, A. B., Chen, C. Y., & Edington, D. W. (2008). The association of worker productivity and mental health: A review of the literature. *International Journal of Workplace Health Management*, *1*(2), 78–94.
6. Choudhary, M. (2023). Mindfulness and well-being: Mindfulness-based interventions for promoting well-being and its impact on cognitive, emotional, and physiological processes. In: *Lloyd Business Review*, (pp. 1–18).
7. Chaudhary, R. R., & Bagga, R. (2018). Work Life Imbalance and Psychosocial Tribulations among Working Women. *International Journal of Management Excellence, 10,* 1323–1333.
8. Cloud, H., & Townsend, J. S. (1996). *Boundaries: When to Say Yes*. Strand Publishing.
9. Cvenkel, N., & Cvenkel, N. (2020). Work-life balance and well-being at work: Strategies for individual and organisational health and potential. In: *Well-Being in the Workplace: Governance and Sustainability Insights to Promote Workplace Health*, (pp. 243–261).
10. Desai, A. K., Desai, A. K., Rush, J., Naveen, L., & Thaipisuttikul, P. (2011). Nutrition and nutritional supplements to promote brain health. In: *Enhancing Cognitive Fitness in Adults: A Guide to the Use and Development of Community-Based Programs*, (pp. 249–269).
11. Frangou, S. (2016). *Women in Academic Psychiatry*. Department of Psychiatry, Icahn School of Medicine at Mount Sinai: New York, USA.
12. Greeson, J. M. (2009). Mindfulness research update: 2008. *Complementary Health Practice Review*, *14*(1), 10–18.
13. Guiliana, J. V., & Ornstein, H. (2023). Time Management in the healthcare practice and delegation strategies. *Healthcare Administration Leadership & Management Journal*, *1*(2), 75–77.
14. Haleem, A., Javaid, M., Suman, R., & Vaishya, R. (2022). Exploring the capabilities of modern technologies for health care. *Apollo Medicine, 19*, 37–40.
15. Halteren, A. V., & Gay, V. C. (2015). Continuous digital health. *IEEE Internet Computer, 19*, 8–9.
16. Harkey, J., Young, J., Carter, J. J., & Demoratz, M. J. (2017). Supporting the support system: How assessment and communication can help patients and their support systems. *Professional Case Management, 22*, 174–180.

17. Hayashi, E., Rau, M., Neo, Z. H., Tan, N., Ramasubramanian, S., & Paulos, E. (2012). TimeBlocks: Mom, can I have another block of time. In: *Proceedings of the SIGCHI Conference on Human Factors in Computing Systems*, (pp. 1713–1716).
18. Henrietta, H. M. (2023). A comprehensive review on human health, promoting the well-being of teaching professionals. *International Journal of Environment, Engineering and Education*, *5*(2), 79–86.
19. Hessing, M. (1994). More than clockwork: Women's time management in their combined workloads. *Sociological Perspectives, 37*, 611–633.
20. Heredia, L., Gasol, L., Ventura, D., Vicens, P., & Torrente, M. (2017). Mindfulness-based stress reduction training program increases psychological well-being, and emotional regulation, but not attentional performance. A pilot study. *Mindfulness & Compassion*, *2*(2), 130–137.
21. Hooda, V. S., Muley, P. A., Muley, P. P., Anjakar, A., & Bandre, G. (2024). Effect of exercise on depression, anxiety and mood: A narrative review. *Journal of Clinical & Diagnostic Research*, *18*(1), 1–3.
22. Jenkins, C. L. (1997). Women, work, and caregiving: How do these roles affect women's well-being. *Journal of Women & Aging*, *9*(3), 27–45.
23. Kamath, V., & Ganguly, S. (2020). Are periodic health checkups useful or necessary. *APIK Journal of Internal Medicine*, *8*(2), 51–55.
24. Kamel, P. L. (2006). Nutritional assessment and requirements. *Dysphagia, 4,* 189–195.
25. Keita, M. A. (2016). Digital technology and health: Evaluating the impact of mobile health-tracking applications on patients well-being. *Munich Personal Re PEc Archive,* 1–21.
26. Majini, D. K., & Bella, J. (2023). CreatingBoundaries to maintain a healthy work-life balance. *International Journal of Multidisciplinary Research in Arts, Science and Technology*, *1*(3), 24–30.
27. McDonald, A., & McDonald, A. (1999). Understanding community care: A guide for social workers. In: *Monitoring and Review,* (pp. 86–98).
28. Morava, A., & Sui, Y. (2019). Who's monitoring the health-monitoring applications. *Health Science Inquiry*, *10*(1), 57.
29. Mousa, M., Boyle, J., Skouteris, H., Mullins, A. K., Currie, G., Riach, K., & Teede, H. J. (2021). Advancing women in healthcare leadership: A systematic review and meta-synthesis of multi-sector evidence on organisationalinterventions. *EClinicalMedicine*, *39*, 101084.
30. Omar, N., Ahamat, A., Sidek, S., Al-shami, S. A., Aripin, M. A., & Aris, M. (2019). The benefits and challenges of practicing work-life balance among women entrepreneurs. *International Journal of Innovative Technology and Exploring Engineering 9(*1), 2028–2033
31. Orel, N. A., Landry-Meyer, L., & Spence, M. A. (2007). Women's caregiving careers and retirement financial insecurity. *Adultspan Journal*, *6*(1), 49–62.
32. Prasad, R., & Pandey, A. K. (2012). Sleep hygiene and good sleep habits: A review. *The Indian Journal of Sleep Medicine, 7,* 134–138.
33. Sari, N. P., Setiawan, M. A., Utama, A. H., Mansur, H., & Mohd Yasin, M. H. (2023). Gen Z Indonesia in the era of post-pandemic disruption. *International Journal of Academic Research in Business and Social Sciences*, *13*(7), 791–806.

34. Stones, S. R. (2016). How innovative technologies can support individuals to better self-manage their conditions. *Annals of the Rheumatic Diseases, 75*, 23–23.
35. Sukh, P., & Sharma, B. R. (2023). Application of meditation for stress management. *International Journal of Yogic, Human Movement and Sports Sciences*, *8*(1), 247–249.
36. Sultan, T., & Nag, N. (2020). Work-health balance: Characterizing short-term and long-term impact to health. *Journals at IDEAS*, 1–6.
37. Trepanier, S. (2023). The Art and Science of Delegating Effectively. *Journal of Continuing Education in Nursing, 54*(10), 444–445.
38. Vijayasekar, M., & Bharanitharan, J. (2014). Time management for working women in Chennai. *Available at SSRN 2448538*.
39. Visvalingam, A., Singh Dhillon, J., & Gunasekaran, S. S. (2019). Role of social support in self-management of health. *Journal of Information Technology Management*, *11*(1), 24–41.
40. Whitton, T., Buchanan, G., & Smith, S. (2019). How a mindfulness intervention can improve patients' mental well-being? *Nursing Times*, *115*, 48–51.
41. Zwetsloot, G., & Pot, F. (2004). The business value of health management. *Journal of Business Ethics*, *55*, 115–124.

CHAPTER 19

Female Health: Educating and Outreach

SHWETA KESWANI* and DIPALI SAXENA

*Corresponding author

ABSTRACT

Higher social status, independence, and more decision-making autonomy are all correlated with education. Because they are further inclined to allocate unrestricted funds to expenditures made on human resources, such as food, health, and education, educated women will have more financial power over their families. The millennium development goals could not be met if women were empowered to make decisions about their own health in a setting that is appropriate and supportive of them. Only community-based demand-side programs focusing on improving maternal health and education will be able to achieve this. Numerous studies revealed that women with education were more likely than those without it to support the nation's economic growth. A higher level of education among women benefits the family's health, which in turn drives economic growth. Studies examining middle-income and lower income nations have consistently found favorable results, the effects of female education on the GDP. A study done by the World Bank analyzed the effect of educating girls in several countries and found that more girls having access to education improves the environment for development and economic prosperity. Effective outreach and education on female health require a comprehensive approach that considers cultural sensitivities, accessibility, and ongoing support to make a lasting impact.

Holistic Approaches for Women's Sustainable Health, Volume 2: Advancements, Socioeconomic Impacts, and Innovative Strategies. Junaid Ahmad Malik, Anamika Chauhan, and Megh R. Goyal (Eds)

DOI: 10.1201/9781779641656-23

19.1 INTRODUCTION

19.1.1 INTRODUCTION OF HEALTH

Health is more than just the absence of illness or disability; it is a state of complete mental, social, and physical well-being. Health is a basic human right that is independent of race, religion, political affiliation, economic background, and social standing [28]. Good health must be attained by providing all people with access to medical, psychological, and related knowledge, to the maximum extent feasible [27]. Cooperation and well-informed opinion are essential for the public to actively engage in improving their health. To uphold their duty to safeguard the health of their populace, governments must offer suitable social and health services.

19.1.2 DETERMINANTS OF HEALTH

Determinants of health [26] are elements that affect a person's state of health and well-being. These contributing factors can be categorized further into several broad categories:

- **Biological and genetic factors:** These include a person's genetic makeup, inherited traits, and biological predispositions to certain diseases or conditions. Genetic factors can influence susceptibility to diseases such as cancer, diabetes, and heart disease [26].
- **Behavioral factors:** Behaviors and lifestyle decisions have a big influence on health. These include the following preventative health measures: immunizations and screenings, sexual behaviors, food, exercise, and substance usage (such as tobacco, alcohol, and narcotics).
- **Demographic factors:** Socioeconomic status, revenue, education, employment, and social support networks all play crucial roles in determining health outcomes [26]. People with higher socioeconomic status generally have better access to healthcare, healthier living conditions, and resources to adopt healthier behaviors.
- **Environmental factors:** The well-being, socioeconomic environments where individuals live, work, and play can affect health. Environmental determinants include exposure to pollutants, access to clean air and water, housing conditions, availability of healthy food options, and access to recreational spaces.

- **Healthcare access and quality:** One important factor influencing health is accessibility to its services, which may be confined to cost, availability, and treatment. Poorer health outcomes might arise from delayed diagnosis and treatment of illnesses caused by a lack of access to healthcare.
- **Public policy and interventions:** Government policies and interventions, such as public health initiatives, regulations, and laws, can influence health at the population level. These include policies related to healthcare, education, transportation, urban planning, and environmental protection.

Understanding and addressing these determinants holistically is necessary for excelling in population health. Public health efforts often focus on addressing social and economic inequalities, improving access to healthcare, promoting healthy behaviors, and creating supportive environments for health-promoting choices.

19.1.3 IMPORTANCE OF ADEQUATE HEALTH FOR FEMALE

Since women are the cornerstone of a family's overall health, improving their access to quality treatment can benefit both children and families as well as their general health [15]. Female health and family health, and community are closely intertwined. In 2011, females continued to face gender inequality [16]. Gender equality is still an elusive objective, especially in the developing world, despite efforts over the past century to eliminate the health and social disparities between women and men [16]. Despite accounting for two-thirds of global working hours, women only make up 10% of global income [7]. This demonstrates the inequality that women face and makes up less than 1% of all property on Earth. Less access to education for women and girls exists in many nations, despite the fact that education is a key indicator of well-being [25]. Poverty is synonymous with marginalization and disempowerment, in addition to hunger and illness. Correspondingly, many females experience abuse and violation of other human rights [23].

Global health systems are failing women and girls, who have unique health requirements [14]. Women's health has emerged as a critical priority in today's world, according to the WHO, although the data on this topic are scant and frequently untrustworthy [14].

According to a UNICEF study estimates that complications that are totally preventable account for nearly 810 deaths of women per day. This is mostly because there are not enough accessible and reasonably priced healthcare systems. The US Bureau of Labor Statistics states that women make up 77.6% of the workforce in social assistance and health care [13]. It will be easier for this group of people to achieve SDG 3 (Good health and well-being) if we invest in them by giving them access to safe spaces, nondiscriminatory opportunities, and quality healthcare systems.

19.1.4 IMPORTANCE OF EDUCATED FEMALE AND ITS ROLE IN SUSTAINABLE DEVELOPMENT GOALS

Encyclopedically, there is still a gender difference in educational achievement despite a net rise in registrations. Education for girls is generally viewed as having lower significance than education for boys in numerous nations [18]. Compared to one in six males, it is projected that one in five girls of primary school age are not enrolled. Education is an important predictor of well-being and has a direct positive impact on women [22]. The rate of child mortality is advanced in homes where the mother has the smallest level of education across all countries with dependable data (WHO, 2009). Also, because knowledge affects availability, it has a significant impact on the quantum of sickness and mortality within a society. Approximately, 597 million women and 352 million men were illiterate worldwide in 1996 [8].

Not only must elementary education be addressed, but secondary and postsecondary education as well. Women will benefit from higher primary and secondary education rates in terms of employment, well-being, and a reduction in social alienation. Higher marriageable ages, lower fertility and mortality rates, improved maternity care, and a lower chance of HIV/AIDS infection are all linked to secondary education [7].

19.2 SUSTAINABLE DEVELOPMENT GOALS AND WOMEN

Females play a variety of roles in sustainable development, and their views must be heard at all levels. They frequently take care of their families first, have original thoughts and viewpoints, and frequently initiate change on many fronts. A study conducted by the University of Wisconsin-Madison confirmed that females make up half of the world's population and work nearly two-thirds of the hours that people work. Because they make up such a large section of the population, women are not only directly involved in achieving development goals but also, occasionally more so than men and boys, are greatly impacted by social, political, and economic challenges.

Gender equality also touches on the social, economic, and environmental pillars of sustainable development. These dimensions have equal and interrelated importance [18]. The effective pursuit of sustainable development necessitates the full and equal engagement of females in all respects of policy creation and decision-making. In the past, women and girls dominated topics that directly affected them. These mostly include child marriage, violence against women, reproductive and maternal health, etc. It turned out to be an error [4]. One critical component that is often overlooked in the pursuit of sustainable development on the environmental, economic, and social fronts is the inclusion of women in the process of making decisions.

It is a right to equal access to education. Achieving this right is essential to tackling some of the most urgent issues of our day, such as violence against women, climate change, and a lack of access to healthcare [23]. Numerous obstacles stand in the way of girls realizing their entitlement to an education. These problems include damaging customs, financial obstacles, and societal and gender conventions. Unrealized human potential and gender inequality endure in some nations because of stigmas associated with women's and girls' education. Because of gender discrimination, which keeps many women behind, the world is also held back [17].

The 2030 Agenda for sustainable development defines clearly that every single one of the 17 goals depends on educating and empowering women and girls [14]. Educated females can play an important role in improving sustainable development goals (SDGs).

19.2.1 REDUCED POVERTY AND HUNGER (SDG 1 AND SDG 2)

Families and the next generation can escape the cycle of poverty by pursuing an education that leads to gainful work. An individual's salary rate for females increased by 10–15% for each extra year of basic education and by 25% for each additional year of secondary school, according to a World Bank study. In addition, a mother's family cares for her 90% of her earnings, which aids in rescuing a home from starvation and poverty [24].

19.2.2 IMPROVED HEALTH AND WELL-BEING (SDG 3)

Females with higher levels of education are better able to give their kids better nutrition and educational support. Children who are well-educated and in good health contribute more to society [21]. A UNESCO study found that there would be a 15% decrease in child fatalities if all women had only completed their primary education. Globally, child mortality would be reduced by half and about three million lives saved if every woman completed an education [18]. According to the same UNESCO study, maternal fatalities would drop by 60% and roughly 98,000 lives may be preserved if all mothers were to get an elementary education [2, 24].

19.2.3 QUALITY EDUCATION CAN EMPOWER FEMALE (SDG 4)

Women who receive a high-quality education are better equipped to take care of themselves, enhance their chances of finding jobs and taking on leadership roles, and make better judgments regarding their general well-being and health. As a result, individuals can actively participate in societies [24, 27].

19.2.4 GENDER EQUALITY (SDG 5 AND SDG 10)

Gender norms, wage discrimination, income inequality, and gender-based violence are the major causes of objectification manifestation. Increasing women's and girls' access to education increases their chances of realizing their full potential, asserting their rights as humans, and contributing to people [8]. Females with education lead to the upcoming generation of female frontrunners and have made major progress in closing the gender gap. Educating women and girls is widely acknowledged as being crucial to the equality in gender.

- **Empowerment:** Education empowers females by providing them with awareness, skills, and confidence. Female with advanced levels of education participates in family and community decision-making, which increases their autonomy and agency [28].
- **Economic opportunities:** Education opens up economic prospects for females and girls, enabling them to access higher paying jobs, entrepreneurship opportunities, and leadership positions. In addition to helping individual women, this economic empowerment advances the general development and prosperity of the economy [20].
- **Health and well-being:** Educated women tend to have better health outcomes for themselves and their families. They utilize healthcare services, adopt healthier behaviors, and make informed choices about reproductive health and family planning, resulting in decreased rates of maternal and infant mortality and enhanced general health [25].
- **Decreased gender-based violence:** By raising understanding of legal rights and safeguards, encouraging critical thinking abilities to question harmful gender norms, and offering channels for obtaining resources and support, education can operate as a preventive measure against gender-based violence.
- **Breaking the cycle of poverty:** Future generations are impacted by female education. Females who are educated are likely to invest in the education and well-being of their children, breaking the cycle of intergenerational poverty and contributing to the long-term development of families and communities.
- **Social and political participation:** Education enhances women's ability to engage in civic and political processes, advocating for their rights and interests, and contributing to democratic governance and social change. Well-educated women can participate in community development initiatives, grassroots movements, and political leadership roles [13].

In due course, supporting women's education is a wise development strategy that has enormous advantages for people on an individual, family, community, and societal level, in addition to being a question of human rights and social justice. Societies can unleash the potential of half of their population and build more inclusive and prosperous futures for all by advancing gender equality via education.

19.2.5 SANITATION, CLEAN WATER, AND WOMEN'S AND GIRLS' EDUCATION ARE ALL STRONGLY RELATED (SDG 6)

- **Health and hygiene:** To be healthy and avoid waterborne infections, one must have access to clean water and sanitary facilities [27]. When female have access to clean water and sanitation, they are healthier, which in turn allows them to attend school regularly without being hindered by illnesses or the burden of caring for sick family members.
- **Education attendance:** Throughout the world, girls are responsible for fetching water for their families, which can be a time-consuming task. Girls may spend hours every day fetching water when there are not any clean water sources close to their homes or schools, which leaves them with little energy or time for study [27]. Girls are more likely to attend school consistently if there is access to sanitary facilities and clean water near communities and schools.
- **Menstrual hygiene management:** Absence of access to sanitary facilities and clean water can pose significant challenges for girls managing menstruation, leading to absenteeism from school [27]. When schools provide clean and private toilets, handwashing facilities, and menstrual hygiene supplies, girls are better able to manage their periods with dignity and attend school regularly.
- **Empowerment and economic opportunities:** Education is a key determinant of women's empowerment and economic participation. When girls can attend school regularly, they are more likely to acquire knowledge and skills that can help them secure better-paying jobs and contribute to economic development. Having access to sanitary facilities and clean water supports girls' education by removing barriers to attendance and improving overall well-being [29].
- **Community development:** Reducing poverty and promoting sustainable development depend on having access to clean water and sanitary facilities. When communities have reliable access to sanitary facilities and clean water, they are better able to thrive economically, socially, and environmentally, leading to improved living standards and opportunities for education for all, including women and girls.

Addressing SDG 6 (clean water and sanitation) and SDG 4 (education) in an integrated method is crucial for achieving sustainable development and advancing gender equality. By ensuring access to sanitary facilities and clean water, especially for females, we can promote their education, empowerment, and well-being, leading to more inclusive and resilient societies.

19.2.6 ENCOURAGING GIRLS AND WOMEN CAN HAVE AN IMPACT ON ACCESSIBLE, PURE ENERGY (SDG 7)

Accessible, pure energy, that is used to brighten a child's homework lamp or a woman's sewing machines for her business, is the driving force behind sustainable development. Since females are the main energy managers in households, the absence of current energy sources has serious repercussions for them. By assisting households in making knowledgeable decisions about energy-related issues, women's empowerment can have a significant impact on SDG 7 [19, 24]. Moreover, ladies with education are more likely to be creative thinkers who develop novel concepts like dependable contemporary energy services.

19.2.7 EDUCATION FOR WOMEN AND GIRLS INCREASES ECONOMIC GROWTH AND ACCESS TO RESPECTABLE JOBS (SDG 8)

According to a World Bank analysis of 100 nations, the income growth rate per year of each country increases by 0.3 percentage points for every 1 percentage point growth in the secondary education of females. For instance, India's GDP would increase by $5.5 billion if there were a 1% increase in the number of girls enrolled in secondary school. A female's chances of arriving in the formal economy, where she can anticipate better working conditions, enhanced rights at work, and social safeguards, are increased, and wage discrepancies are decreased with education [29].

19.2.8 INFRASTRUCTURE, INDUSTRY, AND INNOVATION ALL DEVELOP WHEN FEMALES RECEIVE AN EDUCATION (SDG 9)

Education for females can foster an atmosphere that promotes creativity, entrepreneurship, and innovation. Additionally, participation in science-based research and invention benefits support sustainable development, and educating girls in science, technology, engineering, and mathematics (STEM) courses increases the number of sustainable industries [3, 20].

19.2.9 RESPONSIBLE CONSUMPTION RISES WHEN WOMEN AND GIRLS RECEIVE EDUCATION (SDG 12)

Females can contribute significantly to lowering consumption when they have access to knowledge about climate change adaptation. Additionally, they can strengthen the resiliency within the surroundings. UNICEF stated that educating females is the best strategy to empower societies in the fight against climate change [24].

19.2.10 EDUCATING FEMALE RAISES AWARENESS OF CLIMATE ACTION AND ENVIRONMENTAL WELL-BEING (SDG 13, SDG 14, AND SDG 15)

Among the groups most susceptible to the consequences of climate change are women and girls. Additionally, they are the most potent change agents. Giving women and girls pertinent information about the environment and climate change enables them to support development to be sustained in their local communities [24].

19.2.11 PEACE, FAIRNESS, AND ROBUST INSTITUTIONS ARE THE RESULTS OF EDUCATED FEMALES (SDG 16)

To attain justice, peace, and robust establishments, females must be involved in the process. It is necessary to eradicate gender discrimination before all women can enjoy these fundamental rights. Because they are better aware of their rights, educated women and girls are more inclined to fight for justice and address discrimination, including gender-based violence (GBV) and other forms of discrimination [16]. Additionally, they are involved in their communities as leaders and citizens. There is an urgent need to increase awareness regarding female education worldwide. We are all impacted by the 132 million girls in elementary and secondary school who do not attend school. The examples above are just a few of the ways that achieving the SDGs through female education can help us achieve sustainable development on a global scale.

19.3 GLOBAL SCENARIO OF HEALTH AND EDUCATION FOR FEMALES

The global scenario of health and education for females has seen significant progress in recent decades, but continues to face challenges in many parts of the world. Here is an overview:

Health

- **Progress:** There have been improvements in maternal and child health, with reductions in maternal mortality rates and child mortality rates globally. In many areas, there is now greater access to healthcare services, including family planning and reproductive healthcare.
- **Challenges:** Disparities persist, with women and girls in low-income and marginalized communities facing greater barriers to accessing healthcare services. Maternal mortality remains high in some regions, like Africa and Asia.

Education

- **Progress:** Globally, girls' access to education has improved significantly, as seen by rising elementary, secondary, and university enrollment rates. More girls are enrolling in and finishing their education as a result of efforts to close the gender gap in education.
- **Challenges:** Disparities in access to education still exist despite advancements, especially in rural and underdeveloped areas. Cultural norms, child marriage, gender-based violence, and inadequate school infrastructure are just a few of the obstacles that girls currently face. Disparities in learning outcomes between boys and girls, particularly in STEM disciplines, raise concerns about the quality of education.

19.3.1 GLOBAL INITIATIVES AND EFFORTS

- International organizations, governments, and nongovernmental organizations (NGOs) have implemented various initiatives to address the health and education needs of females globally. These initiatives focus on promoting gender equality, empowering women and girls, improving access to healthcare services, enhancing reproductive rights, and increasing educational opportunities.

- SDGs, particularly SDG 3 and SDG 4, include targets aimed at improving the health and education outcomes of females worldwide [33]. Efforts to achieve these goals involve multisectoral collaborations, policy reforms, investments in infrastructure and human resources, and community engagement.
- Persistent gender inequalities, discriminatory practices, cultural norms, and socioeconomic disparities continue to hinder progress in health and education for females globally.
- Conflict, displacement, natural disasters, and humanitarian crises disproportionately affect females, disrupting access to healthcare and education and exacerbating existing vulnerabilities.

There have been significant improvements in the health and education of females on a global scale, but challenges persist, requiring sustained efforts and investments to achieve equality, well-being, and empowerment for females worldwide.

According to UNICEF estimates, 129 million females globally do not attend school. The proportion of males and females participating in basic and secondary school worldwide is getting close to parity (male 90% and female 89%). In low socioeconomic countries, girls' rate of secondary school completion is still inadequate, with only 36% of them completing secondary school as compared to 44% of boys who complete secondary school.

Gender bias, poverty, violence, and child marriage can have an impact on girls' goals and self-perceptions of their societal duties [8]. These factors can also lead to inequalities in labor market participation and occupational segregation.

Girls' health and well-being are suffering as a result of COVID-19, and many face the possibility of not going back to school when classes resume. Based on existing evidence, there has been a rise in the incidence of violence against women and girls during the pandemic, endangering their general well-being, safety, and health.

19.3.2 INDIAN SCENARIO OF HEALTH AND EDUCATION OF FEMALE [22]

19.3.2.1 LITERACY AND EDUCATION

- According to the 2011 Census, 72.98% of Indians are literate overall, with females having a literacy rate of 64.63% and males having an 80.9% rate. Over the past ten years, rural ladies have experienced the greatest increase in literacy (24%).

- At the primary school level, from 2012–2013, the gross enrolment ratio (GER) of a female child is greater than male child. When we get to higher educational levels, such as upper elementary, secondary, and higher secondary for both males and girls, we notice a declining tendency in GER. The higher secondary level female GER in 2021–2022 was 58.2 (compared to 39.4 in 2012–2013). Furthermore, at higher education levels, there is little variation in the GER of the male and female populations. At this point in 2020–2021, the female GER of 26.7 was somewhat higher than the male GER of 26.7.
- Around 3.1% of girls and 4.5% of males, according to the 75th Round July 2017–June 2018 of NSS, are enrolled under technical or professional programs. 8.3% of men and 6.3% of women in metropolitan areas are enrolled in technical or professional programs.
- Of the major subjects offered by universities, medicine had the highest proportion of female students per 100 male students (157.1), afterward, arts and social sciences (111.6), science (89.1), business (85.9), and engineering and technical (38.7).

19.4 INEQUALITIES FOR FEMALES

19.4.1 CULTURAL AND TRADITIONAL BELIEFS

Cultural and traditional beliefs can significantly contribute to inequalities, particularly concerning gender, ethnicity, religion, and socioeconomic status. Here are some ways in which cultural and traditional beliefs can perpetuate inequalities:

- **Gender roles and expectations:** Many cultures have deeply ingrained beliefs regarding the roles and responsibilities of males and females. Males are typically expected to be the main breadwinners and decision-makers, while women are frequently assigned domestic chores and caring tasks [5, 12]. These rigid gender norms limit opportunities for women and girls in education, employment, and leadership positions, perpetuating gender inequalities.
- **Child marriage and early marriage:** Cultural practices like child marriage and early marriage, often driven by economic,

social, and cultural factors, disproportionately affect girls and perpetuate gender disparities. Child brides are more likely to drop out of school, experience early pregnancies, face health risks, and lack autonomy and agency in decision-making [4].

- Harmful traditional practices: Some social practices, like female genital mutilation, involuntary marriage, honor killings, bride price, and dowry, perpetuate violence, discrimination, and inequalities against females. These practices violate rights of human rights, undermine women's health and well-being, and reinforce patriarchal structures [4, 12].
- Stigmatization of marginalized groups: Cultural beliefs and stereotypes contribute to the marginalization and stigmatization of certain groups, including ethnic minorities, indigenous communities, people with disabilities, individuals, and religious minorities [12]. Discriminatory attitudes and practices based on ethnicity, religion, or caste can limit access to education, healthcare, service engagement, and social services, perpetuating inequalities and exclusion [4].
- Barriers to education: Cultural beliefs and norms may prioritize boys' education over girls' education or discourage certain groups from pursuing education, particularly girls, children with disabilities, or marginalized communities. Gender-based discrimination, early marriage, child labor, and lack of access to schools that accommodate cultural or linguistic diversity can hinder educational opportunities and perpetuate inequalities [4, 12].

Addressing inequalities rooted in cultural and traditional beliefs requires comprehensive strategies that promote human rights, gender equality, social justice, and cultural sensitivity. This includes legal reforms, community engagement, education, awareness-raising, empowerment programs, and efforts to challenge harmful norms and stereotypes while respecting cultural diversity and traditions.

19.4.2 DISCRIMINATION AND GENDER-BASED VIOLENCE

Discrimination and GBV for females are pervasive and multifaceted issues that have serious consequences for individuals, families, communities, and societies. Here is an overview of discrimination and GBV faced by females:

19.4.2.1 TYPES OF DISCRIMINATION

- **Structural discrimination:** Institutionalized discrimination in laws, policies, and systems that perpetuate inequalities based on gender. This includes unequal access to education, employment, healthcare, and political participation [15].
- **Interpersonal discrimination:** Prejudice, bias, and mistreatment experienced by individuals in their interactions with others based on gender. This can manifest as harassment, bullying, stereotyping, and exclusion [15].
- **Intersectional discrimination:** Overlapping forms of discrimination based on intersecting identities, which compound the experiences of marginalization and exclusion [15].

19.4.2.2 GENDER-BASED VIOLENCE

- **Physical violence:** Any violent act, including assault, battery, domestic abuse, and femicide, that results in bodily harm or injury.
- **Emotional and psychological violence:** Verbal abuse, threats, intimidation, coercion, and manipulation that undermine a person's emotional well-being and autonomy.
- **Economic violence:** Controlling finances, withholding resources, and economic exploitation are forms of power and control over females.

19.4.2.3 CAUSES AND CONTRIBUTING FACTORS

- **Patriarchal societies:** Societal structures, norms, and beliefs that prioritize men's power, authority, and control over women and reinforce gender inequalities.
- **Gender stereotypes:** Deeply ingrained cultural beliefs and expectations about the roles, behaviors, and capabilities of men and women, which perpetuate gender-based discrimination and violence.
- **Social and economic disparities:** Inequalities in access to resources, opportunities, and services based on gender, ethnicity, socioeconomic status, and other factors that increase vulnerability to discrimination and violence.

- **Norms of masculinity:** Expectations placed on men to demonstrate dominance, aggression, and control, which can contribute to the perpetration of violence against women and reinforce harmful gender dynamics.

19.4.2.4 CONSEQUENCES

- **Physical health effects:** Injuries, disabilities, chronic health conditions, and reproductive health problems resulting from GBV.
- **Social and economic costs:** Disruption of education, employment, and social relationships, economic dependence, poverty, and barriers to accessing services and support.

Addressing discrimination and GBV against females requires comprehensive approaches that involve legal reforms, policy interventions, community mobilization, education, awareness-raising, empowerment programs, and support services for survivors. It also requires challenging underlying social norms, promoting gender equality, and fostering cultures of respect, dignity, and nonviolence. Violence and gender inequality are intricate cycles that influence one another rather than existing in opposition to one another [5].

19.4.3 DISPARITIES BETWEEN WOMEN AND MEN

Even though men and women face many of the same health issues, women's health needs to get special attention because of these differences. Due to advantages in both biology and behavior, women typically outlive males [16]. However, in some environments, most notably in regions of Asia, gender-based discrimination overcomes these benefits, resulting in a lower or equal life expectancy for women at birth. Furthermore, women do not always live longer, healthier lives. Certain illnesses are unique to women, and only they may have detrimental effects. Pregnancy and childbirth are two examples of these that are biological and social processes rather than disorders that need medical attention. Both men and women are somewhat impacted by other conditions.

19.4.4 SOCIAL NORMS AND STEREOTYPES

Gender stereotyping hinders women's rights from being implemented effectively, and addressing harmful and incorrect stereotypes will require serious attention from all of us—treaty bodies, special procedures, states parties, civil society, academics, and many others—to move beyond recognition of this fact. The report "Gender Stereotyping as a Human Rights Violation" was commissioned by OHCHR.

19.4.5 INEQUALITIES WITHIN COUNTRIES

Social and economic issues within nations, such as access to education, household income, and place of residence, have an impact on the health of females. Females who live in affluent homes tend to use health care services more frequently and have lower mortality rates than those who live in the poorest households in practically all nations. These disparities exist in the industrialized world as well, not just in poor nations. Many of the health issues that adult women deal with have childhood roots. Because girls may play a reproductive role in the future and because poor nutrition for women has long-term effects, it is especially vital to consider their nutritional health [15]. The best possible physical, social, and emotional development for children can be achieved by preventing child abuse and neglect and by providing a nurturing environment in the early years of life. Additionally, these will lessen the likelihood of dangerous behaviors and a heavy burden of illness, such as substance abuse and mental health issues in later life.

19.5 INACCESSIBILITY OF EDUCATION AND HEALTH FOR FEMALES

19.5.1 SOCIOCULTURAL BARRIERS

Social norms, a lack of social security, a big and unprotected informal sector, male-dominated societies with improper behavior toward spouses, restricted access to resources and education, and sociocultural hurdles are some of the sociocultural obstacles that prevent women from achieving economic empowerment [1, 2]. Other barriers include cultural restrictions, limited access to education and economic prospects, poverty, and lack of decision-making power in family matters [9–11]. These barriers hinder women's ability for decision-making processes, pursue entrepreneurship, and control over resources, thereby limiting their economic empowerment. Enforcing gender-responsive laws and policies, promoting women's enablement through labor market interventions and support for the informal sector, educating the public about equal rights for women, and granting access to resources, education, digital inclusion, and social protection are some suggestions for overcoming these obstacles. Additionally, women's participation in self-help groups and wage labor can enhance their decision-making capacity within the family.

19.5.2 ECONOMIC BARRIERS

Economic barriers in education and health for girls are significant obstacles that limit their access to essential services and opportunities. Here are some key economic barriers:

19.5.2.1 COST OF EDUCATION

- **School fees:** Many families, particularly in low-income and marginalized communities, struggle to afford school fees, uniforms, books, and other educational expenses. This often leads to girls being prioritized for household chores or early marriage instead of attending school.
- **Transportation:** Distance to school and lack of affordable transportation options can pose challenges for girls, especially in rural areas, where schools may be far from their homes. Families may be unable to cover transportation costs, leading to reduced school attendance or dropout rates.
- **Hidden costs:** Additional expenses such as exam fees, school supplies, and extracurricular activities can further strain household budgets and prevent girls from accessing education.

19.5.3 CHILD LABOR AND ECONOMIC PRESSURES

- **Household responsibilities:** Girls are often expected to take on domestic chores and caregiving responsibilities within their households, limiting their time and energy for schooling.

- **Economic contributions:** In many communities, girls are viewed as sources of labor or income for their families. As a result, they may be pressured to engage in child labor, informal work, or early marriage to alleviate financial burdens.

19.5.4 HEALTHCARE COSTS AND ACCESS

- **Medical expenses:** Families may struggle to afford healthcare services, medications, and treatment for their daughters, particularly in regions with limited healthcare infrastructure and high out-of-pocket expenses.
- **Menstrual hygiene products:** The cost of menstrual hygiene products, such as pads or menstrual cups, can be prohibitive for many families. Lack of access to affordable menstrual hygiene products can result in school absenteeism and health risks for girls.
- **Transportation and distance:** Similar to education, lack of transportation and long distances to healthcare facilities can impede girls' for healthcare services, particularly in pastoral areas.

19.5.5 POVERTY AND SOCIOECONOMIC INEQUALITIES

- **Income inequality:** Families living in poverty often prioritize basic needs such as food, shelter, and clothing over education and healthcare expenses. Limited financial resources may force families to make difficult decisions regarding their daughters' education and health.
- **Socioeconomic barriers:** Discrimination and marginalization based on socioeconomic status can exacerbate economic barriers, further limiting opportunities for girls from disadvantaged backgrounds.

Addressing economic barriers in education and health for girls requires comprehensive strategies aimed at reducing poverty, promoting gender equality, affordable and quality education, and healthcare services [2]. This includes targeted interventions such as scholarships, cash transfers, school feeding programs, community-based healthcare initiatives, and efforts to address social norms and economic disparities that perpetuate inequalities. Additionally, policies and programs should prioritize the needs of girls from marginalized and vulnerable populations to ensure inclusive and equal education and health services for all.

19.6 EARLY MARRIAGES

Early marriage poses significant barriers to girls' accessibility to education and health. Here is how it happens.

19.6.1 EDUCATION

- **Interrupted schooling:** Early marriage often leads to girls dropping out of school or being unable to attend school regularly. Once married, girls may be expected to assume domestic responsibilities, care for children, or relocate to their husband's home, all of which disrupt their education.
- **Limited educational opportunities:** Early marriage limits girls' opportunities for further education and skill development. Without completing their education, girls are less likely to acquire the knowledge and skills necessary for economic empowerment, independence, and participation in decision-making processes.
- **Negative impact on health and well-being:** Lack of education resulting from early marriage has implications for females' health, including higher risks of maternal mortality, complications during childbirth, and limited access to healthcare services.

19.6.2 HEALTH

- **Reproductive health risks:** Early marriage often leads to early and unplanned pregnancies, which pose significant health risks for girls, including complications during pregnancy and childbirth, higher rates of maternal mortality, and negative outcomes for newborns.

- **Limited access to healthcare:** Access to healthcare treatments may be impeded for married females by social isolation, economic reliance, and a lack of autonomy. They may also experience difficulties in seeking reproductive healthcare, family planning services, and prenatal care.
- **Violence and abuse:** Girls who are married at a young age are at greater risk for intimate partner violence, including physical, sexual, and emotional abuse. These experiences can have profound effects on their physical and mental health, further exacerbating barriers to accessing healthcare services.

Addressing early marriage as a barrier to girls' accessibility to education and health requires comprehensive and multisectoral approaches that address underlying social, cultural, economic, and legal factors. Some strategies include:

- **Legislative reforms:** Enacting and enforcing laws that set minimum age requirements for marriage, as well as policies that protect girls' rights to education and healthcare.
- **Community engagement:** Engaging communities, religious leaders, and traditional authorities to challenge harmful practices and norms that perpetuate early marriage and promote girls' rights to education and health.
- **Education and awareness:** Providing education and awareness programs for parents, families, and communities about the harmful consequences of early marriage on female health, education, and overall well-being.
- **Access to support services:** Ensuring the availability of support services for girls at risk of or affected by early marriage, including counseling, legal assistance, reproductive healthcare, and educational opportunities.
- **Empowerment programs:** Implementing programs that empower girls with information, skills, and resources to make informed decisions about their lives, including their education, health, and future aspirations.

Even if the number of early weddings has decreased, India continues to be a country where early marriages are commonplace and account for 30% of all early marriages worldwide. Thus, comprehending its effects is crucial to achieving global goals for gender equality. Early marriage is associated with a downward trend in life satisfaction for women, as demonstrated by data collected before marriage and up until age 22, when the most recent survey was conducted [9].

By addressing early marriage and its impact on girls' accessibility to education and health through an amalgamation of legal reforms, community engagement, education, and empowerment programs, societies can promote gender equality, protect girls' rights, and improve their overall well-being.

19.7 REACHING OUTREACH: THE POTENTIAL KEY

19.7.1 HEALTH: FOCUS ON WOMEN'S REPRODUCTIVE HEALTH [25]

The reproductive health of women includes a broad diversity of physical, emotional, and social well-being factors related to the female reproductive system. It includes aspects such as menstruation, contraception, fertility, pregnancy, childbirth, postpartum care, menopause, and the prevention and management of reproductive health issues and diseases. To focus on women's reproductive health, it is important to address various aspects comprehensively.

- **Access to healthcare:** Ensuring that females have access to comprehensive healthcare services, including preventive care, screenings, family planning services, and treatment for reproductive health issues.
- **Education and awareness:** Providing accurate and comprehensive education about reproductive health, including menstruation, contraception options, sexually transmitted infections (STIs), fertility, pregnancy, childbirth, and menopause. This education should be accessible to women of all ages and backgrounds.
- **Contraception:** Ensuring access to a wide range of contraception options and education about their use to empower women to make choices for reproductive health and family planning.
- **Maternal health:** Improving maternal health by providing quality prenatal care, skilled attendance during childbirth, and postpartum care to reduce maternal mortality and morbidity.
- **Prevention and treatment of reproductive health issues:** Addressing reproductive health issues such as infertility, menstrual

disorders, STIs, cervical cancer, uterine fibroids, endometriosis, and polycystic ovary syndrome through prevention, early detection, and treatment.

- **Sexual and reproductive rights:** Advocating for women's sexual and reproductive rights, including the right to make autonomous decisions about their bodies, the right to safe and legal abortion services, and protection from coercion and violence.
- **Menstrual health:** Promoting menstrual health and hygiene, including access to affordable menstrual products, adequate sanitation facilities, and education to combat menstrual stigma and taboos.
- **Psychosocial support:** Providing psychosocial support for women experiencing reproductive health challenges, including infertility, pregnancy loss, postpartum depression, and menopausal symptoms.
- **Research and innovation:** Fostering innovation and research in women's reproductive health to close service gaps, increase medical understanding, and create novel therapies and technology.

By addressing these various aspects, we can promote the holistic well-being of women and ensure that they have the resources, support, and agency to make informed decisions about their reproductive health throughout their lives.

19.7.2 MENTAL HEALTH AWARENESS [25]

Focusing on mental health awareness for women is crucial given the unique challenges and vulnerabilities they may face. Here is a comprehensive approach:

- **Education and awareness:** Promote education and awareness campaigns to destigmatize mental health issues among women. This can involve community outreach, online resources, and educational programs in schools and workplaces.
- **Early intervention and screening:** Encourage routine mental health screenings for women during healthcare visits, particularly during key life stages such as adolescence, pregnancy, postpartum, and menopause. Early identification of mental health issues can lead to timely intervention and support.

- **Mental health services:** Ensure equitable access to mental health services for women of all backgrounds. This includes affordable counseling, therapy, psychiatric care, support groups, and helplines. Addressing barriers such as cost, transportation, and stigma is crucial.
- **Culturally competent care:** Provide culturally competent mental health care that acknowledges and respects the diverse experiences and needs of women from different cultural, racial, ethnic, and religious backgrounds.
- **Trauma-informed care:** Implement trauma-informed approaches in mental health services, recognizing the prevalence of trauma among women, including experiences such as domestic violence, sexual assault, and childhood abuse.
- **Maternal mental health:** Prioritize maternal mental health by offering comprehensive screening, support, and treatment services during pregnancy and the postpartum period. Addressing conditions like postpartum depression and anxiety is essential for the well-being of both mother and child.
- **Peer support networks:** Help create community-based programs and peer support networks so that women can meet and relate to others who have similar experiences and provide understanding and support to each other.
- **Workplace mental health:** Promote mental health awareness and support in the workplace by implementing policies that prioritize employee well-being, offering employee assistance programs, and reducing stigma around seeking help for mental health issues.
- **Self-care and coping skills:** Empower women with tools and resources for self-care and coping skills to manage stress, improve resilience, and maintain good mental health. This can include mindfulness practices, relaxation techniques, and stress management strategies.
- **Collaboration and advocacy:** Adoptive collaboration among healthcare workers, community organizations, advocacy groups, policymakers, and individuals to advocate for improved mental health services and policies that prioritize women's mental health needs.

By adopting a multifaceted approach that addresses the social, cultural, and systemic factors influencing women's mental health, we can work toward promoting mental well-being and resilience across diverse communities.

19.7.3 EDUCATION [6, 25]

Closing gender gaps in education: It is crucial for achieving equality and fostering social and economic development. Here are several strategies that can help address this issue:

- **Equal access:** Ensure equal access to education for both boys and girls. This includes removing barriers such as distance to schools, cultural norms, and economic constraints that may disproportionately affect one gender.
- **Early childhood education:** Investing in early childhood education programs that are accessible to all children, regardless of gender, can help lay the foundation for educational success and reduce disparities from the outset.
- **Teacher training and gender sensitivity:** Provide teacher training programs that promote gender sensitivity and awareness. Teachers should be equipped to challenge gender stereotypes, provide inclusive learning settings, and encourage girls to pursue traditionally male-dominated fields like science and technology.
- **Curriculum review:** Review and update curricula to ensure they are gender-sensitive and inclusive. This includes incorporating diverse perspectives, histories, and achievements of both genders, as well as ensuring that learning materials are free from gender bias.
- **Safe and helpful surroundings:** Create harmless and helpful learning surroundings that are free from discrimination, harassment, and violence. Addressing issues such as bullying and sexual harassment is essential to ensuring that all students, regardless of gender, feel safe and valued at school.
- **Family and society involvement:** Engage families and communities in female education. This can involve raising awareness about the value of female education, providing support for girls' schooling, and challenging harmful gender norms and practices.
- **Role models and mentoring:** Foster the visibility of female role models in education and other fields to inspire girls and challenge gender stereotypes. Establish mentoring programs that connect girls with successful female professionals who can offer guidance and support.

- **Data collection and monitoring:** Collect disaggregated data on enrollment, retention, and performance by gender to monitor development and pinpoint places in need of assistance. Keeping an eye on gender disparities in educational achievements is crucial to creating policies and initiatives that work.
- **Policy and advocacy:** Advocate for policy reforms and investments in girls' education at the nation at large. Governments, NGOs, and other stakeholders should work together to prioritize closing gender gaps in education and ensure that resources are allocated accordingly.

By implementing these strategies and promotion of a supportive and comprehensive learning atmosphere, we can work toward closing gender gaps in education and empowering all individuals to reach their full potential.

19.7.4 STEM EDUCATION FOR GIRLS [27]

Promoting STEM female education is essential to address disparities between males and females in these fields and ensure that girls have equal opportunities to pursue careers in STEM-related fields. The following are a few options that may be fruitful in the promotion of STEM education for girls:

- **Timely exposure:** Introduce girls to subjects at an early age via hands-on activities, experiments, and games. Early exposure can help spark interest and curiosity in STEM fields and lay the foundation for future learning.
- **Role models:** Highlight the achievements of female role models in STEM fields to inspire girls and demonstrate that they can succeed in these areas. Encourage female scientists, engineers, and technologists to serve as mentors and role models for girls interested in STEM.
- **Inclusive curriculum:** Ensure that STEM curricula are inclusive and accessible to all students, regardless of gender. Incorporate diverse perspectives, examples, and applications of STEM concepts to make the subject matter relevant and engaging for girls.

- **STEM clubs and programs:** Establish STEM clubs, afterschool programs, and extracurricular activities specifically targeted at girls. These programs can provide additional support, resources, and encouragement for girls interested in STEM.
- **Teacher training:** Provide professional development and training for teachers to enhance their capacity to effectively teach STEM subjects in a way that is engaging and inclusive for all students. Teachers should be equipped with strategies to support girls' participation and achievement in STEM.
- **Parental engagement:** Engage parents and families to support girls' interest and involvement in STEM education. Provide resources, information, and encouragement to parents to help them support their daughters' STEM learning both inside and outside the classroom.
- **Addressing stereotypes:** Challenge gender stereotypes and biases that may discourage girls from pursuing STEM subjects or careers. Encourage the idea that STEM is for everybody and encourage girls to defy stereotypes and pursue their interests and passions in these fields.
- **Partnerships and collaborations:** Foster partnerships between schools, universities, businesses, and community organizations to provide girls with access to STEM resources, mentors, internships, and real-world experiences. Collaboration with STEM professionals and industry partners can help girls see the relevance and potential applications of STEM in their future careers.

By implementing these strategies and creating a supportive and inclusive environment, we can help girls experience their interests and excel in STEM education and careers, contributing to greater diversity and innovation in these fields.

19.7.5 SKILL DEVELOPMENT AND VOCATIONAL TRAINING [24]

Skill development and vocational training programs tailored for women are key to promoting gender equality, economic empowerment, and social inclusion. Here is how such programs can be beneficial and what considerations should be kept in mind:

- **Addressing gender disparities:** Women often face barriers such as limited access to education, cultural norms, and discrimination in the labor market. Skill development and vocational training programs can help address these disparities by providing women with the opportunity to gain marketable skills and enter traditionally male-dominated fields.
- **Flexible training options:** Many women juggle multiple responsibilities, including caregiving and household duties. Offering flexible training options such as part-time courses, evening classes, or online learning can make it easier for women to participate in vocational training programs while managing their other responsibilities.
- **Life skills training:** In addition to technical skills, vocational training programs for women should also include life skills training. This may cover topics such as financial literacy, entrepreneurship, communication skills, and self-confidence building, which are essential for success in both the workplace and personal life.
- **A secure and encouraging setting:** Creating a safe and supportive learning environment is critical for the success of women in vocational training programs. This includes ensuring that training facilities are accessible, free from harassment, and equipped with facilities such as childcare arrangements for women with young children.
- **Role models and mentoring:** Providing women with access to a mentor who is female and who has succeeded in their chosen areas can be inspiring and empowering. Mentorship programs can offer guidance, support, and encouragement to women as they navigate their career paths.
- **Employment placement and support services:** Vocational training programs should include job placement assistance and support services to help women transition from training to employment successfully. This may involve networking opportunities, resume writing workshops, interview preparation, and ongoing career counseling.
- **Engagement of community and family:** Engaging the support of families and communities is essential for the success of women in vocational training programs. Community outreach efforts, awareness campaigns, and initiatives to change societal attitudes

toward women's employment involvement can help create a more supportive environment.

- **Government policies and funding:** Governments play an important role in promoting gender equality through policies that support women's education, training, and employment opportunities. This may include allocating funding for targeted skill development programs for women, implementing gender-responsive policies, and monitoring progress toward gender equality goals.
- **Measuring impact and success:** It is essential to monitor and evaluate the impact of skill development and vocational training programs for women to ensure their effectiveness and identify areas for improvement. Tracking indicators such as employment rates, income levels, and career advancement can help assess the success of these programs in empowering women economically.

Skill development and vocational training programs tailored for women are essential for promoting gender equality, empowering women economically, and creating more inclusive and diverse workplaces.

19.7.6 DIGITAL LEARNING AND ACCESS

Digital learning has the potential to greatly benefit women by increasing access to education, skill development, and vocational training opportunities. Here is how digital learning can be leveraged to promote education and empowerment among women:

- **Flexibility and convenience:** Digital learning platforms offer flexibility and convenience, allowing women to access educational resources from anywhere at any time. This is particularly beneficial for women who may have caregiving responsibilities or limited mobility, enabling them to balance learning with other obligations.
- **Affordability:** Digital learning can be more cost-effective than traditional classroom-based education, as it eliminates the need for transportation, accommodation, and other associated expenses. This affordability makes education more accessible to women, especially those from marginalized communities or low-income backgrounds.

- **Tailored content:** Digital learning platforms can offer tailored content that addresses the specific needs and interests of women. This may include courses on topics such as women's health, gender studies, entrepreneurship, leadership, and career development, empowering women to pursue their interests and aspirations.
- **Skill development:** Digital learning provides women with opportunities to develop valuable skills that are in demand in the modern workforce. Whether it is learning coding, digital marketing, graphic design, or project management, acquiring these skills can enhance women's employability and economic independence.
- **Empowerment through knowledge:** Access to education and information empowers women to make well-informed choices regarding their personal life, employment, health, and finances. Digital learning equips women to advocate for themselves, pursue their goals, and challenge social norms and barriers.
- **Community and support networks:** Digital learning platforms often facilitate the creation of online communities and support networks where women can connect with peers, mentors, and experts. These communities provide a supportive environment for learning, collaboration, and networking, fostering a sense of belonging and empowerment.
- **Addressing barriers to education:** Digital learning can help overcome traditional barriers to education faced by women, such as geographic isolation, cultural restrictions, and lack of access to quality educational institutions. By leveraging technology, women can access a wide range of educational resources regardless of their location or background.
- **Digital literacy:** Engaging in digital learning enhances women's digital literacy skills, enabling them to navigate technology confidently and effectively. This is increasingly important in today's digital world, where digital literacy is a prerequisite for participation in many aspects of society and the economy.
- **Government and NGO initiatives:** Governments and NGOs play a role in promoting digital learning and improving access for women. This may involve initiatives such as providing subsidies for internet access and devices, offering digital literacy training programs, and supporting the development of localized digital learning content.

Digital learning has the potential to promote education, skill development, and empowerment among women. By addressing barriers to access and providing tailored learning opportunities, digital platforms can help unlock the full potential of women and contribute to greater gender equality and social inclusion.

19.7.7 COMMUNITY OUTREACH PROGRAMS [27]

Health camps for women are essential initiatives aimed at addressing the unique health needs and challenges faced by women. These camps typically provide various medical services, screenings, consultations, and educational sessions tailored specifically for women's health issues. Here is a breakdown of what such health camps might involve:

- **Medical screenings:** Health camps often offer screenings for various health conditions that are prevalent among women. This may include screenings for breast cancer, cervical cancer, osteoporosis, diabetes, hypertension, and STIs.
- **Reproductive health services:** Many women's health camps provide reproductive health services such as family planning consultations, access to contraceptives, prenatal care, and post-natal care. These services are crucial for promoting maternal and child health.
- **Education and awareness programs:** Health camps typically include educational sessions on topics like nutrition, menstrual hygiene, sexual health, and preventive care. These sessions aim to empower women with knowledge about their bodies and health, enabling them to make informed decisions.
- **Consultations with healthcare professionals:** Women attending health camps often have the opportunity to consult with healthcare professionals, including gynecologists, obstetricians, nutritionists, and general practitioners. These consultations allow women to address specific health concerns and receive personalized advice.
- **Access to resources and referrals:** Health camps may also provide access to resources such as informational pamphlets, educational materials, and referrals to other healthcare services or specialists as needed. This ensures that women can continue to receive appropriate care beyond the scope of the health camp.

- **Community engagement and support:** Organizers of women's health camps often prioritize community engagement and support by involving local leaders, community health workers, and women's groups. This helps create a supportive environment where women feel comfortable seeking healthcare services and information.
- **Specialized services:** Depending on the target population and local needs, women's health camps may offer specialized services such as mental health screenings, vaccinations, screening for domestic violence, and access to reproductive health products like sanitary pads.

Overall, health camps for women play a vital role in encouraging women's health, preventing diseases, and addressing healthcare disparities. By providing accessible and comprehensive healthcare services, these camps contribute to improving the overall well-being of women and their communities.

19.8 CONCLUSION

Educating and conducting outreach on female health is crucial for empowering women to make informed decisions about their well-being. Here is a comprehensive plan for conducting educational programs and outreach initiatives focused on female health.

19.8.1 NEEDS ASSESSMENT

To determine the unique health issues and knowledge gaps among the target demographic of women, conduct a detailed needs assessment. Gather data through surveys, focus groups, and interviews to understand prevalent health issues, knowledge levels, cultural beliefs, and barriers to accessing healthcare.

19.8.2 TAILORED EDUCATIONAL MATERIALS

Develop culturally sensitive and linguistically appropriate educational materials on a wide range of female health topics, including:

- **Reproductive health:** Menstruation, pregnancy, contraception, and menopause.
- **Breast health:** Breast self-examination, breast cancer awareness, and mammography.
- **Sexual health:** STI prevention, safe sex practices, and consent.
- **Mental health:** Stress management, depression, anxiety, and self-care.
- **Nutrition and physical activity:** Healthy eating habits, exercise, and weight management.

19.8.3 COMMUNITY WORKSHOPS AND SEMINARS

Organize interactive workshops and seminars on female health topics in collaboration with local healthcare providers, community centers, and women's organizations. Invite experts, including doctors, nurses, nutritionists, psychologists, and social workers, to facilitate discussions and provide accurate information. Address myths, misconceptions, and cultural taboos surrounding female health issues in a respectful and nonjudgmental manner.

19.8.4 PEER EDUCATION PROGRAMS

Train peer educators from within the community, especially among youth and women's groups, to disseminate information about female health. Equip peer educators with the knowledge and skills to conduct informal discussions, peer-to-peer support sessions, and outreach activities in their neighborhoods. Foster a supportive environment where women feel comfortable sharing their experiences and seeking advice from trusted peers.

19.8.5 HEALTH MELAS AND SOCIETY PROGRAMS

Contribute in health melas, festivals, and other public events to reach a broader audience of women. Set up informational booths offering educational materials, demonstrations, and interactive activities related to female health. Deliver no cost health screenings, such as BP checks, BMI assessment, and basic gynecological examinations, to encourage participation and early detection of health issues.

19.8.6 DIGITAL OUTREACH

Utilize digital platforms, like social media, websites, and mobile apps, to disseminate educational content and engage with women online. Create engaging multimedia content, such as educational videos, podcasts, and webinars, to deliver health information in an accessible format. Facilitate online support groups and discussion forums where women can connect with peers, ask questions, and share resources.

19.8.7 COLLABORATION AND PARTNERSHIPS

Collaborate with local healthcare providers, clinics, hospitals, schools, religious institutions, and community leaders to maximize outreach efforts. Forge partnerships with government agencies, NGOs, and corporate sponsors to secure funding, resources, and logistical support for educational initiatives. Pool together expertise and resources from diverse stakeholders to create comprehensive and sustainable female health programs.

19.8.8 EVALUATION AND FEEDBACK

Evaluate the impact of educational and outreach activities through pre- and postprogram assessments, surveys, and focus group discussions. Solicit feedback from participants to assess the relevance, effectiveness, and accessibility of educational materials and activities.

Use evaluation findings to refine strategies, address gaps, and improve the quality of future educational initiatives.

By implementing this plan, organizations and communities can effectively educate and engage women in promoting their health and well-being, ultimately contributing to healthier and empowered communities.

KEYWORDS

- **development**
- **economic growth**
- **education**
- **health indicators**
- **maternal health**
- **gender**
- **inequalities**
- **gender discrimination**
- **global health**
- **sustainable development goals**
- **universal health coverage**

REFERENCES

1. Alban, A., & Andersen, N. B. (2007). HIV/AIDS' spread and impact on other health-related millennium development goals. *Danish Medical Bulletin*, *54*(2), 163–166.
2. Beaglehole, R. Reddy, S., & Leeder, R. (2007). Poverty and human development: The global implications of cardiovascular disease. *AHA Journal; Circulation, 116,* 1871–1873.
3. Bobek, V., Schachl, A., & Horvat, T. (2023). The impact of women's economic empowerment on the rise of female entrepreneurship and human capital in South Africa. *International Journal of Diplomacy and Economy, 9*(1), 23–56.
4. Dahal, P., Joshi, & Swahnberg, K., (2022). A qualitative study on gender inequality and gender-based violence in Nepal. *BMC Public Health*, *22*, 2005.
5. Global Reporting Initiative. (2009). Embedding gender in sustainability reporting: A practitioner's guide. www.globalreporting.org; (accessed on 19 October 2024).
6. Green Jobs and Women Workers. (2009). Employment, equity, equality (ITUC report). www.sustainlabour.org/dmdocuments/en255f; (accessed on 19 October 2024).
7. Grown, C., Gupta, G., & Kes, A. (2009). *Taking Action: Achieving Gender Equality and Empowering Women. Task Force on Education and Gender Equality*. UN Millenium Project. UNDP publication. https://www.undp.org/publications/taking-action-achieving-gender-equality-and-empowering-women; (accessed on 19 October 2024).

8. Hausmann, R., Tyson, L. D., & Zahidi, S. (2009). Geneva: World Economic Forum (The Global Gender Gap Report). www.weforum.org/pdf/gendergap/report2009.pdf; (accessed on 19 October 2024).
9. Kanji, S., Carmichael, F., Darko, C., Egyei, R., & Vasilakos, N. (2024). The impact of early marriage on the life satisfaction, education and subjective health of young women in India: A longitudinal analysis. *The Journal of Development Studies, 60*(5), 705–723.
10. Kerk, V., Guert, & Manuel, A. (2008). A comprehensive index for a sustainable society: The SSI—The sustainable society index. *Journal of Ecological Economics, 66*(2), 228–242.
11. Marmot, M., Friel, S., Bell, R., Tanja, A., & Taylor, S. (2008). Closing the gap in a generation: Health equity through action on the social determinants of health. *Lancet Public Health, 372*(9650), 1661–1669.
12. Mehnas, R., Jabeen, N., Akhtar, S., & Yaqoob, M. (2013). Cultural barriers in women empowerment in the rural areas of Faisalabad. *Afro Asian Journal of Anthropology and Social Policy, 4*(1), 1.
13. Murthy, P., & Smith, C. (2010). Women's global health and human rights. *Jones and Bartlett Publishers,* (pp. 519–532).
14. Patricia, M., Davidson, Tessa, D., Rosely, C., Campbell, J., Hoch Leitner, M., Messias, D, Brown, H., Teitelman, A, Sindhu, S., Reessman, K., Richter, S., Sommers, M., Schaeffer, D., Stringer, M., Sampsell, C., Anderson, D., & Tuazon, J., Cao, Y., Covan, E. (2011). The health of women and girls determines the health and well-being of our modern world: A white paper from the international council on women's health issues. *Health Care Women International, 32(*10), 870–886.
15. Read, J. N. G., & Gorman, B. K. (2010). Gender and health revisited. In: *Handbook of the Sociology of Health, Illness, and Healing: A Blueprint for the 21st Century*, (pp. 411–429). Springer New York: New York, NY.
16. Read, J., & Gorman, B. (2010). Gender and health inequality. *Annual Review of Sociology, 36,* 371–386.
17. Rosenfield, A., Min, C., & Bardfield, J. (2009). Women's global health. *Journal of Pharmaceuticals Sciences Jones and Bartlett Publishers, 98*(1), 43–45.
18. Shaw, D. (2006). Women's right to health and the Millennium development goals: Promoting partnerships to improve access. *International Journal of Gynecology & Obstetrics, 94*, 207–215.
19. Stevens, C. (2009). Special issue on gender and sustainable development. *International Journal of Innovation and Sustainable Development*, *4*(2-3), 93–96.
20. The World Bank. (2010). Gender equality as smart economics, www.worldbank.org/gender; (accessed on 19 October 2024).
21. Tomoko, Kodama, T., Osawa, S., Matosuka, S., Yokoyama, T., & Asami, M. (2021). Progress and challenges for achieving UN Sustainable Development Goal 3 (SDG 3). *Journal of National Institute of Public Health. 70*(3), 224–234.
22. Vikaspedia, (2023). Status of women in India. 2022. https://vikaspedia.in/social-welfare/women-and-child-development/women-development-1/status-of-women-in-india; (accessed on 19 October 2024).
23. Wahid, F., Jaffri, M., Ullah, H., & Khan, I. (2020). Economic empowerment of women in socio-cultural perspectives in federally administrative Tribal Area

(Pakistan): A case study of Kurram Agency. *Review of Economic and Development Studies (READS), 6*(2), 257–266.

24. Wonder Foundation. (n.d.). Why educating women and girls is key to achieving SDGs, https://wonderfoundation.org.uk/educating-women-and-girls-sdgs/; (accessed on 19 October 2024).
25. World Health Organization. (n.d.). Women and health: Today's evidence tomorrow's agenda. https://iris.who.int/handle/10665/44168; (accessed on 19 October 2024).
26. World Health Organization. (2024). Determinants of health, https://www.who.int/news-room/questions-and-answers/item/determinants-of-health; (accessed on 19 October 2024).
27. World Bank. (n.d.). Girls education, https://www.worldbank.org/en/topic/girlseducation; (accessed on 19 October 2024).
28. World Health Organization. (2017). Health is a fundamental human right, https://www.who.int/news-room/commentaries/detail/health-is-a-fundamental-human-right; (accessed on 19 October 2024).
29. Bobbitt-Zeher, D. (2007). The gender income gap and the role of education. *Sociology of Education, 8*(1), 1–22.

CHAPTER 20

Advancements in Research and Future Landscape of Female Health

SWATI SHARMA and NISHA RANA*

*Corresponding author

ABSTRACT

This chapter offers a comprehensive overview of advancements and challenges in women's health, spanning historical inequities to emerging technologies and future directions. It highlights past disparities in research and healthcare, emphasizing efforts by organizations like the National Institutes of Health to address them. The chapter covers various aspects of women's health, including reproductive health, mental health, chronic diseases, and emerging technologies. It discusses prevalent conditions like polycystic ovarian syndrome and mental health challenges, stressing the importance of access to services and stigma reduction. Additionally, it addresses inequalities in medical knowledge and treatment across chronic diseases, underlining the need for sex-specific guidelines. Emerging technologies such as telehealth, genetic testing, and fertility treatments are also explored for their potential to revolutionize healthcare for women. Despite advancements, persistent challenges like funding gaps and gender inequality are acknowledged. The chapter advocates for holistic approaches and partnerships to effectively address these issues, particularly in underserved communities. Lastly, it outlines future directions, emphasizing increased research investment and diverse representation. It envisions a future where precision medicine leads to tailored treatments, ultimately enhancing the quality of life for women.

Holistic Approaches for Women's Sustainable Health, Volume 2: Advancements, Socioeconomic Impacts, and Innovative Strategies. Junaid Ahmad Malik, Anamika Chauhan, and Megh R. Goyal (Eds)

DOI: 10.1201/9781779641656-24

20.1 INTRODUCTION

Others realized in the 1970s and 1980s that women were not gaining the same advantages from the significant advancements in biological science and healthcare. A significant contributing aspect to this disparity was an astounding ignorance about ailments that are specific to them or are more common among them. The public was seeking answers to numerous injustices, chronic illnesses, and new health issues, and society was changing quickly. In response, the National Institutes of Health (NIH) expanded in breadth, ambition, and scale [39].

The Working Group on Women's Health Issues was founded by a group of forward-thinking executives in the US Public Health Service, and its report and recommendations set the path for further studies aimed at resolving the disparity and enhancing women's health [50].

Women's health is a broad and complex area that includes social, emotional, and physical dimensions. It explores understanding and resolving the unique health requirements and obstacles that women encounter in their lifetimes [3]. The significance of enhancing women's well-being in the modern era has gained attention in recent years as it addresses a wide variety of issues specific to women, including reproductive health, hormone imbalances, and concerns about female anatomy [6]. Women have a variety of health challenges, including high morbidity rates for illnesses, including cervical and breast cancer [25].

Poverty, prejudice, and restricted access to healthcare are just a few of the factors that exacerbate preexisting health issues. In 2020, about 800 women lost their lives due to pregnancy- and childbirth-related avoidable causes per day. It was shocking to learn that at this time, a mother died every two minutes. Nearly 95% of these fatalities occurred in lower-middle-income countries in 2020 [51]. To improve women's health in the 21st century, a thorough and multidimensional strategy is essential.

Research on women's health too frequently concentrates only on sexual and reproductive health, even though cancer and cardiovascular disease are the two leading causes of mortality for women globally. Despite their influence on women's health, health researchers seldom study gender disparities and the crucial role of sociocultural variables, such as discrimination and unequal power relationships with men. In addition to biological differences, social influences also have a role in how women feel illness compared to men. Although there are many sex variations in illness, they are not well understood and understudied. Women, particularly pregnant women, are consistently underrepresented in clinical trials, and male mice are frequently the only ones used in animal model investigations [5]. Inequitable healthcare and a lack of awareness of sex differences will persist if medical research disregards the biology of women.

20.2 HEALTH AND NUTRITIONAL STATUS OF INDIAN WOMEN

There has been a suggestion that the traditional traditions and prevalent culture in India are contributing to the declining health and nutritional status of Indian women. In general, Indian women are more susceptible to nutritional deficiency, particularly when they are pregnant or nursing. It has been noted that the mother's nutritional state has a greater overall influence on birth weight than do other variables [15]. It has been observed that pregnant women living in rural areas where they consume less food than is advised [17], and as a result, low-birth-weight babies are typically delivered to undernourished and ill moms. Pregnant women and teenage girls had the highest rate of anemia, followed by nursing mothers. According to epidemiological research, at least 120 million women in less developed nations are underweight, and 50% of pregnant women globally are anemic [35].

An estimated 60% of women in South Asia are underweight. Teenagers who are pregnant, particularly those who are underweight, are more likely to experience obstructed labor and other obstetric difficulties [24]. Thus, ignorance of prenatal healthcare has detrimental effects on both the mother and the unborn child. The moms' nutritional condition and general health were significantly impacted by receiving appropriate and suitable instruction. The necessary actions should be taken to inform women about the value of healthcare in promoting safe deliveries and healthy pregnancies [52].

20.3 THE CHALLENGES WITH THE WOMEN'S HEALTH

In spite of extensive research and advancements over the past few decades, there are still numerous challenges facing women's health:

20.3.1 REPRODUCTIVE HEALTH

20.3.1.1 THE INFLUENCE OF POLYCYSTIC OVARY SYNDROME

Depending on the used diagnostic criteria and the population under study, up to 21% of women of reproductive age may be affected by polycystic ovarian syndrome (PCOS), the most common endocrine illness in this group [8, 19]. Menstrual irregularities, polycystic ovaries, and/or hyper-androgenism are common characteristics among women diagnosed with PCOS [32, 34]. According to patient reports of their physical, social, and emotional well-being [13], health-related quality of life (HRQoL) is negatively impacted by the health burden of PCOS overall [38]. HRQoL is a significant outcome in the context of treating and managing chronic diseases [16]. In fact, when comparing data from healthy populations with those of PCOS-afflicted women, a continuously worse HRQoL has been seen [4].

Numerous studies have documented the health advantages of raising physical activity (PA) levels in a variety of groups, including those with PCOS [31, 47]. Furthermore, increasing PA or participation in exercise programs may also enhance HRQoL, especially for those with long-term illnesses like cancer [23], chronic respiratory disorders [18], osteoarthritis or rheumatoid arthritis [30], and other chronic ailments. It is interesting to note that the majority of research comparing the PA levels of PCOS-affected women to healthy controls found no statistically significant differences in energy expenditure between the PCOS-affected and healthy control groups, despite the fact that PCOS-affected women had worse physical and mental health [36, 42 ,48]. Even so, despite PCOS's high incidence, little is known regarding PA's possible mediating function in the disorder's psychological and somatic symptoms.

20.3.2 MENTAL HEALTH

Another issue connected with women's health is mental health [43]. In addition to being far more likely to suffer from posttraumatic stress disorder (PTSD), women are twice as likely as men to feel stress, hopelessness, and melancholy. Women who are intimately abused by their partners are more likely to suffer from anxiety, despair, and PTSD. In addition, a lot of women experience issues with eating disorders, body image, and other mental health issues related to expectations and social pressures. In order to address mental health crises, the government and medical professionals must work more to make mental fitness services, such as counseling and therapy, easily accessible. Furthermore, educational programs that emphasize mental health and reduce stigma might help increase awareness of mental health concerns and motivate more individuals to seek treatment as soon as possible [20].

20.3.3 CHRONIC DISEASES

Women's morbidity and mortality are adversely affected by disparities in medical knowledge and treatment in a number of prevalent disease categories, including autoimmune illnesses, mental illness, endocrine disorders, and cardiovascular disease [7]. Women experience poor health for nine years longer on average than men due to these disparities. For instance, there are differences between the experiences of men and women with heart attacks in terms of symptoms, age at onset, successful therapies, and overall results [37]. However, it is frequently not reported against sex-specific criteria when using troponin blood tests to detect myocardial infarction [12]. For women, the accuracy of diagnosis rises by 42% when such limits are applied [33]. Even though men are more likely than women to have diabetes, women are more likely than men to die from diabetes-related causes and to experience its complications, which include a 27% higher excess risk of stroke and a 44% higher excess risk of coronary heart disease [41]. However, despite the fact that clinical recommendations are not usually sex-specific, women are less likely than men to receive the care that is advised [45].

20.3.4 HORMONAL IMBALANCE

Women's health is continuously and profoundly impacted by hormonal imbalance [44]. Among the many symptoms include irregular menstruation periods, acne, weight gain, and infertility, to name just a few. PCOS is a common condition. Ovarian cysts, irregular menstruation, and infertility are associated with each other. Healthcare professionals themselves need to be capable of and educated about the appropriate diagnosis and treatment of illnesses like PCOS or endometriosis in order to identify and address these problems. Additionally, more investigation is required to identify the illnesses' causes, which may lead to the development of novel remedies and enhance everyone's health [2, 40].

20.4 EMERGING TECHNOLOGIES AND INNOVATIONS

The extent of the obstacles to women's health can no longer be compared to the incredible progress made in the medical field, which has produced amazing changes and an abundance of beneficial, life-changing outcomes for women's health. These advancements, which range from sophisticated treatment strategies to advanced diagnostic procedures and preventative measures, promise to improve patient outcomes and quality of life [14]. Women's healthcare has undergone a revolution thanks to the present revolutionary skills in illness diagnosis, therapy, and prevention. Among them are:

20.4.1 DIGITAL AND TELEHEALTH TECHNOLOGIES

Women's healthcare results are being revolutionized by digital and health technology, including wearables and smartphone applications. Women may precisely track their health and stay on top of any chronic diseases they may have, thanks to state-of-the-art monitoring technologies. Because of its convenience, it is a great option for those who live in rural or distant places, have busy job schedules and childcare responsibilities, or both [27]. In addition, telehealth makes it possible for patients to interact securely with medical professionals from anywhere in the world, giving them the ability to get care right from home. They may also manage their health more proactively and productively, while they are at a distance, thanks to the availability of remote healthcare services. As a result, telehealth and digital technologies are giving women a special chance to take charge of their healthcare, which will improve results overall [1, 9, 29].

20.4.2 GENETIC TESTING

The detection and treatment of hereditary disorders, especially those that impact women, have been transformed by genetic testing. In recent years, genetic testing for mutations in the *BRCA1* and *BRCA2* genes, which raise the risk of ovarian and breast cancers, has become more accessible and affordable. These mutations now allow women to take preventative steps to lower their risk of acquiring cancer, such as regular screenings and prophylactic surgery [49].

20.4.3 FERTILITY TREATMENTS

Approximately 10% of couples experience infertility, yet many women are now able to conceive thanks to advancements in reproductive technologies. The most effective method of reproduction has been *in vitro* fertilization (IVF), whose success rate has been steadily improving over time. But the quality of the eggs and sperm determines how well IVF works, and some women may not be able to create viable eggs because of age or medical issues. Egg freezing and donor egg programs have been popular choices in recent years for women who wish to preserve their fertility or are having difficulties becoming pregnant with their own eggs [11].

20.4.4 PREGNANCY AND CHILDBIRTH MANAGEMENT

A woman's pregnancy and delivery are extremely important life events. Modern labor and delivery techniques, prenatal diagnosis and treatment, and childbirth have improved maternal and child safety. Consider amniocentesis, ultrasounds, and prenatal screening as examples. These procedures exist and are used to identify and monitor possible difficulties, which opens the door to interventions like bed rest or medication to treat conditions like gestational diabetes or preeclampsia. Furthermore, many expecting moms report having a more comfortable birth experience thanks to epidurals and other kinds of pain treatment during labor and delivery [10].

20.4.5 BREAST CANCER SCREENING

Being the second leading cause of cancer-related deaths worldwide, breast cancer poses a serious threat to women everywhere [28]. Thanks to technology, we can combat its destructive consequences thanks to technological developments. Modern mammography and digital breast tomosynthesis (DBT) are examples of advanced care techniques that have arisen to improve the precision of tumor detection, especially in patients with thick breasts. As a result, DBT is suggested by specialists at the American College of Radiology as the best screening method for high-risk populations. The effective use and integration of this three-dimensional imaging method is only one of many achievements in the fight against the deadly disease known as breast cancer in women; it gives affected persons even more encouragement and hope for a speedy recovery [26].

20.4.6 SEXUAL HEALTH MANAGEMENT

It is important for women to take care of their sexual health. Sexually transmitted infections (STIs) and other issues like them continue to have a significant influence on women's health. Better results have been achieved as a result of advancements in STI therapy; the majority of common infections may now be treated with antibiotics and antiviral medications. Treatments like hormone treatment, psychotherapy, and medication have been demonstrated to be effective in controlling signs and symptoms related with sexual dysfunction and STIs. Sexual dysfunction can be caused by psychological or physical causes [2].

20.5 CHALLENGES

A lack of attention is being placed on addressing these issues despite the well-documented health transition that has led to an increase in the number of women's noncommunicable disease-related deaths and disabilities, including cancers, injuries, mental disorders, and suicide. The health of women who are past reproductive age is neglected because funding agencies, donor organizations, and academic bodies have not yet embraced the life-course agenda for women's health. Worldwide, women supply the majority of healthcare, whether in the official healthcare system, the unofficial sector, or the home. However, women's healthcare requirements are not properly fulfilled, particularly in rural and underdeveloped areas. In terms of biology, the environment, and society, gender disparity increases women's susceptibility to specific dangers and lowers their chances of positive results. Special attention to these issues requires separate program that will not be associated with men's health. The projection of health data from men results in unequal access to information and healthcare services, as well as an underestimation of the signs, severity, and effects of disease. Women's health is impacted by their domestic responsibilities, including smoking exposure and restricted physical labor. The answers to these problems lie not in medical health but rather in interdepartmental collaboration and a comprehensive approach to public health [22].

20.6 FUTURE DIRECTION

Numerous medical developments will enable more accurate and customized tests that consider lifestyle, medical history, and genetic composition. In addition, comprehensive sexual and reproductive health services like family planning will be provided, along with early diagnosis and intervention strategies for a variety of ailments like breast cancer, cervical cancer, cardiovascular diseases, and mental health issues [44], planning for the future, using contraceptives, and preventing STIs [21]. It is essential to prioritize funding for studies that address women's health issues while also considering a varied range of age groups, ethnic backgrounds, and socioeconomic statuses. These findings may result in more potent and successful medications that specifically address the ways in which gender affects the onset, course, and efficacy of certain treatments [46].

20.7 SUMMARY

Over the past few decades, significant strides in biological science and healthcare have not equally benefited women, revealing gaps in addressing their unique health needs. The NIH and the Working Group on Women's Health Issues have aimed to rectify these disparities. Women's health encompasses a broad spectrum, including reproductive health, chronic illnesses, mental health, and nutritional status, particularly among vulnerable groups like Indian women, who face malnutrition and anemia. Despite advancements, challenges persist in areas like reproductive health (e.g., PCOS), mental health, chronic diseases, and hormonal imbalances, often exacerbated by sociocultural and economic factors [7].

Emerging technologies and innovations, such as digital health, genetic testing, advanced fertility treatments, improved pregnancy management, and sophisticated cancer screening methods, promise to transform women's healthcare. However, addressing the broader social determinants of health and ensuring equitable healthcare access remain critical. Future efforts must prioritize diverse and inclusive research, comprehensive health services, and interdepartmental collaboration to improve women's health outcomes globally.

KEYWORDS

- **chronic disease**
- **healthcare technologies**
- **women's health**
- **mental health**
- **reproductive health**
- **health disparities**

REFERENCES

1. Ajayi, K. V., Wachira, E., Onyeaka, H. K., Montour, T., & Olowolaju, S. (2022). The use of digital health tools for health promotion among women with and without chronic diseases: Insights from the 2017–2020 health information national trends survey. *JMIR Mhealth Uhealth, 10*(8), e39520.
2. Allshouse, A., Pavlovic, J., & Santoro, N. (2018). Menstrual cycle hormone changes associated with reproductive aging and how they may relate to symptoms. *Obstetrics and Gynecology Clinics of North America, 45*(4), 613–628.
3. Armah, D., van der Wath, A. E., Yazbek, M., & Naab, F. (2022). Development of holistic health care interventions for women with infertility: A nominal group technique. *Holistic Nursing Practice, 36*(2), 85–92.
4. Asdaq, S. M. B., Jomah, S., Hasan, R., Al-Baroudi, D., Alharbi, M., Alsubaie, S., Buhamad, M. H., Alyahya, B., & Al-Yamani, M. J. (2020). Impact of polycystic ovary syndrome on eating behavior, depression and health related quality of life: A cross-sectional study in Riyadh. *Saudi Journal of Biological Sciences*, *27*(12), 3342–3347.
5. Assadpour, E., & Van Spall, H. G. (2023). Pregnant and lactating women should be included in clinical trials for cardiovascular disease. *Nature Medicine*, *29*(8), 1897–1899.

6. Becker, N. V., Moniz, M. H., Tipirneni, R., Dalton, V. K., & Ayanian, J. Z. (2021). Utilization of women's preventive health services during the COVID-19 pandemic. *JAMA Health Forum*, *2*(7), e211408.
7. Bill & Melinda Gates Foundation, National Institutes of Health. (2023). Women's health innovation opportunity map: 50 high-return opportunities to advance global women's health R&D.
8. Boyle, J. A., Cunningham, J., O'Dea, K., Dunbar, T., & Norman, R. J. (2012). Prevalence of polycystic ovary syndrome in a sample of Indigenous women in Darwin, Australia. *The Medical Journal of Australia*, *196*(1), 62–66.
9. Cantor, A. G., Nelson, H. D., Pappas, M., Atchison, C., & Hatch, B. N. (2023). Telehealth for women's preventive services for reproductive health and intimate partner violence: a comparative effectiveness review. *Journal of General Internal Medicine*, *38*(7), 1735–1743.
10. Carrandi, A., Hu, Y., Karger, S., Eddy, K. E., Vogel, J. P., & Harrison, C. L. (2023). Systematic review on the cost and cost-effectiveness of mHealth interventions supporting women during pregnancy. *Women and Birth*, *36*(1), 3–10.
11. Carson, S. A., & Kallen, A. N. (2021). Diagnosis and management of infertility: A review. *JAMA*, *326*(1), 65–76.
12. Chapman, AR., Fujisawa, T., & Lee, K. K. (2019). Novel high-sensitivity cardiac troponin I assay in patients with suspected acute coronary syndrome. *Heart*, *105*, 41.
13. Colwell, K., Lujan, M. E., Lawson, K. L., Pierson, R. A., & Chizen, D. R. (2010). Women's perceptions of polycystic ovary syndrome following participation in a clinical research study: Implications for knowledge, feelings, and daily health practices. *Journal of Obstetrics and Gynaecology Canada*, *32*(5), 453–459.
14. Corey, L., Vezina, A., & Gala, R. B. (2020). Using technology to improve women's health care. *Ochsner Journal, 20*(4), 422–425.
15. Dharmalingam, A., Navanethan, K., Krishnakumar, C. S. (2010). Nutritional status of mothers and low birth weight in India. *Maternal and Child Health Journal*, *14*(2), 290.
16. Dokras, A., Stener-Victorin, E., Yildiz, B. O., Li, R., Ottey, S., Shah, D., Epperson, N., & Teede, H. (2018). Androgen Excess-Polycystic Ovary Syndrome Society: Position statement on depression, anxiety, quality of life, and eating disorders in polycystic ovary syndrome. *Fertility and Sterility*, *109*(5), 888–899.
17. Durrani, A. M., & Rani, A. (2011). Effect of maternal dietary intake on the weight of the newborn in Aligarh city, India. *Nigerian Medicine Journal*, *52*, 177–181.
18. Eichenberger, P. A., Diener, S. N., Kofmehl, R., & Spengler, C. M. (2013). Effects of exercise training on airway hyperreactivity in asthma: A systematic review and meta-analysis. *Sports Medicine*, *43*(11), 1157–1170.
19. ESHRE, & ASRM Group. (2004). Consensus on diagnostic criteria and long-term health risks related to polycystic ovary syndrome. *Fertility and Sterility, 81*(1), 19–25.
20. Fauk, N. K., Merry, M. S., Mwanri, L., Hawke, K., & Ward, P. R. (2022). Mental health challenges and the associated factors in women living with hiv who have children living with hiv in indonesia: a qualitative study. *International Journal of Environmental Research and Public Health, 19*(11), 6879.

21. Fowler, T., Garr, D., Mager, N. D. P., & Stanley, J. (2020). Enhancing primary care and preventive services through Interprofessional practice and education. *Journal of General Internal Medicine, 9*(1), 12.
22. Framing Women's Health Issues in 21st Century India. (2016). *A Policy Report The George Institute for Global Health India*. The George Institute for Global Health, India.
23. Fuller, J. T., Hartland, M. C., Maloney, L. T., & Davison, K. (2018). Therapeutic effects of aerobic and resistance exercises for cancer survivors: A systematic review of meta-analyses of clinical trials. *British Journal of Sports Medicine*, *52*(20), 1311–1311.
24. Ghosh-Jerath, S., Devasenapathy, N., Singh, A., Shankar, A., & Zodpey, S. (2015). Ante natal care (ANC) utilization, dietary practices and nutritional outcomes in pregnant and recently delivered women in urban slums of Delhi, India: An exploratory cross-sectional study. *Reprod Health*, *12*, 20.
25. Ginsburg, O., Bray, F., Coleman, M. P., Vanderpuye, V., Eniu, A. (2017). The global burden of women's cancers: A grand challenge in global health. *Lancet*, *389*(10071), 847–860.
26. Goh, Y., Chou, C. P., Chan, C. W., Buhari, S. A., Hartman, M. S. W. et al. (2022). Impact of contrast-enhanced mammography in surgical management of breast cancers for women with dense breasts: A dual-center, multi-disciplinary study in Asia. *European Radiology*, *5*, 1–2.
27. Goldstein, K. M., Zullig, L. L., Dedert, E. A., Alishahi Tabriz, A., Brearly, T. W. (2018). Telehealth interventions designed for women: An evidence map. *Journal of General Internal Medicine*, *33*(12), 2191–2200.
28. Grimm, L. J., Avery, C. S., Hendrick, E., & Baker, J. A. (2022). Benefits and risks of mammography screening in women ages 40 to 49 years. *Journal of Primary Care & Community Health*, *13*, 21501327211058322.
29. Karim, J. L., & Talhouk, A. (2021). Person-generated health data in women's health: Protocol for a scoping review. *JMIR Research Protocols*, *10*(5), e26110.
30. Kelley, G. A., Kelley, K. S., & Hootman, J. M. (2015). Effects of exercise on depression in adults with arthritis: A systematic review with meta-analysis of randomized controlled trials. *Arthritis Research & Therapy*, *17*(1), 21.
31. Kite, C., Parkes, E., Taylor, S. R., Davies, R. W., Lagojda, L., Brown, J. E., Broom, D. R., Kyrou, I., & Randeva, H. S. (2022). Time to load up–resistance training can improve the health of women with polycystic ovary syndrome (PCOS): A scoping review. *Medical Sciences*, *10*(4), 53.
32. Kyritsi, E. M., Dimitriadis, G. K., Kyrou, I., Kaltsas, G., & Randeva, H. S. (2017). PCOS remains a diagnosis of exclusion: A concise review of key endocrinopathies to exclude. *Clinical Endocrinology*, *86*(1), 1–6.
33. Lee, K. K., Ferry, A. V., Anand, A., et al. (2019). High-STEACS Investigators. Sex-specific thresholds of high-sensitivity troponin in patients with suspected acute coronary syndrome. *Journal of the American College of Cardiology*, *74*, 43.
34. Lizneva, D., Suturina, L., Walker, W., Brakta, S., Gavrilova-Jordan, L., & Azziz, R. (2016). Criteria, prevalence, and phenotypes of polycystic ovary syndrome. *Fertility and Sterility*, *106*(1), 6–15.

35. Mallikharjuna Rao, K., Balakrishna, N., Arlappa, N., Laxmaiah, A., & Barhmam, G. N. V. (2010). Diet and nutritional status of women in India. *Journal of Human Ecology*, *29*(3), 165–170.
36. Mario, F., do Amarante, F., Toscani, M., & Spritzer, P. (2012). Lean muscle mass in classic or ovulatory PCOS: Association with central obesity and insulin resistance. *Experimental and Clinical Endocrinology & Diabetes*, *120*(9), 511–516.
37. Millett, E. R. C., Peters, S. A. E., & Woodward, M. (2018). Sex differences in risk factors for myocardial infarction: Cohort study of UK Biobank participants. *BMJ*, *363*, k4247.
38. Moghadam, Z. B., Fereidooni, B., Saffari, M., & Montazeri, A. (2018). Measures of health-related quality of life in PCOS women: A systematic review. *International Journal of Women's Health*, *10,* 397–408.
39. National Institutes of Health Office of Research on Wo-men's Health. (2021). Report of the National Institutes of Health: Opportunities for research on women's health.
40. Navarro-Pardo, E., Holland, C. A., & Cano, A. (2018). Sex hormones and healthy psychological aging in women. *Front Aging Neurosci*ence, *9*, 439.
41. Peters, S. A., Huxley, R. R., & Woodward, M. (2014). Diabetes as a risk factor for stroke in women compared with men: Systematic review and meta-analysis of 64 cohorts, including 775,385 individuals and 12,539 strokes. *Lancet*, *383*, 80.
42. Rodino, I. S., Byrne, S., & Sanders, K. A. (2016). Obesity and psychological wellbeing in patients undergoing fertility treatment. *Reproductive Biomedicine Online*, *32*(1), 104–112.
43. Srivastava, K. (2012). Women and mental health: Psychosocial perspective. *Indian Psychiatry Journal*, *21*(1), 1–3.
44. Stolp, H., & Fox, J. (2015). Increasing receipt of women's preventive services. *J. Womens Health (Larchmt)*, *24*(11), 875–881.
45. The Lancet Diabetes Endocrinology. (2017). Sex disparities in diabetes: Bridging the gap. *The lancet. Diabetes & Endocrinology*, *5*, 839.
46. Van Hagen, L. J., Muntinga, M., Appelman, Y., & Verdonk, P. (2021). Sex- and gender-sensitive public health research: An analysis of research proposals in a research institute in the Netherlands. *Women & Health, 61*(1), 109–119.
47. Wang, Z., Groen, H., Cantineau, A. E. P., van Elten, T. M., Karsten, M. D. A., van Oers, A. M., Mol, B. W. J., Roseboom, T. J., & Hoek, A. (2021). Dietary intake, eating behavior, physical activity, and quality of life in infertile women with PCOS and obesity compared with non-PCOS obese controls. *Nutrients*, *13*(10), 3526.
48. Warburton, D. E., & Bredin, S. S. (2017). Health benefits of physical activity: A systematic review of current systematic reviews. *Current Opinion in Cardiology*, *32*(5), 541–556.
49. Watts, K. J., Meiser, B., Mitchell, G., Kirk, J., Saunders, C., et al. (2012). How should we discuss genetic testing with women newly diagnosed with breast cancer? Design and implementation of a randomized controlled trial of two models of delivering education about treatment-focused genetic testing to younger women newly diagnosed with breast cancer. *BMC Cancer*, 12, 320.
50. Women's health. (1985). Report of the Public Health Service Task Force on women's health issues. *Public Health*, *100*, 73–106.
51. World Health Organization (WHO) (2023). Maternal mortality.

52. Yazdkhasti, M., Pourreza, A., Pirak, A., & Abdi, F. (2015). Unintended pregnancy and its adverse social and economic consequences on health system: A narrative review article. *Iranian Journal of Public Health,* 44(1), 12–21.

CHAPTER 21

Healthcare Needs for Female Sexual Dysfunctions

NEELESH KUMAR MAURYA* and ZOOMI SINGH

*Corresponding author

ABSTRACT

Sexual health is a fundamental component of women's overall well-being, encompassing physical, emotional, and social aspects. However, a significant portion of the female population experiences sexual dysfunction. This chapter emphasizes the importance of understanding the prevalence, unique needs of affected women, and healthcare access disparities to effectively address these concerns. Research suggests that 43–51% of women encounter at least one sexual dysfunction in their lifetime. Common issues include decreased libido, arousal difficulties, orgasmic dysfunction, and dyspareunia (pain during intercourse). The development of these dysfunction may be the result of a complicated interaction of biological, psychological, social, and relational variables. Women's sexual health needs vary based on cultural, religious, and personal backgrounds. Healthcare providers need to understand and customize their approach to each woman's unique context. Unfortunately, women often face significant barriers to seeking help for sexual problems. Addressing the challenges for sexual disorders necessitates a multifaceted approach encompassing holistic strategies such as lifestyle modifications and open communication with partners. Additionally, psychiatric counseling and interventions facilitated by healthcare professionals, who adopt a holistic perspective, are crucial elements for successful treatment. Fostering open

Holistic Approaches for Women's Sustainable Health, Volume 2: Advancements, Socioeconomic Impacts, and Innovative Strategies. Junaid Ahmad Malik, Anamika Chauhan, and Megh R. Goyal (Eds)

DOI: 10.1201/9781779641656-25

communication with partners is essential to maintaining cooperation and support throughout the intervention process.

21.1 INTRODUCTION

Since the World Health Organization released the definition of sexual health in 1975 (which included the following components, such as autonomy, pleasure, freedom from coercion and violence, and a positive contribution to overall well-being [54]), there has been a substantial amount of progress made in the knowledge of sexual health. Most definitions [26] in the literature reflect these basic principles that emphasize the importance of autonomy, pleasure, the absence of compulsion and violence, and positive contributions to general well-being [29]. These principles are significant benchmarks that can be utilized by both physicians and researchers. In accordance with the fundamental idea that sexual health is an essential sign of overall health conditions [29], this chapter focuses primarily on the development of good sexual functions in females. Even though sexual health involves a wide array of topics, including contraception and sexually transmitted infections, the primary focus of this chapter is on addressing the specific requirements that women have under these circumstances. As a result of the fact that a significant number of adult women in the United States do not have access to the appropriate medical counsel, support, or care to completely address the challenges that they are experiencing with their sexual health, it is disheartening to discover that this is the situation. For women who are suffering from symptoms such as painful sexual activity, a decrease in desire or pleasure, and/or difficulty with orgasmic experiences, this is the scenario that they find themselves in.

Female sexual dysfunction (FSD) includes a variety of sexual issues, such as permanent or recurring lack of sexual fantasies and desires, inability to achieve or sustain lubrication, and genital congestion for enjoyable sexual activity. The difficulty or delay in orgasm after sexual stimulation is called female orgasmic dysfunction causing genital pain before, during, or after sexual activity. Sometimes, these dysfunctions co-occur causing a complicated interaction that affects sexual well-being [7, 38]. Hormonal changes after menopause can worsen FSD or cause new symptoms in unaffected women [4, 7].

This chapter highlights holistic approach to healthcare needs under various scenarios contributing to FSDs, including reduced libido, orgasmic dysfunction, pain disorders, vaginal dryness, low self-esteem, relationship issues, and underlying health conditions. The chapter includes herb formulations and plant-based medicines.

21.2 FSD: A MULTIFACETED IMPACT ON WELL-BEING

Although it is possible for adult women of any age to experience disturbing sexual health concerns [7], yet women under transition from menopause to postmenopause are more likely to experience FSD conditions. According to the North American Menopause Society [42], this widespread menopause disorder is known as genitourinary syndrome of menopause (GSM) that occurs when vulvar and vaginal atrophy occur simultaneously. According to the North American Menopause Society [42], common symptoms include postcoital bleeding, vaginal irritation or itchiness, genital dryness, and sexual pain throughout menopause. These symptoms frequently continue to be present throughout the menopause stage. These symptoms have the potential to have substantial impact on woman's sexual activity, intimate relationships, lifestyle, and emotional well-being [38]. It is important to note that the consequences of GSM on the quality of life of women are comparable to those of illnesses, such as arthritis, chronic obstructive pulmonary disease, asthma, or irritable bowel syndrome [38].

21.2.1 COMPLEXITIES OF FSD

Female sexuality is a rich tapestry, but it can be disrupted by various challenges leading to FSD. This spectrum of difficulties disrupts the intricate interplay of desire, arousal, lubrication, orgasm, and ultimately a woman's well-being [7]. Manifestations range from low libido to painful intercourse (dyspareunia), difficulty achieving orgasm, and hormonal fluctuations during life stages such as menopause [38]. Understanding FSD's multidimensionality requires acknowledging the complex interplay of biopsychosocial factors [7], such as:

- **Biological factors:** Hormonal changes due to medical conditions, neurological complications, or natural life stages can disrupt physical responses [7].
- **Psychological factors:** Stress, anxiety, and past traumas can significantly impact desire and arousal [7].
- **Social factors:** Relationship dynamics, communication, intimacy, and partner compatibility all influence sexual satisfaction [7].

21.2.2 SEXUAL DISORDERS AND FEMALE WELL-BEING: A MULTIFACETED IMPACT

- Sexual disorders can profoundly impact women, extending beyond the physical act of sex to influence physical health, emotional well-being, and overall quality of life [3, 16]. A closer look at some key areas is given as follows:
- **Physical health:** Discomfort and pain during sexual activity or difficulties with orgasm can lead to physical disengagement and contribute to disorders such as the GSM, which is characterized by chronic dryness and irritation that further compromise sexual function and well-being [37].
- **Emotional well-being:** Frustration, anxiety, and distress often accompany sexual dysfunction. Issues such as low libido, body image concerns, or orgasm difficulties can erode self-esteem and trigger feelings of inadequacy or dissatisfaction [48].
- **Interpersonal relationships:** Sexual disorders can strain relationships. Communication breakdowns, emotional distance, and avoidance of sexual activity may result, creating tension and conflict [34]. Partners may also experience frustration, adding complexity.
- **Mental health:** Persistent sexual problems can contribute to mental health challenges such as depression and anxiety. The emotional burden and societal stigma surrounding sexual difficulties can exacerbate existing mental health concerns [12].

- **Quality of life:** Sexual disorders can significantly diminish a woman's overall quality of life. The impact extends beyond the bedroom, affecting daily activities, social interactions, and the ability to find joy and satisfaction in various aspects of life [16].
- **Negative experiences** related to sexual function can contribute to poor self-esteem and body image issues. Women may feel disconnected from their bodies, leading to a negative self-perception that transcends sexuality [49].
- **Overall well-being:** Sexual health is intricately linked to overall well-being. Unattended sexual disorders can contribute to a sense of unfulfillment and hinder a woman's ability to lead a healthy, balanced life [44].

21.2.3 IMPORTANCE OF ADDRESSING FSD

Sexual disorders are significant public health concern, affecting up to 45% of women globally [25]. Their impact transcends the realm of sexual function, profoundly affecting women's physical health, emotional well-being, and overall quality of life [16]. Recognizing and addressing this issue is crucial for following reasons:

1. **Broad and interconnected consequences:**
    - **Physical health:** Sexual disorders can cause physical discomfort (painful sex, dryness), contribute to conditions such as GSM [37], and negatively impact a woman's sexual function and overall well-being [16].
    - **Emotional well-being:** These difficulties can trigger emotional distress, anxiety and frustration, erode self-esteem, and lead to feelings of inadequacy or dissatisfaction [49].
    - **Interpersonal relationships:** Sexual disharmony can strain communication, intimacy, and connection within relationships, potentially leading to conflict and emotional distance [34].
    - **Mental health:** Persistent sexual problems are often associated with depression and anxiety [12, 13]. The emotional burden and societal stigma surrounding sexual health can further exacerbate existing mental health challenges.

- **Quality of life:** Sexual difficulties can significantly diminish a woman's overall quality of life, impacting daily activities, social interactions, and the ability to find joy and fulfillment in various aspects of life [16].

2. **Beyond the individual:**
   - Unaddressed sexual disorders can have negative repercussions for partners and families, leading to relationship conflict and frustration and potentially impacting family dynamics.
   - The economic burden of sexual dysfunction can be significant, with increased healthcare costs and lost productivity [44].
   - Societal stigma surrounding sexual health can prevent women from seeking help, perpetuating the cycle of negative impact and hindering progress toward gender equality and sexual well-being for all.

21.3 REDUCED LIBIDO IN WOMEN

Libido (also known as sexual desire) refers to the psychological and biological drive toward sexual activity. Several factors (such as hormones, neurotransmitters, emotions, relationships, cultural expectations, and personal experiences) can influence libido [7]. While there is no single "normal" level of libido, a significant and persistent decrease in sexual desire (hypoactive sexual desire disorder) can impact an individual's well-being and interpersonal relationships [4]. Factors affecting libido are given as follows:

- **Hormonal changes:** Fluctuations in hormones such as estrogen, testosterone, and progesterone can significantly impact libido, particularly during life stages (such as puberty, pregnancy, postpartum, and menopause).
- **Medical conditions:** Chronic illnesses, thyroid disorders, neurological conditions, and certain medications can affect libido [13].
- **Psychological factors:** Stress, anxiety, melancholy, challenges related to body image, and previous traumatic experiences can have a negative impact on sexual desire [48].
- **Substance use:** Alcohol, drugs, and smoking can negatively influence libido [12].

- **Relationship issues:** Communication problems, intimacy difficulties, and relationship conflict can contribute to reduced libido [33].

21.3.1 MAINTAINING LIBIDO

- **Addressing underlying medical conditions:** Consulting a healthcare professional to identify and manage any medical conditions impacting libido is crucial.
- **Managing stress and anxiety:** Implementing stress reduction techniques such as mindfulness, yoga, or exercise can be beneficial [5].
- **Improving communication and intimacy:** Open and honest communication with partners about sexual desires and concerns can strengthen the relationship and enhance intimacy [31].
- **Prioritizing sleep and a healthy lifestyle:** Sleep deprivation and unhealthy lifestyle choices can negatively impact energy levels and sexual desire. Maintaining a healthy diet, regular exercise, and adequate sleep can improve overall well-being and support a healthy libido [22].
- **Exploring self-pleasure:** Learning about and experiencing self-pleasure can increase sexual knowledge, body positivity, and overall sexual satisfaction, potentially boosting desire [23].
- **Professional help:** Consulting a sex therapist or mental health professional can provide individual or couples therapy to address specific concerns, improve communication, and develop strategies for enhancing sexual desire and satisfaction [35].

21.4 ORGASMIC DISORDERS IN WOMEN

An orgasm (referred to as a climax) is the intense physiological and emotional sensation of pleasure that marks the peak of sexual activity. It involves a complex interplay of hormonal, neurological, and muscular responses, characterized by changes in heart rate, breathing, muscle tension, and blood flow [11]. Often described as a wave of intense pleasure that culminates in physical and emotional release, the experience of orgasm varies greatly among individuals.

Female orgasmic disorders refer to the persistent difficulty or inability to achieve orgasm during sexual activity, despite adequate stimulation and arousal. These difficulties can manifest in following ways:

- **Primary orgasmic disorder:** Never having experienced an orgasm [7].
- **Secondary orgasmic disorder:** Previously experiencing orgasms but no longer being able to do so [30].
- **Situational orgasmic disorder:** Only being able to achieve orgasm in specific situations, such as with masturbation but not with partner sex [24].

Orgasm is the result of a complex interaction between following factors, including those that are physical, psychological, and social [16]:

- **Physical factors:** Hormonal changes such as those associated with menopause, certain medications [13], and neurological conditions can impact orgasm potential. Genital sensitivity and blood flow to the area can also play a role [22].
- **Psychological factors:** Stress, anxiety, depression, body image issues, and past sexual trauma can all inhibit sexual responsiveness and make reaching orgasm difficult [49].
- **Social factors:** Relationship dynamics, communication about sexual needs and desires, and cultural expectations related to sex can all influence orgasmic experiences [34].
- **Sexual techniques and knowledge:** Lack of familiarity with one's own body and effective stimulation techniques, as well as inadequate communication with partners about preferences, can hinder orgasm achievement [23].

21.5 IMPACT OF LOW SELF-ESTEEM ON FEMALE SEXUAL HEALTH

Lack of self-esteem is characterized by emotions of inadequacy, insecurity, and self-doubt. When someone has low self-esteem, she has a negative perception of herself, which is characterized by sensations [9] that are due to critical self-evaluations, a poor body image, and a lack of confidence in one's own abilities and values. These characteristics describe this condition. At some point in a lifetime, this person will, without fail, be confronted with the experience of questioning her own abilities. On the other hand, persistent and pervasive low self-esteem can have a considerable impact on many elements of life, including but not limited to sexual health [33]. Following factors can contribute to low self-esteem in women:

- **Societal expectations and beauty standards:** Societal pressures to conform to unrealistic beauty ideals can lead to negative body image and feelings of inadequacy, impacting sexual confidence and enjoyment [20].
- **Past experiences:** Experiences of sexual trauma, abuse, or negative body comments can have long-lasting consequences, influencing self-perception and sexual well-being [19].
- **Relationship dynamics:** Unhealthy relationships characterized by criticism, insecurity, or a lack of intimacy can contribute to feelings of worthlessness and inadequacy, impacting sexual assertiveness and satisfaction [6].
- **Mental health conditions:** Conditions such as depression or anxiety can exacerbate negative self-perceptions and hinder healthy self-esteem development, affecting sexual expression and fulfillment.
- **Comparison with others:** Social media and societal pressures to compare oneself to others can fuel feelings of inadequacy and negatively impact self-worth, including in the sexual domain.

Low self-esteem can have a profound impact on women's sexual health in following ways:

- **Sexual function:** Negative self-perceptions and body image concerns can lead to difficulties with arousal, lubrication, and orgasm function [48].
- **Sexual desire:** Feeling unattractive or unworthy can diminish sexual desire and motivation for sexual activity [39].
- **Intimacy and communication:** Insecurity and self-doubt can hinder open communication about sexual needs and preferences, limiting intimacy and creating relationship strain [34].

- **Sexual pleasure:** Negative self-image can limit the ability to experience and enjoy sexual pleasure fully [23].
- **Sexual risk behaviors:** In some cases, low self-esteem can lead to engaging in risky sexual behaviors as a means of validation or acceptance.

21.6 IMPACT OF VAGINAL DRYNESS ON FEMALE HEALTH

Vaginal dryness (also known as GSM in postmenopausal women) is a sexual disorder characterized by a decrease in vaginal lubrication and thinning of the vaginal lining [2]. This can lead to discomfort, pain, and irritation during sexual activity, as well as other symptoms affecting daily life. Postmenopausal women prefer the term GSM because it emphasizes the urogenital system, while nonmenopausal women can still use vaginal dryness. Vaginal dryness affects a significant portion of women across various life stages given as follows:

- **Postmenopausal women:** Up to 50% of women experience GSM after menopause due to declining estrogen levels.
- **Younger women:** Vaginal dryness can also occur in younger women due to factors such as birth control pills, hormonal imbalances, certain medications, or medical conditions according to National Health Service.
- **Cancer survivors:** Women treated for cancer with hormonal therapies or radiation can experience vaginal dryness as a side effect [1].

Vaginal dryness can significantly impact women's quality of life in following ways:

- **Physical discomfort:** Pain, burning, itching, and irritation during sexual activity or daily activities such as wearing tight clothing can significantly affect well-being [39].
- **Psychological distress:** Frustration, anxiety, and low self-esteem can arise from difficulties with sexual intimacy and feeling different from one's partner's expectations [48].

- **Relationship strain:** Communication challenges and decreased intimacy can strain relationships with partners [33].
- **Reduced sexual satisfaction:** Diminished lubrication and pleasure can negatively impact sexual enjoyment and satisfaction [23].

Common symptoms and manifestations of dry vagina are given as follows:

- **Decrease in estrogen production after menopause causes dryness and irritation in the vagina and vulva (a hallmark symptom of GSM):** The vaginal tissues become thinner, less elastic, and less lubricated, leading to discomfort and irritation.
- **Discomfort during sexual activity:** Pain, burning sensations, and difficulty with penetration can occur due to vaginal dryness and decreased elasticity. Sexual activity may become less pleasurable or even painful.
- **Difficulty in inserting tampons or using other vaginal products:** Like discomfort during sex, dryness and irritation can make it difficult to insert tampons or use other vaginal products comfortably.
- **Frequent urination due to irritation:** The vulva and urethra (urinary opening) are located close together. Irritation in the vulva can irritate the urethra, triggering a frequent urge to urinate.
- **Bleeding after sexual activity:** Due to the thin and fragile vaginal tissues, sexual activity can sometimes cause minor spotting or bleeding [40].

21.7 SEXUAL DISORDERS IN WOMEN

Several sexual disorders in women can arise from following contributing factors:

1. **Hormonal changes during menopause:** Menopause marks a significant decline in ovarian function and sex hormones, particularly estrogen. This decline plays a significant role in several sexual disorders, such as:

- **Vaginal dryness:** Estrogen helps maintain vaginal lubrication and elasticity. Its decline leads to thinning of the vaginal lining, decreased lubrication, and discomfort during sex.
- **Decreased libido:** Estrogen also modulates sexual desire and arousal. Lower levels can lead to a reduced interest in sexual activity [13].
- **GSM** encompasses a range of symptoms affecting the urogenital system due to estrogen deficiency, including vaginal dryness, pain, and irritation [42].

2. **Estrogen declines beyond menopause:**
    - **Medications:** Certain medications, such as antihistamines and antidepressants, can have side effects that affect sexual function, including vaginal dryness, decreased libido, and difficulty with orgasm [48].
    - **Medical conditions:** Chronic illnesses such as diabetes, thyroid disorders, and neurological conditions can also impact sexual function through hormonal imbalances and nerve damage [13].
3. **Changes in vaginal tissue:**
    - **Pregnancy and childbirth:** During pregnancy and postpartum, hormonal changes and physical stretching of the vaginal tissues can temporarily affect sexual function and sensitivity [34].
    - **Aging:** Normal aging processes can also lead to gradual changes in vaginal tissue, making it less elastic and more susceptible to irritation.
4. **Other life stages and medical conditions:**
    - **Postpartum:** Beyond immediate physical changes, postpartum depression and anxiety can further impact sexual desire and enjoyment [49].
    - **Breastfeeding:** Lactation and prolactin levels can temporarily suppress libido in some women [33].

- **Psychological factors:** Stress, anxiety, depression, and past trauma can significantly inhibit sexual response and desire [13].
- **Relationship dynamics:** Communication issues, intimacy challenges, and partner factors can contribute to sexual difficulties [33].

21.8 IMPACT OF CANCER TREATMENTS ON SEXUAL HEALTH IN WOMEN

This section explores the physical, psychological, and emotional factors that play a crucial role in female sexual health under cancer treatment.

21.8.1 PSYCHOLOGICAL AND EMOTIONAL FACTORS

- **Changes in body image:** Cancer treatments, particularly surgery and radiation, can lead to physical changes that can negatively impact body image and self-esteem, affecting sexual confidence and desire [39].
- **Fear of intimacy and recurrence:** Concerns about pain, discomfort, or the potential recurrence of cancer can create anxiety and fear around sexual activity, leading to avoidance or decreased enjoyment [15].
- **Depression and anxiety:** The emotional stress of cancer diagnosis and treatment can contribute to depression and anxiety, further impacting sexual desire and function [13].
- **Loss of control and vulnerability:** Cancer treatment can often involve a loss of control over one's body, which can negatively impact sexual feelings and intimacy [33].

21.8.2 STRESS

The chronic stress associated with cancer diagnosis and treatment can significantly impact sexual functioning. Stress hormones can interfere with libido, arousal, and orgasm, leading to difficulties with sexual enjoyment and satisfaction [13].

21.8.3 ANXIETY

Anxiety about cancer recurrence, pain during sex, or partner expectations can create a negative cycle of anxiety and avoidance, further hindering sexual desire and response [15].

21.8.4 RELATIONSHIP DYNAMICS

Open communication and understanding from partners are crucial during and after cancer treatment. However, communication challenges, changes in roles and responsibilities within the relationship, and partner anxieties can all contribute to difficulties with sexual intimacy [33].

21.9 DEVASTATING PSYCHOSOCIAL FACTORS OF SEXUAL DISORDERS IN WOMEN: UNDERSTANDING AND SUPPORT

Sexual disorders in women can have profound and far-reaching psychosocial consequences, impacting not only their physical health but also their emotional well-being, relationships, and social experiences. Following is a closer look at these impacts.

21.9.1 EFFECT ON SEXUAL SATISFACTION

- **Frustration and disappointment:** Difficulty in experiencing pleasure and orgasm can lead to frustration, disappointment, and feelings of inadequacy among women and their partners [33].
- **Reduced self-esteem and confidence:** Sexual difficulties can negatively impact women's self-esteem and confidence, particularly in their sense of attractiveness and desirability [13].
- **Loss of intimacy and connection:** Sexual difficulties can create barriers to intimacy and emotional connection within relationships, leading to feelings of isolation and disconnection [15].

21.9.2 RELATIONSHIP ISSUES AND COMMUNICATION

- **Communication challenges:** Discussing sexual problems can be difficult and embarrassing, leading to communication breakdown and emotional strain within relationships [33].
- **Misunderstandings and resentment:** Lack of understanding and support from partners can lead to resentment and blame, further exacerbating relationship difficulties [15].
- **Potential for relationship breakdown:** In severe cases, unaddressed sexual problems can contribute to relationship dissatisfaction and even breakdown [13].

21.9.3 EMOTIONAL WELL-BEING

- **Depression and anxiety:** Sexual difficulties can be a source of significant emotional distress, contributing to depression, anxiety, and feelings of low self-esteem [13].
- **Shame and guilt:** Societal stigma and misconceptions surrounding female sexuality can lead to feelings of shame and guilt, further hindering women from seeking help [33].
- **Reduced quality of life:** Ultimately, sexual difficulties can significantly impact women's overall quality of life, affecting their happiness, well-being, and sense of fulfillment [15].

21.9.4 SOCIAL STIGMA AND MISCONCEPTIONS

- **Silence and taboo:** Sexual dysfunction in women is often shrouded in silence and taboo, leading to a lack of open discussion and understanding [33].
- **Misconceptions and stereotypes**: Myths and stereotypes about female sexuality can further stigmatize women experiencing sexual difficulties, making it harder for them to seek help [13].

- **Need for education and awareness**: Challenging societal stigma and promoting education about female sexuality are crucial for creating a supportive environment where women can openly discuss and address sexual difficulties [15].

21.10 EFFECTIVE TREATMENT OPTIONS FOR FEMALE SEXUAL DISORDERS

Understanding the causes and impacts of sexual disorders in women is crucial, but finding the right treatment path is equally important. This section explores various treatment options, their efficacy, safety, and potential side effects.

21.10.1 LIFESTYLE MODIFICATIONS

- **Stress management:** Techniques such as yoga, meditation, and relaxation exercises can help manage stress, a key contributor to sexual dysfunction [13].
- **Healthy diet and exercise:** Maintaining a healthy weight and engaging in regular physical activity can improve overall health and sexual function [49].
- **Pelvic floor muscle exercises:** Kegel exercises can strengthen the pelvic floor muscles, potentially improving sensation and control during sex [33].
- **Communication and relationship therapy:** Open communication with partners and, if needed, seeking professional relationship therapy can address communication challenges and foster intimacy [15].

21.10.2 OVER-THE-COUNTER LUBRICANTS AND MOISTURIZERS

- Water-based lubricants can address vaginal dryness and discomfort during sex and can improve the sexual enjoyment [40].
- Moisturizers can alleviate vulvar and vaginal dryness, providing relief from irritation and soreness [2].

21.10.3 HORMONE THERAPY

- **Estrogen-based therapies:** Topical creams, vaginal rings, and low-dose oral therapy can be effective for alleviating vaginal dryness and improving libido associated with hormonal decline, particularly in postmenopausal women.
- **Hormone replacement therapy (HRT):** Systemic HRT with estrogen and progesterone can address various menopausal symptoms, including sexual dysfunction, but carries potential risks such as increased blood clot risk and breast cancer [49].

21.10.4 HOLISTIC APPROACH TO MANAGING SEXUAL DISORDERS IN WOMEN

Sexual disorders in women are multifaceted and can significantly impact their physical, emotional, and relational well-being. Thankfully, a holistic approach that goes beyond managing symptoms can empower women to reclaim their sexual health and overall sense of well-being. Some key aspects of a holistic approach are given below.

21.10.4.1 PATIENT-CENTERED COMMUNICATION

- **Open and honest communication:** Building trust and fostering safe spaces for women to discuss sensitive sexual concerns with their healthcare providers is crucial for accurate diagnosis and personalized treatment [13].
- **Shared decision-making:** Involving women in treatment choices empowers them and increases adherence to the plan [15].

21.10.4.2 PERSONALIZED TREATMENT PLANS

- **Acknowledging individual needs:** There is no "one-size-fits-all" approach. Recognizing individual experiences, preferences, and the specific causes of the sexual disorder is key to successful management.

- **Multifaceted interventions:** A combination of medical interventions, such as hormone therapy or lubricants, alongside lifestyle modifications such as stress management and pelvic floor exercises, may be necessary [2].
- **Continuous monitoring and adjustments:** Regularly assessing progress and adapting the treatment plan based on individual responses ensures optimal outcomes [12].

21.10.4.3 INTEGRATING PHYSICAL AND EMOTIONAL CARE

- **Recognizing the interconnection:** Sexual health encompasses both physical and emotional well-being [33]. Addressing underlying psychological factors such as anxiety or depression alongside physical interventions can significantly improve sexual function [2].
- **Psychotherapeutic approaches:** Integrating therapies such as cognitive–behavioral therapy can help address negative thoughts and beliefs about sex, enhancing sexual response and enjoyment [15].

21.10.4.4 ADDRESSING UNDERLYING CAUSES

- **Identifying and managing medical conditions:** Underlying medical conditions or medications can contribute to sexual dysfunction. Treating or adjusting these factors can be crucial for successful management [42].
- **Cancer-related sexual problems:** For women facing cancer-related sexual difficulties, addressing emotional distress and concerns about recurrence alongside physical therapies can improve sexual well-being [49].
- **Relationship dynamics:** Partner involvement and open communication can be essential in addressing relationship dynamics or partner anxieties that may contribute to sexual difficulties [15].

21.10.4.5 FAMILY AND COMMUNITY SUPPORT

- **Emotional understanding and encouragement:** The role of family and community support systems in offering emotional understanding, encouragement, and practical assistance can significantly impact women's ability to cope with sexual dysfunction [33].
- **Partner involvement:** Open communication and partner support are crucial for addressing relationship dynamics and anxieties that may contribute to sexual difficulties [2].
- **Support groups and communities:** Sharing experiences and accessing resources with other women experiencing similar challenges can empower individuals and reduce feelings of isolation [15].

21.11 INTEGRATIVE MEDICINE FOR SEXUAL HEALTH

Holistic approach for integrative medicine combines conventional therapies with complementary and alternative medicine, and it has gained prominence as a comprehensive healthcare approach. This method encompasses a diverse range of practices and therapies, offering promising avenues for enhancing sexual health. By considering not only the physical aspects but also the mental and emotional well-being of individuals, integrative medicine provides a holistic approach to achieving a fulfilling and balanced sexual life. The incorporation of nutrition, exercise, sleep, stress management, and mental wellness is pivotal in promoting sexual health within this framework.

21.11.1 ROLE OF NUTRIENTS FOR SEXUAL HEALTH

Dietary optimization is a cornerstone of sexual health within an integrative medicine framework. Tables 21.1 and 21.2 indicate the benefits of nutrients/herbs/supplements on sexual health. Fruits and vegetables, abundant in antioxidants, combat oxidative stress in the genitourinary system, potentially mitigating its detrimental effects on sexual function [45]. Omega-3 polyunsaturated fatty acids (PUFAs) (prevalent in fish and nuts) can enhance blood flow, a key physiological factor for optimal sexual response [53]. Furthermore, a balanced diet promotes hormonal homeostasis, influencing libido and sexual performance through its regulatory effects on sex hormone production [27].

- Antioxidants (fruits, vegetables, nuts, and seeds) protect cells from damage and may improve blood flow [8, 18].
- Omega-3 fatty acids (walnuts, flaxseeds, and fatty fish): Diets abundant in omega-3 PUFAs might improve endothelium function, which may in turn contribute to an increase in blood flow. According to researchers, these PUFAs display anti-inflammatory properties and have the potential to exert mood-regulating effects [18, 28].
- Vitamin D (fatty fish, eggs, and fortified dairy product) may help regulate hormone levels and boost mood [21].
- Zinc (oysters, beef, chickpeas, and pumpkin seeds) supports healthy hormone production and may improve libido and sexual function [41, 51].
- Iron (lean meat, poultry, beans, and lentils) transports oxygen throughout the body, which is crucial for energy production and sexual function [10, 43].
- Folic acid (green leafy vegetables, lentils, and fortified grains) supports cell growth and development [14, 46].

TABLE 21.1 Sexual Healthy Foods

Nutrients	Food Sources	Benefits of Sexual Health	References
Antioxidants	Fruits (berries, citrus), vegetables (broccoli, spinach), nuts, and seeds	Protect cells from damage, improve blood flow, and reduce inflammation	[8, 18]
Folic acid	Green leafy vegetables, lentils, and fortified grains	Support cell growth and development and reduce the risk of birth defects	[14, 46]
Iron	Lean meat, poultry, beans, and lentils	Transport oxygen throughout the body, improve energy levels, and support sexual function	[10, 43]
Omega-3 fatty acids	Fatty fish (salmon, tuna), flaxseeds, and walnuts	Improve blood flow, reduce inflammation, and enhance mood	[18, 28]
Vitamin D	Fatty fish, eggs, and fortified dairy products	Regulate hormone levels, boost mood, and improve immune function	[21]
Zinc	Oysters, beef, chickpeas, and pumpkin seeds	Support healthy hormone production, improve libido, and enhance sexual function	[41, 51]

TABLE 21.2 Herbs and Supplements for Female Sexual Health

Herbs/Supplements	Potential Benefits
Ashwagandha	Reduce stress and anxiety, improve mood, and boost energy
L-arginine	Improve blood flow and enhance sexual response
Maca	Improve libido, reduce fatigue, and support hormonal balance
Panax ginseng	Enhance blood flow, improve energy levels, and support sexual function

21.11.2 EXERCISE

Regular physical activity is closely linked to improved sexual health within the integrative medicine paradigm. Exercise increases blood flow, reduces stress, and enhances self-confidence [32]. Activities such as yoga and strength training contribute to flexibility and stamina, fostering a more satisfying sexual life [47]. The release of endorphins during exercise further enhances mood and desire [36].

21.11.3 MENTAL WELL-BEING

The integrative medicine approach intricately connects mental well-being to sexual health. Depression and anxiety can interfere with multiple aspects of sexual functioning, including desire, arousal, and orgasm [3, 35], highlighting the importance of seeking therapy or counseling when necessary to address mental health issues and enhance sexual satisfaction.

21.11.4 ADDRESSING HORMONAL IMBALANCE

This may involve using herbal medicines, vitamins, or dietary changes to support healthy hormone production and balance. A qualified healthcare professional should guide the use of herbs for hormonal issues [17].

21.11.5 IMPROVING BLOOD FLOW

Certain herbal medicines, massage therapy, or acupuncture may enhance circulation, which can benefit sexual function in some cases. Research on the effectiveness of these approaches is ongoing [17, 50].

21.11.6 REDUCING STRESS AND ANXIETY

Techniques such as meditation, yoga, or stress management interventions can address psychological factors that contribute to sexual problem [52].

21.12 SUMMARY

A complete analysis of the varied nature of FSD is presented in this chapter. The contents highlight the enormous impact that sexual dysfunction has on the physical, emotional, and relational well-being of women. An examination of the intricacies of female sexuality, which is impacted by a variety of elements, including biological, psychological, and social influences, is presented. The need to resolve sexual issues to enhance the overall quality of life is emphasized throughout the chapter. The numerous forms of FSD (such as decreased libido, difficulties in attaining orgasm, and vaginal dryness) are among the key topics that are being investigated. The work also investigates the far-reaching effects that FSD has on the lives of women, including the effects it has on their physical health, mental well-being, relationships, and self-esteem. In addition to this, it detects probable underlying reasons of sexual dysfunction, such as changes in hormone levels, physical disorders, psychological variables, and the dynamics of relationships. Several different treatment options are discussed in the chapter to meet these issues. These include hormone therapy, lifestyle adjustments, and over-the-counter remedies. Additionally, literature emphasizes the need to take a holistic approach. This chapter places an emphasis on the significance of creating novel treatments, individualized treatment plans, and tackling the stigma that is associated with sexual health. In the end, the statement advocates for a holistic approach to the sexual health of women, which includes the incorporation of sexual health into primary care and the undertaking of long-term research to get an understanding of the progression of sexual health during woman's lifetime. By focusing on these aspects, future study can contribute to the enhancement of the sexual health and well-being of women worldwide.

KEYWORDS

- **arousal difficulties**
- **diminished libido**
- **holistic approach in women**
- **orgasmic challenges**
- **pain during intercourse**
- **sexual disorders**

REFERENCES

1. American Cancer Society. (2023, January 11). Vaginal dryness after cancer treatment. https://www.nm.org/healthbeat/healthy-tips/treating-vaginal-dryness-after-breast-cancer
2. American College of Obstetricians and Gynecologists. (2023, February). Vaginal dryness. https://www.acog.org/clinical/clinical-guidance/practice-bulletin/articles/2018/06/prevention-of-infection-after-gynecologic-procedures
3. American Congress of Obstetricians and Gynecologists. (2015). Female sexual dysfunction. https://www.acog.org/clinical/clinical-guidance/practice-bulletin/articles/2019/07/female-sexual-dysfunction
4. American Psychiatric Association (APA). (2013). *Diagnostic and Statistical Manual of Mental Disorders*, 5th ed., APA: Arlington, VA, USA.
5. American Psychiatric Association. (2017). Stress disorders. In: *Diagnostic and Statistical Manual of Mental Disorders* (5th ed., online). https://dsm.psychiatryonline.org/doi/book/10.1176/appi.books.9780890425596
6. Ayala, G., & Follette, V. C. (2015). The impact of intimate partner violence on sexual health. *American Journal of Public Health*, *105*(11), 2267–2274.
7. Basson, R., & Leiblum, S. R. (2004). Female sexual dysfunction. *The Lancet*, *363*(9421), 1805–1811.
8. Basu, A., Mukhopadhyay, S., & Ghosh, S. (2010). Antioxidant potential of fruits: An in vitro evaluation. *Current Pharmaceutical Biotechnology*, *11*(1), 41–48.
9. Baumeister, R. F., Heatherton, T. F., & Tice, D. M. (1994). Physical attractiveness and social acceptance: Influence of perceived attractiveness on social interaction and self-evaluation. *Journal of Personality and Social Psychology*, *66*(3), 577–593.
10. Brown, W. D., Inder, W. J., Lipton, A., Theobald, A. E., Watts, C., & Kingwell, E. (2015). The effects of iron deficiency on sexual function in women. *The Cochrane Database of Systematic Reviews*, (7), CD004731.
11. Carney, S. E., Bancroft, J., & Janssen, E. (2004). The psychological and interpersonal dynamics of female orgasm. *Journal of Sex Research*, *41*(2), 141–150.

12. Clayton, A. H., Jang, K. J., Luo, Z., & Jeon, S. Y. (2009). Sexual dysfunction and depression in women: A bidirectional relationship. *The Journal of Clinical Psychiatry*, *70*(6), 854–861.
13. Clayton, A. H., Jang, K. J., Luo, Z., Desai, M., & Goldstein, I. (2009). The association between sexual dysfunction and mental health in a nationally representative sample of US women. *Journal of Women's Health*, *18*(2), 201–208.
14. Czeizel, A. E., Dudas, S., Pop, J. A., & Surjan, I. (2014). Periconceptional folic acid supplementation and congenital anomalies. *The New England Journal of Medicine*, *370*(17), 1687–1695.
15. Denham, S. W., Duncan, S. L., & Wright, D. M. (2016). Sexual health and quality of life after cancer treatment: A review of the literature. *Annals of Palliative Medicine*, *5*(2), 114–124.
16. Dennerstein, M. (2019). Sexual health and well-being in women. Australian and New Zealand. *Journal of Obstetrics and Gynaecology*, *59*(2), 142–147.
17. Ernst, E., & Pittler, M. H. (2000). Efficacy of herbal medicine for the treatment of sexual function problems: A systematic review. *Archives of Internal Medicine*, *160*(17), 2499–2506.
18. Esposito, K., Nappo, R., Di Palo, C., Giugliano, D., Maiorino, M., Melillo, G., & Menzione, A. (2014). Effects of a Mediterranean diet on endothelial function in overweight subjects with type 2 diabetes. *Diabetes Care*, *37*(1), 201–208.
19. Feingold, A. (1994). Masturbation and sexual identity crisis in female sexual dysfunction. *Journal of Sex & Marital Therapy*, *20*(2), 127–136.
20. Fredrickson, B. L., & Roberts, T.-A. (1998). Objectification theory: Toward understanding women's lived experiences and mental health risks. *Psychology of Women Quarterly*, *22*(2), 173–206.
21. Giugliano, D., Esposito, K., Märker, S., Mendes, E., Cowie, C. C., Taddei, S., & Schwartz, E. (2013). Vitamin D supplementation and cardiometabolic risk in overweight or obese subjects with type 2 diabetes: A randomized trial. *Annals of Internal Medicine*, *159*(8), 507–515.
22. Goldstein, I., Meston, C. M., Davis, S. R., Trapido, E. M., Kerns, L. M., Raphaelson, Y., & Levine, S. B. (2000). Blood flow to the sexual organs in women during sexual activity. *Journal of Urology*, *163*(3), 805–810.
23. Herbenick, D. (2010). Self-reported orgasm problems among US women: Prevalence, correlates, and associations with health and relationship satisfaction. *Journal of Sexual Medicine*, *7*(11), 3707–3721.
24. Herbenick, D., Reece, J., Sanders, S. A., & Fortenberry, K. (2017). Why some women have difficulty orgasming during partnered sex: A review of explanations and a proposed model. *The Journal of Sexual Medicine*, *14*(3), 301–310.
25. International Society for Sexual Medicine. (2015). Female sexual dysfunction management. *The Journal of Sexual Medicine*, *13*(2), 153–167.
26. Jacobi, A. E. (2014). The evolving definition of sexual health. *Journal of Sexual Medicine*, *11*(7), 1630–1633.
27. Jarrous, A. E., Khalil, M. H., & Kandalaft, N. M. (2018). The role of diet in male and female sexual health. *Clinical Nutrition Experimental*, *16*, 1–10.
28. Kiecolt-Glaser, J. K., Belanger, A. J., & Patterson, T. L. (2013). Omega-3 fatty acids and mental health. *Current Opinion in Psychiatry*, *26*(1), 48–53.

29. Laumann, E. O., Paik, A., & Xuan, C. N. (1999). Sociodemographic differences in sexual dysfunction in the United States: Results from a national probability sample. *Journal of Sex Research*, *36*(1), 51–61.
30. Leiblum, S. R. (2010). Principles and techniques of sex therapy. In: *Oxford Handbook of Couples and Family Therapy* (pp. 271–289). Oxford University Press: New York.
31. Lenzi, A., Lombardo, V., Spera, G., Francavilla, S., & Paolini, S. (2018). The effect of exercise on sexual function in women: A systematic review with meta-analysis. *Journal of Sexual Medicine, 15*(10), 1421–1432.
32. Lindau, S. T., & Berman, L. (2004). Sexual health: A model for primary care. *Primary Care Clinics in Office Practice*, *31*(4), 741–755.
33. Loewenson, R. J. (2015). *Human Sexuality: An Integrated Approach*, 7th ed., Routledge: London.
34. Loewenson, R. J. (2015). The impact of female sexual dysfunction on relationships. *Sexual Medicine Reviews*, *3*(1), 60–67.
35. McMahon, M. M., Shin, C. H., & Jang, J. Y. (2018). The bidirectional relationship between depression and sexual dysfunction: A review of the evidence. *Current Psychiatry Reports*, *20*(11), 98–105.
36. Meeks, G. D., Dishman, R. K., & Thompson, R. W. (2011). Exercise, endorphins, and sexual function. *Mayo Clinic Proceedings*, *86*(5), 403–410.
37. Nappi, G. (2014). Vulvar and vaginal atrophy: A multifaceted approach to a common problem. *Climacteric*, *17*(5), 551–558.
38. Nappi, G., & Moggi, M. (2004). Vulvar and vaginal atrophy in postmenopausal women: Management with local estrogen therapy. *Maturitas*, *48*(Suppl 1), S23–S30. https://www.sciencedirect.com/science/article/pii/S1743609515304318
39. Nappi, G., & Moggi, R. (2000). Vulvovaginal atrophy: A review of the effects on female sexual function. *Menopause International*, *6*(3), 104–108.
40. Nettleton, S., Vahvi, M., & Bates, G. (2013). Zinc supplementation for asthma prevention in children. *Cochrane Database of Systematic Reviews*, *2013*(2), CD006597.
41. Newson, L., Kirby, M., Stillwell, S., Hackett, G., Ball, S., & Lewis, R. (2023). Position statement for management of genitourinary syndrome of the menopause (GSM). *British Society for Sexual Medicine.*
42. North American Menopause Society (NAMS). (2013). Management of symptomatic vulvovaginal atrophy: 2013 position statement of The NAMS. *Menopause*, *20*(9), 888–902 (quiz 903-4), online. doi: 10.1097/GME.0b013e3182a122c2. PMID: 23985562.
43. O'Brien, S., Weinberg, E. D., & Sturgeon, A. E. (2013). The prevalence of anemia in women with chronic fatigue syndrome and fibromyalgia. *Journal of Clinical Medicine*, *2*(2), 217–221.
44. Reed, B. D. (2014). The economics of female sexual dysfunction. *The Journal of Sexual Medicine*, *11*(7), 1682–1690.
45. Saleh, A. T., & Agarwal, A. (2002). Oxidative stress and male infertility: From laboratory to the clinic. *Journal of Andrology*, *23*(7), 737–753.
46. Scott, J. M., Moretti, M., Piscopo, S., Abdalla, S., Zhu, H., Roberts, C. A., & Messerlian, S. (2012). Folic acid supplementation for the primary prevention of

cardiovascular disease and stroke: A meta-analysis of randomized controlled trials. *JAMA of Internal Medicine*, *172*(12), 927–935.

47. Silva, A. M., Teixeira, L. C., & Carioca, A. A. (2017). Yoga for sexual health of women: A systematic review. *International Journal of Women's Health*, *9*, 337–347.
48. Taylor, S. E., Davis, M. C., & Guay, A. T. (2017). Women's sexual health: A review of the effects of sexual dysfunction on quality of life. *Psychotherapy and Psychosomatics*, *86*(3), 130–143.
49. Taylor, S. E., LeClerc, P. L., Rogers, R. W., & Biggs, T. A. (2017). *Social Psychological Foundations of Health.* McGraw-Hill Education: New York.
50. Vickers, A. J., Zollmann, C., & Linde, K. (2004). Massage for promoting relaxation and wellbeing. *The Cochrane Database of Systematic Reviews*, *2004*(4), CD000383.
51. Walsh, L. P., Wessells, K. R., Klein, S. L., & Connelly, K. A. (2014). Effects of combined zinc and creatine supplementation on muscle performance and hormones in athletes. *Journal of Strength and Conditioning Research*, *28*(1), 166–175.
52. Wang, C., Tian, Y., & Liu, J. (2014). Mindfulness-based interventions for improving sexual health: A systematic review and meta-analysis. *International Journal of Women's Health*, *6*, 1031–1042.
53. Wong, D. S., Lopez, V., & Lin, Y. T. (2015). The role of dietary omega-3 fatty acids in male sexual dysfunction. *Asian Journal of Andrology*, *17*(5), 715–721.

CHAPTER 22

Cancer in Females: Diagnostics, Treatment, Posttreatment, and a Case Study

PRIYA AND POONAM JOSHI*

*Corresponding author

ABSTRACT

A disease marked by the violent growth and the proliferation of abnormal cells, often resulting to the invasion of healthy tissues within the body, is explained as cancer. It is frequently mentioned as a neoplasm or malignant tumor. Globally, the second main cause of death is found to be cancer, accountable for one in six deaths (estimated 9.6 million deaths in 2018). Among women, the most recurrent cancers include breast, colorectal, cervical, lung, and thyroid cancer. The most prevalent types of cancer in men are lung, colorectal, stomach, liver, and prostate cancer. Cancer screening and detection with many imaging modalities are available. However, the main focus in this chapter is on X-ray-based, magnetic field-based, and ultrasound wave-based techniques. Other than imaging, aberrant DNA methylation is recognized as one of the earliest and most typical cause of malignant cell transformation and tumors of various localization. Two major breakthroughs have transformed cancer treatment paradigms: First, targeting actionable alterations in oncogene-driven cancers and second, optimizing treatment delivery through immune checkpoint inhibitors. The symptoms experienced in cancer are insomnia, fatigue, and cognitive impairment by psychological and physical manifestations. This chapter highlights the particulars on neoplastic diagnostics, treatments,

Holistic Approaches for Women's Sustainable Health, Volume 2: Advancements, Socioeconomic Impacts, and Innovative Strategies. Junaid Ahmad Malik, Anamika Chauhan, and Megh R. Goyal (Eds)

DOI: 10.1201/9781779641656-26

and posttreatment while discussing the case study of patients with breast cancer. Prospective research should focus on identifying effective interventions that can be administered directly to a larger number of patients.

22.1 INTRODUCTION

Cancer is a devastating condition, triggered by abnormal and uncontrollable cellular mitosis that invades nearby tissue. It is found to be the second foremost reason of demise, besides cardiovascular diseases. Globally, millions of people are identified with cancer every year, and about 10 million people lose their lives due to this disease. Deaths from cancer all over the globe are projected to keep up rising, with an estimate of 12 million deaths by 2030. Cancer affects the health of our human society. Cancer emerges via a sequence of mutations in genes that affect the normal cell functioning. Some chemical substances have a potential of forming gene with mutations or cancerous cells, known as carcinogens. For example, smoking involves several carcinogenic compounds that is the reason behind lung cancer. Unfortunately, it is a variety of disease that affects at the tissue level, and it a major challenge to provide a success rate of treatment for this [1].

Recent data shows that lung cancer is the most prevalent in both genders, constituting 11.6% of all cases, while breast cancer (BC) affects females at the same rate. Among men, prostate cancer accounts for 7.1% of cases. Colorectal cancer ranks third with respect to diagnosis (6.1%) but second in relation to mortality (9.2%). Prediction suggests a projected 60% rise in mortality from rectal cancer and 71.5% rise in mortality from colon cancer by 2035 [2].

Around 100 form of malignancies affect humans, unique to itself traits and impact. Etiological factors such as tobacco use, obesity, poor diet, excessive use of alcohol, lack of physical exercises, exposure to carcinogens or ionizing radiations, and environmental pollutants are the causes of cancer in today's life. Lifestyle choices, such as not smoking, maintaining a healthy weight, limited alcohol consumption, and proper and balanced diet, can reduce the risk of cancer occurrence. Vaccination against various infectious diseases plays a role in prevention. For cancers such as cervical and colorectal cancer, early detection through screening is necessary. Cancers also contribute a small percentage to inherited genetic defects [3].

How cancerous cell is different from a normal cell?

- Accumulation of multiple chromosomes in cancerous cells, duplications, or deletion of chromosomes leads to mutations in cancerous cells.
- Cancerous cells also trick the immune system to defend themselves from the attack, as the abnormal cells are eliminated by the immune system.
- Cancerous cells ignore the signals, which normally tells a cell to stop from growing, that is, apoptosis (Figure 22.1).
- Cancerous cells invade the nearby tissues and the other body regions (metastasis), whereas normal cells, on encounter with the other cells of the body, stop to grow.
- Cancerous cells rely on various kind of nutrients, unlike normal cells. Additionally, cancerous cell forms their energy from nutrients in a different form, unlike normal cell, which make the cancerous cells grow even rapidly.
- Normal cells grow only when they receive such signals, whereas cancerous cells grow in the absence of such signals.
- For the supply oxygen and nourishment for the growth, cancerous cells manipulate the blood vessels to grow toward tumors.

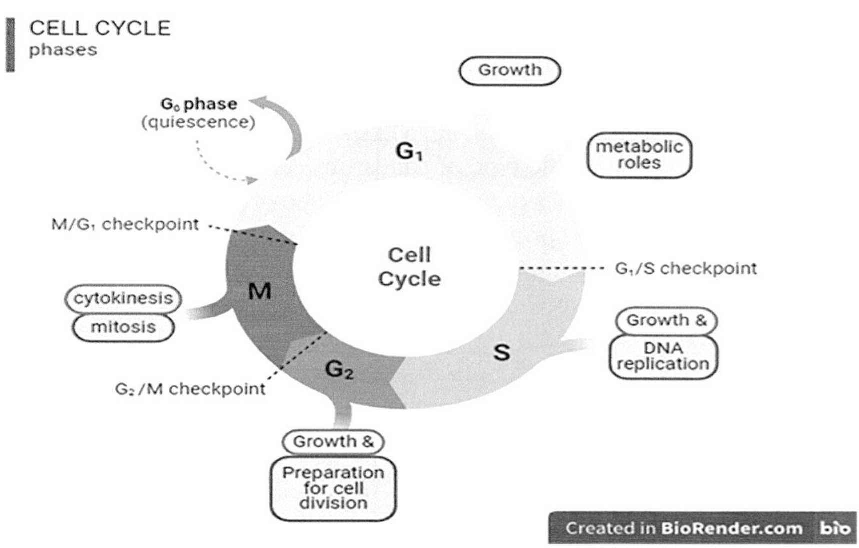

FIGURE 22.1 Representation of cell cycle.

The researchers have taken the advantage of the cancer's abnormal behavior, where the cancer cells strongly rely on the mentioned actions; so, the therapies have been developed that targets these abnormal actions such as some therapies block the blood vessels from growing toward the tumors, which starve the tumor from the needed nourishment [4].

22.2 TYPES OF GENES RESPONSIBLE FOR THE OCCURRENCE OF CANCER

Genomic maintenance genes, cellular oncogenes, and antioncogenes are the "drivers" of cancer. Cellular oncogenes play their role in healthy cell growth and cell division. When the specified genes undergo alteration or perform more actively than normal, they undergo a change into genes that promote cancer-promoting genes called oncogenes, enabling cells to proliferate and endure beyond their normal limits. Antioncogenes happen to be responsible in consideration of controlled cell proliferation as well as division, and any alteration in these may lead to uncontrolled division of normal cells. Damaged DNA is fixed by DNA repair genes. Cell mutations tend to develop changes in chromosomes, and the addition or deletion of chromosomal parts leads to mutations that cause cells to become cancerous. There are molecular changes that lead to cancer, and based on this, cancer treatments are available that target gene mutations. Some of the treatment can be administered to individuals with cancer who have been diagnosed with specified targeted mutations, regardless of the cancer's origin.

The process where the cancer spreads to different areas of the body from the original location is known as metastasis. Metastatic cancer is a same type of cancer or have same type of cancerous cells from primary cancer. A metastatic cancer cells have the same presence of specific chromosome changes, as of original or primary cancer. Metastatic cancer causes severe damage to the bodily functions, and most patients die from the same.

Some tissue changes in the body may develop into cancer if not treated at an early stage. Not every change in tissue is a cancer. However, the mentioned series of terms refers to tissue changes that are not considered cancer, but in some cases are monitored because they could develop into cancer over time.

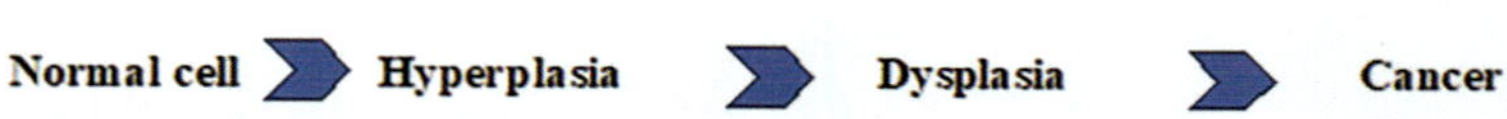

How is cancer developed from normal cell?

Hyperplasia is a term for the condition where the cells within the tissue grow rapidly than normal and build up the extra cells, even though under a microscope they look normal. It is led by chronic irritation. Dysplasia is a severe condition than the former. It also involves formation of additional cells, but they look abnormal and their arrangement in a tissue. Generally, more abnormal cells or tissue looks, greater chances are of it developing into a cancer. Mostly, dysplasia does not develop into cancer, but in some cases, it is required to be treated and observed for the prevention and control of cancer, for example, dysplastic nevus can convert into a melanoma if not monitored or treated well in few cases. There is a condition of stage 0 cancer in which the anomalous cells do not invade the neighboring tissue, unlike the cancer cell does [5].

22.3 TOTAL NUMBER OF CANCERS

The International Agency for Research on Cancer (IARC), World Health Organization, GLOBOCAN, and the American Cancer Society are the main international cancer reporting agencies that exist till date. They focus on the research and the recent trends observed in the diseases. The globe has been burdened by the incidence of different types of cancer. IARC has Global Cancer Observatory, which records the incidences and deaths related to cancer [6].

Figure 22.2 shows the global cancer data chart.

According to the recent data (January 2022), there are about 100 different types of cancers, and these cancers affect the distinct parts of the body differently; they have also different treatment approaches and prognoses [7]. There are many types of cancer, named accordingly from where it arises. The familiar types of cancers are bladder, blood, bone cancer (sarcoma), brain cancer (glioblastoma, meningioma, and others) as well as nonmelanoma of skin, squamous cell carcinoma and basal cell carcinoma, esophageal, ovarian, pancreatic, prostate, renal, soft-tissue sarcoma, testicular cancer, and thyroid.

The statistics of cancer for India were documented by National Cancer Registry Programme of the National Centre for Disease Informatics and Research under the auspices of the Indian Council of Medical Research. These statistics were compiled from the data collected from hospital-based cancer registries (approximately 236) and population-based cancer

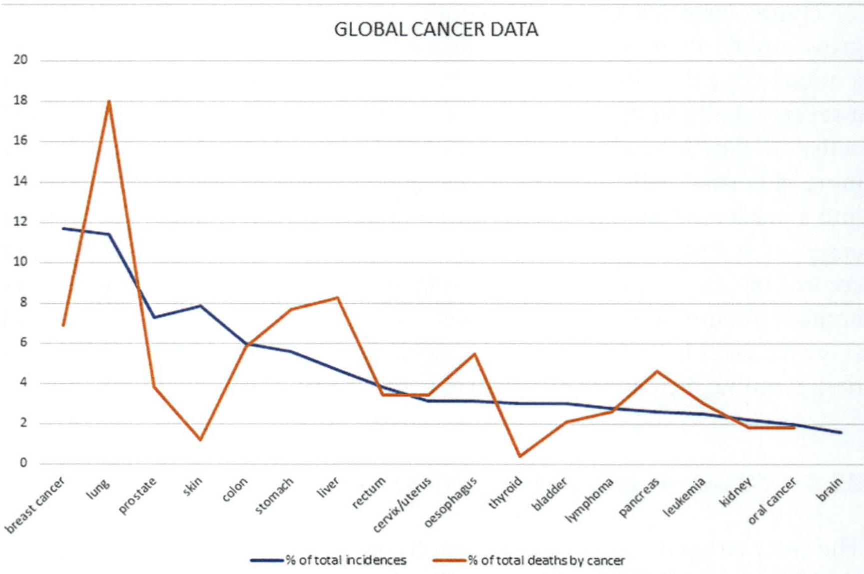

FIGURE 22.2 Data on percentage of total incidences and total deaths for various types of cancers.

registries (approximately 36) [8]. Projected cases of cancer in India were approximately 1.4 million in year 2020, leading to 0.85 million deaths. As per reported data, cancer in India were breast, lung, cervix and uteri, and also tongue. The sex-based incidences were also reported, with male patients of 679,421 and female patients of 712,758 [8, 9]. Breast and uteri cancer were reported to be most common type of cancers in females in India. The increase in incidence reports with BC in women concludes with a concern for health agencies to take necessary action in order to control and generate essential medical care facilities. The most prominent cancers in males were lung, mouth, esophagus, stomach, and nasopharynx. The cancer, which is in general agreement with the trend line of global data, is lung cancer and considered as leading type of cancer to be repeated around the cities. The conjectural association of the lung cancer with air pollution and tobacco smoking in the cities is consistent along with this trend. The population-based cancer registry data demonstrated the association of third of cancer incidences with tobacco use in India. Avoiding tobacco use has been emphasized for the preventive measures for most of the cancers in India. Therefore, on comparing India and US cancer statistical data indicates few similarities, but significant differences regarding to the prevalence of cancer types [10].

This chapter discusses diagnostics, treatment, and posttreatment for cancers in females. Finally, it presents a case study of a cancer in a woman.

22.4 DIAGNOSIS OF CANCER: ADVANCEMENTS AND APPROACHES

- **Smart technology**: It is used to analyze clinical imaging and pathology information, aiding in cancer diagnosis and prognostication. They assist pathologist and radiologist in addressing subtle patterns and features in tissue samples/graphics that may not be perceptible to an individual's eye, enhancing diagnostic precision [15].
- **Early diagnosis as well as screening**: Early diagnosis requires notably less investment and is proportionally simple to implement compared to cancer screening. However, this motion is likely less fruitful in declining cancer burden compared to screening. Population awareness concerning the typical cancers with their early symptoms is required for implementation of early diagnosis. Also, training of frontline healthcare providers discerns the preliminary signs and punctually alludes the symptomatic individual to relevant diagnostic testing. There has been a rising prominence on screening programs for various cancer, as these screening involves imaging techniques such as colonoscopy, mammography, pap smears, and prostate-specific antigen test. Furthermore, advancements in genetic testing have enabled for the identification of an individual with higher genetic risk of certain cancer allowing earlier and more site targeted screening [11].
- **Histopathology and biopsy**: Biopsy stays as a crucial part of cancer diagnosis, which allows examination of tissue samples through a microscope to validate the presence of cancerous cells and diagnose their grade and type. Recent trends involve the use of minimal invasive approaches such as needle biopsies and liquid biopsies, which present less invasive techniques over conventional surgical biopsies. The analysis of biomarkers, that

is, exosomes, extracellular DNA, and circulating tumor cells exist in body fluids such as blood and urine, falls under liquid biopsy. These tests are noninvasive, which offer the information about tumor genetics and help observe treatment response and disease progression [13].

- **Imaging technology**: CT scans, PET scans, and MRIs have significantly improved over time in their potential to characterize and detect the tumor. Diagnostic imaging modalities, namely, dynamic contrast-enhanced MRI along with diffusion-weighted imaging focus on functionality, present valuable information about the tumor behavior and biology [12].
- **Molecular and genetic analysis**: For personalized cancer treatment, molecular profiling of tumors has been increasingly set off to be important. Approaches such as next-generation sequencing offer analysis of tumor's genetic makeup, recognizing specific mutations/biomarkers that may lead the way for treatment decisions. Genetic alterations and protein expression have been assessed by using fluorescence *in situ* hybridization and immunohistochemistry [14].
- **Multidisciplinary approach**: Oncologists, surgeons, radiologists, pathologists, and other specialists contribute to ensure accurate diagnosis and treatment planning; all are involved in multidisciplinary team for cancer diagnosis. Experts from various disciplines discuss varies cases and treatment plans and have come to standard practice in many healthcare settings (tumor boards) [16].

22.5 TREATMENT OPTIONS FOR CANCER

- **Seven-minute cancer treatment** is an injectable cancer treatment that takes only 7 min to administer that was introduced by the National Health Service, England. This is notably faster than the current intravenous (IV) infusion treatment, which takes 1 hour. Atezolizumab (TelCentris) treats cancer patients, including lung cancer and BC. Though this accelerates the treatment, it also liberates precious time for healthcare providers [26].

- **Combination therapy** in cancer treatment involves combination of multiple treatment modalities to attain best results. Combination of chemotherapy with either targeted therapy or immunotherapy can increase treatment efficacy and prevail over the resistance mechanism. Furthermore, the concept of adjuvant therapy and neoadjuvant has gained momentum, at which treatments such as chemotherapy and radiation are given before or after surgery to enhance the outcomes and reduce the recurrence risk [21].
- **CRISPR and gene editing technology** is used for the precise modification of genes. Researchers are investigating its ability for cancer treatment, involving correcting genetic defects and enhancing immune responses [22, 40, 41].
- **Epigenetic therapy** is a modification of epigenetics in cancer treatment development, as the drugs targeting these modifications such as DNA methylation inhibitors are being explored as potential alternatives [24].
- **Immunotherapy** is an innovative strategy for cancer therapy, harnessing the body's immune system to detect as well as combat cancerous cells. Checkpoint inhibitors (adoptive cell therapies and cancer vaccines) encompass in immunotherapy strategies that have shown better results in treating cancers such as melanoma, lung cancer, and certain hematological malignancies. The key development includes checkpoint inhibitors that block protein, which inhibits immune responses, allowing T cells to distinguish and strike cancerous cells; In CAR-T therapy, genetically modified T cells are infused back in the recipient to aim specific cancerous cells; also, cancer vaccines stimulate the immunological system to identify and destroy cancerous cells [19].
- **Minimal invasive techniques**: Laparoscopic- and robotic-assisted surgeries have emerged as popular alternative in the treatment of cancer for its minimally invasive technique. The techniques offer advantages over conventional open surgeries, less duration stays at hospital, rapid recovery time, and reduced post-operative pain [20].
- **Nanotechnology**: Nanoparticles are designed to deliver drugs to the cancer cells/tumors directly. This approach enhances

effectiveness of drug and reduces toxicity toward healthy tissues and cells [23].

- **Particle beams and liquid radiotherapy**: Carbon ion therapy and lutetium-177 PSMA therapy provide precise tumor targeting with minimal damage to nearby tissues [25].
- **Personalized medicine and vaccines**: Recent trends emphasize precision/personalized medicine, which includes tailoring treatment strategy based on the specific feature of an individual tumor. Molecular profiling of tumors, for example, next-generation sequencing, offers oncologists to analyze and recognize specific genetic mutations/biomarkers, which maneuver cancer growth. It helps in planning and selecting targeted treatment that is more effective and less harmful than conventional options of chemotherapy. The key treatment includes poly(ADP-ribose) polymerase inhibitors, which are effective for certain cancers with BRCA mutations, and epidermal growth factor receptor (EGFR) inhibitors, which are used in lung cancer for patients with EGFR mutations. Personalized cancer vaccines are made based on patient tumor-specific antigens, as these vaccines prompt the immunological defense system to identify and combat neoplastic cells [17].
- **Radiation therapy**: Advancements have been done in radiation therapy technology; these approaches allow more precise targeting of cells and tumors, minimizing the damage to healthy tissues in the surroundings, which results in evolved treatment outcomes with less side effects [21].
- **Survivorship and supportive care**: As active cancer treatments are provided, there is an increasing trend of supportive care and survivorship programs with the objective of improving the well-being of cancer patients. These services address emotional, physical, and psychological needs and requirements of the patients throughout their cancer journey, which has pain management, nutritional support, counseling, and rehabilitation services [23].
- **Targeted therapy treatment**: Drugs are designed to specifically target the cancerous cells by interfering with the specific pathways followed by cancer growth and progression. Monoclonal

antibodies and small molecule inhibitors fall under this category. For example, tyrosine kinase inhibitors target selected enzymes involved in cell signaling, whereas immune checkpoint inhibitors target proteins, which inhibit the immune response against cancerous cells [18].

22.6 POSTTREATMENT OPTIONS FOR CANCER

Monitoring, sustaining overall health, and recovery are critical phases that are focused during the postcancer treatment. This stage of posttreatment may encompass following activities:

- **Esthetic postcancer care**: Esthetic treatments reduce the appearance and discomfort of keloids, surgical scars, lymphedema, fibrosis, pigment disorders, and alopecia as a demerit of cancer therapies. Dermal fillers, botulinum toxin, and laser treatments are common.
- **Emotional well-being**: Cancer treatment is emotionally exhausting. Seek help and support from family, friends, or therapist. Join support groups to connect with others who experienced the same events.
- **Financial and legal considerations**: Review the health insurance coverage, analyze financial implications, and consider legal documents such as wills and advance directives.
- **Habit modifications**: The chances of recurrence are reduced with the help of balanced diet and physical workouts, as it contributes to enhance overall health. Diet and physical activity contribute to improve overall health and lower the risk of recurrence. It is advisable to embrace a nutritionally comprehensive regimen rich, cutoff the alcohol consumption, and quit smoking to mitigate the related risks. Additionally, incorporating stress busting techniques such as breathing exercises, yoga, meditation, and art therapy for stress management.
- **Medicines**: Combination therapy and hormone therapy are prescribed and continued for a while. Potential side effects or unusual symptoms are reported. Attend rehabilitation sessions for physical or speech therapy, if needed.

- **Review sessions**: Regular posttreatment visits/checkups are vital as they enable monitoring for any indications of recurrence or any other cancer. Cancer specialists propose blood test, scans, and schedule regular visits.
- **Screening for other cancers**: Few of the cancer survivors are at the elevated risk for advancing other types of cancers. Mammograms, colonoscopies, and skin checks are some regular screenings, which must be done.
- **Sexual health and fertility**: Consult for sexual health, intimacy, and fertility with personal healthcare team. In some cases, cancer can affect fertility.
- **Stay informed and celebrate life**: Celebrate milestones, learn survivorship, and embrace a life postcancer. Each day is a new achievement [27].
- **Vaccinations**: Stay up to date with vaccinations for flu shots and pneumonia vaccines. Consult your healthcare incharge for recommendations.

22.7 TYPES OF CANCERS: AN EXAMPLE OF A BC

Carcinogenesis is considered as a multifactorial process, as primarily it is stimulated by environmental factors and genetic predispositions. The major cause of death worldwide is oncologic mortality, which is alarmingly rising annually. Moreover, mammary carcinoma is the fifth cause of oncologic mortality and currently utmost prevalently worldwide cancer occurrence with an estimation of 2.3 million recent incidences worldwide based on the GLOBOCAN data 2020. Preventive behavioral procedures along with screening programs are essential related to a potential minimization of incidence rate of mammary carcinoma plus application of early treatment. Presently, Breast Health Global Initiative is accountable for developing appropriate approaches along with directives to come up with satisfactory mammary carcinoma control globally [28].

Breast cancer is prevailing identified cancer among females globally, with an approximate range of 2.26 million new occurrences in 2020. In the United States, BC is prevalent to take in consideration for 29% of all recent cancer incidence in women. From the data of 2020, high development index (HDI) countries had topmost age-standardized incidence rates, while it had been much greater than 200% in low and medium HDI countries. BC is reported to be cause of 684,996 deaths worldwide. Females diagnosed with BC in an affluent nation will thrive, whereas the reverse is truth for females in economically disadvantaged country. In 2020, ratio of BC mortality to incidence was 0.30 globally, as a benchmark for 5-year survival rates. Current scenario represents that by 2030, international counts of newly diagnosed occurrences will hit 2.7 million yearly, and death numbers will be 0.87 million. The BC incidence in low and medium countries is to be expectedly increased because of the westernization of lifestyles, cancer detection, and better cancer registration [29].

22.7.1 CONTRIBUTING FACTORS IN BC (TABLE 22.1)

TABLE 22.1 Contributing Factors: Alterable and Unalterable

Alterable Factors	Unalterable Factors
• Alcohol intake	• Density of the tissues of breast
• Diethylstilbesterol	• Genetic mutations
• Excessively illumination by synthetic light	• Ancestry of either breast of ovarian cancer
• Exposure to chemicals	• Ethnicity/Race
• Hormone replacement therapy	• Female sex
• Intake of processed food in excess	• Pregnancy or breastfeeding
• Insufficient vitamin supplementation	• Menopause/Menstrual period
• Obese/obesity	• Ancient background of BC
• Physical activity	• Previous background of radiation therapy
• Smoking	• Noncancerous breast diseases
• Other drugs	• Older age

There is a crucial need to understand the distinction between the alterable and unalterable contributing factors (Table 22.1) in aid of developing targeted prevention strategies and interventions aimed at reducing the impact of BC. Unalterable factors are not controlled or changed by individual actions/interventions; they are typically inherent circumstances or characteristics, which contribute to risk of disease but are beyond control. On the other hand, modifiable factors can be modified and controlled through interventions, actions, or lifestyle adjustments; these factors are within an individual control and effort to mitigate the factors, which potentially reduce the risk of developing BC. While nonmodifiable factors cannot be altered, but focusing and addressing on modifiable risk factors through lifestyle adjustments and actions can potentially assist lowering the likelihood of developing BC as well as improve health outcomes [30].

22.7.2 BC CLASSIFICATION [39–41]

- **Benign tumor**: Further evaluation is conducted to assess the risk factors and the additional tests or imaging, if necessary.
- **Malignant tumor**: The process is proceeded toward the histopathological examination to determine its specific characteristics. Histopathological examination includes testing for hormone receptors [estrogen receptor (ER)], human epidermal growth factor receptor2 (HER2), progesterone receptors (PRs), and other prognostic markers. The malignant tumor is sorted as invasive [infiltrating ductal carcinoma (IDC)] and noninvasive (ductal carcinoma *in situ*) type based on its spread and behavior with the tissue of the breast [31]. **Noninvasive subtypes** include intraductal carcinoma, confined within the ducts of the breasts, and other subtypes are rare or less common noninvasive subtypes of BC. The noninvasive BCs are confined within the milk ducts and have not invaded the surrounding breast tissues [32]. Ductal carcinoma is the commonly occurring subtype of invasive BC, which includes IDC as well as other less variants. IDC is identified as the malignant cells extending past the ducts present within breast into the neighboring breast tissue. Invasive lobular carcinoma arises from the lobules present in the breast which have its variants. Variants are tubular carcinoma (characterized by clear-cut tubular structures), medullary carcinoma (characterized by well-confined tumor with lymphatic infiltrate), mucinous carcinoma (identified by mucin producing tumor cells), cribriform carcinoma (identified by tumor cells arranged in glandular structures with punched out spaces), micropapillary carcinoma (small papillary structures lacking fibrovascular core), and all other variants [33].

22.7.3 BC TREATMENT STRATEGIES

- **Surgery** (lumpectomy and mastectomy) is a chief surgical process for the breast tumor excision. Alternatively, it is termed as lumpectomy, partial or segmental mastectomy, quadrantectomy, and wide local excision; it enables the BC resection with consequently breast-conserving oncoplastic surgery. The complete breast resection associated with immediate breast reconstruction is termed as mastectomy. Dissection of axillary lymph node and biopsy of sentinel lymph node entail the extraction of affected lymph nodes. BC surgery is more associated to enhance esthetic outcomes, lower emotional distress of patients, and reduce postoperative complications. However, BC surgery has seen profoundly favorable for the cancer patients but those who have been handled with respective procedure commonly exhibit an inclination for an additional necessity of a complete mastectomy [34].
- **Chemotherapy**: Comprehensive therapy for BC might be neoadjuvant or adjuvant. Secondary BC can take advantage of this. Neoadjuvant chemotherapy is employed in local progressive BC, inflammatory BC, and for regression BC; larger tumors or in small tumors with inferior molecular subtype prognostication (HER2), able to support to discern prognostics as well as predictive markers of response, could be administered via IV or by mouth. Carboplatin, cyclophosphamide, capecitabine/5-fluorouracil, taxanes such as docetaxel and paclitaxel, and anthracyclines such as doxorubicin and epirubicin are some of the medication deliveries included in contemporary management [35]. Chemotherapy shows effective outcomes; however, its use often leads to unintended consequences such as nausea, diarrhea, hair loss, oral lesions, fatigue, increased susceptibility to infections, bone marrow suppression, anemia, neuropathy, cardiomyopathy, cognitive impairment, and hand foot syndrome. Disturbance of menstrual cycle and fertility issues in young women have been observed. Electrochemotherapy is a special type of chemotherapy, which can be used for BC that has spread to skin, but it is unavailable at most of the clinics and is quite uncommon [36].

- **Radiation therapy** is a localized intervention for BC, normally needed postchemotherapy or surgical treatment. This has to be done to guarantee the elimination of malignant cells and decreasing all chances of BC relapse. It is considered to be favorable for the distantly advanced and inoperable BC. BC-specific radiotherapy is differentiated as intraoperative radiation therapy. Radiation-induced skin discoloration, lethargy, and lymphedema along with irritation are few side effects seen in the BC patients [37].
- **Hormonal therapy** is used in preoperative or postoperative treatment in individuals with luminal molecular subtype BC, also potent in BC reappearance/metastasis. The treatment seeks to reduce estrogen levels and hinder the stimulation of cancer cells by estrogen. Hormone therapy associated with chemotherapy results in decrease in mortality rates among BC patients. Drugs include tamoxifen and toremifene as well as fluvastatin; drugs that decrease estrogen levels include aromatase inhibitors such as anastrozole and letrozole [38].
- **Biological therapy** (also known as targeted therapy) can be provided as neoadjuvant treatment before surgical intervention or like adjuvant treatment after surgical procedure.

It is prevalent in HER2-positive BC patients. Key pharmaceuticals are deruxtecan, lapatinib, neratinib, and epratuzumab. In luminal, HER2-negative subtype of BC, premenstrual women get everolimus-target of rapamycin inhibitor with exemestane, whereas postmenopausal females get palbociclib/ribociclib (CDK 4–6 inhibitor) concurrently, associated alongside the hormonal therapy. Two penultimate medications alongside (1) abemaciclib and (2) everolimus are likely suitable in estrogen-positive BC and HER2-negative BC. Denosumab is certified for metastasis, while atezolizumab is sanctioned in triple-negative BC [39, 41].

22.8 A CASE STUDY: A NEW MANAGEMENT APPROACH IN A SCENARIO OF REGIONALLY ADVANCED BC [40, 41]

22.8.1 CASE REPORT

A 59-year-old male patient, having a prominent left breast lump and bulging axillary lymph nodes (IDC), has been neglecting this lump and has denied all diagnostic regimen. He consented for an extended radical mastectomy postadjusting the diagnostic evaluation and agreed to visit a psychiatrist during the treatment. Lymph node metastasis along with advanced IDC along with lymph node metastasis was demonstrated by histopathology. HER2, PR, as well as triple-positive for ER is engaged here. Postoperative therapy involved Herceptin, tamoxifen, and radiation therapy.

22.8.2 BACKGROUND

Ductal carcinoma is an infrequent disease. The reason for diagnostic delay and its combative behavior is the unawareness about this infrequent malignance, which leads to poor prognosis. This case study describes an old male patient aged 59 years that is unwilling to go through diagnosis process for patient care.

22.8.3 HISTORY

An old man of age 59 years, who completed elementary school, presented at an operative facility with secretion from a lump in the left breast. The lump had reportedly increased in dimension over the course of a year. The patient described attempting to cauterize the mass multiple times without any improvements. The patient avoided seeking medical attention until experiencing pain and noticing a putrid discharge. He has a health background of poorly managed *diabetes mellitus* but denies any psychological condition, anabolic steroids use, alcohol consumption, or drug use. He has been smoking two packs of cigarettes daily for the past 30 days. There is no record of radiation exposure events and no health background of malignancies in the family tree.

22.8.4 DESCRIPTION

The person seemed healthy, displaying typical male-bodily hair distribution, zero signs of enlarged breast tissue, and 36.9 kg/m^2 body mass index. Upon medical evaluation of axilla and left breast, firm, reddened, ulcerated lump of nearly 9 × 5 cm^2 was observed within subareolar area. The mass distorted the left nipple, but no discharge was noted. The patient had a normal body temperature. Evaluation of the ipsilateral axilla revealed a distended, movable lymph node. Examination of the breast on the right side yielded standard findings.

22.8.5 LAB INVESTIGATION

The hepatic function assessment revealed following results:

- Total protein: 48 g/L
- Albumin: 28 g/L
- Alkaline phosphatase: 87 IU/L
- Aspartate aminotransferase: 42 U/L
- Alanine aminotransferase: 38 U/L
- Amylase and lipase: 56 and 37 U/L, respectively
- Conjugated bilirubin and total bilirubin: 2.3 and 5.9 μmol/L
- Cancer antigen 19-9: 7 IU/mL
- Prostate-specific antigen: 1.9 ng/mL
- Carcinoembryonic antigen: 2.2 ng/mL

The values were in the expected limits. Similarly, levels of tumor markers were within typical parameters. Additionally, the remaining laboratory findings were inconclusive.

22.8.6 IMAGING

Ultrasound examination and mammography of the breast were attempted but deemed impractical because of severe discomfort and soreness in the left breast; even though it was provided with potent pain relief medications, yet the patient declined imaging examinations. Additionally, the patient did not adhere to recommendations for further diagnostic evaluation, including computed tomography (CT) of thoracic, abdominal, and pelvic region, coupled with a bone scan, for metastatic assessment. Psychiatric consultation was also sought because of the patient's diagnosis of anxiety disorder. The patient's apprehension stemmed from a belief that biopsies performed during mammography or ultrasound could potentially exacerbate the illness. Use of oral alprazolam was initiated to alleviate anxiety, along with counseling and psychotherapy. In the end, the patient consented to engage in imaging without direct physical contact between the breast lesion and the equipment. Left-sided breast CT scans revealed a necrotic exophytic mass with associated skin thickening, along with cortical thickening (enhanced ipsilateral axillary lymph node). No distant metastases were detected on CT, and a bone scan gave negative findings for bone metastases.

22.8.7 TREATMENT

Preoperative diagnostic histopathology was not conducted. The medical symptoms, along with CT scans findings, served as the basis for diagnosing metastasis to the ipsilateral axillary lymph node along with regionally advanced breast tumor/cancer. Yet, there was no grade, histological type, as well as receptor status available; preoperative chemotreatment was not feasible for the treatment. Consequently, mastectomy was proposed to the patient. For the treatment of axillary metastasis, axillary dissection was advised. The pectoralis major muscle and the mass were discovered not to be connected, during an extended radical mastectomy. Axillary dissection (level I and II) was carried out, and the skin graft was not required for closing the wound.

22.8.8 POSTOPERATIVE HISTOPATHOLOGY

The histopathological assessment of the breast operative resection specimen demonstrated IDC with dermal deposits along with lymphovascular invasion. It is classified as grade 3 tumor and measured $8 \times 8 \times 6$ cm^3. The margins of the operative resection were clear of tumor cells. Metastatic deposits in one out of 19 lymph nodes dissected were unveiled in axillary lymph nodes analysis. Intense positivity for estrogen receptor at 70%, progesterone receptor at 50%, and HER2 positivity at 3+ were indicated in a biomarker analysis via immunotherapy. The breast carcinoma was categorized as stage IIIB.

22.8.9 ADJUVANT THERAPY

Patient was directed for both a clinical oncologist along with a radiation oncologist for additional treatment. Herceptin and epratuzumab, associated by radiation therapy to the axilla along with thoracic wall, as well as treatment with tamoxifen for a minimum of 5 years, were included in the postoperative plan. Additionally, the patient was recommended to consult with a genetic counselor regarding testing for *BRCA* gene mutations.

22.8.10 DISCUSSION

The delay and failure in seeking medical care can show consequences in the patient being clinically identified with advanced BC. Because of delayed medical intervention, person in case study presented with stage IIIB regionally advanced BC, which had already spread to the axillary lymph nodes. Various elements may contribute to this delay, including sufficient awareness about BC, geographical distance from medical facilities, lack of understanding, apprehension of consequences, intense faith in conventional remedies, limited knowledge and education, and financial constraints. In the scenario of this patient, three factors led to this delayed presentation: (1) a conviction in conventional remedies, (2) a basic grade of education, as well as (3) unawareness about the condition.

All prevalent psychiatric conditions observed in individuals with BC typically included anxiety disorders along with depression. These mental health challenges manifested at various stages throughout the course of the illness. In the present case, the patient's interaction with the psychiatrist upon admission to the hospital partially facilitated cooperation with the clinical team. Nevertheless, owing to the advanced stage of the disease and apprehensions about its progression, the psychotherapy session of the patient was brief.

The established protocol for assessing individuals with breast carcinoma typically involves mammograms and ultrasound examinations of the axilla and the breasts. Initially, patient's intense misconception regarding potential spread of BC through biopsy and physical contact with medical apparatus hindered adherence to the typical diagnostic procedure. Nonetheless, given the advanced stage of tumor, characterized by sizable ulcerating breast mass as well as an enlarged lymph node in same area, along with the necessity for mastectomy, mammography, ultrasound was also foregone. Instead, CT imaging studies were employed to delineate the extent of the BC as well as its impact on axillary region.

In men, IDC represents the predominant form of BC. Because of the typically small size of male breast, cancerous cells often infiltrate locally and covertly, with a tendency to affect the pectoralis major muscle. Mastectomy coupled with radiotherapy is the preferred course of action to ensure comprehensive tumor removal. However, in this case, there was no evidence of pectoralis muscle involvement based on findings of CT scan or surgical evaluation. Furthermore, mastectomy specimen's histological examination revealed negative margins, indicating successful removal of the tumor.

This patient was diagnosed with HER2-positive IDC of the breast. Cases of HER2-positive BC has typical protocol that involves initiating neoadjuvant chemotherapy with Herceptin, which has shown a 40% rise within the scope of pathological complete response. Research indicates that combining Herceptin with epratuzumab in preoperative setting may further enhance the complete response rate by 60%, with demonstrated long-term benefits in respect of improved overall survival. However, due to the patient's refusal of a preoperative diagnosis biopsy, the histological type of tumor and receptor status could not be determined before surgery. Consequently, the treatment strategies were modified for the patient; surgical intervention was provided as the primary therapy, along with HER2-based chemotherapy in postoperative setting.

22.8.11 CONCLUSION

Breast carcinoma in males poses an uncommon yet formidable challenge for clinicians primarily because of low awareness among patients and the tendency for it to be diagnosed at an advanced stage. Raising community education about male BC is crucial to prompt timely medical consultation, prevent the development of axillary and distant metastases, and ensure diagnosis when treatment is most effective. Identifying and addressing factors contributing to delayed medical attention is vital for improving patient outcomes. Physicians should acknowledge the benefits of involving psychiatric support early in the management of patients who may deny or misunderstand their condition, potentially impacting decision-making abilities. In complex situations, maintaining flexibility in the treatment plan is essential to navigate challenges effectively. As demonstrated in this case, modifications to the diagnostic process and treatment strategy can be implemented safely while adhering as closely as possible to established guidelines, with the goal of achieving the best possible outcome for the patient.

22.9 SUMMARY

Advancements in female cancer diagnostics have significantly transformed the early detection, management, and treatment of cancer targeting women, specifically breast, cervical, and ovarian cancers. The improvements have greatly enhanced survival statistics and patient life satisfaction. Mammography continues to serve as the primary method for prompt detection in breast malignancy diagnostics. Computational mammography provides superior imaging potential, allowing for clearer visualization of abnormalities. Moreover, tomosynthesis, also known as three-dimensional mammography, offers even more detailed imaging of the breast by capturing multiple slices. This advancement enhances detection rates and declines the occurrence of false positives. MRI and ultrasound are widely used alongside mammography, specifically for females with high breast density or for those individuals with more likelihood of maturing the malignancy. Introduction of human papillomavirus (HPV) and pap smear test has revolutionized cervical cancer diagnostics. The HPV test detects high-risk strains of the virus that causes cervical cancer, often used along with the pap smear for a more thorough screening procedure. The pap smear involves examination of cervical cells under a microscope and has been critical for cervical cancer in bringing down its mortality and incidence. The cotesting approach has improved the stratification of patients based on their risk, enabling more personalized checkups and intervention.

Ovarian cancer is a silent killer due to its lack of symptoms at the early stages and has conventionally been challenging to diagnose. Advancements in imaging techniques such as MRI and ultrasound have enhanced the detection of ovarian masses. Also, hematological analysis that measures cancer antigen levels, though not specific to ovarian cancer, is used along with imaging procedures to identify potential malignancies. Recent trends in biomarker research and the identification of genetic mutations, such as BRCA1 and BRCA2, have improved risk assessment and early detection approaches. Advancements in molecular diagnostics and genomics have potentially impacted female cancer diagnostics, especially through next-generation sequencing as it allows for detailed analysis of genetic mutations driving cancer. This has led to the development of personalized treatment strategies modified to the tumor's genetic profile. Liquid biopsies involve detection of ctDNA within the blood that provides noninvasive practice to monitor disease progression and treatment response in real time. Furthermore, artificial intelligence and machine learning potentially enhanced cancer diagnostics by exactly assessing extensive sum of imaging information, aiding in early detection of cancer stages. Innovations in molecular and genetic testing, as well as in imaging technologies associated with artificial intelligence, have collectively enhanced the early detection of cancer, personalized treatments, and patient care, providing more effective diagnostic tools for the future.

KEYWORDS

- **cancer**
- **malignant tumor**
- **neoplasm**
- **proto-oncogenes**
- **tumor**

REFERENCES

1. Aldossary, M. Y., Alquraish, F., & Alazhri, J. (2019). A case of locally advanced breast cancer in a 59-year-old man requiring a modified approach to management. *The American Journal of Case Reports*, *20*, 531–538.
2. Alrushaid, N., Khan, F. A., Al-Suhaimi, E. A., & Elaissari, A. (2023). Nanotechnology in cancer diagnosis and treatment. *Pharmaceutics*, *15*(3), 1025–1038.
3. Asadzadeh, Z., Safarzadeh, E., Safaei, S., Baradaran, A., Mohammadi, A., Hajiasgharzadeh, K., Derakhshani, A., Argentiero, A., Silvestris, N., & Baradaran, B. (2020). Current approaches for combination therapy of cancer: The role of immunogenic cell death. *Cancers*, *12*(4), 1047–1055.
4. Banys-Paluchowski, M., Untch, M., Krawczyk, N., Thurmann, M., Kühn, T., Sehouli, J., Gasparri, M. L., de Boniface, J., Gentilini, O. D., Stickeler, E., Ditsch, N., Rody, A., Paluchowski, P., & Blohmer, J. U. (2023). Current trends in diagnostic and therapeutic management of the axilla in breast cancer patients receiving neoadjuvant therapy: Results of the German-wide Noggo Monitor 24 survey. *Archives of Gynecology and Obstetrics*, *307*(5), 1547–1556.
5. Berdzuli, N. (2023). Breast cancer: From awareness to access. *BMJ*, *380*, 290.
6. Bhushan, A., Gonsalves, A., & Menon, J. U. (2021). Current state of breast cancer diagnosis, treatment, and theranostics. *Pharmaceutics*, *13*(5), 723–728.

7. Brady, M. S., Garfein, C. F., Petrek, J. A., & Brennan, M. F. (1994). Post-treatment sarcoma in breast cancer patients. *Annals of Surgical Oncology*, *1*, 66–72.
8. Chhikara, B. S., & Parang, K. (2023). Global Cancer Statistics - 2022: The trends projection analysis. *Chemical Biology Letters*, *10*(1), 451–451.
9. Crosby, D., Bhatia, S., Brindle, K. M., Coussens, L. M., Dive, C., Emberton, M., & Balasubramanian, S. (2022). Early detection of cancer. *Science*, *375*(6586), EAAY9040.
10. Debela, D. T., Muzazu, S. G., Heraro, K. D., Ndalama, M. T., Mesele, B. W., Haile, D. C., Kitui, S. K., & Manyazewal, T. (2021). New approaches and procedures for cancer treatment: Current perspectives. *SAGE Open Medicine*, *9*, e20503121211034366.
11. Eckhert, E., Lansinger, O., Ritter, V., Liu, M., Han, S., Schapira, L., & Kurian, A. W. (2023). Breast cancer diagnosis, treatment, and outcomes of patients from sex and gender minority groups. *JAMA Oncology*, *9*(4), 473–480.
12. Emre, N., & Yılmaz, S. (2023). Sleep quality, mental health, and quality of life in women with breast cancer. *Indian Journal of Cancer*, 2022. doi: 10.4103/ijc.IJC_859_20. PMID: 36861698.
13. Ferlay, J., Colombet, M., Soerjomataram, I., Parkin, D. M., Piñeros, M., Znaor, A., & Bray, F. (2021). Cancer statistics for the year 2020: An overview. *International Journal of Cancer*, *149*(4), 778–789.
14. Guida, J. L., Green, P., Clague-DeHart, J., Eshraghi, L., Laurita, N., O'Connell, M., & Love, S. (2023). The Health of Women (HOW) Study: Web-based survey of breast cancer risk factors, diagnosis, and treatment. *Journal of Cancer Survivorship*, *17*(5), 1445–1451.
15. He, Z., Chen, Z., Tan, M., Elingarami, S., Liu, Y., Li, T., Deng, Y., He, N., Li, S., Fu, J., & Li, W. (2020). A review on methods for diagnosis of breast cancer cells and tissues. *Cell Proliferation*, *53*(7), e12822.
16. Hussain, S., Mubeen, I., Ullah, N., Shah, S. S. U. D., Khan, B. A., Zahoor, M., Ullah, R., Khan, F. A., & Sultan, M. A. (2022). Modern diagnostic imaging technique applications and risk factors in the medical field: A review. *BioMed Research International*, *2022*(1), e5164970.
17. Iqbal, M. J., Javed, Z., Sadia, H., Qureshi, I. A., Irshad, A., Ahmed, R., Malik, K., Raza, S., Abbas, A., Pezzani, R., & Sharifi, J. (2021). Clinical applications of artificial intelligence and machine learning in cancer diagnosis: Looking into the future. *Cancer Cell International*, *21*(1), 270–280.
18. Kirkby, K. J., Kirkby, N. F., Burnet, N. G., Owen, H., Mackay, R. I., Crellin, A., & Green, S. (2020). Heavy charged particle beam therapy and related new radiotherapy technologies: The clinical potential, physics and technical developments required to deliver benefit for patients with cancer. *The British Journal of Radiology*, *93*(1116), e20200247.
19. Köpke, M. M., Aktas, B., & Ditsch, N. (2023). Recommendations for the diagnosis and treatment of patients with early breast cancer. *Current Opinion in Obstetrics and Gynecology*, *35*(1), 67–72.
20. Lau, K. H., Tan, A. M., & Shi, Y. (2022). New and emerging targeted therapies for advanced breast cancer. *International Journal of Molecular Sciences*, *23*(4), e2288.
21. Madu, C. O., Wang, S., Madu, C. O., & Lu, Y. (2020). Angiogenesis in breast cancer progression, diagnosis, and treatment. *Journal of Cancer*, *11*(15), 4474–4481.

22. Majchrzak-Celińska, A., Warych, A., & Szoszkiewicz, M. (2021). Novel approach to epigenetic therapies: From drug combinations to epigenetic editing. *Genes*, *12*(2), 208–215.
23. Matthews, H. K., Bertoli, C., & de Bruin, R. A. (2022). Cell cycle control in cancer. *Nature Reviews Molecular Cell Biology*, *23*(1), 74–88.
24. Mutebi, M., Anderson, B. O., Duggan, C., Adebamowo, C., Agarwal, G., Ali, Z., Bird, P., Bourque, J. M., DeBoer, R., Gebrim, L. H., Masetti, R., Masood, S., Menon, M., Nakigudde, G., Ng'ang'a, A., Niyonzima, N., Rositch, A. F., Unger-Saldaña, K., Villarreal-Garza, C., Dvaladze, A., & Eniu, A. (2020). Breast cancer treatment: Phased approach to implementation. *Cancer*, *126*, 2365–2378.
25. Nenclares, P., & Harrington, K. J. (2020). The biology of cancer. *Medicine*, *48*(2), 67–72.
26. Obeagu, E. I., & Obeagu, G. U. (2024). Breast cancer: A review of risk factors and diagnosis. *Medicine*, *103*(3), e36905.
27. Pilleron, S., Soto-Perez-de-Celis, E., Vignat, J., Ferlay, J., Soerjomataram, I., Bray, F., & Sarfati, D. (2021). Estimated global cancer incidence in the oldest adults in 2018 and projections to 2050. *International Journal of Cancer*, *148*(3), 601–608.
28. Rehm, J., Shield, K. D., & Weiderpass, E. (2020). Alcohol consumption. A leading risk factor for cancer. *Chemico-Biological Interactions*, *331*, e109280.
29. Sarhadi, V. K., & Armengol, G. (2022). Molecular biomarkers in cancer. *Biomolecules*, *12*(8), 1021–1028.
30. Sathishkumar, K., Chaturvedi, M., Das, P., Stephen, S., & Mathur, P. (2022). Cancer incidence estimates for 2022 & projection for 2025: Result from National Cancer Registry Programme, India. *Indian Journal of Medical Research*, *156*(4&5), 598–607.
31. Saxena, M., van der Burg, S. H., Melief, C. J., & Bhardwaj, N. (2021). Therapeutic cancer vaccines. *Nature Reviews Cancer*, *21*(6), 360–378.
32. Seidler, S. J., & Huber, D. E. (2020). Overview of diagnosis and treatment of breast cancer in young women. *EC Gynaecology*, *2*, 18–25.
33. Senan, E. M., Alsaade, F. W., Al-Mashhadani, M. I. A., Theyazn, H. H., & Al-Adhaileh, M. H. (2021). Classification of histopathological images for early detection of breast cancer using deep learning. *Journal of Applied Science and Engineering*, *24*(3), 323–329.
34. Siegel, R. L., Miller, K. D., Wagle, N. S., & Jemal, A. (2023). Cancer statistics, 2023. *Cancer Journal for Clinicians*, *73*(1), 17–48. doi: 10.3322/caac.21763. PMID: 36633525.
35. Soerjomataram, I., & Bray, F. (2021). Planning for tomorrow: Global cancer incidence and the role of prevention 2020–2070. *Nature Reviews Clinical Oncology*, *18*(10), 663–672.
36. Sund, M., Garmo, H., Andersson, A., Margolin, S., Ahlgren, J., & Valachis, A. (2023). Estrogen therapy after breast cancer diagnosis and breast cancer mortality risk. *Breast Cancer Research and Treatment*, *198*(2), 361–368.
37. Wang, L., Wang, T., Zhang, Y., Kang, X., Ouyang, X. K., Yu, X., Chen, T., Li, W., & Mei, L. (2024). Biomimetic nanosystems harnessing NIR-II photothermal effect and hypoxia-responsive prodrug for self-amplifying and synergistic tumor treatment. *Nano Today*, *57*, e102395.

38. Xu, Y., Gong, M., Wang, Y., Yang, Y., Liu, S., & Zeng, Q. (2023). Global trends and forecasts of breast cancer incidence and deaths. *Scientific Data, 10*(1), 334–341.
39. Yang, L., Ning, Q., & Tang, S. S. (2022). Recent advances and next breakthrough in immunotherapy for cancer treatment. *Journal of Immunology Research*, *2022*(1), e8052212.
40. Zhang, H., Qin, C., An, C., Zheng, X., Wen, S., Chen, W., Liu, X., Lv, Z., Yang, P., Xu, W., Gao, W.,& Wu, Y. (2021). Application of the CRISPR/Cas9-based gene editing technique in basic research, diagnosis, and therapy of cancer. *Molecular Cancer*, *20*, 1–22.
41. Zubair, M., Wang, S., & Ali, N. (2021). Advanced approaches to breast cancer classification and diagnosis. *Frontiers in Pharmacology*, *11*, e632079.

CHAPTER 23

Blood Cancers in Females: Types, Causes, Risks, and Treatment with Traditional Plant Medicines

JYOTI SRIVASTAVA and POONAM JOSHI*

*Corresponding author

ABSTRACT

Cancer is highly prevalent in the world and affects millions of people, including females. The common blood cancer types are leukemia, lymphoma, and myeloma. It is believed that hematologic malignancies result from a combination of genetic and environmental influences. The risk of developing specific types of blood cancer has been connected to factors such as smoking, exposure to radiation, and contact with chemicals. The management and therapy of cancer that control survivance and death of malignant cells are the most salient strategies. Synthetic and semisynthetic antineoplastic agents kill the cancerous cell, but certain natural substances, such as plants, cause apoptotic pathways in cancer cells to become inhibited. Vinca alkaloids, Texans, podo phytotoxin, and camptothecins have been medically used as plant-derived antileukemic agents. This book chapter discusses alkaloids obtained from *Catharanthus roses*, that is, vinca alkaloids, which are either obtained from nature or semisynthetic isolated from the plant with pink periwinkles *Roseus catharanthus* G. Don. Although various vinca alkaloids have undergone extensive testing, only leurocristine, vinblastine, and vinorelbine (brand name: vinca leucoblastine sulfate) have been approved for use in the United States.

Holistic Approaches for Women's Sustainable Health, Volume 2: Advancements, Socioeconomic Impacts, and Innovative Strategies. Junaid Ahmad Malik, Anamika Chauhan, and Megh R. Goyal (Eds)

DOI: 10.1201/9781779641656-27

23.1 INTRODUCTION

Unrestricted or inappropriate proliferation of the cells that demolish body tissue is also known as malignant tumors. Many malignant tumors start from the bone marrow (myeloid tissue). Blood cancer is one of them. Blood cancer, also called leukemia, influences tissue production and function, inhibiting the body's ability to fight illness. Stem cells, which are found in bone marrow, have three types of blood cells, namely, erythrocytes, leukocytes, and thrombocytes. In many cases of blood cancer, the abnormal and uncontrolled growth of hepatocytes occurs [1].

Acute leukemia: It is an aggressive and fast-growing white blood cell (WBC) cancer. Large numbers of white blood cells are produced and enter the bloodstream. Blood cell production spirals out of control. Immature cells produced by the bone marrow grow into leukemia WBCs known as lymphoblasts. These aberrant cells cannot operate correctly and can accumulate, crowding out good cells [2]. Leukemia is of the following types:

- **Acute myeloid leukemia (AML)** is an intense form of carcinogenesis. There is no direct cause for this, but some causes are genetic mutation, smoking, family history, and myelofibrosis [3]. Symptoms include loss of platelets, red blood cells, WBCs; an increase in the number of tumor cells; headache; neutropenia; gum bleeding. Nonspecific symptoms are fever, sweating, headache, stroke, an increase in lymph nodes, deep vein thrombosis, and frequent infections.
- **Acute lymphatic leukemia** is also known as acute lymphoblastic leukemia. "Acute" means leukemia progresses swiftly and, if not cured and managed, it may become fatal after some time. The term "lymphocytic" refers to developing lymphocytes (a kind of WBC) from its immature stages [4, 5]. These originate in bone marrow. Leukemia cells typically exhibit rapid entry into the bloodstream, with the ability to disseminate to different parts like testicles, central nervous system (CNS), and spleen. Tumors may arise in these organs and may move to bone marrow.
- **Acute megakaryoblast leukemia**, potentially fatal type of leukemia, in which aberrant proliferation of malignant

megakaryoblasts damages different organs. In a lineage of precursor cells that create platelets, megakaryoblasts are the most immature. These cells develop into promegakaryocytes and then megakaryocytes, which release platelets into the bloodstream. For appropriate blood clotting, platelets are essential. Although proliferating and tissue-damaging malignant megakaryoblasts are often the main cells, promegakaryocytes, and megakaryocytes, their equally malignant progeny contribute differently to the malignancy [6, 7]. AML is thought to have acute megakaryoblastic leukemia as a subtype. To be more precise, it falls under French–American–British classification's AML-M7 category according to the World Health Organization's 2016 classification [8].

- **Chronic lymphocytic leukemia:** It can also be called small lymphocytic lymphoma (SLL). It is a slow-growing cancer or also a treatable cancer [9]. Symptoms are fever, sudden weight loss, lymph node enlargement, frequent infections, and hemolytic anemia.
- **Chronic myeloid leukemia (CML)** is some sort of carcinogenesis that forms in the bone marrow, which occurs in the cells, and then after metastasis, it reaches out to the blood, which spreads affecting other organs of the body uncontrolled. It is uncommon in children. CML is caused by a genetic abnormality that cannot be inherited. It is produced by the swapping of DNA molecules across chromosomes, which results in the development of a gene known as BCR-Abl. This gene generates the BCR-ABL protein, which is the major cause to proliferate and divide uncontrollably and spread throughout the body [10, 11]. This type has three phases, namely, (1) chronic: it is the earliest and easiest to treat, which might not have symptoms sometimes. (2) Accelerated: In this stage, there is an increase in the quantity of cancerous cells present in the bone marrow and bloodstream. As a result, the individual may experience symptoms like pyrosis, exhaustion, sweating at night, decreased appetite, reduction in weight, unexplained bruising, and discomfort in the bones. (3) Plastic: In this stage, cancer cells overrun the remaining healthy blood cells and platelets, causing more severe symptoms, such as recurrent

infections, spontaneous bleeding, enlarged glands, skin tumors, and bone discomfort [12, 13].

- **Chronic myelomonocytic leukemia (CMML)** is an uncommon kind of blood cancer. The blood's monocyte count is immoderate in CMML. Among the WBCs are monocytes. CMML is distinguished by the World Health Organization as a myeloproliferative and myelodysplastic disease, a category of blood malignancies [14]. Due to the possibility of both myeloproliferative disorders (MPNs) and myelodysplastic disorders (MDS) traits in its patients, CMML is a distinct illness with distinct curative options. Symptoms are low platelet counts, which might create infections that do not improve, such as nosebleeds or bruising that happens readily; stomach (abscess) splenic swelling causing pain; decrease in weight; decrease in hunger; perspiring, redness, bumps on the skin; muscle and bone aches and pains.
- **Childhood leukemia** is the most prevalent kind of tumor occurring in juveniles and teenagers. Bone marrow produces aberrant WBCs. They displace healthy cells from circulation as they move swiftly. This increases the body's vulnerability to infection and other issues [15, 16]. Despite how difficult it is for a child to suffer from cancer, it is encouraging to know that most kids and teenagers with childhood leukemia can get effective treatment. Several forms of pediatric leukemia are (1) acute lymphocytic leukemia: three out of every four pediatric leukemia cases are caused by ALL. (2) Leukemia with acute myelogenous (AML): The second prevalent kind of juvenile blood cancer is AML [17, 18]. (3) Mixed or hybrid lineage leukemia combines characteristics of AML and ALL.
- **Juvenile myelomonocytic leukemia** is neither acute nor chronic, and it primarily affects youngsters under the age of four. Symptoms are coughing, shortness of breath, fatigue, and pale skin [19].
- **Hairy cell leukemia** is an infrequent type of leukemia that involves mature B-cells generated by the V600 metamorphosis of the BRAF gene. The root of hairy cell leukemia is unspecified. It is caused by exposure to tobacco, radiation, and chemicals. Lung

invasion is a symptom of hairy cell leukemia. It might be difficult to distinguish between infection and malignant involvement in cases of hairy cell leukemia [20].

- **Large granular lymphocytic leukemia:** Approximately 10–15% of the total peripheral blood mononuclear cells in individuals without any health issues consist of large granular lymphocytes (LGLs) [1]. The natural killer (NK) cell lineage, which accounts for 85% of these cells, is followed by the CD3+ T-cell lineage, which accounts for 15% of them. Based on their cytology, LGLs are medium to large cells with azurophilic granules that are coarse and have eccentric nuclei and copious cytoplasm (Figure 23.1). Cytotoxic CD8+ T cells that have been primed with antigens are known as T-cell LGLs. LGLs from the innate immune system, known as NK cells, can cytotoxically act in a manner that is not constrained by the major histocompatibility complex [21].
- **Mast cell leukemia:** Mastocytosis is identified by the unusual multiplication and accumulation of mast cells in several organs. The WHO has revised the diagnostic criteria and classification, which now includes seven different disease variants, such as hidden mastocytosis, mast cell leukemia (MCL), extracutaneous astrocytoma, aggressive splenic margin (ASM), as well as mast cell sarcoma, which are all distinct clinical entities within the spectrum of mastocytosis. Major and minor features are used to describe SM, with the diagnosis requiring the presence of at least one of the above criteria, either major or minor. Subtypes are distinguished based on the level of disease aggression, involvement of non-MC lineages, and MC burden (C results). Clinical presentation can vary widely, from asymptomatic with benign characteristics to progressively aggressive with a lack of diagnosis [22].
- **Lymphoma** is a kind of cancer of the blood that develops when lymphocytes or WBCs proliferate unchecked. Immune system components that aid in the defense against infections are called lymphocytes. Thanks to the lymphatic system, lymph is carried throughout the body by lymphocytes. The glands called lymph nodes, which are distributed throughout the body, are where this

fluid flows. Accordingly, medical professionals may describe lymphoma as an immune system cancer [23].

- **Burkitt lymphoma:** Burkitt lymphoma can begin in the lymph nodes (as an extremely aggressive form of non-Hodgkin lymphoma [NHL]) and then move to the blood as well as bone marrow, or it can develop in the bone marrow and blood without ever showing signs of lymph node involvement. Previously, leukemia and lymphoma were defined by the numerous blasts (typically 25%) and the existence or absence of an extramedullary tumor mass at the time of early appearance. More recently, the lymphoma stages have been recognized by the WHO classification, including the lymphoma and leukemic stages [24].
- **CNS lymphoma:** The differential diagnosis of individuals presenting with localized neurologic impairments or increasing encephalopathy accompanied by enhancing abnormalities on brain imaging may include CNS cancer, a rare kind of NHL. When there is immunosuppression or when corticosteroids are used, imaging characteristics and differential diagnosis concerns may change. Leptomeninges, the eye, and brain parenchyma are among the anatomic locations impacted by CNS lymphoma. It is unusual for CNS lymphoma to first present as systemic, peripheral nerve, or spinal cord involvement [25].
- **Diffuse large B-cell lymphoma (DLBCL)**: The initial description of the disease was documented in 1969. Among adults, it stands out as the extremely prevalent form of lymphoid cancer. The current annual occurrence rate of NHL in the United States and Europe varies from 15–20 cases per 100,000 individuals. DLBCL constitutes about 31% of all NHL cases in Western countries, as indicated by data from the WHO [26].
- **Double-hit lymphoma (DHL):** September 2017 saw the release of the WHO's revised fourth edition categorization system for hematological and lymphoid tissue tumors. B-cell lymphoma of high grade is an entity that is described by this classification. There are two different kinds of mature B-cell lymphomas within this category. A MYC rearrangement, together with a few

additional specific chromosomal rearrangements, is required to identify DHL [27].

- **Follicular lymphoma:** Follicle center cells, often an amalgamation of centrocytes and centroblasts, are the basis for the malignancies known as follicular lymphomas. Although there are follicles, diffuse patches may occur and could potentially be dominant.
- **Zone lymphoma:** The phrase "nodal marginal-zone B-cell lymphoma," or "monocytoid lymphoma," and the "indolent lymphoma of MALT type," today known as "MALT lymphoma" were proposed to be included under the REAL classification as early as the 1990s. These two lymphoma subtypes appeared to be closely related [28]: (1) Hodgkin lymphoma (HL)—The tumor microenvironment of HL, a kind of B-cell lymphoma, contains both malignant and immunological effector cells. HL can affect the elderly, although it is more common in adolescents and young people [29]. (2) MALT lymphoma—B-cell lymphoma HL is classified by a prominent concentration of immune effector cells present in the tumor microenvironment along with a limited population of malignant cells. Adolescents and children are more likely to see HL, while older people can still be impacted [30].
- **Mantle cell lymphoma** is found in lymph nodes but can be found anywhere in the body including bone marrow, spleen, and GI tract, it stems from abnormal WBCs that decided to take a different pattern instead of becoming an infection-fighting WBC cancer underlying biology of that cell is one of disordered cell-cycle regulation that means the cell proliferates or it goes from 1–2 to 4–8 and so on with less regulation and typical WBC over time those accumulate and have lymphoma [31].
- **Nodal marginal zone lymphoma** develops in lymph nodes and B cells and comes in a category of non-Hodgkin lymphoma. It is an infrequent type of lymphoma, found in two out of 100 cases, mostly in patients who are suffering from hepatitis C [32].
- **Nodular lymphocyte-predominant Hodgkin lymphoma (NLPHL):** Typically, early-stage NLPHL patients have peripheral lymph node involvement and no symptoms. In contrast to conventional HL, late and frequently recurrent relapses have

been extensively documented; nevertheless, the overall prognosis is good, and NLPHL-related fatalities are quite rare. Owing to the rarity of the condition, the majority of data about the natural history of NLPHL and its care comes from retrospective series or the assessment of subsets included in more extensive randomized controlled HL trials; very few prospective studies are available. A distinct clinical registry was established, and NLPHL was withdrawn from bigger HL clinical trials after 1993 by the European Organisation for Research and Treatment of Cancer and the Groupe d'Études des Lymphomes de l'Adulte research groups. Conversely, NLPHL patients have usually been included as a part of the (German Hodgkin study group) [33].

- **NHL** is a collection of disorders that are associated with malignancies of lymphocytes, a kind of WBCs that exhibit an expansion of lymph nodes., low blood count, and bone marrow it can affect someone's body in a variety of ways one can just be from a mass effect of a lump growing big and causing some kind of either discomfort or other anatomical problem, it can also affect blood count because it a blood cell that can fill up the bone marrow space. WBCs are made and make the normal blood cell count very low, and since they are immune cells, they can also affect the functioning of the immune system; people are also potentially at increased risk for infections [34].
- **Peripheral T-cell lymphoma (PTCL)** is a form of lymphoma of T cells that typically originates in the lymph nodes. It is very diverse and heterogenous and difficult to diagnose and classify, determining which T-cell lymphoma any given patient has. It is much more prominent as compared to B-cell lymphoma is a fact that PTCL tends to affect the organs outside of the lymphatic lymph nodes and the lymphatic system would call them extra nodal and affect the gastrointestinal system (bleeding from your bowels, abdominal pain, respiratory issues, etc.) [35].
- **Skin lymphoma (cutaneous lymphoma):** Skin-derived lymphoma is the second-most prevalent type of NHL that occurs outside of the lymph nodes. This review looks at how radiation therapy is used to treat cutaneous lymphomas nowadays, allowing for recent developments in technology, systemic treatments, and

innovative radio-enhancing treatments. A review is conducted on contemporary low-dose and combination techniques, as well as modern complete skin electron beam radiation. Over the past 50 years, radiotherapy has continued to be the most effective treatment for cutaneous lymphoma [36].

- **SLL** is an immunological cancer that grows slowly. It is a non-Hodgkin lymphoma that affects the infection-fighting WBCs known as B cells. In 2016, the WHO classified the two malignancies as the same illness, and they are treated similarly. The sole distinction between each cancer is its location within the body [37].
- **Splenic marginal zone lymphoma (SMZL):** SLL, like CLL, is a type of NHL. In 2016, the WHO classified the two malignancies as the same illness, and they are treated similarly. The sole distinction between these two cancers is their location in the body. A unique and well-studied B-cell malignancy affecting the spleen and other organs are called SMZL. The WHO has recognized SMZL as an entity; however, its histogenesis is yet unknown.
- The first diagnosis of SMZL was made either by morphologic and immunophenotypic characterization of circulating neoplastic cells, including splenic lymphoma with villous lymphocytes, or by histopathologic study of surgically excised spleens that revealed SMZL. It is now clear that, whereas the two entities have different circulating cell appearances, they share the same pathophysiology foundation. A bone marrow biopsy can also be used to make the diagnosis if typical intrasinusoidal bone marrow infiltrates in SMZL with or without villous lymphocytes are seen. This feature is extremely useful since it enables a clear diagnosis, preventing a needless splenectomy. O'Reilly's retrospective study of a large group of patients with splenomegaly indicated that in the case of splenomegaly of unknown cause, the invasive technique of choice for individuals with hematologic correlations may be a bone marrow biopsy [38].
- **Triple-hit lymphoma (THL):** Immune system tissues can develop into a severe malignancy known as triple-hit lymphoma (THL). B-lymphocytes are WBCs affected by malignancy. NHL is the type that it is. Approximately 2% of B-cell lymphomas are

THLs, which are extremely uncommon. Men are significantly more likely to have it, and it mostly affects older people. Two further categories of provocative NHL are linked to THL. Rarely, follicular lymphoma, a kind of indolent lymphoma with a sluggish growth rate, may be the precursor of THL. Even while these tumors frequently include gene alterations, "triple-hit" lymphomas contain three gene mutations rather than simply one. THL is frequently researched with DHL, which is characterized by mutations in two genes.

- **Multiple myeloma** is a hematologic malignancy that originates from abnormal plasma cells. It begins when the bone marrow produces aberrant plasma cells, which divide into additional myeloma cells. Myeloma cells produce abnormal forms of antibodies known as paraproteins or monoclonal proteins, which do not act. Myeloma lowers the amount of normal immune cells and normal antibodies, which is why individuals with myeloma acquire more infections. Large amounts of abnormal antibodies or paraproteins can thicken the blood and cause headaches or vertigo. Additionally, myeloma cells swarm the bone marrow, making it difficult for other blood types to proliferate [39, 40].

This chapter focuses on types, risks, and causes of blood cancer in females, and treatment with traditional plant medicines.

23.2 TRADITIONAL NATURAL MEDICINES TO TREAT BLOOD CANCER (TABLE 23.1) AND BIOACTIVE COMPOUNDS (TABLE 23.2)

TABLE 23.1 Uses of Traditional Medicines for Treatment of Blood Cancer

Disease	Traditional Remedies	References
Acute erythroid leukemia	Herbal teas (e.g., ginger tea, green tea), dietary supplements (e.g., vitamin C, iron)	[41]
Acute lymphoblastic leukemia (ALL)	Essiac tea, Astragalus root, cat's claw	[41]
Acute megakaryoblastic leukemia	Herbal remedies for supporting bone marrow health and immune function	[41]
Acute myeloid leukemia (AML)	Chinese herbal formulations, Reishi mushroom extract	[42]

TABLE 23.1 *(Continued)*

Disease	Traditional Remedies	References
Acute promyelocytic leukemia (APL)	*Aloe vera* gel, curcumin (turmeric extract)	[42]
Burkitt lymphoma	Essiac tea, turmeric, mistletoe extract, Astragalus root, medicinal mushrooms	[45]
Central nervous system (CNS) lymphoma	*Ginkgo biloba*, Ginseng, *Polygala tenuifolia*, herbal formulas for cognitive function	[46]
Childhood leukemia	Supportive care, nutritional support, emotional support	[44]
Chronic lymphocytic leukemia (CLL)	Echinacea, garlic, ginger, dietary changes (e.g., Mediterranean diet)	[43]
Chronic myeloid leukemia (CML)	Gleevec (imatinib)-targeted therapy, dietary adjustments, acupuncture	[43]
Chronic myelomonocytic leukemia (CMML)	Traditional Chinese herbal medicine, dietary changes, mind-body practices	[43]
Diffuse large B-cell lymphoma (DLBCL)	Reishi (*Ganoderma lucidum*), Turkey tail (*Trametes versicolor*), herbal remedies for immune support	[47]
Double-hit lymphoma	Astragalus root, green tea extract, herbal supplements	[47]
Erdheim-Chester disease	Interferon-alpha, chemotherapy, steroids	[55]
Follicular lymphoma	Astragalus root, *Codonopsis pilosula*, *Atractylodes macrocephala*, herbal remedies for immune support	[47]
Gray-zone lymphoma	Adaptogenic herbs (e.g., ashwagandha, rhodiola), herbal teas	[48]
Hairy cell leukemia (HCL)	Cladribine (2-CdA)—chemotherapy, interferon-alpha, splenectomy	[44]
High-grade B-cell lymphoma, not otherwise stated	Echinacea, Licorice root, cat's claw, herbal teas	[48]
Hodgkin lymphoma	Ayurvedic herbal formulations, traditional Chinese herbal remedies, supportive care	[48]
Langerhans cell histiocytosis	Rosemary, Ginseng, sage	[55]
Large granular lymphocytic leukemia (LGLL)	Supportive care, symptom management, immune-boosting therapies	[44]
MALT lymphoma	Turmeric, ginger, herbal teas, dietary adjustments	[49]

TABLE 23.1 *(Continued)*

Disease	Traditional Remedies	References
Mantle cell lymphoma	Astragalus root, medicinal mushrooms, dietary changes	[49]
Mast cell leukemia (MCL)	Symptom management, supportive care, avoidance of triggers (e.g., certain foods, medications)	[45]
Mastocytosis	Boswellia, mast cell stabilizers	[55]
Monoclonal gammopathy of undetermined significance	Supportive care, regular monitoring, dietary changes	[54]
Myelodysplastic syndromes (MDS)	Chinese herbal medicine, acupuncture, nutritional supplements	[53]
Myelodysplastic/ myeloproliferative neoplasms (MDS/MPN overlap)	Supportive care, symptom management, nutritional support	[54]
Myeloproliferative neoplasms (MPN)	Gleevec (imatinib)-targeted therapy, dietary adjustments, acupuncture	[54]
Nodal marginal zone lymphoma	Various traditional remedies	[54]
Nodular lymphocyte-predominant Hodgkin lymphoma (NLPHL)	Various traditional remedies	[50]
Non-Hodgkin lymphoma	Echinacea, garlic, ginger, herbal teas	[50]
Peripheral T-cell lymphoma (PTCL)	Various traditional remedies	[51]
Polycythaemia vera (PV) Essential thrombocythaemia (ET) Myelofibrosis	Phlebotomy (for PV), aspirin (for ET), supportive care	[54]
Small lymphocytic lymphoma (SLL)	Echinacea, green tea extract, mind–body practices	[51]
Splenic marginal zone lymphoma	Supportive care, symptom management, dietary adjustments	[52]
Triple-hit lymphoma	Herbal remedies for immune support, nutritional supplements	[52]
Waldenström macroglobulinaemia (WM)	Dietary modifications (e.g., low-fat diet), herbal supplements (e.g., turmeric)	[52]

TABLE 23.2 Detailed Study for Bioactive Compounds in Traditional Plant Medicines

Plant	Bioactive Compounds	Leukemia cells Lines	MOA	References
Basella alba/malabar spinach	β-Sitosterol terpenoids	The cell lines U937 and Jurkat	Anticancer of the blood and magnification inhibition	[56]
Blumea lacera/among mahabo	Terpenoids, tannins, corticosteroids, gums, alkaloids	Raji, U937	Antiproliferation	[57]
Catharanthus roseus/ sadabahar	Alkaloids: vinorelbine, vinblastine, vindesine, vincristine, etc.	P1534 and L1210 leukemia cells	Karyokinesis inhibitors apprehend the demise of a cell dividing up which is the source of the fatalness of cells	[57]
Coreopsis lanceolata/ lanceleaf coreopsis, lanceleaf tickseed, lanceleaf coreosis	Flavonoids: flavanone, aurones 4, methoxylanceoletin, and chalcones	Acute promyelocytic leukemia (APL) line (leukemia HL-60 cells)	Antiproliferation and programmed cell death induction	[57]
Ferulago angulate/chavir (in Persian)	β-Pinene α-Pinene	Raji, PBMC cell lines, and HL-60 cell lines	Antiproliferation, programmed cell death, autophagocytosis, and cell death	[57]
Ficus deltoid/mistletoe, rusty leafed bush fig	Flavonoids, terpenoids, tannins, phenol, lignans, proanthocyanins, coumarins, and alkaloids	HL60 cell line	Programmed cell death induction	[58]
Houttuynia cordata Thunb/ fishwort, chameleon plant, heart leaf	Flavanones	L1210, acute T lymphocytic leukemic Molt-4 cells, and HTLV 1	Endoplasmic reticulum stress pathway-mediated activation of apoptosis and antiproliferation	[58]
Litchi chinensis Sonn/lychee, litchee, litchi	Phenols, flavonoids, polysaccharides, and tannins	Promonocytic (human myeloid leukemia cell line), HL-60, and K562 cell lines	Induction of programmed cell death and antiproliferation	[59]
Nyctanthes arbor-tristis/ tree of sadness, the night of jasmine, seri gading	Phenols: phenol, (dimethyl ethyl), hydroxyproline oxide	Chronic lymphocytic leukemia, Jurkat T cells, and CML	Antiproliferation and apoptosis induction	[60]

TABLE 23.2 *(Continued)*

Plant	Bioactive Compounds	Leukemia cells Lines	MOA	References
Olea europaea/olive tree	Phenols, caffeic acid, and vanillic acid	Jurkat, K562 cells line, and HL60 cell line	Cell cycle arrest, activation of apoptosis, and differentiation	[61]
Salvia officinalis/sage	Flavonoids	U937, immortalized myelogenous leukemia, KG-1A cell line (promyeloblast macrophage)	Antimigratory, and antiangiogenic	[61]
Scutellaria baicalensis/ Chinese skullcap	Flavonoid, baicalein, and wogonin	M2 (AML-M2) cell line, HL-60, NB-4 (acute promyelocytic leukemia), THP-1 (human leukemia monocytic cell line), lymphoma cell lines, the NALM-6 cell line (human peripheral blood)	Inhibition of growth results in a dose–response relationship in cellular respiration, cell cycle arrest, and death	[61]
Tithonia diversifolia/tree marigold, Mexican sunflower, Mexican tournesol, Japanese sunflower, notable chrysanthemum	Flavonoids, phenols, tannins, and terpenoids	Anti-K562 (lymphoblasts cells), L1210 (mouse lymphocytic leukemia cell line), Raji and U937 leukemia cells, and HL-60 cell line	Cytotoxic	[61]
Willows tree/sallows and osiers	Salicin	ALL and AML cell lines, human promyelocytic leukemia cells	Apoptosis is induced by the destruction of deoxyribonucleic acid, opposition to proliferation	[62]

23.3 SUMMARY

Considering that over half of all medications now in use come from plants, it is obvious that effective cancer treatments can be found by looking at natural sources, particularly plants. Discord of natural materials, including plants, used to be an intensive procedure. However, by employing contemporary methods, the search for plant active complexes has quickened recently. Recycling of herbal plants is the outcome of this—the resurgence of medications derived from herbs, particularly for the treatment of cancer. Over 60 herbal complexes are now being researched as anticancer medications.

KEYWORDS

- **anticancer agents**
- **apoptosis**
- **blood cancer**
- **leukemia**
- **lymphoma**
- **myeloma**

REFERENCES

1. Abdullah, S. (2024). The prevention of multi-drug resistance in cancers through the application of nanotechnology-based targeted delivery systems for combination therapies involving Traditional Chinese medicine. *Pharmacological Research-Modern Chinese Medicine, 2024,* e100386.
2. Barista, I., Romaguera, J. E., & Cabanillas, F. (2001). Mantle-cell lymphoma. *The Lancet Oncology*, *2*(3), 141–148.
3. Barosi, G. (2014). Essential thrombocythemia vs. early/ prefibrotic myelofibrosis: Why does it matter? *Best Practice & Research Clinical Haematology*, *27*(2), 129–140.
4. Bomken, S. N., & Vormoor, H. J. (2009). Childhood leukemia. *Paediatrics and Child Health*, *19*(8), 345–350. doi: 10.1016/j.paed.2009.04.003
5. Brockmueller, A., Samuel, S. M., Mazurakova, A., Büsselberg, D., Kubatka, P., & Shakibaei, M. (2023). Curcumin, calebin A and chemo-sensitization: How are they linked to colorectal cancer? *Life Sciences*, *318*, e121504.

6. Cesaro, S., Ljungman, P., Mikulska, M., Hirsch, H. H., von Lilienfeld-Toal, M., Cordonnier, C., Meylan, S., Mehra, V., Styczynski, J., Marchesi, F., Besson, C., Baldanti, F., Masculano, R. C., Beutel, G., Einsele, H., Azoulay, E., Maertens, J., de la Camara, R., ECIL 9, & Pagano, L. (2022). Recommendations for the management of COVID-19 in patients with hematological malignancies or hematopoietic cell transplantation. In *2021 European Conference on Infections in Leukemia* (ECIL-9). *Leukemia*, *36*(6), 1467–1480.
7. Connors, J. M., Cozen, W., Steidl, C., Carbone, A., Hoppe, R. T., Flechtner, H. H., & Bartlett, N. L. (2020). Hodgkin lymphoma. *Nature Reviews Disease Primers*, *6*(1), 61–69.
8. Dave, S. S., Fu, K., Wright, G. W., Lam, L. T., Kluin, P., Boerma, E. J., & Staudt, L. M. (2006). Molecular diagnosis of Burkitt's lymphoma. *New England Journal of Medicine*, *354*(23), 2431–2442.
9. De Kouchkovsky, I., & Abdul-Hay, M. (2016). Acute myeloid leukemia: A comprehensive review and 2016 update. *Blood Cancer Journal*, *6*(7), e441.
10. DiNardo, C. D., Erba, H. P., Freeman, S. D., & Wei, A. H. (2023). Acute myeloid leukemia. *The Lancet*, *401*(10393), 2073–2086.
11. Dores, G. M., Anderson, W. F., Curtis, R. E., Landgren, O., Ostroumova, E., Bluhm, E. C., & Linet, M. S. (2007). Chronic lymphocytic leukemia and small lymphocytic lymphoma: Overview of the descriptive epidemiology. *British Journal of Haematology*, *139*(5), 809–819.
12. Fleischer, T., Chang, T. T., Chiang, J. H., Sun, M. F., & Yen, H. R. (2017). Improved survival with integration of Chinese herbal medicine therapy in patients with acute myeloid leukemia: A nationwide population-based cohort study. *Integrative Cancer Therapies*, *16*(2), 156–164.
13. Frazer, R., Irvine, A. E., & McMullin, M. F. (2007). Chronic myeloid leukemia in the 21st century. *The Ulster Medical Journal*, *76*(1), 8–15.
14. Fu, Y. S., Chen, T. H., Weng, L., Huang, L., Lai, D., & Weng, C. F. (2021). Pharmacological properties and underlying mechanisms of curcumin and prospects in medicinal potential. *Biomedicine & Pharmacotherapy*, *141*, e111888.
15. George, B. P., Chandran, R., & Abrahamse, H. (2021). Role of phytochemicals in cancer chemoprevention: Insights. *Antioxidants*, *10*(9), 1455–1461.
16. Ghojogh, M., Kor, Y., & Rafiemanesh, H. (2015). Leukemia in Iran: Epidemiology and morphology trends. *Asian Pacific Journal of Cancer Prevention*, *16*(17), 7759–7763.
17. Gupta, A., Gehlot, S., & Gupta, R. (2023). Microscopy cancer cell imaging in b-lineage acute lymphoblastic leukemia. In: *State of the Art in Neural Networks and Their Applications* (pp. 1–28). Academic Press: New York.
18. Halton, J. M., Nazir, D. J., McQueen, M. J., & Barr, R. D. (1998). Blood lipid profiles in children with acute lymphoblastic leukemia. *Cancer: Interdisciplinary International Journal of the American Cancer Society*, *83*(2), 379–384.
19. Hawkes, E. A., Grigg, A., & Chong, G. (2015). Programmed cell death-1 inhibition in lymphoma. *The Lancet Oncology*, *16*(5), e234–e245.
20. Heise, T., Villar-Lopez, M., & Salaverry, O. (2023). Person-centered traditional medicine. In: *Person Centered Medicine* (pp. 665–684). Springer International Publishing: Cham.

21. Hibner, U., Benhamou, L. E., Haury, M., Cazenave, P. A., & Sarthou, P. (1993). Signaling of programmed cell death induction in WEHI-231 B-lymphoma cells. *European Journal of Immunology*, *23*(11), 2821–2825.
22. Hjalgrim, H., & Jarrett, R. F. (2020). Epidemiology of Hodgkin lymphoma. In: *Hodgkin Lymphoma: A Comprehensive Overview* (pp. 3–23). SpringerLink.
23. Ivachtchenko, A. V., Kiselyov, A. S., Tkachenko, S. E., Ivanenkov, Y. A., & Balakin, K. V. (2007). Novel mitotic targets and their small-molecule inhibitors. *Current Cancer Drug Targets*, *7*(8), 766–784.
24. Jaskulska, A., Janecka, A. E., & Gach-Janczak, K. (2020). Thapsigargin—From traditional medicine to anticancer drug. *International Journal of Molecular Sciences*, *22*(1), 4–9.
25. Joseph, E., Lawal, A. U., Ubaidullah, A., & Kado, S. (2024). Health implication and nutritional value of baobab leaves in Katsina state - Nigeria using instrumental neutron activation analysis. *International Journal of Applied Science and Research*, *7*(4), 98–114.
26. Kantarjian, H., Kadia, T., DiNardo, C., Daver, N., Borthakur, G., Jabbour, E., & Ravandi, F. (2021). Acute myeloid leukemia: Current progress and future directions. *Blood Cancer Journal*, *11*(2), 41–51.
27. Komiljonova, O. (2024). The use of ginger for medicinal diseases based on traditional medicine. *Central Asian Journal of Education and Innovation*, *3*(1), 203–211. doi: 10.5281/zenodo.10521581.
28. Kumar, D., Jain, N., Khurana, A., Mittal, S., Satapathy, S. C., Senkerik, R., & Hemanth, J. D. (2020). Automatic detection of white blood cancer from bone marrow microscopic images using convolutional neural networks. *IEEE Access*, *8*, 142521–142531.
29. Küpeli-Akkol, E., Genç, Y., Karpuz, B., Sobarzo-Sánchez, E., & Capasso, R. (2020). Coumarins and coumarin-related compounds in pharmacotherapy of cancer. *Cancers*, *12*(7), 1959–1962.
30. Kuruppu, A. I., Paranagama, P., & Goonasekara, C. L. (2019). Medicinal plants commonly used against cancer in traditional medicine formulae in Sri Lanka. *Saudi Pharmaceutical Journal*, *27*(4), 565–573.
31. Law, B. Y. K., Mok, S. W. F., Wu, A. G., Lam, C. W. K., Yu, M. X. Y., & Wong, V. K. W. (2016). New potential pharmacological functions of Chinese herbal medicines via regulation of autophagy. *Molecules*, *21*(3), 359–363.
32. LeBlanc, M. R., LeBlanc, T. W., Yang, Q., McLaughlin, J., Irish, K., & Smith, S. K. (2023). A mobile app to support self-management in patients with multiple myeloma or chronic lymphocytic leukemia: Pilot randomized controlled trial. *JMIR Cancer*, *9*(1), e44533.
33. Lewis, W. D., Lilly, S., & Jones, K. L. (2020). Lymphoma: Diagnosis and treatment. *American Family Physician*, *101*(1), 34–41.
34. Lichetman, M. A. (2010). Obesity and the risk for a haematological malignancy: Leukemia, lymphoma, or myeloma. Oncologist, 15(10), 1083–1101, online; doi: 10.1634/theoncologist.2010-0206. PMID: 20930095.
35. Linendoll, N., Murphy-Banks, R., Sae-Hau, M., Rodday, A. M., DiFilippo, C., Jain, A., Reinhart, C., Rapkin, B., Weiss, E., & Parsons, S. K. (2023). Evaluating the role of financial navigation in alleviating financial distress among young adults with a

history of blood cancer: A hybrid type 2 randomized effectiveness-implementation design. *Contemporary Clinical Trials*, *124*, e107019.

36. Lister, A., Abrey, L., & Sandlund, J. T. (2002). Central nervous system lymphoma. *ASH Education Program Book*, *2002*(1), 283–296.
37. Madhan, S., Dhar, R., & Devi, A. (2024). Plant-derived exosomes: A green approach for cancer drug delivery. *Journal of Materials Chemistry B*, *12*(9), 2236–2252. doi: 10.1039/d3tb02752j. PMID: 38351750.
38. Maher, T., Ahmad Raus, R., Daddiouaissa, D., Ahmad, F., Adzhar, N. S., Latif, E. S., Abdulhafiz, F., & Mohammed, A. (2021). Medicinal plants with anti-leukemic effects: Review. *Molecules*, *26*(9), 2741–2748.
39. Mardiana, S., & Gill, S. (2020). CAR T cells for acute myeloid leukemia: State of the art and future directions. *Frontiers in Oncology*, *10*, 697–703.
40. Marrero, R. J., & Lamba, J. K. (2023). Current landscape of genome-wide association studies in acute myeloid leukemia: A review. *Cancers*, *15*(14), 3583–3588.
41. Minhas, L. A., Kaleem, M., Farooqi, H. M. U., Kausar, F., Waqar, R., Bhatti, T., Aziz, S., Won Jung, D., & Mumtaz, A. S. (2024). Algae-derived bioactive compounds as potential nutraceuticals for cancer therapy: A comprehensive review. *Algal Research*, *2024,* e103396.
42. Morris, S. L. (2012). Skin lymphoma. *Clinical Oncology*, *24*(5), 371–385.
43. Mwirigi, A., Dillon, R., & Raj, K. (2017). Acute leukemia. *Medicine*, *45*(5), 280–286.
44. Newell, L. F., & Cook, R. J. (2021). Advances in acute myeloid leukemia. *BMJ, 375*n2026. https://doi.org/10.1136/bmj.n2026
45. Paillassa, J., Cornet, E., Noel, S., Tomowiak, C., Lepretre, S., Vaudaux, S., Dupuis, J., Devidas, A., Joly, B., Petitdidier-Lionnet, C., Haiat, S., Mariette, C., Thieblemont, C., Decaudin, D., Validire-Charpy, P., Drenou, B., Eisenmann, J. C., Uribe, M. O., Olivrie, A., Touati, M., Lambotte, O., Hermine, O., Karsenti, J. M., Feugier, P., Vaillant, W., Gutnecht, J., Lippert, E., Huysman, F., Ghomari, K., Boubaya, M., Levy, V., Riou, J., Damaj, G., Tanguy-Schmidt, A., Hunault-Berger, M., & Troussard, X. (2020). Analysis of a cohort of 279 patients with hairy-cell leukemia (HCL): 10 years of follow-up. *Blood Cancer Journal*, *10*(5), 62–70.
46. Pan, X., Shen, Q., Zhang, C., Zhang, X., Li, Y., Chang, Z., & Pang, B. (2023). Coicis semen for the treatment of malignant tumors of the female reproductive system: A review of traditional Chinese medicinal uses, phytochemistry, pharmacokinetics, and pharmacodynamics. *Frontiers in Pharmacology*, *14*, e1129874.
47. Pelcovits, A., & Niroula, R. (2020). Acute myeloid leukemia: A review. *Rhode Island Medical Journal*, *103*(3), 38–40.
48. Phuoc, V., Sandoval-Sus, J., & Chavez, J. C. (2019). Drug therapy for double-hit lymphoma. *Drugs in Context*, *8*, 2019-8-1.. doi: 10.7573/dic.2019-8-1.
49. Puri, A., Mohite, P., Maitra, S., Subramaniyan, V., Kumarasamy, V., Uti, D. E., & Atangwho, I. J. (2024). From nature to nanotechnology: The interplay of traditional medicine, green chemistry, and biogenic metallic phyto-nanoparticles in modern healthcare innovation and sustainability. *Biomedicine & Pharmacotherapy*, *170*, e116083.
50. Puumala, S. E., Ross, J. A., Aplenc, R., & Spector, L. G. (2013). Epidemiology of childhood acute myeloid leukemia. *Pediatric Blood & Cancer*, *60*(5), 728–733.

51. Rai, K. R., Holland, J. F., Glidewell, O. J., Weinberg, V., Brunner, K., Obrecht, J. P., Preisler, H. D., Nawabi, I. W., Prager, D., Carey, R. W., Cooper, M. R., Haurani, F., Hutchison, J. L., Silver, R. T., Falkson, G., Wiernik, P., Hoagland, H. C., Bloomfield, C. D., James, G. W., Gottlieb, A., & Kaan, S. K. (1981). Treatment of acute myelocytic leukemia: A study by cancer and leukemia group B. *Blood*, *58*(6), 1203–1212.
52. Raina, R., Gondhi, N. K., Chaahat, Singh, D., Kaur, M., & Lee, H. N. (2023). A systematic review on acute leukemia detection using deep learning techniques. *Archives of Computational Methods in Engineering*, *30*(1), 251–270.
53. Rodriguez-Galindo, C., & Allen, C. E. (2020). Langerhans cell histiocytosis. *Blood, The Journal of the American Society of Hematology*, *135*(16), 1319–1331
54. Rose-Inman, H., & Kuehl, D. (2017). Acute leukemia. *Hematology/ Oncology Clinics*, *31*(6), 1011–1028.
55. Sevgi, E., Dag, A., Kızılarslan-Hançer, Ç., Atasoy, S., Kurt, B. Z., & Aksakal, Ö. (2021). Evaluation of cytotoxic and antioxidant potential of *Dittrichia viscosa* (L.) Greuter used in traditional medicine. *Journal of Ethnopharmacology*, *276*, e114211.
56. Sharma, A. N., Dewangan, H. K., & Upadhyay, P. K. (2024). Comprehensive review on herbal medicine: Emphasis on current therapy and role of phytoconstituents for cancer treatment. *Chemistry & Biodiversity*, *21*(3), e202301468.
57. Singh, R., Shaik, S., Negi, B. S., Rajguru, J. P., Patil, P. B., Parihar, A. S., & Sharma, U. (2020). Non-Hodgkin's lymphoma: A review. *Journal of Family Medicine and Primary Care*, *9*(4), 1834–1840.
58. Sivakumar, T. (2023). Traditional medicine, phytochemicals and pharmacological applications of common plants in the Cucurbitaceae family: An extensive review. *Journal of Xidian University*, *17*(7), 758–767.
59. Spina, V., Khiabanian, H., Messina, M., Monti, S., Cascione, L., Bruscaggin, A., Spaccarotella, E., Holmes, A. B., Arcaini, L., Lucioni, M., Tabbò, F., Zairis, S., Diop, F., Cerri, M., Chiaretti, S., Marasca, R., Ponzoni, M., Deaglio, S., Ramponi, A., Tiacci, E., & Rossi, D. (2016). The genetics of nodal marginal zone lymphoma blood. *The Journal of the American Society of Hematology*, *128*(10), 1362–1373.
60. Terwilliger, T., & Abdul-Hay, M. J. B. C. J. (2017). Acute lymphoblastic leukemia: A comprehensive review and 2017 update. *Blood Cancer Journal*, *7*(6), e577.
61. Tomizawa, D., Miyamura, T., Imamura, T., Watanabe, T., Moriya Saito, A., Ogawa, A., Ogawa, A., Takahashi, Y., Hirayama, M., Taki, T., Deguchi, T., Hori, T., Sanada, M., Ohmori, S., Haba, M., Iguchi, A., Arakawa, Y., Koga, Y., Manabe, A., Horibe, K., Ishii, E., & Koh, K. (2020). A risk-stratified therapy for infants with acute lymphoblastic leukemia: A report from the JPLSG MLL-10 trial. *The Journal of the American Society of Hematology*, *136*(16), 1813–1823.
62. Zhu, J. Y., Lavrik, I. N., Mahlknecht, U., Giaisi, M., Proksch, P., Krammer, P. H., & Li-Weber, M. (2007). The traditional Chinese herbal compound rocaglamide preferentially induces apoptosis in leukemia cells by modulation of mitogen-activated protein kinase activities. *International Journal of Cancer*, *121*(8), 1839–1846.

Index

C

D

G

H

I

S

U

V

W

X

Y

For Product Safety Concerns and Information please contact our EU representative GPSR@taylorandfrancis.com Taylor & Francis Verlag GmbH, Kaufingerstraße 24, 80331 München, Germany